Imaging of the Scrotum

Textbook and Atlas

Imaging of the Scrotum
Textbook and Atlas

Editors

Hedvig Hricak, M.D., Ph.D.
Professor of Radiology, Urology, and Radiation Oncology
Department of Radiology
University of California
San Francisco, California

Bernd Hamm, M.D.
Professor of Radiology
Department of Radiology
Charité, Humboldt-Universität
Berlin, Germany

Bohyun Kim, M.D.
Department of Diagnostic Imaging
Samsung Medical Center
Seoul, Korea

Raven Press New York

Raven Press Ltd., 1185 Avenue of the Americas, New York, New York 10036

Printed and bound in Singapore

Library of Congress Cataloging-in-Publication Data

Hricak, Hedvig.
Imaging of the scrotum: textbook and atlas/authors, Hedvig Hricak, Bernd Hamm, Bohyun Kim.—1st ed.
p. cm.
Includes bibliographical references and index.
ISBN 0-7817-0153-8
1. Scrotum—Imaging. 2. Scrotum—Imaging—Atlases. I. Hamm, Bernd, Prof. Dr. II. Kim, Bohyun. III. Title.
[DNLM: 1. Testicular Diseases—diagnosis—atlases. 2. Scrotum—pathology—atlases. 3. Diagnostic Imaging—methods—atlases. WJ 17 H873i 1995]
RC897.H75 1995
616.6'70754—dc20
DNLM/DLC
for Library of Congress 94-33651

The material contained in this volume was submitted as previously unpublished material, except in the instances in which credit has been given to the source from which some of the illustrative material was derived.

Great care has been taken to maintain the accuracy of the information contained in this volume. However, neither Raven Press nor the editors can be held responsible for errors or for any consequences arising from the use of the information contained herein.

9 8 7 6 5 4 3 2 1

Contents

Contributors

Peter R. Carroll, M.D. *Associate Professor, Department of Urology, University of California, San Francisco, California*

Mailine H. Chew, M.D. *Associate Clinical Professor, Departments of Medicine and Radiology, Davies Medical Center, San Francisco, California*

Klaus-Peter Dieckmann, M.D. *Associate Professor, Department of Urology, Albertinen Hospital, Hamburg, Germany*

Franz Fobbe, M.D. *Associate Professor, Department of Radiology, Klinikum Benjamin Franklin, Freie Universität, Berlin, Germany*

Ruth B. Goldstein, M.D. *Associate Professor, Department of Radiology, University of California, San Francisco, California*

Bernd Hamm, M.D. *Professor, Department of Radiology, Charité, Humboldt-Universität zu Berlin, Berlin, Germany*

Hedvig Hricak, M.D., Ph.D. *Professor of Radiology, Urology, and Radiation Oncology, Department of Radiology, University of California, San Francisco, California*

Bohyun Kim, M.D. *Department of Diagnostic Imaging, Samsung Medical Center, Seoul, Korea*

Wolfgang Kramer, M.D. *Department of Urology, Goethe-Universität, Frankfurt, Germany*

Bruce L. McClennan, M.D. *Professor, Mallinckrodt Institute of Radiology, St. Louis, Missouri*

Eugene T. Morita, M.D. *Associate Clinical Professor, Department of Radiology, University of California, San Francisco, California*

David C. Price, M.D. *Professor, Department of Radiology, University of California, San Francisco, California*

Preface

Although the scrotum is a superficial structure, its clinical examination frequently fails to provide a specific diagnosis because the patient's clinical history and physical findings are similar in many conditions. Cross-sectional imaging studies, ultrasound, computed tomography, magnetic resonance imaging, or nuclear medicine studies, when added to the clinical examination, have significantly refined the diagnostic approach in scrotal disease.

In this age of constantly rising health care expenditures resulting in the demands for cost control, duplication of diagnostic imaging procedures must be eliminated and a logical algorithmic diagnostic approach should be adopted. *Imaging of the Scrotum* provides a streamlined assessment of scrotal pathology, starting with the simplest and least expensive imaging technique—ultrasound. There is, at times, a need for computed tomography, magnetic resonance imaging, and nuclear medicine. The indications for these techniques need to be defined.

The book is subdivided into two parts: a textbook and an atlas. The textbook is classically organized in presenting the clinical and imaging findings of the different scrotal disorders. The epidemiology and clinical presentation of the most commonly encountered scrotal diseases are described and correlated with their imaging features.

Scrotal ultrasound, considered an extension of the physical examination, confirms the clinical presumptive diagnosis and provides relevant additional information. In most clinical problems, ultrasound supplies sufficient information for the correct diagnosis. Other imaging modalities, except in the staging of testicular cancer, should be used only as problem-solving approaches. This is why both the textbook and atlas heavily emphasize the ultrasound findings.

The atlas, with its 130 cases, allows self-instruction in analyzing and interpreting the imaging findings (including ultrasound, nuclear medicine, magnetic resonance imaging, computed tomography and angiography) of the scrotum. Readers can use the atlas to test and improve their understanding of scrotal imaging diagnosis through practical exercises. Each case report includes the clinical findings, images with short descriptions, and the final diagnosis.

The atlas cases were primarily selected on the basis of their clinical relevance and frequency, and no attempt was made to study the entire spectrum of scrotal pathology. To intensify the learning process, the cases are arranged at random and not according to their clinical picture or classification.

Imaging of the Scrotum will be helpful to all clinicians dealing with scrotal diseases.

Acknowledgments

We thank our contributors for providing us with valuable input, Johnette Coleman for her tireless administrative assistance, and Katherine Pitcoff for a stellar job of editing. We wish to express our gratitude to Prof. Gretchen Gooding, M.D., for the generous support in providing interesting case material. We would also like to thank Springer-Verlag and Hippokrates Verlag who have generously given their permission to reprint many of the photographs in this text from *Sonographische Diagnostik des Skrotalinhalts* (Hamm © 1991 Springer-Verlag, Berlin-Heidelberg), and from *Das Akute Skrotum: Bibliothek fur Kinderchirurgie* (Waldschmidt, Hamm, and Schier © 1990 Hippokrates Verlag, Stuttgart).

Imaging of the Scrotum

Textbook and Atlas

CHAPTER 1

Anatomy and Embryology

EMBRYOLOGY

The embryologic development of the testes has a direct bearing on the understanding of the anatomical structure of the scrotal contents. Differentiation of the male gonads begins at 7 weeks of gestation. Before this time, proliferation of the coelomic epithelium and consolidation of the underlying loose mesenchyme lead to development of the **genital ridges** at the dorsal wall of the primitive abdominal cavity, lateral to the base of the mesentery on both sides (Fig. 1.1A). These ridges give rise to the **sex cords,** which are formed by ingrowth of coelomic epithelial cells. The precursors of spermatogenic cells are the **primordial (primitive) germ cells.** The germ cells develop in the yolk sac and then migrate into the differentiating tissue of the sex cords by active, ameboid movements (1). The first primordial germ cells can be detected in the sex cords at 6 weeks of gestation (2). During the seventh week, the epithelium of the sex cords becomes detached from the dorsal coelomic epithelium and forms a fine mesenchymal layer. Initially, this provides only a loose partition, but later it becomes the tight and fibrous **tunica albuginea.** After incorporation of the primordial germ cells, the sex cords—originally rather unstructured—acquire a parallel arrangement and form delicate compartments consisting of epithelial columns and surrounding mesenchyme (Fig. 1.1B). These structures, termed **seminiferous cords,** are the precursors of the tubuli seminiferi (**seminiferous tubules**). They undergo pronounced elongation and finally are arranged in a horseshoelike pattern. On the gonadal surface opposite the coelom, the **hilus,** which will become the **rete testis,** develops as a fine meshwork of thin cellular strands that is closely associated with the seminiferous cords (Fig. 1.1B). The former coelomic epithelial cells within the seminiferous cords differentiate into **Sertoli cells (supporting cells)** (3). **Leydig cells (interstitial cells)** arise in the mesenchyme surrounding the seminiferous cords and show marked proliferation during the third to fifth months of gestation. Pronounced testosterone secretion by these cells induces the male development of the indifferent gonads (4–6).

By the sixth week of gestation, the **mesonephros** has developed adjacent to the genital ridges (7) (Fig. 1.1A). It extends cranially beyond the gonadal structures and joins the **mesonephric** or **wolffian duct** in a caudal direction. By the eighth week, the glomeruli and most tubules of the mesonephros atrophy and disappear. The tubules of the middle portion are retained, however, and form a connection with the hilus of the primordial gonad (Fig. 1.1B). They later develop into the **efferent ductules,** which in turn open into the mesonephric duct. Frequently, some mesonephric tubules persist cranial to the fusion site of the wolffian duct and the gonadal hilus, giving rise to the so-called **appendix epididymis (stalked hydatid of Morgagni)** seen in adults. Under the influence of testosterone produced by the interstitial cells, the mesonephric duct differentiates into the efferent duct of the gonads (**the epididymis**). The future epididymis starts developing by a pronounced elongation and convolution of the duct below the site where it joins the efferent ductules. In the tail portion of the epididymis, the wolffian duct becomes coated by a muscular layer and passes into the deferent duct (**ductus or vas deferens**) (3). The duct courses caudad and opens into the cloaca adjacent to the müllerian ducts. The latter undergo regression in the male fetus and leave, as their remains, the **prostatic utricle.**

Although the structural-anatomic development of the testis and epididymis is completed at the end of the fourth month of gestation, the two organs also undergo a subsequent, and concomitant, anatomic–topographic development and further internal maturation.

TESTICULAR DESCENT

The testes require a temperature 2° to 4°C below the average body temperature for spermatogenesis and hormone production. This environment is achieved by their

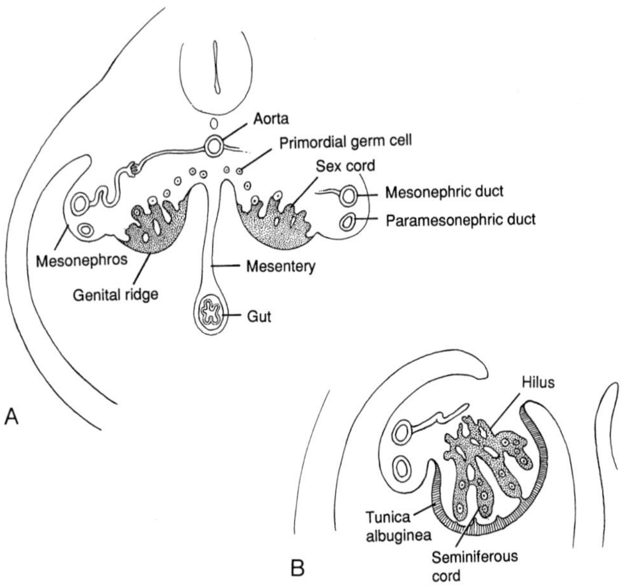

FIG. 1.1. Normal development of the male gonad (transverse anatomic cross section through the lumbar region). **(A)** A 6-week embryo, demonstrating indifferent gonad with the primitive sex cords. **(B)** An 8-week embryo, showing development of the tunica albuginea, seminiferous cords, and hilus. The hilus later becomes the rete testis.

extra-abdominal position, resulting from testicular descent. During fusion of the gonad with the mesonephric tubules, the caudal **genitoinguinal ligament** develops at the lower gonadal pole. This structure passes directly below the coelomic epithelium in the direction of the future inguinal region and ends in the mesenchyme of the scrotal swellings (3). The genitoinguinal ligament develops into the **gubernaculum testis** through mesenchymal consolidation. During the second month of gestation there is rapid growth of the embryo, but the gubernaculum testis does not expand. Because it is attached to the gubernaculum, the gonad is thus passively drawn to the inguinal region in a caudal direction. During its passage, the testis pulls along the blood vessels and lymphatics developing at the level of its original position. This accounts for the fact that the testicular arteries and veins branch off the lumbar aorta and vena cava/renal vein, respectively. During the third month of gestation two symmetric evaginations, the **vaginal processes,** develop in the caudal—ventral part of the coelomic cavity. The vaginal processes pass along the gubernaculum and extend into the scrotal swellings. The testes themselves remain in their position above the internal inguinal ring until the seventh month, and actual descent through the inguinal canal begins at approximately 36 weeks of gestation. At the time of birth they usually reach their final position in the scrotum, where they are invested by the two walls of the processus vaginalis, resulting in parietal and visceral serous layers (8). The narrow, tubular connection of the processus vaginalis with the abdominal cavity is usually obliterated but may occasionally persist and give rise to a congenital inguinal hernia (**open processus vaginalis**). Incomplete obliteration leads to the formation of a **funiculocele.**

Although the mechanisms regulating testicular descent are not completely understood (8–12), the contribution of hormonal regulation by maternal gonadotropins and testosterone secreted by the fetal testes are confirmed (9). Biomechanical and neurogenic mechanisms (10) are also involved in this process. The condition resulting from incomplete testicular descent at the time of birth is referred to as **cryptorchidism.** It occurs in approximately 5% of full-term boys and is much more common (10% to 30%) in premature infants. Since delayed spontaneous descent occurs in many of these infants within the first year after birth, the incidence of cases requiring treatment for undescended testis is only 0.7% to 1.8% at the beginning of the second year of life (13).

ANATOMY OF THE INTRASCROTAL CONTENTS

The scrotum is formed by fusion of the two scrotal swellings which gives rise to an outer cutaneous ridge, or raphe, and an inner septum dividing the entire scrotum into two separate pouches—one for each testis, epididymis, and lower spermatic cord (funiculus spermaticus) with corresponding blood vessels and lymphatics (Fig. 1.2) (14–15). The coverings of testes consist of at least six layers: skin, dartos tunic, external spermatic fascia, cremasteric layer, internal spermatic fascia, tunica vaginalis. The characteristic wrinkled appearance of the scrotal skin results from the muscular layer. The testis and epididymis are surrounded by the **cavum serosum testis** (the cavity of the tunica vaginalis) which contains a small amount of serous fluid (Fig. 1.2). The covering of the cavum serosum testis is formed by parietal and visceral leaves of tunica vaginalis, an extension of the peritoneum. The testis is attached to the scrotal skin inferiorly by the gubernaculum testis, allowing mobility of the testis within the scrotal sac. This mobility serves to protect the testis against traumatic injury. The testicular parenchyma is encapsulated by the inelastic tunica albuginea, from which numerous fibrous partitions, the **septula testis,** extend vertically into the parenchyma dividing the organ into approximately 200 to 250 compartments, the **lobuli testis** (Fig. 1.3). Each of these lobules contains up to four **seminiferous tubules** (tubuli seminiferi).

Seminiferous Tubules

Each seminiferous tubule is a self-contained, convoluted system of interconnected canals. The two ends of each tubule often combine to form a straight tubule (**tubulus rectus**) before draining into the rete testis (Fig. 1.3) (16). Histologically, 15% of a normal tubule consists of

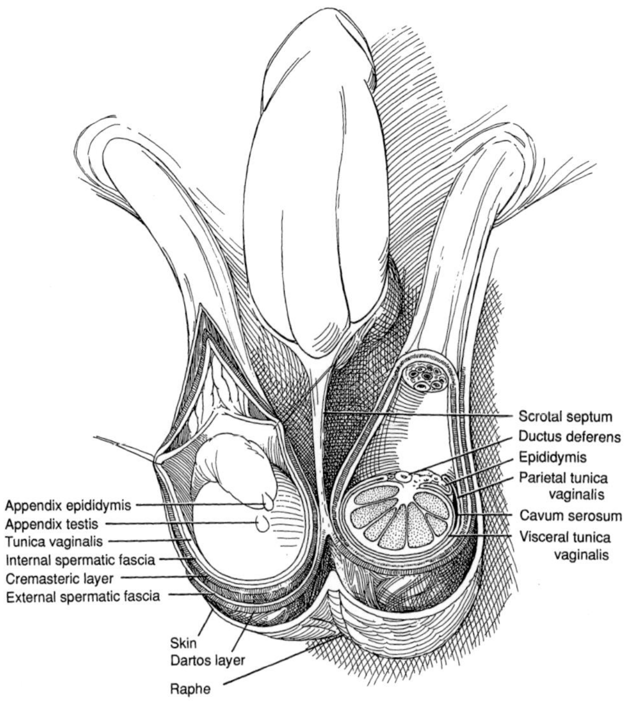

FIG. 1.2. Normal anatomy of the scrotum. On the right side, the testis and epididymis have been exposed by the longitudinal incision of tunica vaginalis. On the left side, cross section of testis demonstrates axial relationship among multiple compartments, mediastinum testis, and epididymis. Note the coverings of the testes.

supporting Sertoli cells. The other cellular components are germ cells at different stages of maturation. The tubular lumen, which functions in uptake and transport of the sperm-containing fluid, does not develop before puberty. The androgen-producing Leydig cells are located in the interstitial tissue around the tubules. A histologic cross-section shows an average of 4 Leydig cells around each tubule in adults.

Rete Testis

The rete testis is an irregularly anastomosing network of tubules situated dorsocranially in the area of the gonadal hilus. Histologically, the cavernous system is lined by cuboidal epithelium and partly by squamous epithelium. The rete testis functions like a sponge that continuously takes up the stream of sperm-containing fluid. Numerous exchange processes occur at the large contact surface between the walls of the rete testis and the intraluminal fluid (16). The 10 to 15 efferent ducts from the rete testis empty into the ductus epididymis (Fig. 1.3).

Mediastinum Testis

The mediastinum testis, which consists of the supporting connective tissue (an invagination of the tunica albuginea) and the rete testis, also contains two branches of the testicular artery as well as the centripetal veins and lymphatics from the lobules, which join in this area to form larger draining vessels (17–18).

Epididymis

The highly convoluted and spiraled ductus epididymis forms a compact organ only 2 to 3 cm in length (16). Straightened, the ductus would be approximately 3 to 4 m long (19). Like the testis, the epididymis has a lobulated structure, which results from connective tissue septula given off by the outer connective tissue capsule of the organ. The ductus epididymis is lined with a bilaminar epithelium and has an outer coat consisting of connective tissue and a layer of smooth muscle, which becomes thicker toward the vas deferens.

The epididymis as a whole is situated dorsally on the testis like a saddle and is macroscopically subdivided into the head (caput epididymis or globus major), the body (corpus epididymis), and the tail (cauda epididymis or globus minor) (Fig. 1.3). On the head of the epididymis there is a club-shaped appendage about 2 mm long, the so-called **appendix epididymis,** which is a remnant of the mesonephric tubules. This structure is distinct from the **appendix testis** (a similar protuberance off the upper pole of the testis) which is embryologically derived from the müllerian duct (6). Both appendages are referred to as "**hydatids**" by clinicians and may become clinically important in the differential diagnosis of the acute scrotum (appendiceal torsion). The testis and epididymis are anatomically and functionally connected via the mediastinum testis and thin connective tissue structures at the head and tail of the epididymis (**epididymal ligaments**).

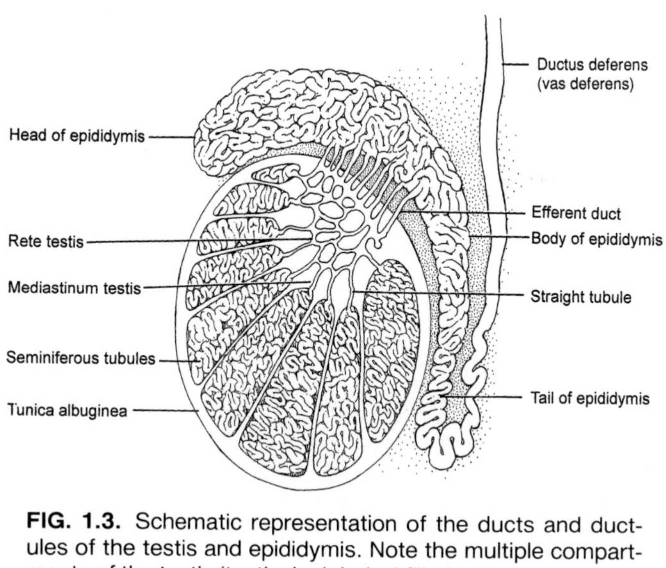

FIG. 1.3. Schematic representation of the ducts and ductules of the testis and epididymis. Note the multiple compartments of the testis (testicular lobules) filled with the seminiferous tubules, and the rete testis and efferent duct, which connect those tubules with epididymis.

The epididymis is involved in maturation, transport, and storage of sperm (19).

Scrotal Circulation

Blood is supplied to the intrascrotal organs by the **testicular (internal spermatic) artery, the deferential artery (artery of the ductus deferens), and the cremasteric (external spermatic) artery.** The right and left testicular arteries arise directly from the anterior aspect of the aorta just inferior to the origin of the renal arteries and descend along the psoas major. Each artery passes the deep inguinal ring to enter the spermatic cord, via which it traverses the inguinal canal to enter the scrotum. **Within the inguinal canal** the testicular artery gives off smaller connecting branches to the cremasteric artery and the deferential artery. Shortly before entering the hilus of the testis, it gives off a separate branch to the epididymis, which supplies the head and body of the epididymis. The epididymal branch again anastomoses with the deferential and cremasteric arteries at the tail of the epididymis.

After giving the epididymal branch, the testicular artery divides into two major branches, the internal testicular artery (outer branch) and the inferior testicular artery (inner branch). This division commonly occurs distal to the inguinal canal but may occur in the spermatic cord or in the retroperitoneum (20). The larger branch, the inferior testicular artery, runs between the testis and the body of the epididymis and enters the testis from the posterior aspect (Fig. 1.4). The internal testicular artery, on the other hand, enters the testis superiorly. After entering the tunica albuginea, both arteries (the capsular arteries) are located within the tunica vasculosa—an anatomic layer beneath the tunica albuginea—giving branches to each lobule (centripetal arteries) (17,21). The centripetal artery running in the septula testis toward the rete testis gives a branch—the centrifugal artery—that reverses direction and courses away from the rete testis.

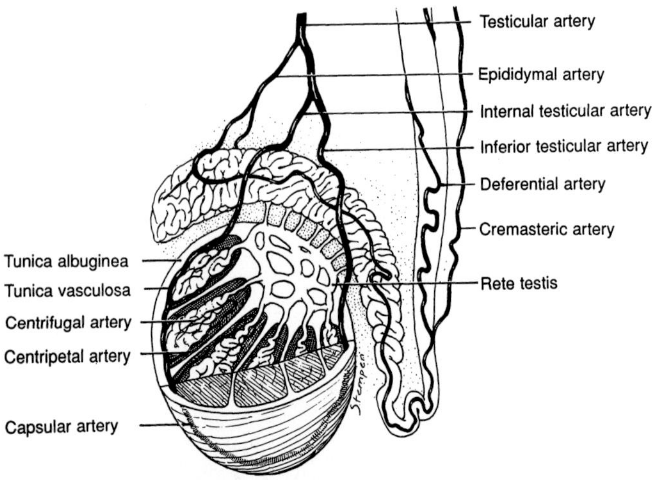

FIG. 1.4. Schematic representation of arterial blood supply to the testis and epididymis.

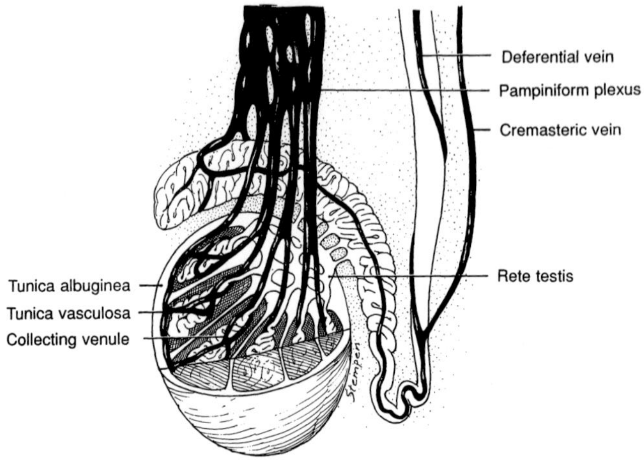

FIG. 1.5. Schematic representation of venous drainage of the testis and epididymis.

The very small deferential artery (originating from superior vesical artery—a branch of internal iliac artery) passes immediately adjacent to the ductus deferens, whereas the funicular vessel bundle comprising the venous pampiniform plexus and the testicular artery is a bit farther away. The third arterial vessel is the small cremasteric artery (originating from inferior epigastric artery—a branch of external iliac artery), which supplies the coverings of the testis and the spermatic cord. Anastomoses between the three arterial vessels of the scrotum are frequent but irregular (14).

Whereas the testis and the anterior part of the epididymis drain into the pampiniform plexus, the blood from the posterior part of the epididymis, the vas deferens, and the paratesticular tissues drains into the cremasteric, deferential, and funicular veins. The cremasteric vein drains into the internal saphenous or the inferior epigastric vein, and the deferential vein, which courses along the vas deferens, drains into the venous plexus of the spermatic cord or the prostatic and vesical plexus (4). The funicular vein drains the posterior part of the epididymis into the inferior epigastric vein.

Venous blood from the seminiferous tubules drains to the pampiniform plexus, either through the mediastinum testis (more commonly) or through veins in the tunica vasculosa (Fig 1.5). The blood flow of collecting venules is centripetal like corresponding arteries. The head and body of the epididymis also drain to the pampiniform plexus, and the tail, like its arterial supply, has an anastomosing loop with the deferential and cremasteric veins (18).

In the spermatic cord, the testicular vein is formed by the joining of the pampiniform plexus veins. Usually, one or two vessels remain on passage through the inguinal canal. Cranial to the internal inguinal ring, the testicular vein commonly has a variety of branches with connections to other retroperitoneal veins (paralumbar, renal-capsule, and iliac veins) (22,23).

Spermatic Cord

A major constituent of the spermatic cord (funiculus spermaticus) are the **ductus deferens (deferent duct)** and accompanying vessels which includes pampiniform plexus, testicular, deferential, and cremasteric arteries. It is the continuation of the ductus epididymis which gradually straightens out as it passes into the ductus deferens. Histologically, the deferent duct has a 1.5-mm-thick muscular layer for active sperm transportation, which gives this duct the typical cylindrical "roll-around" feeling on palpation.

Other components of the spermatic cord are the fibers of the cremaster muscle, nerves, and lymphatics as well as fatty and connective tissue. All of these structures are enveloped by the thin spermatic fascia.

A detailed description of the function of the intrascrotal organs is beyond the scope of this book. The interested reader is referred to the reference list for additional literature.

REFERENCES

1. Neville AM, Grigor KM. Structure, function and development of the human testis. In: Pugh RCB, ed. *Pathology of the testis*. Oxford: Blackwell; 1976:1–37.
2. Teilum G. Embryology of ovary, testis, and genetic ducts. In: Teilum G, ed. Special tumors of ovary and testis and related extragonadal lesions: comparative pathology and histological identification, 2nd ed. Philadelphia: JB Lippincott; 1976:15–30.
3. Sadler TW. Urogenital system. In: Sadler TW, ed. *Langman's medical embryology*, 6th ed. Baltimore: Williams and Wilkins; 1990:260–296.
4. Gondos B. Development of the testis and associated disorders. In: Gondos B, Riddick DH, eds. *Pathology of infertility*. New York: Thieme-Stratton; 1987:219–241.
5. Voutilainen R. Differentiation of the fetal gonad. *Horm Res* 1992:(Supp. 2):66–71.
6. Muller J, Skakkebaek NE. The prenatal and postnatal development of the testis. *Baillieres Clin Endocrinol Metab* 1992;6:251–271.
7. Satoh M. Histogenesis and organogenesis of the gonad in human embryos. *J Anat* 1991;177:85–107.
8. Wensing CJG. The embryology of testicular descent. *Horm Res* 1988;30:144–152.
9. Hadziselimovic F. Embryology of testicular descent and maldescent. In: Hadziselimovic F, ed. *Cryptorchidism: management and implications*. New York: Springer-Verlag; 1983:11–34.
10. Hutson JM, Beasley SW, Bryan AD. Cryptorchidism in spina bifida and spinal cord transection: a clue to the mechanism of transinguinal descent of the testis. *J Pediatr Surg* 1988;23:275–277.
11. Hutson JM, Williams MP, Fallet ME, Attah A. Testicular descent: new insights into its hormone control. *Oxford Rev Reprod Biol* 1990;12:1–56.
12. Nistal M, Paniagua R. Cryptorchidism. In: Nistal M, Paniagua R, eds. *Testicular and epididymal pathology*. New York: Thieme-Stratton; 1984:120–139.
13. Kleinteich B. Klinische problematik. In: Kleinteich B, Hadziselimovic F, Hesse V, Schreiber G, eds. *Kongenitale Hodendystopien*. New York: Thieme-Stratton, 1979:15–107.
14. Williams PL, Warwick R, Dyson M, Bannister LH. Reproductive organs of the male. In: Williams PL, Warwick R, Dyson M, Bannister LH, eds. *Gray's anatomy*, 37th ed. New York: Churchill Livingstone; 1989:1424–1435.
15. Tanagho EA. Anatomy of the lower urinary tract. In: Walsh PC, Retik AB, Stamey TA, Vaughan ED, eds. *Campbell's urology*, 6th ed., vol. 1. Philadelphia: WB Saunders; 1992:40–69.
16. Holstein AF. Die männlichen Geschlechtsorgane. In: Fleischhauer K, ed. *Benninghoff-anatomie: makroskopische und mikroskopische anatomie des menschen*, 13th ed., vol. 2. Urban/Schwarzenberg, Munich 1988:460–514.
17. Jarow JP. Intratesticular arterial anatomy. *J Androl* 1990;11:255–259.
18. Wishahi MM. Anatomy of the venous drainage of the human testis: Testicular vein cast, microdissection and radiographic demonstration. A new anatomical concept. *Eur Urol* 1991;20:154–160.
19. Cosentino MJ, Cockett AT. Structure and function of the epididymis. *Urol Res* 1986;14:229–240.
20. Hinman F, Jr. Testis. In: Hinman F, Jr. Atlas of urosurgical anatomy. Philadelphia: WB Saunders; 1993:471–506.
21. Kormano M, Suoranta H. Microvascular organization of the human testis. *Anat Record* 1971;170:31–39.
22. Fobbe F, Hamm B, Sörensen R, Felsenberg D. Percutaneous transluminal treatment of varicoceles: where to occlude the internal spermatic vein. *AJR* 1987;149:983–987.
23. Riedl P. Radiologic anatomy of the left testicular vein in varicoceles. In: Jecht EW, Zeitler E, eds. *Varicocele and male infertility: recent advances in diagnosis and therapy*. New York: Springer-Verlag; 1982:49–58.

CHAPTER 2

Clinical Examination of the Scrotum

Physical examination of the scrotum is a challenge to the clinician. Although the scrotal contents are superficial and easily palpated, the physical findings and clinical presentations of the various diseases frequently overlap, making definitive diagnosis difficult. Testicular torsion, for example, is misdiagnosed in as many as 50% of cases (1–3). In testicular cancer patients one study found that up to 55% were initially treated for presumed epididymitis, sometimes delaying the correct diagnosis of testicular tumor for more than 9 months (4).

Clinical examination of the scrotum includes history taking, inspection, and palpation, sometimes supplemented by transillumination.

HISTORY

History taking begins with a review of the symptoms (including information about their duration) that led to presentation. It also includes obtaining information about earlier scrotal or testicular diseases or operations, especially a history of cryptorchidism and possible hormone treatment, traumatic events, and inflammation in the scrotal area. Depending on the nature of the presenting symptoms, it may also be important to ask about potency and fertility.

Pain

When scrotal pain is the presenting symptom, information about its nature and temporal course should be obtained. Acute conditions—such as trauma, torsion, and epididymo-orchitis—often cause acute scrotal pain that radiates to the ipsilateral groin. Varicocele and hydrocele, on the other hand, most often cause dull pain without radiation. Inflammatory conditions, such as orchitis or epididymitis, may be accompanied by irritative voiding symptoms, such as dysuria, urinary frequency, or urgency. Fever is also indicative of an inflammatory condition. Renal, retroperitoneal, or inguinal diseases may also cause scrotal pain. A urinalysis should be considered part of the clinical examination.

Painless Testicular Swelling

Patients presenting with painless testicular swelling suggestive of tumor should be questioned regarding the presence of weight loss, malaise, supraclavicular swelling, or gynecomastia. When a testicular tumor is suspected, patient evaluation should include measurement of serum markers, such as human chorionic gonadotropin (HCG), alpha-fetoprotein (AFP), and lactate dehydrogenase (LDH). AFP is elevated in approximately 40% of patients with disseminated nonseminomatous germ cell tumors, and HCG is elevated in approximately 75%. One or both markers is elevated in 85% of patients (4). Of patients with seminomas, only 10% have elevated HCG, except for those with stage III disease, 50% of whom have elevated HCG.

INSPECTION

After history taking, the next step in the clinical examination is inspection of the patient's external genitalia. Inspection is performed with the patient in a comfortable, recumbent position. The ambient temperature should be sufficiently warm to ensure relaxation of the scrotal sac. The scrotum is initially inspected for major volume differences between the right and left side or enlargement of the entire scrotum. It is important to evaluate the scrotal skin, which is wrinkled and hairy under normal conditions. Inflammatory processes of the scrotal contents are typically accompanied by loss of the wrinkled appearance of the scrotal skin as well as erythema, swelling, and hyperthermia. Although isolated diseases of the scrotal skin are rare, atheromas or mycoses may occasionally be seen.

PALPATION

Palpation is performed bimanually and all findings are compared with those in the contralateral hemiscrotum. The presence and position of the testis is determined, as well as its axes (horizontal and vertical), bilaterally. Since the testis is mobile within the scrotum, it is grasped caudally with one hand and gently kept in position for palpation with the fingers of the other hand. The consistency is determined by taking the testis between two or three fingers of the palpating hand. The consistency of normal testes is rubbery. An accurate estimate of size may be facilitated by the use of an orchidometer. Normal testes in the adult measure 15 to 20 cc (5). Size usually indicates interindividual variation and has little bearing on function. However, very small and soft testicles suggest atrophy. Enlargement of the testis with a preserved outer contour is rare, and testicular cancer should be excluded with ultrasonography. Indurations or nodule formation within the testis or at the tunica albuginea are indicative of tumor. When a scrotal mass is palpated, it is crucial to determine whether it arises from the testes, epididymis, or cord structures. Masses arising from the testes are usually malignant, whereas those arising from the epididymis and spermatic cord are usually benign.

Although a specific diagnosis of the testicular tumor cannot be made by palpation alone, sometimes simple palpation can suggest a certain pathology. For example, seminomas are often associated with enlargement of the entire testicular substance. Teratomas and embryonal cell carcinomas, on the other hand, often present as discrete nodular masses within the testis (4).

Epididymis

It is important to evaluate the epididymis, which lies along the posterior aspect of the testis and may swell to the thickness of a finger in the presence of inflammation. Palpation of the epididymis is unpleasant for the majority of patients, even in the absence of inflammation. In patients presenting with epididymitis, tenderness often precludes a thorough examination of the epididymis. As inflammation spreads into the testis, the entire scrotal contents may be painful. However, in the supine position, the pain often can be relieved by elevating the scrotum above the pubic symphysis (*Prehn's sign*). The consistency of the epididymis is evaluated with special attention to cystic and solid lesions.

Spermatic Cord

Examination of the spermatic cord begins with a search for the ductus deferens. Its cordlike shape is easily identified as a firm, cylindrical structure. In patients presenting with fertility disorders, it is important to establish whether the vas deferens is present. Within the spermatic cord it is often possible to palpate the vascular bundle next to the duct as a soft tissue structure. Cystic and solid lesions (spermatic cord tumors) are very rare and can be identified by palpation. Attention must also be paid to varicose dilatation of the pampiniform plexus, a condition known as a *varicocele.* This condition more commonly occurs on the left side, since venous drainage is into the left renal vein. A varicocele is easily recognized with the patient standing, when the engorged varices often occupy an entire hemiscrotum. It may be even more evident if the patient performs a Valsalva maneuver. Varicoceles usually diminishes in size or disappear with the patient supine, but in severe cases they may be readily recognizable in the supine position as well.

Herniation

Finally, with the patient still standing, the inguinal canal openings are examined by insertion of the index finger and invagination of the scrotal skin in the direction of the external inguinal ring. The examining finger is placed through the external ring into the inguinal canal, which can be identified by its sharp-edged fascial borders. In the presence of a hernia, a sudden impulse against the examining finger will be felt when the patient coughs. When the internal and external inguinal canals are widely open, a hernial sac may protrude into the scrotum even at rest. This condition is termed a *scrotal hernia* and generally can be completely repositioned with the patient supine.

TRANSILLUMINATION

The last step of the clinical examination is *transillumination (diaphanoscopy)*. Transillumination is helpful in the evaluation of questionable intrascrotal masses and can be used to distinguish between solid and cystic lesions. With the patient in a dark room, a strong, focused light (e.g., a fiberoptic light) is placed against the scrotal sac dorsally. A cystic lesion, such as a hydrocele or large spermatocele, will transillumine; but light will not be transmitted through a solid tumor. Since approximately 10% of testicular tumors are associated with a reactive hydrocele, however, findings should be carefully evaluated (6). Although sonography provides more detail about the nature of a scrotal mass, transillumination may still yield valuable information in the initial examination of a patient.

REFERENCES

1. Williamson RCN. Torsion of the testis and allied conditions. *Br J Surg* 1976;63:465–476.
2. Cass AS, Cass BP, Veeraraghavan K. Immediate exploration of the unilateral acute scrotum in young male subjects. *J Urol* 1980;124: 829–832.
3. Del Villar RG, Ireland GW, Cass AS. Early exploration in acute testicular conditions. *J Urol* 1972;108:887–888.
4. Einhorn LH, Crawford ED, Shipley WU, Loehrer PJ, Williams SD. Cancer of the testes. In: DeVita VT, Hellman S, Rosenberg SA, eds. *Cancer: principles and practice of oncology*, 3rd ed, vol 1. Philadelphia: JB Lippincott; 1989:1071–1098.
5. Rifkin MD. Measurements of scrotal contents. In: Goldberg BB, Kurtz AB, eds. *Atlas of ultrasound measurements*. Chicago: Year Book; 1990:180–187.
6. Lowe FC, Brendler CB. Evaluation of the urologic patient. In: Walsh PC, Retik AB, Stamey TA, Vaughan ED, eds. *Campbell's urology*, 6th ed, vol 1. Philadelphia: WB Saunders; 1992:307–341.

CHAPTER 3

Imaging Techniques, Anatomy, Artifacts, and Bioeffects

A. Ultrasound

Ultrasound (US) is considered the primary imaging modality in the scrotum because of its high accuracy in differentiating cystic from solid and intratesticular from extratesticular lesions. Low cost, ready availability, and lack of ionizing radiation add to its appeal as a diagnostic tool.

Major indications for ultrasound include

1. Assessment of the origin of intrascrotal masses—assignment of the lesion to the testis, epididymis, or other scrotal structure; and distinction of fluid from solid lesions.
2. Confirmation or exclusion of a testicular tumor when a mass is palpated on clinical exam—US is also the most suitable modality for excluding testicular tumor in the presence of unexplained retroperitoneal lymphadenopathy.
3. Evaluation of the testis when palpation is difficult, as in cases of large hydrocele or painful epididymitis.
4. Assessment of the extent of inflammatory disease and presence or absence of abscess in patients with intrascrotal inflammatory disease.
5. Follow-up of severe intrascrotal inflammatory disease.
6. Evaluation of varicocele, in particular as a workup for infertility patients.
7. Evaluation of etiology of acute scrotal pain, and the differentiation between torsion and inflammatory process.
8. Assessment of scrotum after trauma and evaluation of hematocele and testicular rupture.
9. Location of undescended testis (especially when searching in the area from the internal inguinal ring to the scrotal sac) and detection or exclusion of malignant degeneration of an undescended testis.
10. Evaluation of endocrine abnormality or gynecomastia and demonstration or exclusion of an occult testicular tumor.
11. Carcinophobia, a rare indication, but good documentation of normal morphologic structures provides considerable reassurance to the patient.

TECHNIQUES AND METHODS OF EXAMINATION

Diagnosis should always be based on a combination of sonographic and clinical findings. Palpation and history taking are important parts of the sonographic examination of the scrotum. Palpation before scanning provides a general impression of the anatomic situation, the consistency of the testes, and pathologic alterations. With palpation, small, suspicious abnormalities—not immediately seen on a sonogram—can be identified while scanning. History taking before scanning reduces the imaging time and allows the examiner to ask specific questions that may arise during scanning. The average time required for a sonographic examination of the scrotum, including palpation, history taking, and documentation, is 10 to 15 minutes.

Patient Preparation and Positioning

Scrotal sonography is easiest to perform with the patient in the supine position with the scrotum resting on a towel draped over the abducted thighs. The penis is elevated onto the abdomen and covered with a towel. A special device for supporting the scrotum is not required. Additional scanning in the standing position may be helpful if evaluating for varicoceles or inguinal hernias.

The coupling gel should be applied generously, as the scrotal hair frequently leads to bubble-shaped air inclusions, which degrade the image. Air bubbles can be removed by careful smoothing of the coupling gel. It is important to remember that application of the gel and mechanical manipulations during the examination may provoke a contraction of the cremaster muscle and retraction of the testis into the inguinal canal. This is especially important when examining children or patients with suspected cryptorchidism. When examining neonates and infants, prewarming the coupling gel helps to prevent unnecessary irritation.

Equipment and Scanning Parameters

High-resolution, real-time scanners with frequencies of 5 to 10 MHz should be used for sonographic examination of the scrotum. Either linear-array transducers or sector scanners can be used, but the former yield better spatial resolution in the near field and are preferable.

Either direct-contact scanning or scanning through a water path can be used. Since the flexible water path adapts very well to the convex surface of the testis, it allows better focusing of structures close to the transducer and an easy and nearly compression-free coupling of the transducer to the scrotum (Fig. 3.1). If an electronically focused high-frequency transducer is used, a water path is not usually necessary.

With water path scanning, tumors are not compressed and are seen to their full extent (Fig. 3.2). It may also be helpful in examining patients with a painful and tender scrotum. Instead of a system with a water path as a standoff device, a simple water-filled finger stall (or condom) can be attached in front of the sound-emitting window (Fig. 3.3). The transducer with the water path is freely mobile, and patients can be examined both standing and in the supine position, allowing for palpation during scanning. Some of the newest scanners have a built-in device to increase the distance between the transducer and the scrotal skin (Fig. 3.4). Direct contact scanning is also frequently used. It is often less cumbersome than a water path, and physical examination during scanning is feasible.

The sonographic technique (i.e., overall gain and time gain compensation curve) can best be adjusted on the basis of a longitudinal scan through the unaffected testis. The normal testis has a homogeneous echo texture of medium-level echogenicity throughout (Figs. 3.4 and 3.5). Thereafter, the sonographic examination comprises continuous scanning of the scrotum in both longitudinal and transverse planes. It is important to ensure that the entire testis is scanned. When probes with a narrow window are used, stepwise scanning of the testis is recommended. The longitudinal scan yields a good view of the anatomic boundaries between the testis and the epididymis (Fig. 3.5), whereas the transverse scan allows direct comparison of the echo texture of both testes (Fig. 3.4A). Longitudinal and transverse scans are generally sufficient for complete evaluation. In selected cases, such as patients with very large intrascrotal lesions, scanning from a dorsal or lateral direction may yield additional diagnostic information (Fig. 3.4B). Palpation during scanning may be important to locate small, clinically suspected masses, which would otherwise be difficult to identify on the sonogram.

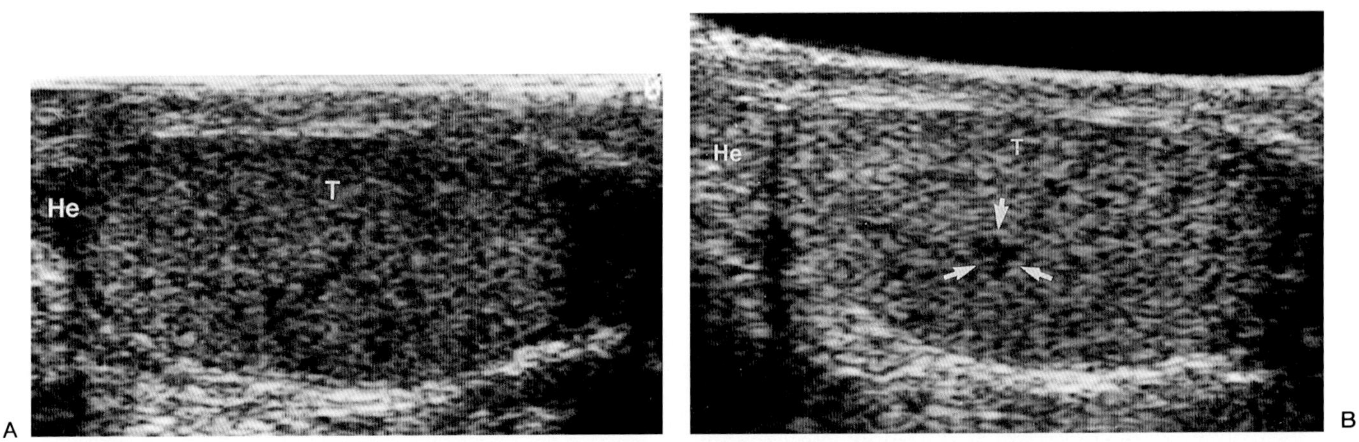

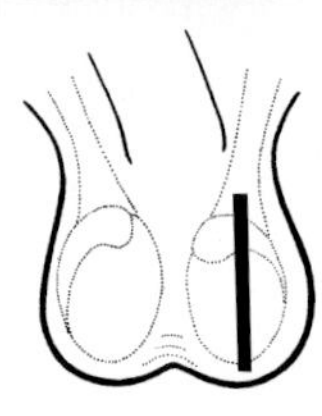

FIG. 3.1. Small (3 mm) mature teratoma in the center of the testis. **(A)** Using a 5-MHz transducer without a water path, the intratesticular lesion is difficult to identify. In addition, there is poor spatial resolution in the ventral parts of the testis (T) and at the interface between the testis (T) and the head (He) and tail of the epididymis. **(B)** Using a 5-MHz transducer with a water path, the small central tumor (*arrows*) is reliably identified.

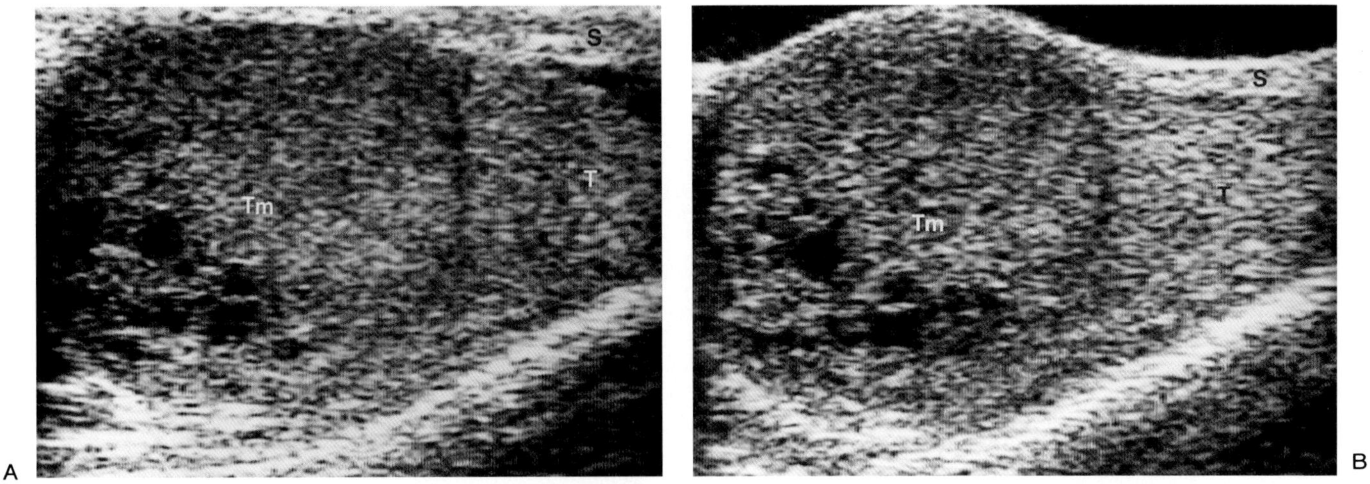

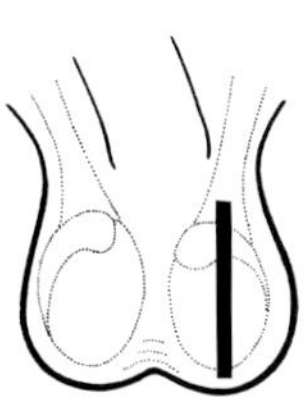

FIG. 3.2. Solid testicular lesion, histologically shown to be a seminoma. Sonogram using a 5-MHz, linear-array transducer without **(A)** and with **(B)** a flexible water path. With the water path the tumor (Tm) is not compressed and there is better visualization of the mass effect (the small, cystlike areas within the tumor correspond to liquefied necrosis of the seminoma). (T, testis; S, scrotal skin)

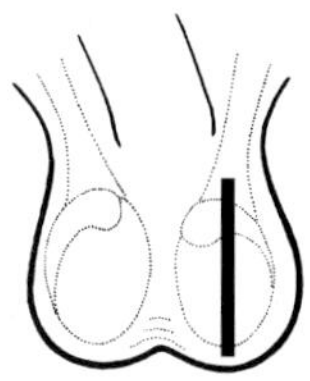

Sonographic findings should be documented with, at a minimum, a longitudinal scan of each testis and a transverse scan of both testes. It is useful to include one or two transverse images of both testes side by side, so that size and echo texture can be compared. Additional documentation depends on the findings and may, in particular, be required in patients who will undergo conservative treatment and are therefore likely to be referred for follow-up.

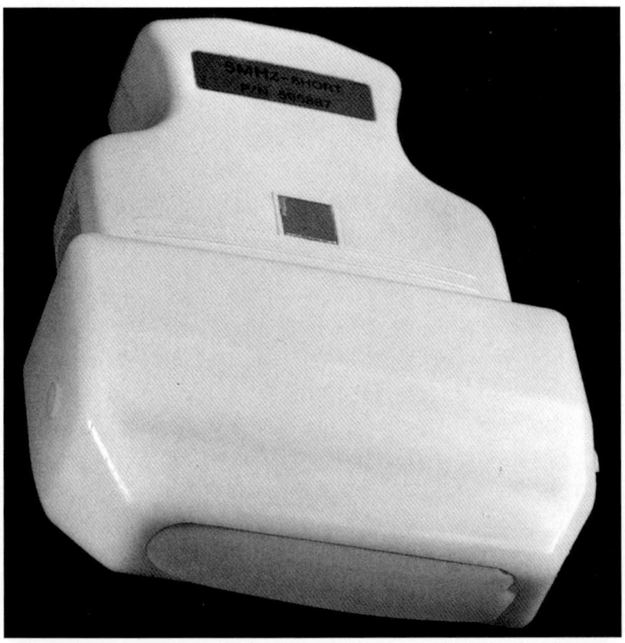

FIG. 3.3. Linear-array transducer with attached water path. The water-filled finger stall used as a stand-off device is kept in position by a Teflon cap.

When a testicular tumor is diagnosed or suspected, ultrasound may be used for preliminary staging by examining the retroperitoneal lymph nodes at the level of and below the renal hili, the lymph node regions to which testicular tumors tend to spread first. Rarely, the lymph node group in the common iliac region is affected. In general, lymph node involvement is better evaluated by computed tomography (CT) or magnetic resonance (MR) imaging (see Chapter 5).

Color-Coded Duplex Sonography

Although Doppler sonography and B-mode sonography were developed separately, they are both based on analysis of the sound waves that are reflected by body structures and return to the transducer. Doppler sonography uses the frequency and phase shifts of the returning sound waves to derive information about the movement of blood. In B-scanning, reflected echoes are processed with respect to their temporal delay and different amplitudes. The temporal delay permits identification of the spatial position of a reflector and the amplitude of the reflected sound wave provides information on the type of tissue.

Combination of B-mode and Doppler sonography poses technical challenges, since the reflected signal from vessel wall and vascular lumen differs by two to three orders of magnitude. In duplex sonography two separate sound sources are used, one to generate the B-mode (gray-scale) image and a second to derive Doppler (flow) information from the relatively low-amplitude signal from intraluminal blood. A major limitation of duplex

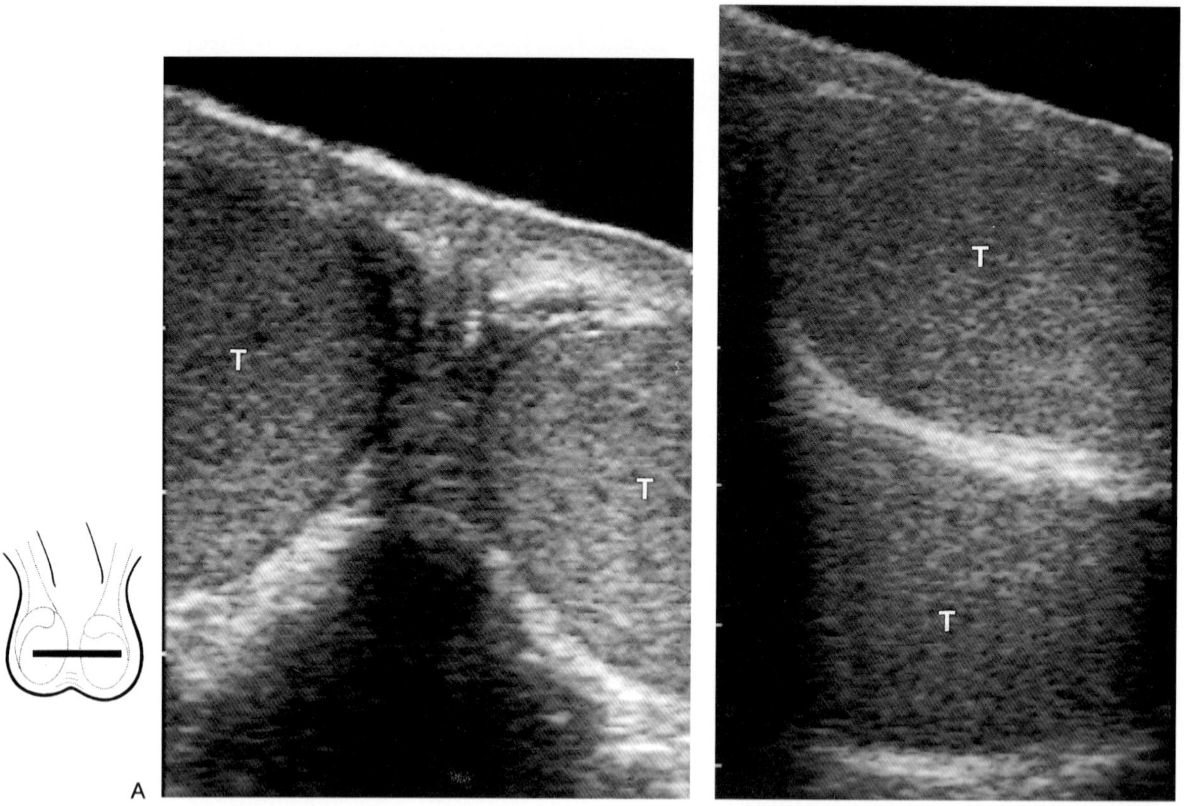

FIG. 3.4. Normal testis, transverse **(A)** and coronal sonograms **(B)** obtained with a built-in device to increase the distance between the transducer and the scrotal skin. Note symmetrical homogeneous echo texture of both testes (T).

sonography is that blood flow information can only be derived from a small volume of tissue at a time.

In color-coded duplex sonography (CCDS) the temporal delay, amplitude, and frequency and phase shifts of the reflected signal are processed simultaneously from all measuring points. Blood flow characteristics, derived from Doppler analysis of the frequency and phase shifts, are displayed in varying shades of red or blue, depending on whether the direction of flow is toward or away from the transducer, respectively. Color shadowing corresponds to mean frequency shift and is roughly proportional to blood flow velocity.

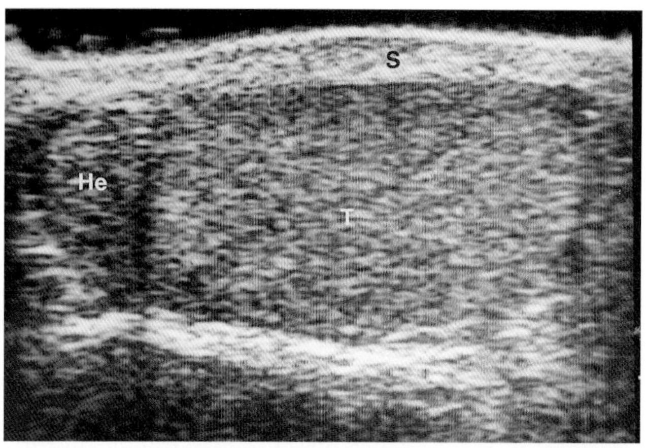

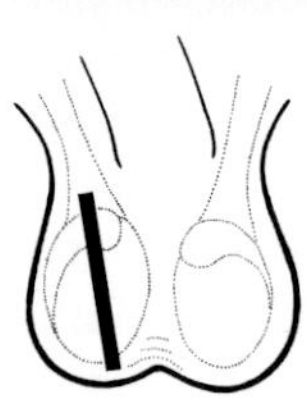

FIG. 3.5. Normal testis and epididymis in adult. Note the homogeneous echopattern of the testicular tissue and good differentiation between the testis (T) and the head of the epididymis (He).

Color-coded duplex sonography (CCDS), however, simultaneously processes the temporal delay and amplitude, and the frequency and phase shifts from all measuring points. Blood flow characteristics are displayed in varying shades of red and blue. The color indicates the direction of blood flow relative to the transducer, and the shading corresponds to the frequency shift (proportional to blood flow velocity). For instance, slow flow toward the transducer is displayed in dark blue, whereas a high-velocity flow away from the transducer appears as light red. In this way there is simultaneous display of real-time images of gray scale tissue structures and blood movement within vessels. Most modern CCDS systems are sensitive enough to register flow signals even from small vessels, which cannot be delineated on the B-scans. Even the slow blood flow in very small organs like the testicles in infants can be observed.

Because the intensity of US reflection is proportional to the fourth power of the transmitted frequency, a higher-frequency transducer is preferred for color Dopp-

TABLE 3.1. *Importance of additional information on perfusion in testicular disorders*

Disorder	Importance*
Inflammation (testis/epididymis)	=
Tumor (testis/epididymis)	−
Torsion (testis/appendix testis)	+
Trauma	+
Varicocele	+

* − means additional information on perfusion is unimportant; = means additional information is only moderately helpful; + means additional information is definitely important.

ler US examinations. Higher-frequency transducers, however, have limited penetrability. A 7.5-MHz transducer is optimal for both sensitive detection of Doppler signals and adequate tissue penetration in the testicle (1). When a 7.5-MHz transducer is employed, frequency shifts as low as 38 Hz can be detected and encoded in color. This corresponds to a calculated flow velocity of 1.25 cm/s at a beam angle of 72°. For better depiction of slow flow in the small vessels, color gain should be maximized to the point just before excessive noise degrades the image. The Doppler scale should be adjusted to increase the sensitivity (1).

The clinical applications for CCDS include any situation in which additional information on testicular perfusion is needed to establish the diagnosis (2), particularly testicular torsion (see p. 111), scrotal trauma (see p. 119), testicular abscess formation (see p. 99), and varicocele (see p. 149). In other scrotal disorders, information on blood flow is of minor importance in diagnosis (Table 3.1) (3).

RELIABILITY OF SCROTAL ULTRASOUND

The value of ultrasound in the diagnostic evaluation of intrascrotal pathology has been investigated in a number of studies (4–15). The studies were performed with high-resolution ultrasound scanners (between 5 and 10 MHz), and all studies attributed the following characteristics to scrotal sonography:

1. High sensitivity in detection of intrascrotal abnormalities.
2. Very good differentiation of testicular from paratesticular lesions.
3. Limited usefulness in distinguishing malignant from benign tumors.

Rifkin et al. studied 289 patients and found that ultrasound had a sensitivity of 98.5% in the detection of pathologic changes and correctly differentiated testicular from paratesticular abnormalities in 99% of cases (4). In the detection of testicular tumors, both London et al. (5) (109 patients) and Fowler et al. (6) (230 patients) reported a 100% sensitivity and 99% specificity. Clinical examination, in contrast, has a sensitivity of only 72% and specificity of 89% in the detection of testicular tumors (6). In addition, London et al. (5) found that ultrasonography provided clinically relevant information in 53% of patients and that 8% were spared surgery based on sonographic findings. Kromann-Andersen et al. (7) calculated the positive predictive value (the probability that a patient with positive findings will actually have the diagnosed disorder) of both clinical examination and scrotal ultrasound in 166 patients and found that it increased from 33% with clinical findings to 53% with ultrasound findings.

Although gray-scale ultrasonography was found to be unsatisfactory in the evaluation of testicular torsion, color-coded Doppler sonography is very helpful in the diagnosis of this condition (2,16–19).

RISKS AND BIOEFFECTS

The reputation of ultrasound as a risk-free procedure is based on the fact that no definite adverse effects have been described to date. Potential damage is of particular importance in connection with a germ-cell organ like the testis, but discussion of this aspect of diagnostic sonography is complicated by the fact that there are no uniform definitions of the units and energies used.

There are several mechanisms by which ultrasonic waves can damage cells, including

1. Absorption of energy in tissue and release of heat (a method used therapeutically at much higher energies than those typically applied in diagnostic ultrasound).
2. Formation of hollow spaces (cavitation) in tissues exposed to ultrasound waves and subsequent damage to cells when the spaces expand or collapse.
3. Direct mechanical action in which transmission of sound waves is associated with acceleration and deceleration processes in tissues. These processes may induce cellular changes, especially in chromosomes.

Intensity, the most important parameter of the US beam, has both spatial and temporal characteristics. For example, energy applied to a large area over a prolonged period of time is less likely to have a deleterious effect on cells than the same amount of energy applied to one discrete point for a short time. Several descriptors have been developed to designate a peak or average value with regard to both space and time. The most widely used parameters for describing tissue exposure are ISATA (spatial average, time average intensity); ISATP (spatial average, time peak intensity); ISPTA (spatial peak, time average intensity); and ISPPA (spatial peak, pulse average intensity).

The unit of measurement for energy is **mWatt**; that for intensity is **mWatt/cm²** (20). **Spatial peak (SP)** refers to the maximum intensity in a plane perpendicular to the beam axis, and **spatial average (SA)** refers to the cross-sectional area of the beam with a cutoff point of 0.25

times the SP intensity (20). SP is usually 2 to 6 times greater than SA for nonfocused transducers and 5 to 50 times greater for focused transducers (20). These notations, which are only a sample of the units used to determine intensity, are complex and a potential source of error when studying the effects of ultrasound. For instance, an ISATA of 5 mW/cm^2 in a commercial transducer results in an ISPTA of 15 mW/cm^2.

The determining factor for tissue damage is the amount of energy applied per area and unit time. Numerous animal studies have been performed to identify a threshold value below which damage can be definitely excluded. Difficulties arise because of the wide range of possible alterations and the problems associated with application of the results to humans. The most frequently quoted safety recommendations on ultrasound safety are published by the the American Institute for Ultrasound in Medicine (AIUM) and were last revised in 1984 (21). These guidelines suggest that no bioeffects are expected when tissue is exposed to an intensity of less than 100 mW/cm^2 (ISPTA) for unfocused US, or less than 1 W/cm^2 for focused US. Even higher intensities are not likely to damage tissue if the time of exposure is limited and if the product of intensity and ultrasonic exposure time is less than 50 $joules/cm^2$. Conventional ultrasound scanners operate at intensities of about 40 mW/cm^2, with peaks of 200 mW/cm^2 (ISPTA). Application of experimental data to the diagnostic setting is limited. In diagnostic applications the continual movement of the examined organ and the transducer result in short time exposures for any specific area.

As yet there is no well-established evidence for potential health risks associated with the diagnostic application of ultrasound (20,22–26).

NORMAL ANATOMY

On sonograms the mature (postpubescent) **testis** is an oval structure with a longitudinal diameter of 3 to 5 cm and a transverse diameter of 2 to 3 cm. The testis, along with the epididymis, decreases in size with advancing age. The normal testis has a homogeneous echo texture of medium echogenicity, similar to the thyroid gland (Figs. 3.4 and 3.5). Normally, the homogeneous appearance is interrupted only by the mediastinum testis and individual testicular septa (Fig. 3.6).

The **mediastinum testis** is displayed as a hyperechoic (echogenic) line extending in a caudocranial direction, becoming slightly thicker in the cranial portion of the testis (Fig. 3.6). It is eccentrically located in the testis beneath the tunica albuginea on the side facing the epididymis. The width of the hyperechoic mediastinum testis varies widely among individuals and may even be different in the right and left testes in the same patient. Neither sonographic visualization of the mediastinum testis nor its width have any diagnostic implications. It should not be mistaken for a pathologic lesion.

The **rete testis**, a major structure in the mediastinum testis, can be seen on US in approximately 18% of normal testes (27). It is characterized by a spectrum of sonographic findings ranging from decreased echogenicity at

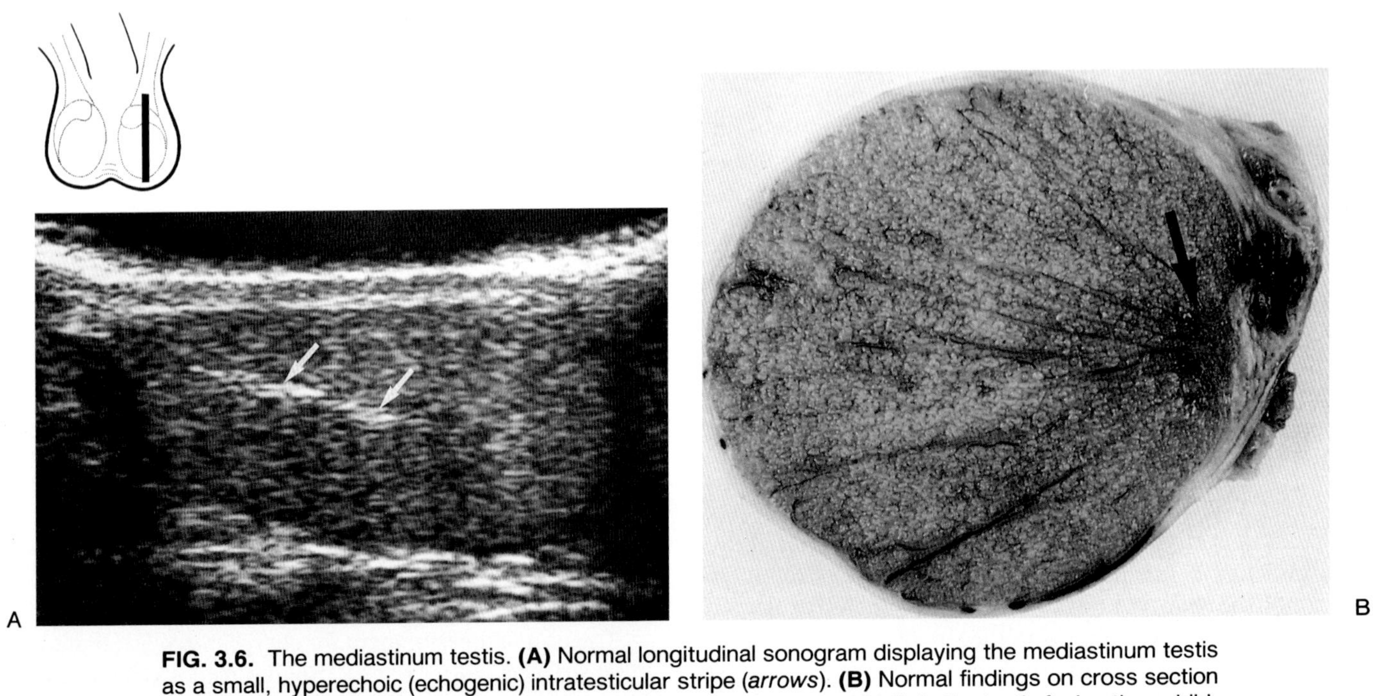

FIG. 3.6. The mediastinum testis. **(A)** Normal longitudinal sonogram displaying the mediastinum testis as a small, hyperechoic (echogenic) intratesticular stripe (*arrows*). **(B)** Normal findings on cross section of macroscopic specimen. The mediastinum testis (*arrow*) lies eccentrically in the testis facing the epididymis. The septula testis run toward the mediastinum testis.

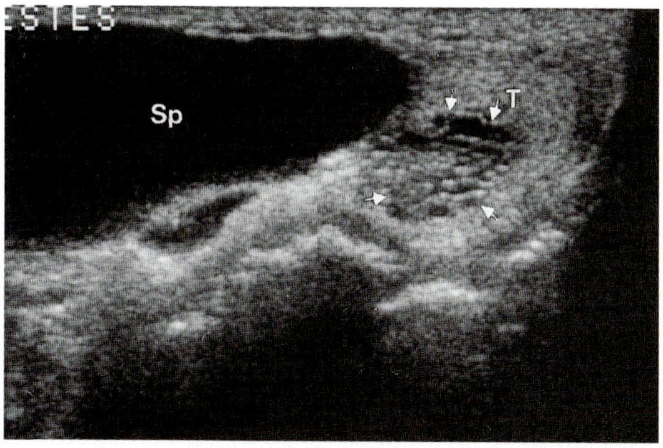

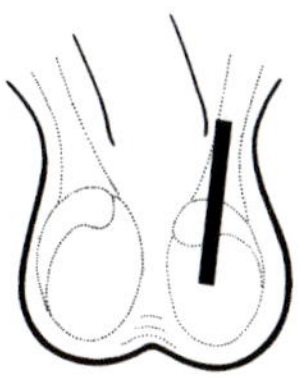

FIG. 3.7. Seminiferous tubular ectasia of the rete testis (*arrows*) and associated spermatocele (Sp). Testis (T)

the testicular hilum to a discrete masslike structure characterized by numerous tiny cysts from which tubular structures extend into the testicular parenchyma (27). The latter is sometimes referred to as seminiferous tubular ectasia of the rete testis (p. 82) (28–30). Tubular ectasia occurs along a continuum from prominence of the rete testis to a masslike structure with resolvable cysts. Prominent rete testes are often the result of a more distal obstruction and therefore are often associated with epididymal cysts or spermatoceles (Fig. 3.7).

Rarely, the **septula testes** are displayed on the sonogram. They appear as delicate linear structures, sometimes identified indirectly by refractory shadowing. These shadows disappear upon slight compression or when the scan direction is changed.

In about 10% of normal testes, one or two vessels are seen as a tapering curvilinear hypoechoic structure with or without echogenic borders (Fig. 3.8) (31). These represent intratesticular arteries and veins and can be identified easily by pulsed or color Doppler sonography.

In rare instances, multiple, tiny speckled echos can be seen diffusely throughout the testis. This condition, called testicular microlithiasis, is discussed in detail on p. 84. It is commonly associated with undescended testis or testicular tumor, most commonly seminoma, but may occur without any associated disease. The clinical significance is not completely understood, although many believe these findings suggest a premalignant condition. These patients should be carefully evaluated for associated diseases.

The **tunica albuginea**, which surrounds the testicular tissue like a capsule, is usually not recognized as a separate structure.

The **epididymis** is an elongated structure situated dorsally on the testis. By rotating the testis and epididymis slightly, the latter may be viewed in a position lateral to

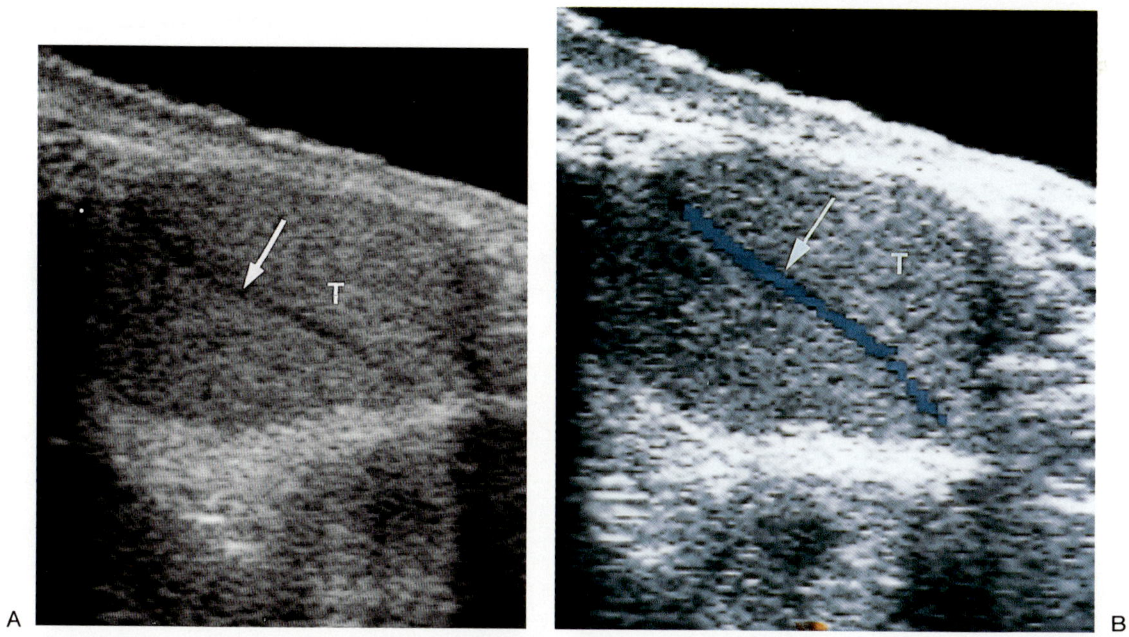

FIG. 3.8. Intratesticular vessel (*arrow*) which traverses through the testis (T). **(A)** Gray-scale and **(B)** color-coded duplex sonography.

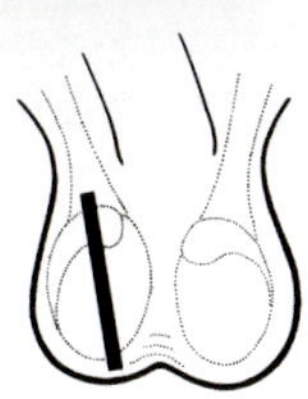

the testis. The length of the epididymis has no diagnostic significance, but it is important to be able to delineate the testis precisely from the epididymis, which is easiest on a longitudinal scan. Sonographic differentiation of the epididymis from the testis is also facilitated by scattering the sound beam at the oblique interface of the convex surfaces of the upper and lower poles of the testis, producing a hypoechoic line between the testicular tissue and the head and tail of the epididymis (Fig. 3.9). The epididymal head (**globus major**) (Fig. 3.9) is seen as a small, caplike structure located on the upper pole of the testis. It may vary in shape (triangular, crescent, or droplike), and its diameter ranges from 5 to 12 mm. The body of the epididymis is slender and flat (approximately 2 to 4 mm in diameter) and may not always be distinguishable from the surrounding paratesticular tissue. The tail of the epididymis (**globus minor**) is approximately 2 to 5 mm, is also flat, and is attached to the lower pole of the testis in a crescentlike manner. Its echo texture is comparable to that of the testis but may sometimes be more dense (more echogenic). The head of the epididymis is usually slightly more echogenic than the body or tail, probably because it contains more tubules and therefore has an increased number of interfaces (32).

The **appendix of the testis** and **appendix of the epididymis** are seldom recognized sonographically, since they are too small (between 1 and 4 mm) to stand out against the surrounding paratesticular tissue. In patients with a hydrocele, they may be visualized as small, stalked appendages at the upper pole of the testis.

The testis and epididymis are surrounded by the two leaves of the **tunica vaginalis.** The cleftlike space between the leaves of the tunica vaginalis is known as the **cavum serosum testis** and, even under normal physiological conditions, contains small amounts of fluid, most likely seen as a thin (1- to 3-mm) echo-free rim in the area adjacent to the epididymal head (Fig. 3.9). This normal amount of fluid must not be misinterpreted as a hydrocele.

The **spermatic cord**, which contains the ductus deferens, arteries, veins, lymphatics, and nerves as well as fatty and connective tissue, is enveloped by the spermatic fascia. These different anatomic structures give the spermatic cord an inhomogeneous sonographic appearance. It is seen as a long band of varying shape, which can be reliably evaluated in the cranial direction up to the external inguinal ring. The mobility of the cord may be diagnostically useful (e.g., during a Valsalva maneuver). Although the ductus deferens, arteries, lymphatics, and veins cannot be distinguished as individual structures, the veins of the pampiniform plexus are seen as tortuous, hypoechoic lines, 1 to 2 mm in diameter. Nodular alterations of constant shape within the spermatic cord represent pathologic change requiring further evaluation.

The sonographically visualized scrotal coverings are composed of portions of the cremasteric muscle, the external spermatic fascia, the tunica dartos, and the skin. The thickness of the scrotal wall, usually 2 to 8 mm, depends on the state of relaxation or contraction of the cremasteric muscle. The **septum testis** is displayed on transverse scans and can be seen as a vertically oriented structure with dorsal acoustic shadowing.

In **infants and children**, the testis is hypoechoic compared to that of adults [compare Fig. 3.5 (p. 14) with Fig. 3.10]. Nonetheless, the prepubescent, hypoechoic testis should be homogeneous. During puberty (between 9 and 16 years of age) there is a significant increase in testicular echogenicity (Fig. 3.11) (33). This is primarily the result of growth of the seminiferous tubules, which increase in diameter and develop a lumen. The epididymal head can often be identified even in infants. In the postnatal period a physiologic hydrocele may be present, which disappears spontaneously. Sonographic evaluation of the

A

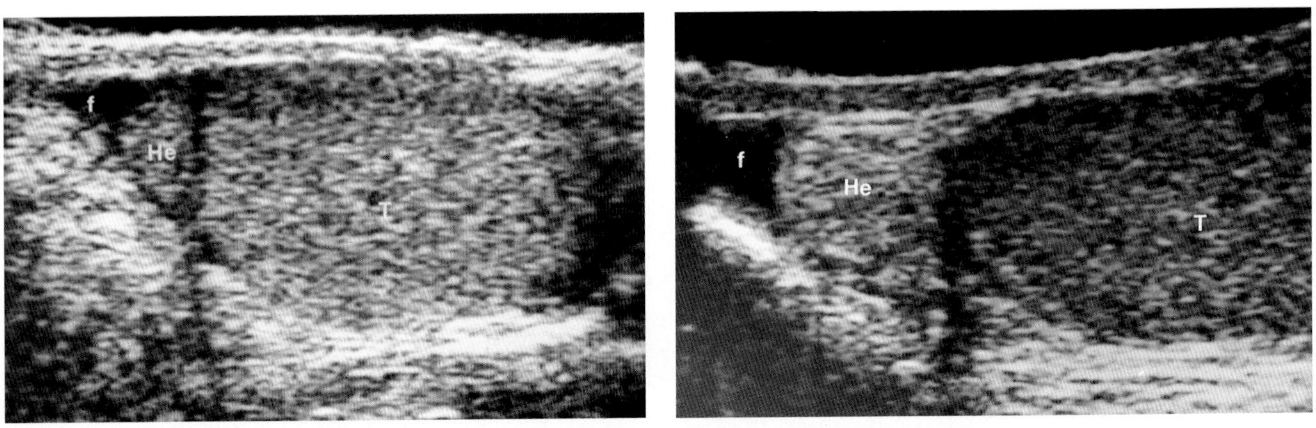

B

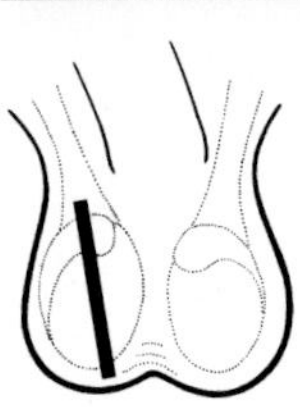

FIG. 3.9. (A), (B) Normal sonogram of the head of the epididymis (He). The head may vary in shape, size, and echogenicity. It is important to delineate the epididymal head from the upper pole of the testis (T). Note the small amount of physiologic fluid (f) within the serous cavity.

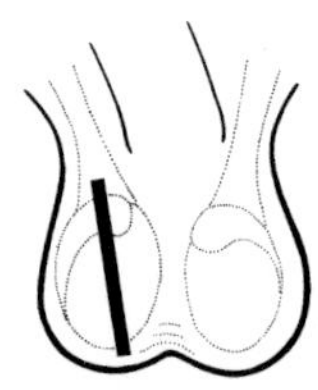

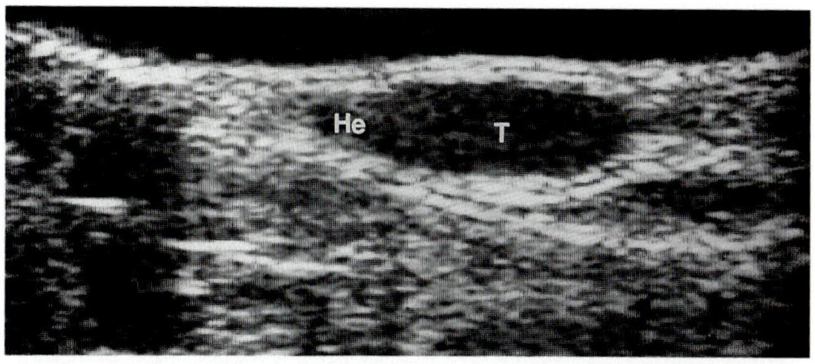

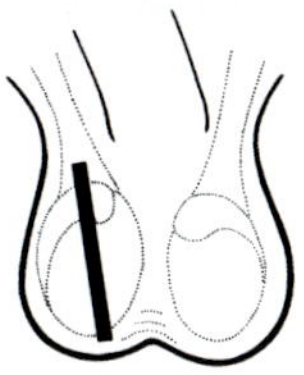

FIG. 3.10. Normal sonogram of the testis of a 7-year-old boy. The testicular tissue (T) is hypoechoic. The epididymal head (He) is seen cranial to the upper pole of the testis.

scrotum during infancy and childhood is often difficult and less reliable than in adults, because of the very small size and mobility of the organs.

In summary, the following features of normal sonographic anatomy are of diagnostic importance:

1. The major characteristic of the normal testis is its homogeneous echo texture of medium-level intensity. It is interrupted by the echogenic stripe of the mediastinum testis. Symmetry in size is more important than absolute size.
2. The epididymis may not be visualized in all its segments, but, in the appropriate clinical setting, an enlargement of the organ is pathologic.
3. The testis should be clearly differentiated from the paratesticular structures (including the epididymis).

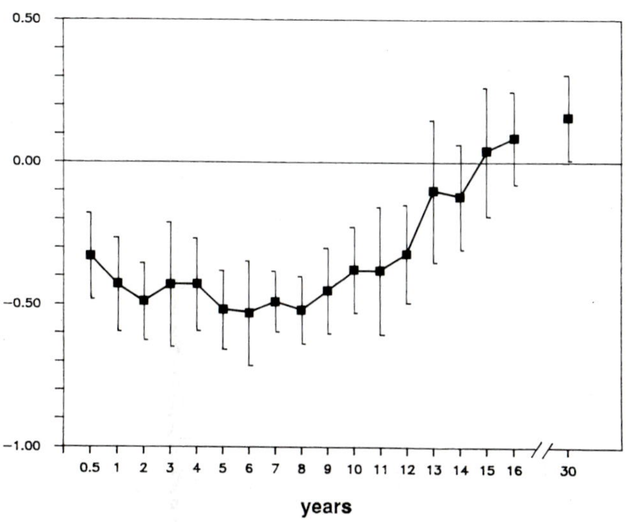

FIG. 3.11. Graphic representation of the age-dependent development of testicular echogenicity relative to a standard. The prepubescent testis is markedly hypoechoic compared to the mature testis. Echogenicity begins to increase at approximately 9 years of age and becomes especially pronounced from 12 to 15 years old. Further changes in the mature testis (i.e., in the age group from 16 to 30 years) do not occur.

4. Not all anatomic structures (e.g., tunica albuginea, ductus deferens) can be recognized sonographically.
5. Hypoechogenicity of the immature testis is a normal finding.
6. Testicular blood flow.

Color-Coded Duplex Sonography (CCDS)

With CCDS, arterial blood flow in the testis and in the spermatic cord is usually demonstrable in normal subjects. However, arterial flow in the epididymis is not depicted, because of smaller vascular sizes and lesser flow. Venous flow can be depicted in the normal scrotum by CCDS.

In the testis capsular and centripetal arteries are seen in most normal subjects, and the centrifugal arteries are also commonly seen (Fig. 3.12) (1). In some men an artery (sometimes along with an accompanying vein) running obliquely from the rete testis through testicular parenchyma can be depicted by CCDS (Fig. 3.8).

On spectral Doppler analysis the testicular artery and its intratesticular branches show low-resistance-type waveforms—broad systolic peak and high diastolic flow (1,34). The waveforms of the supratesticular arteries are variable. In this region the deferential and cremasteric arteries often demonstrate high-resistance waveforms—narrow systolic peaks and low diastolic flow (1,34). As either the testicular, the deferential, or the cremasteric

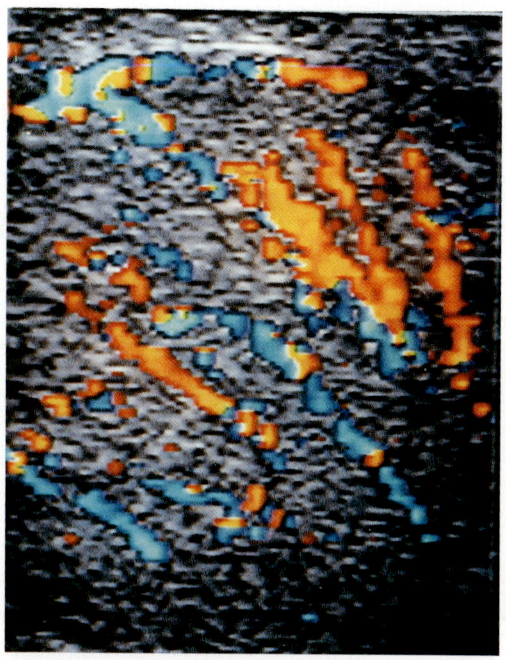

FIG. 3.12. Color-coded duplex sonography demonstrating capsular, centripetal, and centrifugal arteries of the testis.

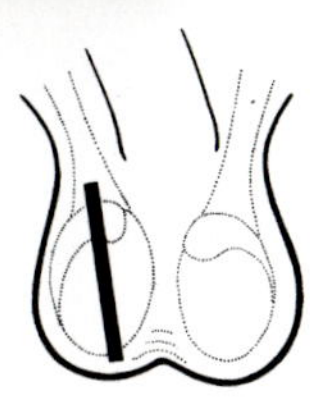

artery can be depicted in the supratesticular region, the flow information should be carefully interpreted, especially for the evaluation of testicular perfusion or paratesticular hyperemia.

Although CCDS may depict blood flow even in a small blood vessel, detection of blood flow in the small normal testes (<1 cm^3) of prepubertal boys is often difficult (35).

ARTIFACTS

Interpretation of ultrasound scans of the scrotum can be impaired by a variety of artifacts. Vertical line artifacts (Fig. 3.13) arise posterior to small air bubbles that persist around scrotal hair after application of the coupling gel. These lines typically extend from the scrotal skin through all tissue structures. The air bubbles producing these artifacts can be eliminated by repeated application and spreading of the coupling gel.

Horizontal hyperechoic line artifacts (Fig. 3.14) result from reverberating echoes from the transducer/water path interface. Such lines are best recognized against the homogeneous background of the testicular parenchyma. They impair the evaluation of the testis and may be mistaken for the mediastinum testis. Typically, these artifacts are seen as hyperechoic, horizontally oriented, fine, smooth lines that also appear in other positions at the same depth when the transducer is moved. These artifacts can be eliminated by reapplying coupling gel between the transducer and the water path or the water path and the scrotum, or, if possible, by eliminating the water path entirely.

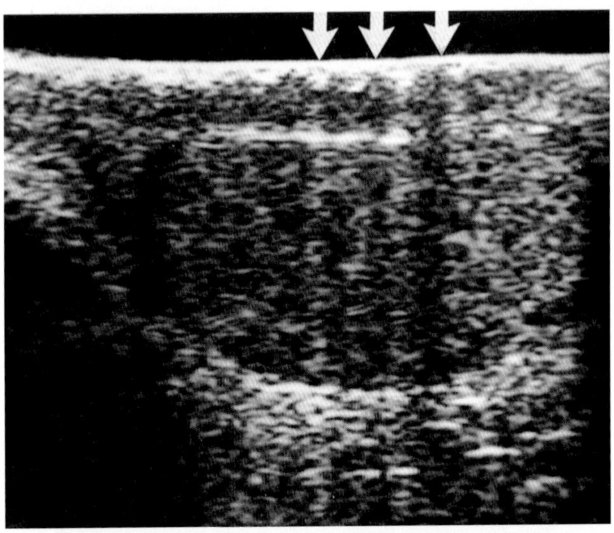

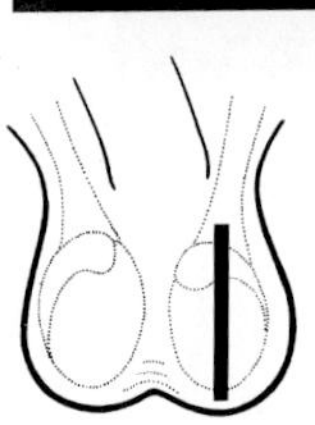

FIG. 3.13. Vertical line artifacts (*arrows*).

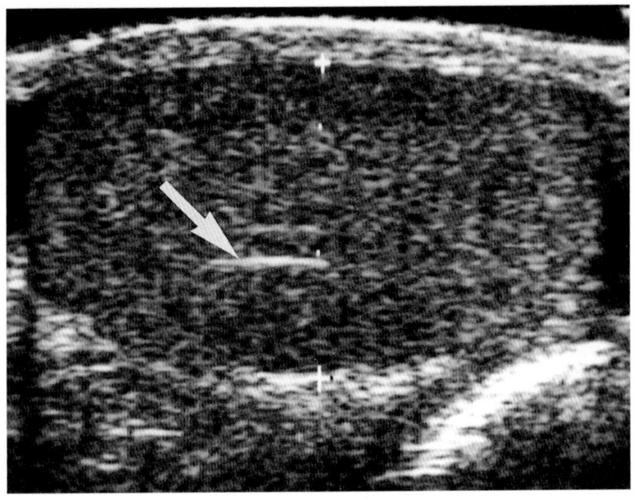

FIG. 3.14. Horizontal line artifacts (*arrow*).

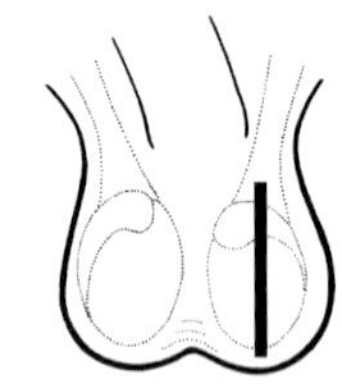

Discrete intratesticular acoustic shadows may occur at any scanning orientation within the testis. These may be refractory shadows produced by the mediastinum testis (easy to identify) or by the obliquely oriented testicular septula (which are not visualized directly). Refractory shadowing is rare, and misinterpretation of these shadows as hypoechoic intratesticular lesions can be avoided

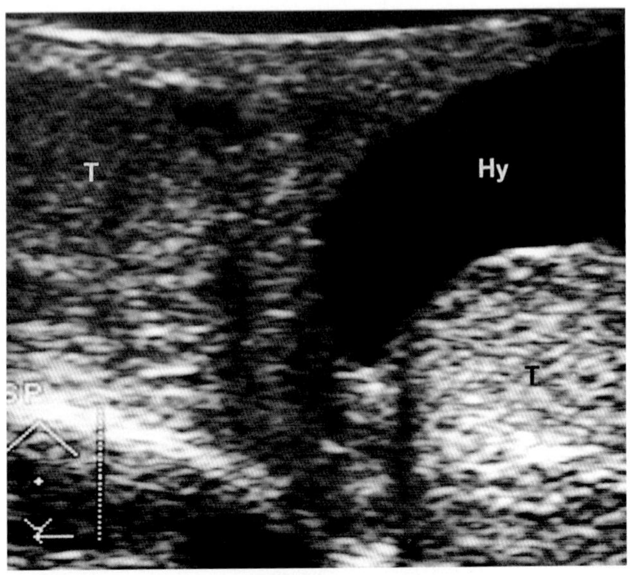

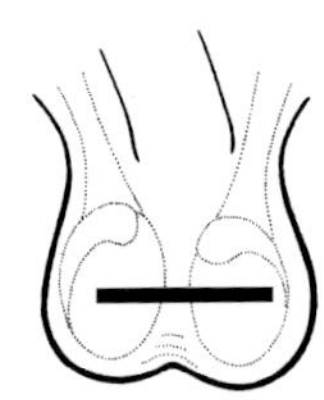

FIG. 3.15. A hydrocele (Hy) in front of the left testis produces a false impression of asymmetrical echogenicity. (T, testes)

by slight compression with the transducer (which makes the shadows disappear) or by scanning the same region with a different scan orientation.

A unilateral hydrocele may also distort sonographic comparison of the two testes by amplifying the echogenicity of the underlying testicle (Fig. 3.15).

VOLUMETRY OF THE TESTIS

The size of the testis is closely related to total count, motility, morphology, and daily production of sperm. Therefore, measurement of testicular volume can be helpful in evaluating male reproductive function (36). Ultrasonographic measurement has been proved to be accurately correlated with actual testicular volume and is preferred over clinical assessment, especially when intrascrotal pathology, such as hydrocele, hematocele, varicocele, or epididymitis, precludes an accurate clinical measurement (36).

Sonographically, the volume of the testis is best calculated as a rotational ellipsoid:

$$V = a \times b \times c \times d$$

where V = volume, a = length, b = height, c = width, and d is a correction factor of 0.52 ($\pi/6$) (34). This method has an error of 15%. Accuracy increases with larger volumes and decreases with smaller volumes. With volumes less than 4 ml the error may be as high as 50% (37). Care must be taken not to compress the testis during sonographic measurement and actually to scan the maximal longitudinal and transverse axes.

Clinically, determination of the size of a normally developed adult testis plays only a minor role. Disorders are primarily identified on the basis of their echo texture; and comparison with the contralateral, normal testis is much more helpful than volume determination. Although volume may be of interest after treatment of cryptorchidism and in patients with a varicocele, conclusive data are not available.

REFERENCES

1. Horstman WG, Middleton WD, Melson GL, Siegel BA. Color Doppler US of the scrotum. *Radiographics* 1991;11:941–957.
2. Middleton WD, Siegel BA, Melson GL, Yates CK, Andriole GL. Acute scrotal disorders: prospective comparison of color Doppler US and testicular scintigraphy. *Radiology* 1990;177:177–181.
3. Mitchell DG. Color Doppler imaging: principles, limitations, and artifacts. *Radiology* 1990;177:1–10.
4. Rifkin MD, Kurtz AB, Pasto ME, Goldberg BB. Diagnostic capabilities of high-resolution scrotal ultrasonography: prospective evaluation. *J Ultrasound Med* 1985;4:13–19.
5. London NJ, Smart JG, Kinder RB, Watkin EM, Rees Y, Haley P. Prospective study of routine scrotal ultrasonography in urological practice. *Br J Urol* 1989;63:416–419.
6. Fowler RC, Chennells PM, Ewing R. Scrotal ultrasonography: a clinical evaluation. *Br J Radiol* 1987;60:649–654.
7. Kromann-Andersen B, Hansen LB, Larsen PN, et al. Clinical versus ultrasonographic evaluation of scrotal disorders. *Br J Urol* 1988;61:350–353.
8. Anderson KA, McAninch JW, Jeffrey RB, Laing FC. Ultrasonography for the diagnosis and staging of blunt scrotal trauma. *J Urol* 1983;130:933–935.
9. Cunningham JJ. Sonographic findings in clinically unsuspected acute and chronic scrotal hematoceles. *AJR* 1983;140:749–752.
10. Gutman H, Golimbu M, Subramanyam BR. Diagnostic ultrasound of scrotum. *Urology* 1986;27:72–75.
11. Jeffrey RB, Laing FC, Hricak H, McAninch JW. Sonography of testicular trauma. *AJR* 1983;141:993–995.
12. Kratzik C, Kuber W, Donner G, Lunglmayr G, Frick J, Schmoller HJ. Impact of sonography on diagnosis of scrotal diseases: a multicenter study. *Eur Urol* 1988;14:270–275.
13. Lupetin AR, King W, Rich PJ, Lederman RB. The traumatized scrotum. Ultrasound evaluation. *Radiology* 1983;148:203–207.
14. Scott RF, Bayliss AP, Calder JF, Garvie WH. Indications for ultrasound in the evaluation of the pathological scrotum. *Br J Urol* 1986;58:178–182.
15. Willscher MK, Conway JF, Daly KJ, DiGiancinto TM, Patten D. Scrotal ultrasonography. *J Urol* 1983;130:931–932.
16. Wilbert DM, Schaerfe CW, Stern WD, Strohmaier WL, Bichler KH. Evaluation of the acute scrotum by color-coded Doppler ultrasonography. *J Urol* 1993;149:1475–1477.
17. Fitzgerald SW, Erickson S, DeWire DM, et al. Color Doppler sonography in the evaluation of the adult acute scrotum. *J Ultrasound Med* 1992;11:543–548.
18. Atkinson GO Jr, Patrick LE, Ball TI Jr, Stephenson CA, Broecker BH, Woodard JR. The normal and abnormal scrotum in children: evaluation with color Doppler sonography. *AJR* 1992;158:613–617.
19. Horstman WG, Middleton WD, Melson GL. Scrotal inflammatory disease: color Doppler US findings. *Radiology* 1991;179:55–59.
20. Hykes DL, Hedrick WR, Starchman DE. Biologic effects. In: Hykes DL, Hedrick WR, Starchman DE. *Ultrasound physics and instrumentation,* 2nd ed. St. Louis: Mosby–Year Book; 1992:190–209.
21. American Institute of Ultrasound in Medicine (AIUM). Safety considerations for diagnostic ultrasound. Bioeffects Committee; 1984.
22. Hagen-Ansert SL. *Textbook of diagnostic ultrasonography,* 3rd ed. St. Louis: Mosby; 1989.
23. Miller DL. A review of the ultrasonic bioeffects of microsonation, gas-body activation, and related cavitation-like phenomena. *Ultrasound Med Biol* 1987;13:443–470.
24. Powis RL, Powis WJ. *A thinker's guide to ultrasonic imaging.* Baltimore: Urban & Schwarzenberg; 1984.
25. *Biological effects on ultrasound: mechanisms and clinical implications.* NCRP Report No 74, Bethesda: National Council on Radiation Protection and Measurements; 1983.
26. Ludwig GD, Struthers FW. *Project M.M. 004, 001,* report 4. US Naval Medical Research Institute; 1949:1.
27. Thomas RD, Dewbury KC. Ultrasound appearances of the rete testis. *Clin Radiol* 1993;47:121–124.
28. Weingarten BJ, Kellman GM, Middleton WD, Gross ML. Tubular ectasia within the mediastinum testis. *J Ultrasound Med* 1992;11:349–353.
29. Brown DL, Benson CB, Doherty FJ, et al. Cystic testicular mass caused by dilated rete testis: sonographic findings in 31 cases. *AJR* 1992;158:1257–1259.
30. Tartar VM, Trambert MA, Balsara ZN, Mattrey RF. Tubular ectasia of the testicle: sonographic and MR imaging appearance. *AJR* 1993;160:539–542.
31. Fakhry J, Khoury A, Barakat K. The hypoechoic band: a normal finding on testicular sonography. *AJR* 1989;153:321–323.
32. Rifkin MD. Scrotal ultrasound. *Urol Radiol* 1987;9:119–126.
33. Hamm B, Fobbe F, Winter S, Dietzel M. Maturation of the testis: ultrasound investigation. The American Roentgen Ray Society, 88th Annual Meeting 1988, *Book of Abstracts, The American Roentgen Ray Society; 1988:*125.
34. Middleton WD, Thorne DA, Melson GL. Color Doppler ultrasound of the normal testis. *AJR* 1989;152:293–297.

35. Atkinson GO, Patrick LE, Ball TI, Stephenson CA, Broecker BH, Woodard JR. The normal and abnormal scrotum in children: evaluation with color Doppler sonography. *AJR* 1992;158:613–617.
36. Behre HM, Nashan D, Nieschlag E. Objective measurement of testicular volume by ultrasonography: evaluation of the technique and comparison with orchidometer estimates. *Int J Androl* 1989;12:395–403.
37. Doernberger V, Doernberger G, Eggstein M. Volumetrie des Hodens mittels Real-time-Sonographie. *Ultraschall Med* 1986;7:300–303.

B. Magnetic Resonance Imaging

Although ultrasonography (US)—because of its relatively low cost, general availability, and accuracy in evaluating intra- and extratesticular pathology—is the initial imaging study for investigation of the testes and other scrotal contents, magnetic resonance (MR) imaging is extremely valuable as a problem-solving modality. It is primarily used when ultrasound is equivocal or suboptimal or when there is a discrepancy between clinical and US findings. Similarly, although computed tomography (CT) is recommended as a primary modality for staging testicular cancer, MR imaging is preferred for follow-up of patients with previous lymph node dissection in whom metallic clip artifacts may degrade the image quality on CT. The major indications for MR imaging of the scrotum include the following:

1. Localization of undescended testis and detection of complications, such as torsion and malignant degeneration. (Although MR imaging is usually recommended when US findings are suboptimal or inconclusive, many physicians now prefer to use MR as a primary modality.)
2. Evaluation of intrascrotal masses, including differentiation between intra- and extratesticular masses and assignment of the lesion to the testis, epididymis, or other scrotal structure. (MR imaging is particularly useful for localization of a diffusely infiltrative intratesticular mass, for extensive bilateral disease, and for characterization of testicular cysts.)
3. Evaluation of the testis when palpation is difficult (e.g., in cases of hydrocele or epididymitis) and in patients with a painful scrotum, in whom US examination is difficult.
4. Staging of testicular cancer and evaluation of primary tumors and lymph node or visceral metastases when iodinated contrast media are contraindicated or when CT findings are questionable (e.g., evaluation of small retrocrural lymph nodes).
5. Follow-up and evaluation of treatment response, especially in patients with previous lymph node dissection in whom clip artifacts degrade CT images.
6. Assessment of the extent of inflammatory disease and determination of the presence or absence of abscess and their follow-up. (MR imaging may be helpful in differentiating orchitis from testicular tumor when US is equivocal.)
7. Evaluation of torsion of the spermatic cord. (MR imaging may be helpful in differentiation from epididymitis when US and/or scintigraphy are equivocal.)
8. Testicular infarcts and vascular injuries.
9. Evaluation of scrotal trauma—demonstration of a hematocele and demonstration or exclusion of testicular rupture. (MR imaging can be useful for differentiation between intratesticular hematoma and tumor.)
10. Evaluation of extratesticular lesions—such as inguinal hernias, hydroceles, varicoceles, or spermatoceles—when US is equivocal.

TECHNIQUES OF EXAMINATION

General Guidelines

A surface coil (usually a circular 12.5-cm [5-inch] coil) is recommended for best results in imaging the testis. Adequate support and positioning of the scrotum under the surface coil are key factors in obtaining good-quality MR images. With the patient in the supine position, the penis is taped against the abdominal wall. Towels or sponges are placed between the thighs to minimize motion artifact, and an additional sheet is placed over the thighs to support the scrotum. The scrotum is then covered by a light cloth, such as gauze, and the surface coil is placed in a flat position, supported and secured. Respiratory compensation is recommended to reduce motion artifact, and, when possible, flow compensation is used.

Both T1- and T2-weighted spin-echo (either conventional or fast spin-echo) sequences are essential. Contrast-enhancement and special techniques, such as fat suppression and gradient-echo, may also be used when further tissue characterization is needed. T1-weighted images provide information about the nature of a fluid collection and the presence or absence of hemorrhage. They are also helpful in localizing undescended testes and enlarged lymph nodes. T2-weighted images contribute to tissue characterization, enabling differentiation of the testes, tunica albuginea, and epididymis; and detection of intratesticular tumors. Since the signal intensity for most intratesticular pathologic conditions (with the exception of cysts and old hematoma) is lower than that of the testes, they are most commonly depicted on T2-weighted images (1).

In addition to transaxial images, sagittal plane images (which can be used as localizers) and/or coronal plane images are recommended. The transaxial and coronal plane images allow direct comparison of the two testes and evaluation of the spermatic cord. Since the testis and adjacent epididymis are movable within the scrotum, it is difficult to predict the ideal plane for identification of the entire epididymis. The epididymis is always demonstrated on transaxial plane images. Coronal plane images usually demonstrate the head of the epididymis, and sagittal plane images sometimes allow demonstration of the entire epididymis.

Optimal coverage is provided by thin sections (4 to 5 mm) with a 1- to 2-mm interslice gap (with a 12.5-cm surface coil) and an 8- to 20-cm field of view.

Special Circumstances

Undescended Testis

Some changes to the routine protocol are necessary for evaluation of undescended testis. In infants a body or head coil may be applied instead of a surface coil. Use of a pelvic multicoil may provide better resolution. Because a distended bladder can displace inguinal structures, the patient is asked to empty the bladder before the study. Using a T1-weighted sagittal localizer, transaxial T1- and T2-weighted images are obtained from the bottom of the scrotum to above the seminal vesicles. Coronal T1-weighted images can be added if the testis is found in the pelvic cavity. The examination should be extended to the lower poles of the kidneys when no testis is seen in the pelvis.

Staging of Testicular Cancer

For staging or posttreatment follow-up of testicular cancer, MR examination should extend from the pubic symphysis to the diaphragm. Transaxial T1- and T2-weighted images are recommended, and IV contrast media should be used only when nodal metastasis is questionable.

RISKS AND BIOEFFECTS

Unlike CT, which carries certain radiation risks, MR imaging is considered a relatively safe imaging modality. Although some biologic effects are caused by the static and gradient magnetic fields and by radiofrequency (RF) radiation, clinical application of static magnetic fields at strengths up to 2.0 T are considered safe and the possible reactions harmless (2).

Static Magnetic Fields

Although there is controversy regarding the effects of static magnetic fields on body and skin temperatures of mammals, recent evidence indicates that exposure to static magnetic fields less than 1.5 T does not affect the skin or body temperature of human subjects (3). Other changes that have been described include electrocardiographic effects (an increase in the amplitude of T-waves) and central nervous system effects (4). However, there is no evidence of irreversible biologic effects from short-term exposure to static magnetic fields of less than 2.0 T (5).

Magnetic Field Gradients

A magnetic field gradient and a moving object in a static magnetic field can induce electric currents. In conductive tissues (e.g., muscle fibers, nerve cells, and blood vessels), electric currents can produce harmful biologic effects, such as skin sensation, muscle contraction, magnetophosphenes (visual light flashes), and cardiac arrhythmias, and fibrillation (6,7). Such effects can occur with high-strength magnetic fields or with the newer echo planar MR imaging. Current recommendations from the FDA suggest that the rate of change of magnetic fields should not exceed 6 T/s or that the fields used should not be sufficiently high to cause peripheral nerve stimulation (by a factor of 3 at least) (8).

Another potential risk is related to the acoustic noise caused by activation and deactivation of gradient magnetic fields and enhanced when higher static and gradient magnetic fields are used (5). Acoustic noise may be associated with a reversible hearing loss, and earplugs or an "antinoise" or destructive interference technique are recommended to minimize acoustic noise.

RF Radiation

The major biologic effects caused by exposure to RF radiation are related to its thermogenic characteristics.

RF radiation can generate heat and can cause elevation of skin and body temperature on MR imaging. The organs most susceptible to injury by the temperature elevation are the testis and the eye. Because elevation of tissue temperature in the testis can adversely affect spermatogenesis, the heating effects of RF radiation, especially in high-field-strength MR imaging, are considered major risks to the testis.

The specific absorption rate (SAR, W/kg) is used to quantify the absorbed energy that causes tissue heating (9). The SAR is defined as the rate of energy absorbed per unit mass of tissue (9). The FDA recommends limiting RF exposure to a whole-body average SAR of less than 0.4 W/kg, a core temperature elevation of less than 1°C, or local exposures of less than 38°C in the head, 39°C in the trunk, and 40°C in the extremities (8). Although fast spin-echo techniques deliver approximately twice the SAR of conventional spin echo, absorbed energy remains within the FDA upper limits. One study, done with fluoroptic thermometry, showed that exposure up to 4.0 W/kg did not increase body temperature significantly and only elevated skin temperature to a degree not believed to be hazardous (10). Another study, which evaluated changes in scrotal skin temperature before and after MR imaging done with a 1.5 T-scanner at a whole-body average SAR ranging from 0.56 to 0.84, showed a significant increase (from 30.8°C to 32.3°C) in average temperature of the scrotal skin (11). Although elevated, scrotal skin temperatures remained below the threshold known to affect spermatogenesis in mammals (i.e., approximately body temperature in human subjects) (11).

Although some reports claim that exposure to RF radiation is associated with an increased incidence of cancer and developmental anomalies (12,13), these findings remain controversial (5).

Metallic Implants and Devices

MR imaging is contraindicated for patients who have electrically, magnetically, or mechanically activated implants, such as cardiac pacemakers, implantable cardiac defibrillators, cochlear implants, neurostimulators, bone-growth stimulators, and implantable drug infusion pumps (5). MR imaging is also contraindicated in patients with ferromagnetic aneurysmal clips. The principal danger in patients with ferromagnetic or metallic biomedical implants or foreign bodies (including various kinds of vascular clips, skin staples, prosthetic heart valves, and orthopedic implants and devices) is associated with dislodgement or movement of the object (14). In addition, such objects may be subject to heating and induction of electrical currents. The major factors affecting these risks include magnetic field strength; the degree of ferromagnetism; geometry, orientation, and location of the object; and the length of time the object has been implanted (14). Ferromagnetic material in a spherical shape, for example, might have a markedly different set of forces than one of a linear, rodlike shape (15).

In addition, ferromagnetic materials produce a variety of artifacts on MR imaging (see later). Like tattoo eyeliner or certain types of eye cosmetics, tattoos in the scrotum and thigh may contain ferromagnetically active pigments, such as iron oxide particles (black or flesh), ferric sulfate (brown), and cobalt chloride (blue) (16,17). These particles act as conductors causing energy absorption or heating in the adjacent tissues. In patients with tattooed eyelids, reversible painless eyelid swelling after MR examination has been reported (16). Patients with tattoos should be screened with a short-gradient echo sequence. If a tattoo is found to cause a metallic artifact, the MR examination can be modified to minimize RF radiation by using gradient-echo technique (rather than spin-echo technique), by reducing the number of phase-encoding steps, or by increasing the distance from the transmit coil (16). In general, patients with nonferromagnetic or minimally ferromagnetic implants or devices can safely undergo MR imaging.

NORMAL ANATOMY

On MR images the normal **testis** appears as a sharply defined oval structure with a homogeneous texture. On T1-weighted images the testis demonstrates intermediate signal intensity, similar to that of the corpora cavernosa or corpus spongiosum and lower than that of subcutaneous fat. On T2-weighted images the testis demonstrates high signal intensity, similar to that of the corpus spongiosum (Fig. 3.16). (Although the signal intensity of the testis may be similar to that of the corpora cavernosa, the latter is influenced by blood flow and varies (18), often demonstrating a lower signal intensity than the testis.) The **tunica albuginea**, a dense, fibrous connective tissue capsule covering the testis, is seen as a thin stripe (less than 1 mm in thickness) of low signal intensity on both T1- and T2-weighted images (Fig. 3.16). The **mediastinum testis** has signal characteristics similar to the tunica albuginea and is seen as a low-signal-intensity stripe (1 to 2 cm long) invaginating into the high-signal-intensity testis. Fine **septula** are often seen as thin linear structures of low signal intensity extending from the mediastinum testis and dividing the testis into lobules. The **rete testis** is an anastomosing network of tubules in the area of the gonadal hilus. When dilated it may be seen on MR and US (Fig. 3.17) (see Chapter 5, under "Seminiferous tubular ectasia of the rete testis"), and demonstrates low signal intensity on T1-weighted MR images and high signal intensity (isointense with or higher than normal testis) on T2-weighted images. It can thus be differentiated from testicular tumor, which usually exhibits low signal intensity on T2-weighted images (19).

The parietal and visceral layers of the **tunica vaginalis** are often separated by a small amount (commonly 1 to 2

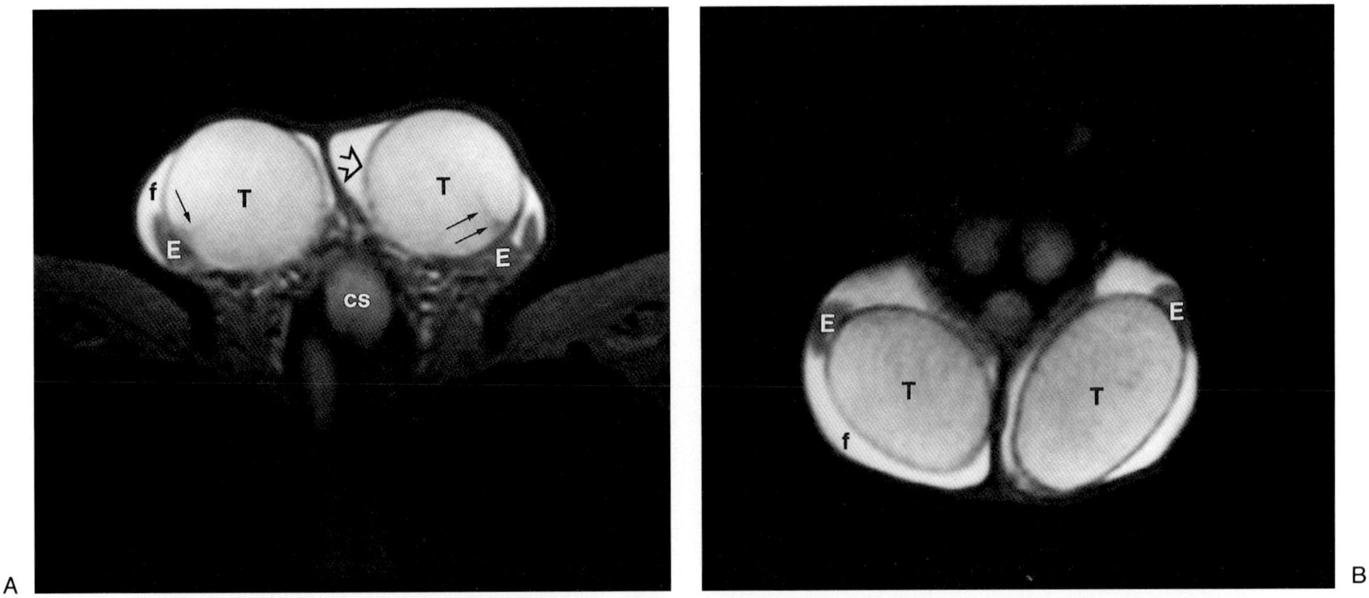

FIG. 3.16. Normal scrotal anatomy. **(A)** Transaxial and **(B)** coronal T2-weighted images. The testes (T) show homogeneous high signal intensity and the epididymis (E) demonstrates low signal intensity. Note low signal intensity tunica albuginea (*open arrow*) and mediastinum testis (*arrows*). (cs, corpus spongiosum; f, fluid collection between layers of the tunica vaginalis [cavum serosum])

ml) of normal serous fluid (**cavum serosum**), which demonstrates medium to low signal intensity on T1-weighted images and high intensity on T2-weighted images (Fig. 3.16). As in a hydrocele, this normal fluid usually surrounds the testis completely, except for the posteromedial bare area.

The signal intensity of the **epididymis** is similar to or slightly lower than that of the testis on T1-weighted images, and much lower than the testis on T2-weighted images (Fig. 3.16). The head, the most commonly seen part of the epididymis, is often surrounded by high-signal-intensity fluid on T2-weighted images. On T2-weighted images the epididymis can be differentiated from adjacent testicular tissue or surrounding fluid by its characteristic signal intensity. Sometimes the **vas deferens** (ductus deferens) can be traced from the tail of the epididymis to the inguinal canal and through the pelvis to the ejaculatory ducts. It demonstrates low signal intensity, but on high-resolution images the signal intensity center can be separated from a low-intensity wall on

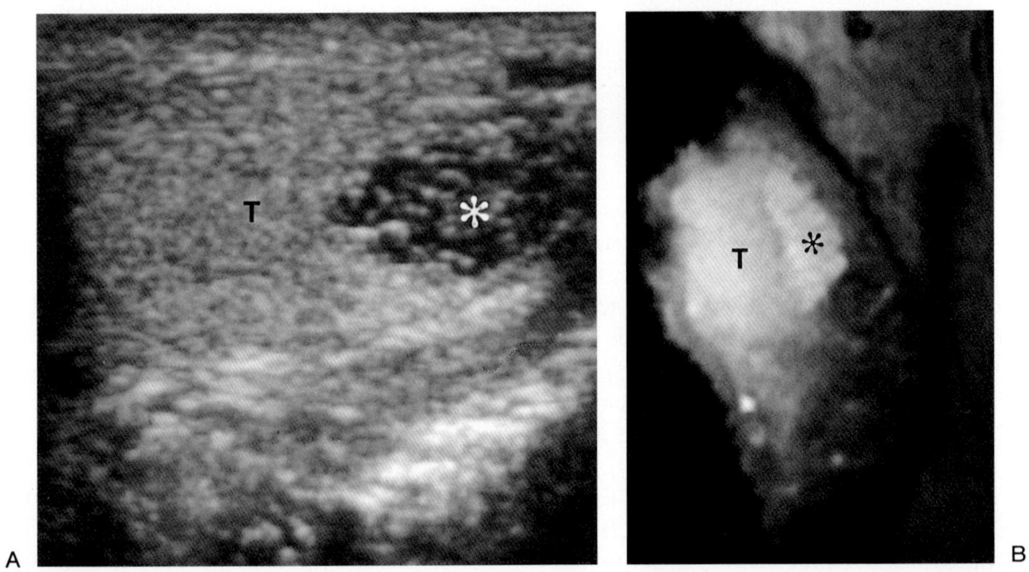

FIG. 3.17. Dilatated rete testis (seminiferous tubular ectasia). **(A)** Ultrasonogram and **(B)** gradient echo MR image. The dilatated rete testis (asterisk) demonstrates a low-level echo on US and high signal intensity on gradient echo image. (T, testis)

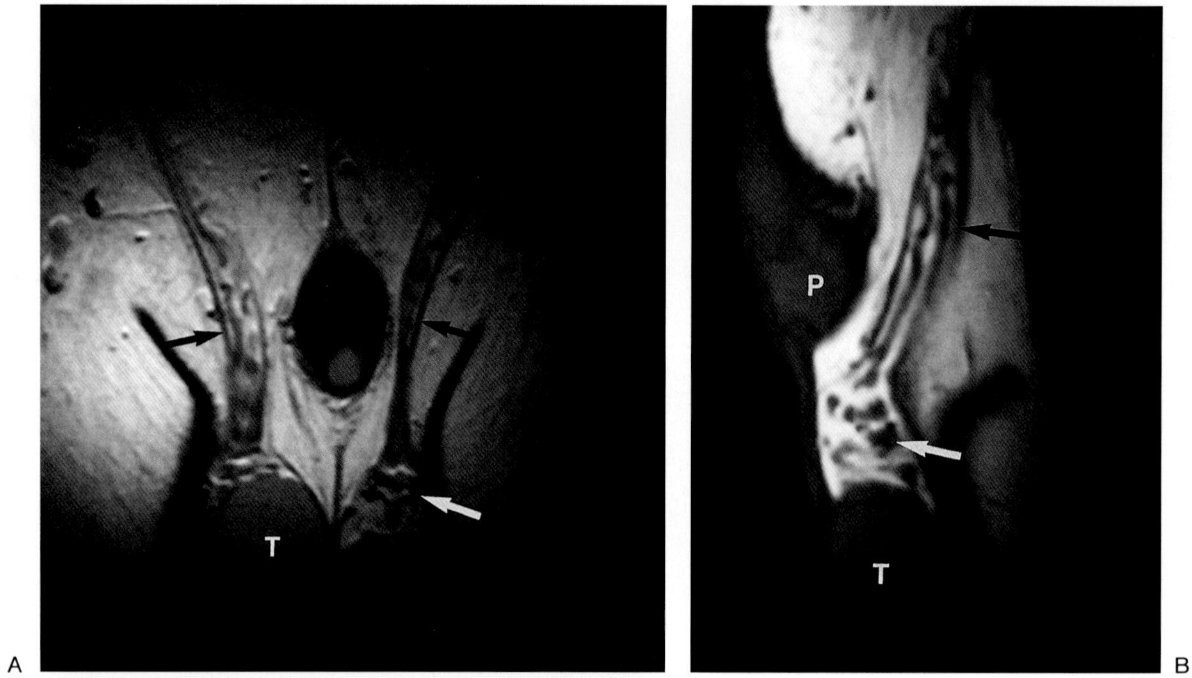

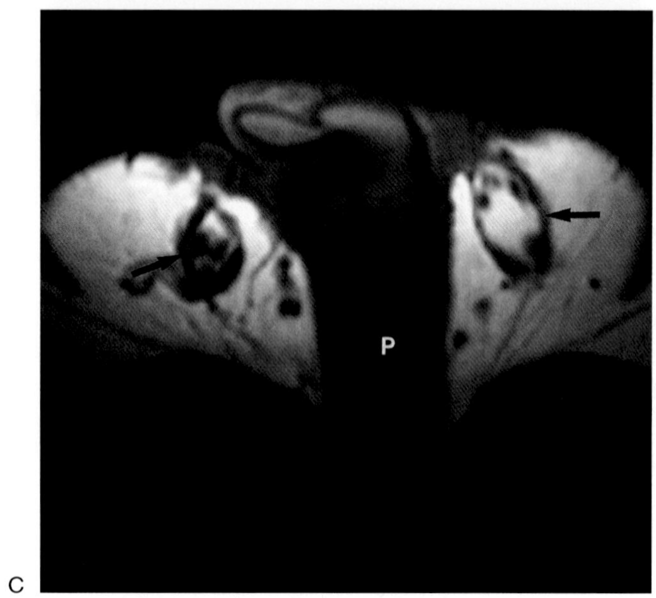

FIG. 3.18. Normal anatomy of the spermatic cord distal to the external inguinal ring. **(A)** Coronal, **(B)** sagittal, and **(C)** transaxial T1-weighted MR images obtained with a surface coil. The spermatic cord (black arrows) is seen as a tubular structure extending from the scrotal neck toward the external inguinal ring. The thick, fibrous wall and linear internal structures (the ductus deferens and vessels) are visualized but not differentiated. (*white arrow*, pampiniform plexus; P, root of the penis; T, testis)

T2-weighted images. The **pampiniform plexus** can be seen as tortuous tubular structures, cephalad to the head of the epididymis, and can sometimes be traced to the inguinal canal (Fig. 3.18). The wall of the plexus is seen as a low-intensity structure on both T1- and T2-weighted images. Because of flow artifacts in the venous plexus, the internal structure is usually seen as serpiginous areas of high signal intensity on T2-weighted images (20).

The **scrotal skin** exhibits medium to high signal intensity on T1-weighted images. Since the dartos muscle and fascia demonstrate low signal intensity on this sequence, they can be separated from the higher-intensity scrotal skin. On T2-weighted images, however, all layers of the scrotum demonstrate low signal intensity.

The vas deferens, pampiniform plexus, respective arteries, veins, and nerves are present within the spermatic cord. The envelope of the **spermatic cord**, which consists of the dartos muscle and several fascial layers, is easily recognizable as a low-intensity ring within the subcutaneous fat (Figs. 3.18 and 3.19). The arteries and veins within the spermatic cord (i.e., pampiniform plexus and testicular and deferential vessels) may be seen as areas of signal void. However, the separate structures within the spermatic cord cannot be identified individually.

Neither the internal nor the external inguinal ring can be demonstrated directly on MR images, and the location of the **inguinal canal** is determined by locating bony and muscular landmarks. The **external inguinal ring** is at or just superior to the upper margin of the symphysis pubis and is bordered on each side by the crura of the aponeurosis of the external oblique muscle. The **internal ring** is demarcated by the inferior epigastric vessels medially and the transversus abdominis muscle laterally and superiorly. Above the level of the internal inguinal ring, two of the main constituents of the spermatic cord, the **ductus deferens** and **testicular vessels**, are located lateral to the inferior epigastric vessels and then diverge. The testicular vessels ascend into the abdomen anterior to the psoas muscle, and the ductus loops behind the inferior epigastric artery, coursing posteriorly and downward to the seminal vesicle (Fig. 3.19D).

Testicular Prosthesis

For cosmetic and psychologic purposes, prosthetic testicles are commonly placed in patients with congenitally absent or surgically removed testes. Because various sili-

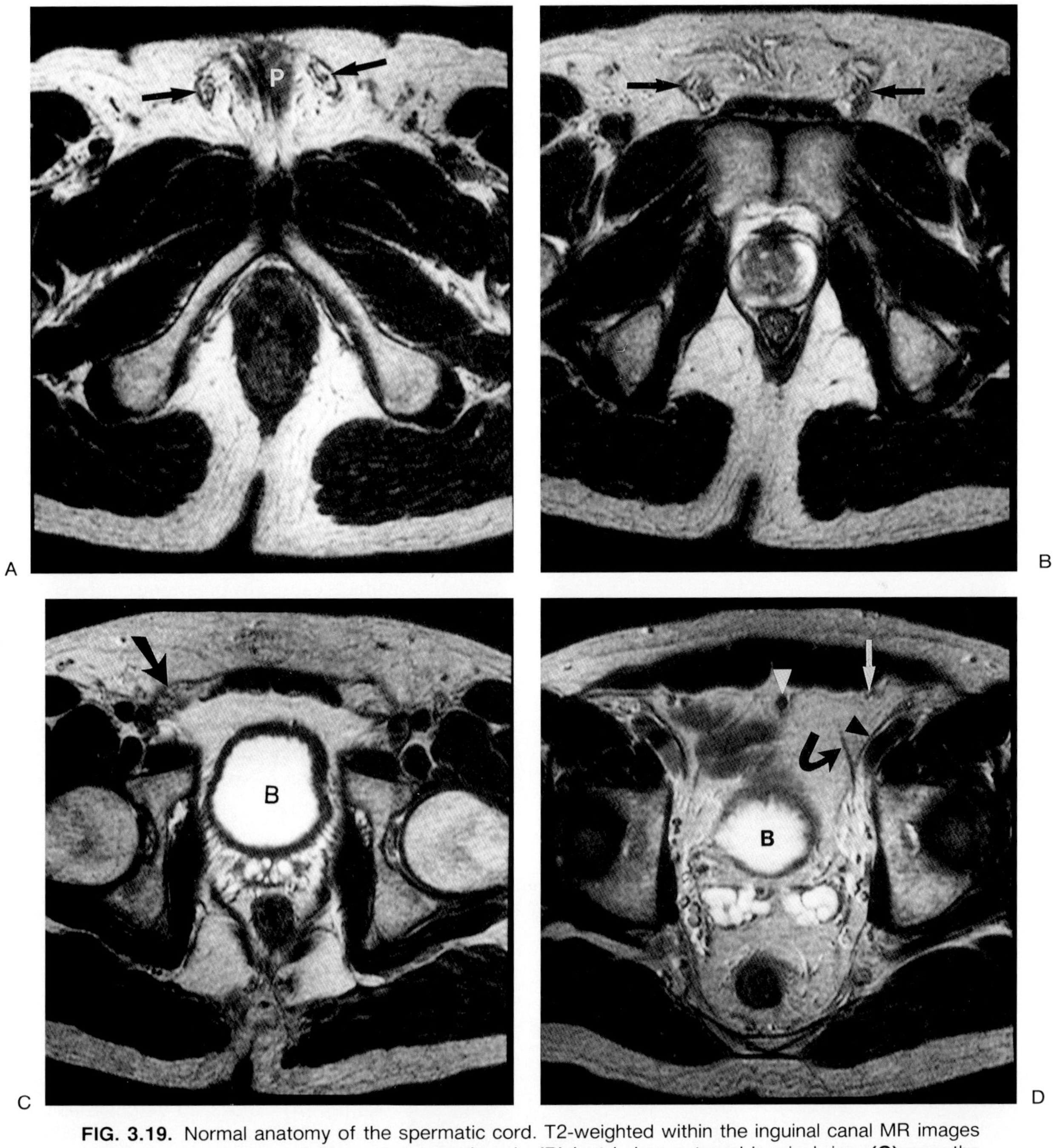

FIG. 3.19. Normal anatomy of the spermatic cord. T2-weighted within the inguinal canal MR images obtained with a body coil **(A)** at the scrotal neck, **(B)** just below external inguinal ring, **(C)** near the external inguinal ring, and **(D)** just above the internal inguinal ring. (*black arrow*, spermatic cord; *white arrow*, inferior epigastric vessels; *black arrowhead*, ductus deferens; *white arrowhead*, median umbilical ligament; *curved arrow*, medial umbilical ligament; B, urinary bladder; P, partially visualized penile shaft)

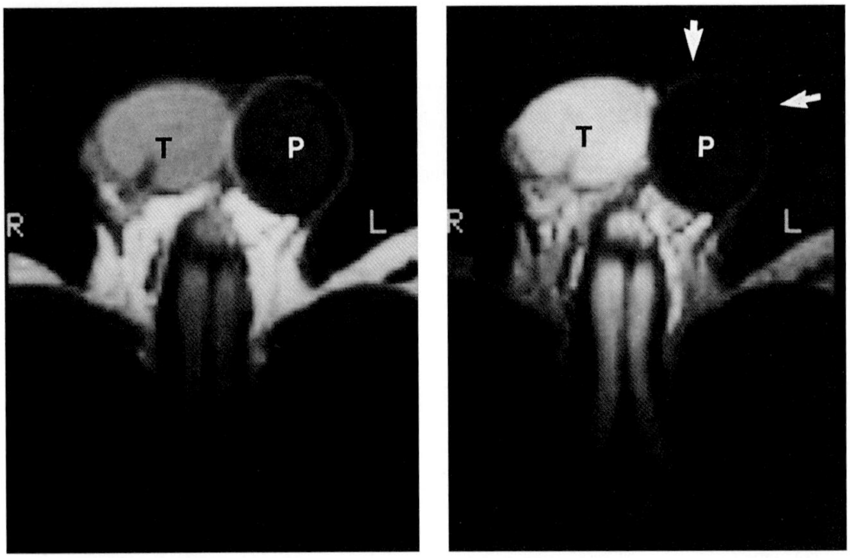

A,B

FIG. 3.20. Fluid-filled testicular prosthesis (P). **(A)** Transaxial T1-weighted and **(B)** T2-weighted images. The testicular prosthesis on the left side demonstrates low signal intensity on both T1- and T2-weighted scans. The chemical-shift artifact (*arrows*) is seen around the prosthesis but not around the normal right testis (T).

con materials are used, the MR appearance differs. Older prostheses are hard in consistency and contain viscous fluid, which demonstrates low signal intensity on both T1- and T2-weighted images (Fig. 3.20). They should not be mistaken for a diffuse pathologic condition replacing the whole testis. Newer prostheses made of solid elastomer have a consistency and MR signal characteristics similar to the normal testis (Fig. 3.21). They demonstrate medium signal intensity on T1-weighted images and high signal intensity on T2-weighted images. They can be differentiated from the normal testis by the presence of a pronounced chemical shift artifact and the absence of other intrascrotal or spermatic cord structures (see Fig. 3.21) (21).

ARTIFACTS

The most common artifacts encountered in testicular MR imaging are motion artifacts and metallic artifacts produced by orthopedic prostheses. In the retroperitoneum surgical clips may produce similar artifacts.

Motion Artifacts

Image quality can be degraded by physiologic motion, such as respiration and blood flow, by movement of the patient's thighs, or by involuntary cremasteric muscle spasm. Motion artifact is intensified in the presence of a large hydrocele (Fig. 3.22). Motion usually causes streak artifacts, increased noise, and edge blurring. Motion artifacts, prominent in the phase-encoding direction, are often severe because of the high signal intensity of subcutaneous fat. Motion artifacts can be minimized by using short repetition and echo times (TR and TE) or fewer matrix elements along the phase-encoding axis (22).

Motion artifacts caused by breathing can be controlled by respiratory gating or respiratory compensation. Respiratory compensation (ROPE, COPE) is preferred because respiratory gating requires longer imaging times and limits the selection of the repetition time.

Vascular motion can cause phase shift artifacts, which also degrade image resolution. Flow artifacts can be eliminated by the use of spatial presaturation or flow compensation technique.

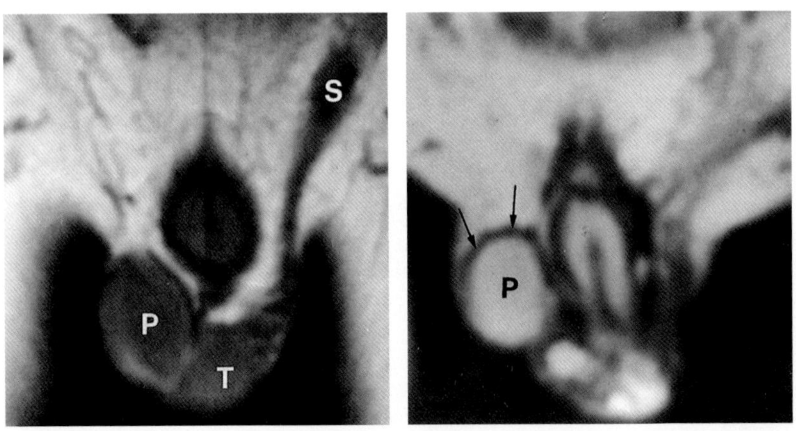

A,B

FIG. 3.21. Solid elastomer testicular prosthesis (P). **(A)** Coronal T1-weighted and **(B)** T2-weighted MR images. The signal intensity of the prosthesis is similar to that of the normal testis (T). The prosthesis can be identified by presence of the chemical-shift artifact (*arrows*) and lack of the spermatic cord. (S, spermatic cord)

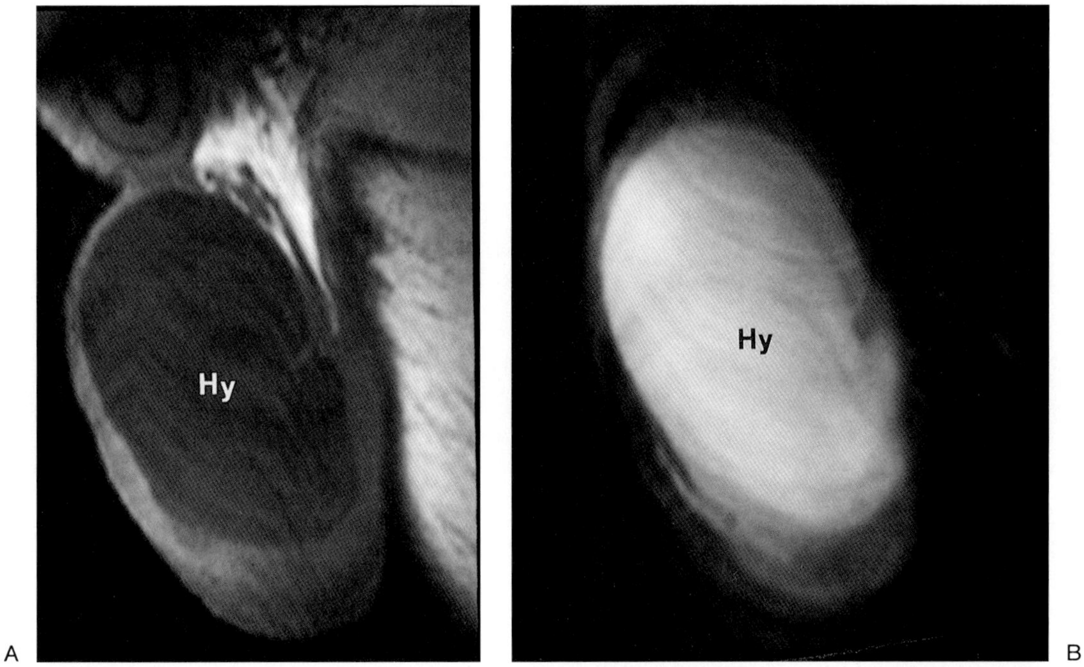

FIG. 3.22. Motion artifacts in presence of hydrocele (Hy). **(A)** Sagittal T1-weighted and **(B)** T2-weighted MR images. Motion artifacts are enhanced in presence of hydrocele, more prominent on the T2-weighted image.

Metallic Artifacts

As with CT, **metallic surgical clips** can cause artifacts on MR images. Although MR image degradation is usually less severe than with CT (Fig. 3.23), some ferromagnetic clips produce larger artifacts than on CT (Fig. 3.24). The severity of an artifact is usually proportional to the degree of ferromagnetism and the mass of the object (23). It is also affected by the shape, orientation, and position of the object in the body. Imaging techniques also affect metallic artifacts (5), which are more prominent with gradient-echo techniques than with spin-echo techniques.

Metallic artifacts may be seen as local distortion of the image or as focal signal void surrounded by a hyperintense halo that fades peripherally (Fig. 3.24). Image distortion is usually caused by ferromagnetic materials that significantly distort the main magnetic field (14). Even

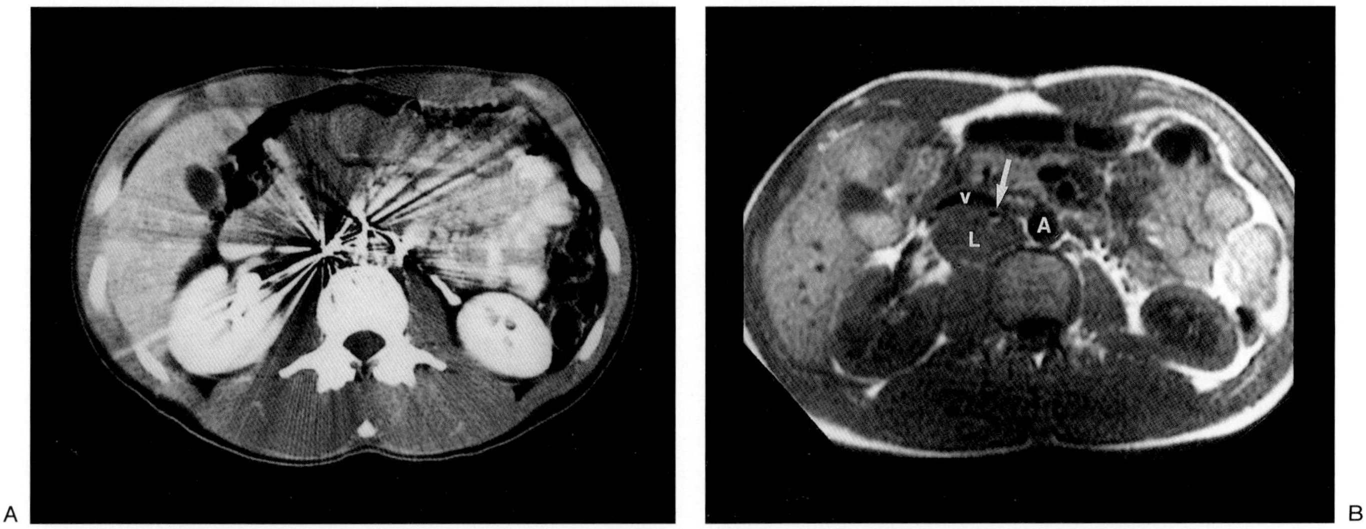

FIG. 3.23. Metallic artifacts caused by surgical clips. **(A)** CT scan and **(B)** T2-weighted MR image of a patient with testicular cancer who underwent RPLND. A large metastatic lymph node (L) in the retrocaval region is seen on MR image but cannot be identified on CT because of extensive metallic artifacts. There is only a small metallic artifact (*arrow*) (nonferromagnetic clip) on the MR scan. (A, aorta; v, inferior vena cava).

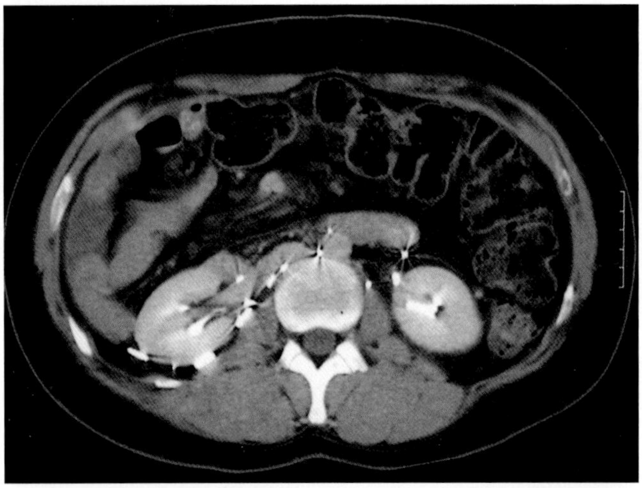

A

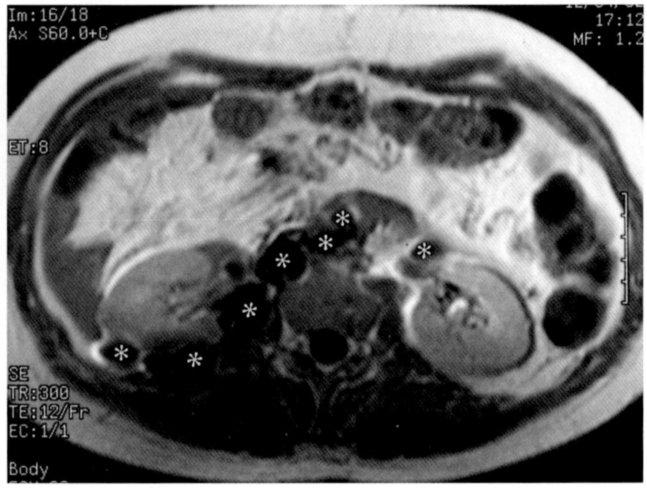

B

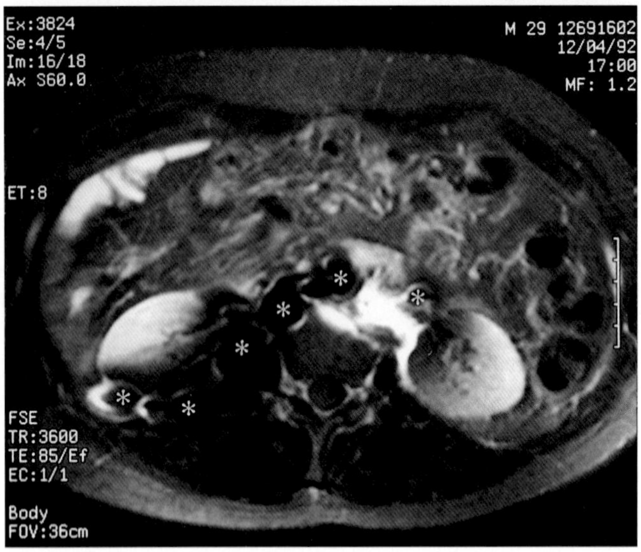

C

FIG. 3.24. Metallic artifacts caused by surgical clips. **(A)** CT scan, **(B)** contrast-enhanced T1-weighted MR image, and **(C)** fat-saturation T2-weighted MR image. Multiple surgical clips posterior to the right kidney and great vessels, and in the left renal parahilar region in a patient with testicular cancer who underwent RPLND. Only mild streak artifacts are seen on the CT scan, but the MR images show larger round areas of signal void with hyperintense rims around the metallic clips (asterisks). Image degradation is more severe on fat saturation images **(C)** as a result of high susceptibility to magnetic field inhomogeneity.

nonferromagnetic metals can produce similar, but less extensive, artifacts when local eddy currents are induced in the objects by RF fields (24). Because these currents are strongly dependent on the shape of the object, the shape of a clip can affect the severity of the artifact. Compressed U-shaped clips are preferred, because artifacts increase when there is a large closed conducting path (24). Although most of these artifacts have characteristic appearances, they are sometimes mistaken for calcifications or hemorrhagic foci.

Both **tantalum** and **stainless steel clips** produce severe artifacts on CT images. However, all nonsteel (i.e., tantalum, titanium, or silver) and some of the stainless steel (austenitic stainless steel, such as high chromium-nickel alloys) clips are nonferromagnetic and do not produce severe artifacts on MR images (24,25). On the other hand, metallic clips outside the imaging slice do not produce artifacts on CT, whereas artifacts may occur on MR images of nearby slices (because the magnetic field homogeneity has been altered in every direction) (26). As mentioned, tattoos in scrotum and thighs can produce unusual artifacts on MR images.

The size of an image artifact is related to the strength of the gradient. Since a strong gradient can increase the noise in an image, the strength of the gradient may need to be reduced to achieve the best possible result (26). Because the orientation of image artifacts depends on the direction of the frequency-encoding axis, artifacts can be reoriented by reversing the gradient or interchanging with the phase-encoding gradient.

In theory, artifacts should be the same on both T1- and T2-weighted images. However, artifacts on T2-weighted images are often more pronounced than those on T1-weighted images, owing to weaker gradients and a lower signal-sampling rate (26).

Wraparound Artifacts (Aliasing)

Because a small field of view is used with a surface coil for testicular MR imaging, structures outside the scrotum (such as the thighs) are also excited and can produce wraparound artifacts. These artifacts occur in both the frequency- and the phase-encoding directions. Artifacts in the frequency axis can be eliminated by using filters. Artifacts in the phase-encoding axis can be eliminated by increasing the field of view (22).

Chemical Shift Artifacts

Chemical shift artifacts occur at water–fat interfaces and appear as a low-intensity band on one side and a high-intensity band on the other. They are seen in the frequency-encoding direction and are more severe with a high-strength magnetic field, a low-strength gradient field, or a narrow bandwidth. These artifacts are often seen around testicular prostheses and may help in detecting them.

Miscellaneous Artifacts

Because of the extreme inhomogeneity of the magnetic field produced by a surface coil, a ring-shaped area of high signal intensity near the conductor of the surface coil may be seen. Other artifacts, such as partial volume averaging, truncation artifacts, or artifacts produced by static electricity (e.g., from a wool blanket) should not degrade testicular MR imaging if properly performed.

REFERENCES

1. Mattrey R, Trambert M. MR imaging of the scrotum and testis. In: Edelman RR, Hesselink JR, eds. *Clinical magnetic resonance imaging.* Philadelphia: WB Saunders; 1990:952–979.
2. Buettner UW. Human interactions with ultra high fields. In: Magin RL, Liburdy RP, Persson B, eds. *Biological effects and safety aspects of nuclear magnetic resonance imaging and spectroscopy.* New York: New York Academy of Sciences; 1992:59–66.
3. Shellock FG, Schaefer DJ, Crues JV. Exposure to a 1.5-T static magnetic field does not alter body and skin temperatures in man. *Magn Reson Med* 1989;11:371–375.
4. Tenforde TS. Magnetic field effects on biological systems: based on the Proceedings of the Biomagnetic Effects Workshop held at Lawrence Berkeley Laboratory, University of California, on April 6–7, 1978. New York: Plenum Press, 1979.
5. Shellock FG. MRI: Biologic effects and safety considerations. In: Higgins CB, Hricak H, Helms CA. *Magnetic resonance imaging of the body,* 2nd ed. New York: Raven Press, 1992;233–265.
6. Reilly JP. Peripheral nerve stimulation by induced electric currents: exposure to time-varying magnetic fields. *Med Biol Eng Comput* 1989;27:101–110.
7. Bernhardt J. The direct influence of electromagnetic fields on nerve and muscle cells of man within the frequency range of 1 Hz to 30 MHz. *Radiat Environ Biophys* 1979;16:309–323.
8. Food and Drug Administration. Magnetic resonance diagnostic device panel recommendation and report on petitions for MR reclassification. *Federal Register* 1988;53:7575–7579.
9. National Council on Radiation Protection and Measurements. Radiofrequency electromagnetic fields: properties, quantities, and units, biophysical interaction, and measurements: recommendations of the National Council on Radiation Protection and Measurements. Washington, DC: National Council on Radiation Protection and Measurements. 1981.
10. Wickersheim KA, Sun MH. Fluoroptic thermometry. *Med Electron* 1987; Feb:84–91.
11. Shellock FG, Rothman B, Sarti D. Heating of the scrotum by high-field-strength MR imaging. *AJR* 1990;154:1229–1232.
12. Pool R. Electromagnetic fields: the biological evidence. *Science* 1990;249:1378–1381.
13. Beers GJ. Biological effects of weak electromagentic fields from 0 Hz to 200 MHz: a survey of the literature with special emphasis on possible magnetic resonance effects. *Magn Reson Imaging* 1989;7: 309–331.
14. Shellock FG, Crues JV. High-field-strength MR imaging and metallic biomedical implants: an ex vivo evaluation of deflection forces. *AJR* 1988;151:389–392.
15. Kanal E. An overview of electromagnetic safety consideration associated with magnetic resonance imaging. In: Magin RL, Liburdy RP, Persson B, eds. *Biological effects and safety aspects of nuclear magnetic resonance imaging and spectroscopy.* New York: New York Academy of Sciences; 1992:204–224.
16. Jackson JG, Acker JD. Permanent eyeliner and MR imaging. *AJR* 1987;149:1080.
17. Lund G, Wirtschafter JD, Nelson JD, Williams PA. Tattooing of eyelids: magnetic resonance imaging artifacts. *Ophthalmic Surg* 1986;17:550–553.
18. Hricak H, Marotti M, Gilbert TJ, et al. Normal penile anatomy and abnormal penile conditions: evaluation with MR imaging. *Radiology* 1988;169:683–690.
19. Tartar VM, Trambert MA, Balsara ZN, Mattrey RF. Tubular ectasia of the testicle: sonographic and MR imaging appearance. *AJR* 1993;160:539–542.
20. Baker LL, Hajek PC, Burkhard TK, et al. MR imaging of the scrotum: normal anatomy. *Radiology* 1987;163:89–92.
21. Semelka R, Anderson M, Hricak H. Prosthetic testicle: appearance at MR imaging. *Radiology* 1989;173:561–562.
22. Lee JKT, Koehler RE, Heiken JP. MR imaging techniques. In: Lee JKT, Sagel SS, Stanley RJ. *Computed body tomography with MRI correlation,* 2nd ed. New York: Raven Press; 1989:61–88.
23. Hricak H. Technical consideration. In: Hricak H, Carrington BM. *MRI of the pelvis: a text atlas.* London: Martin Dunitz; 1991:1–30.
24. Mechlin M, Thickman D, Kressel HY, Gefter W, Joseph P. Magnetic resonance imaging of postoperative patients with metallic implants. *AJR* 1984;143:1281–1284.
25. Barrafato D, Henkelman RM. Magnetic resonance imaging and surgical clips. *Can J Surg* 1984;27:509–512.
26. Romner B, Olsson M, Ljunggren B, et al. Magnetic resonance imaging and aneurysmal clips: magnetic properties and image artifacts. *J Neurosurg* 1989;70:426–431.

C. Computed Tomography

Although limited spatial resolution and the risk of radiation damage to the testis limit the usefulness of computed tomography (CT) in the examination of the scrotum, CT is relatively commonly used for the following:

1. Localization and characterization of an undescended testis (particularly when the testis is likely to be located within the abdomen and not detectable by ultrasound (US) or magnetic resonance imaging [MRI]).
2. Diagnosis of undescended testis associated with torsion or malignant degeneration.
3. Staging of testicular cancer (with emphasis on evaluation of lymph node and distant metastasis) and assessment of response to chemotherapy, radiation therapy, or surgery.

It is less commonly used for evaluation of

1. Extratesticular lesions, such as inguinal hernias, hydroceles, varicoceles, or spermatoceles.
2. Testicular and scrotal trauma.
3. Genital swelling in patients on continuous ambulatory peritoneal dialysis (1,2). (CT examination can be performed following the intraperitoneal instillation of water-soluble contrast media.)
4. Inflammatory conditions, such as scrotal gangrene.

TECHNIQUES OF EXAMINATION

Contrast Media

Adequate administration of both oral and intravenous contrast media is essential to obtain good-quality CT images of the abdomen and pelvis. To achieve sufficient opacification of the distal small bowel and colon, 500 to 1,000 mL of dilute oral contrast media (e.g., diatrizoate meglumine [Gastrografin] or barium sulfate) is administrated 1 to 4 hours before the examination, and an additional 350 to 500 mL of contrast material is given 30 to 45 minutes prior to the study. (When preparing children for evaluation of suspected undescended testes, ingestion of the oral contrast material may be simplified by administering 500 mL of oral contrast at least 1 hour before the examination.) Occasionally, 100 to 300 mL of air and/or dilute contrast material (diazoate sodium [Hypaque]) is administrated through the rectum to improve colonic filling. Complete filling of both small and large bowel with contrast material facilitates differentiation of lymph nodes from bowel loops, which is especially important for staging or follow-up of testicular cancer. Bolus injection of intravenous contrast material with prompt scanning is also necessary to obtain optimal vascular enhancement for the evaluation of lymph node disease and for detection of undescended testes. Oral contrast media may not be necessary for scrotal CT examination.

Imaging Parameters

For the evaluation of undescended testes, contiguous 5-mm sections from the inferior border of the symphysis to the anterior superior iliac spine are needed. If the testes are not visualized in the scrotal sac or inguinal regions, the examination should be extended up to the renal hilus at 10-mm intervals.

CT examination for staging of testicular cancer is usually performed after an orchiectomy, and assessment of retroperitoneal lymph node and visceral metastases requires 10-mm sections from the symphysis pubis to the diaphragm. If CT examination is performed before radical orchiectomy, 5-mm sections through the scrotum can be included.

RISKS AND BIOEFFECTS

Radiation Hazards

Unlike US and MR imaging, which have been deemed to be safe methods for examination of the testes, CT carries certain radiation risks. Even though several radiobiologic studies suggest that ionizing radiation can induce biologic effects, including carcinogenesis, it is very difficult to estimate absorbed doses to individual organs and the ultimate effects of radiation.

The radiation dose from CT examinations is similar to that from many other radiologic studies and is much less than that of some specialized imaging studies (e.g., angiography) (3). The distribution of the absorbed dose of radiation depends upon the amount and the direction of the radiation and on the attenuation of the beam in the body (4). The amount of incident radiation depends on the skin dose and the size of the radiation field (4). Typical skin doses from abdominal CT scans are reported to be 20 to 45 mGy at 10-mm contiguous sections and 20 to 65 mGy at 5-mm contiguous sections (3). (For comparison, the average skin dose delivered with a pelvic AP radiograph is 5.5 mGy (4)). High mAs settings, longer scan times, and contiguous or overlapping slices, needed for high-resolution scans, increase the radiation dose delivered to the patient. Although using thinner CT sections causes less radiation, it requires higher amperage to suppress noise and improve image quality, thereby increasing the overall radiation dose.

In radiography the radiation dose is typically highest at the entrance site and lowest at the exit point. In CT, however, the dose is lowest in the center of the body, and dose distribution is uneven. To standardize the description of absorbed doses from CT examinations, Shope et al. (5) designed the computed tomography dose index (CTDI), and it has been recommended by the Food and Drug Administration (FDA). The CTDI describes the absorbed dose at specified locations (e.g., central axis, 1 cm from the outer surface) in a phantom in the central scan of a series of slices. This index reflects both the primary and the scattered and penumbral doses. It can be used to predict the organ-absorbed dose and to assess the efficiency of CT scanners (6).

The major concern about radiation hazards is related to the risks of somatic effects (e.g., the risk of developing cancer). Relative biologic effectiveness per unit of absorbed dose depends on the types of radiation used and the tissues and organs exposed. Both the International Commission on Radiation Protection (ICRP) (7) and the National Council on Radiation Protection (NCRP) (8) have recommended the use of effective dose equivalents to assess radiation risk, particularly when only a portion of the body is exposed to radiation. The *effective dose equivalent* is the weighted sum of organ doses where the weighting factors account for the different mortality risks from cancer and the risk of severe hereditary effects (8). The tissue weighting factor for testis recommended by ICRP is 0.20, versus 0.12 and 0.01 for bone marrow and skin, respectively (7).

Nishizawa et al. (9) have measured organ doses for a variety of CT scanners for different CT procedures, including chest, upper abdomen, and lower abdomen (pelvis). They also measured the skin dose and calculated the effective dose equivalent for these procedures. The average testis dose from a lower abdominal (pelvic) CT procedure is approximately the same as that for a plain abdominal radiograph (KUB). The effective dose equivalent is higher for a chest CT than for the abdomen because of the organs exposed.

Radiation exposure is of greatest concern in children because of their longer life expectancy and their probable higher sensitivity to radiation (10). In an experimental study done with a simulated pediatric patient phantom (the equivalent of a 6-year-old), the organ-absorbed dose to the testes was found to be 0.77 mGy with abdominal CT examination and 5.4 mGy with a CT examination of the torso (11).

Despite decreases in the last few years in the levels of radiation exposure from an individual CT study, more frequent use of CT has resulted in an increase in collective radiation exposure in the general population. In the United States, CT examinations account for 7% to 8% of the active bone marrow dose delivered by diagnostic radiology procedures (10). Two quantities, gonadal dose and genetically significant dose (GSD), are often used to estimate possible genetic hazards to the population. Gonadal dose is the calculated radiation dose to the testes or ovaries from a certain examination in an individual patient. The GSD is defined as "the dose which, if given to every member of the population, would produce the same genetic detriment as the actual doses received by the various individuals" (4). Calculation of the GSD is based on the number of procedures, the gonadal dose, and the age distribution of the population exposed (especially the number of children expected in that population). The GSD to the U.S. population from diagnostic radiologic procedures is estimated to be about 0.3 mGy and has increased approximately 50% over the last decade (4).

Because of potential radiation hazards, CT examination should be limited to those instances where the information gained is essential for the evaluation and treatment of patients. Every effort should be made to minimize radiation exposure during the examination and to optimize scan parameters (e.g., scan thickness, mAs), especially in children.

NORMAL ANATOMY

On axial CT images the testis is often seen as an ovoid homogeneous region that is isodense with the pelvic muscles (Fig. 3.25). It is difficult to distinguish the epididymis from the testis. The tunica albuginea is seen as a thin, high-density ring structure around the testes (Fig. 3.25). The scrotal septum and outer coverings, including multiple muscle and fascial layers, are seen as isodense structures. Occasionally a small amount of fluid (**cavum serosum**) is seen between the testes and scrotal covering (Fig. 3.25).

The **spermatic cord** extends from the scrotal sac through the subcutaneous fat directly into the inguinal canal. As it passes through the external inguinal ring, it acquires an outer muscle sheath (the transversus abdominis and the internal and external oblique muscles). The **external inguinal** ring is a triangular opening bordered medially and laterally by the crura of the aponeurosis of the external oblique muscle. The **internal inguinal** ring is bordered medially by the inferior epigastric vessels, lat-

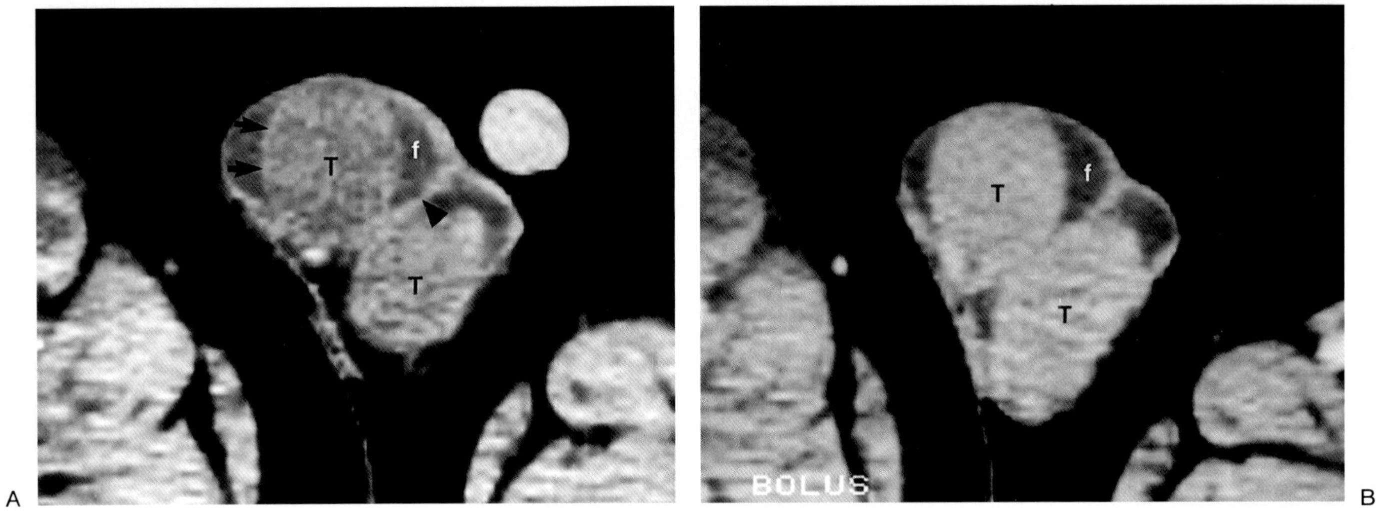

FIG. 3.25. Normal CT scans of the testes (T) both before **(A)** and after **(B)** intravenous bolus injection of the contrast media. Note small amount of fluid collection in the scrotum (f), commonly seen in normal subjects. (*arrows,* tunica albuginea; *arrowhead,* scrotal septum)

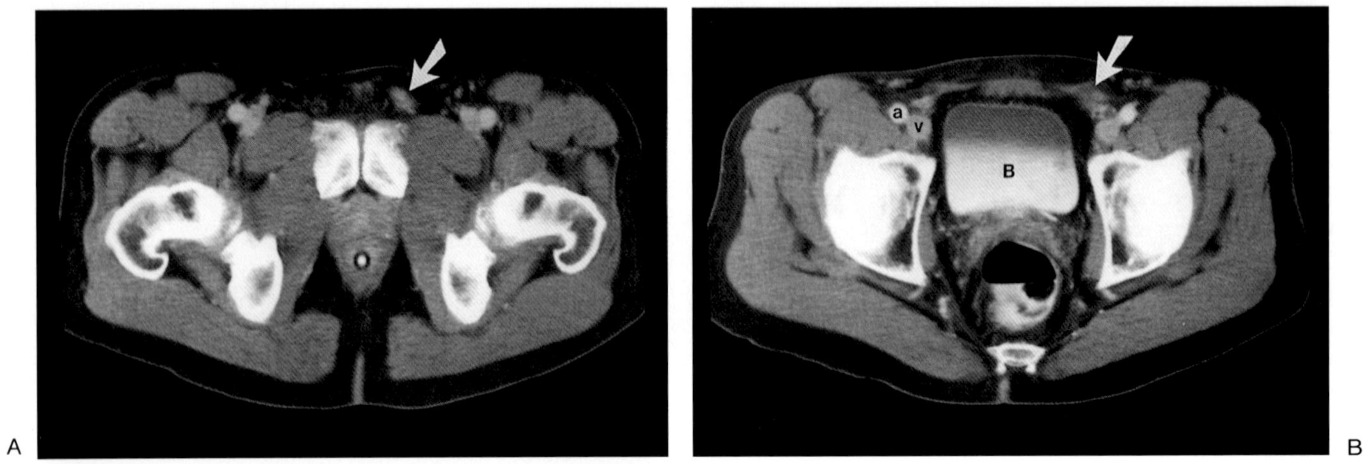

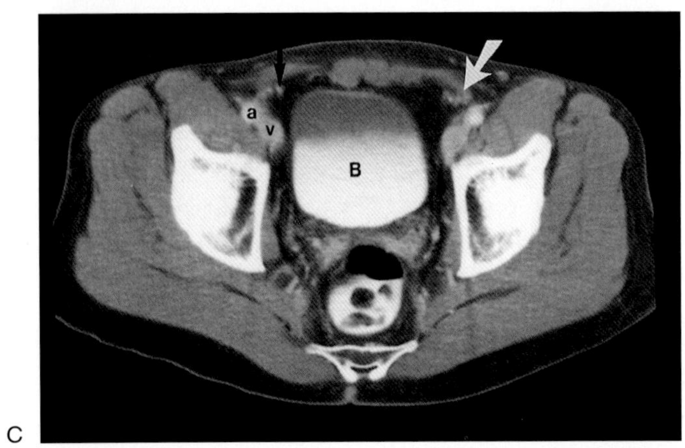

FIG. 3.26. Left spermatic cord (*white arrow*) in patient with right testicular cancer who underwent orchiectomy. The left spermatic cord is seen in the high scrotal region **(A)**, within the inguinal canal **(B)**, and just above the internal inguinal ring **(C)** Note the surgical absence of the cord on the right side. (*black arrow,* inferior epigastric vessels; B, urinary bladder; a and v, iliac vessels)

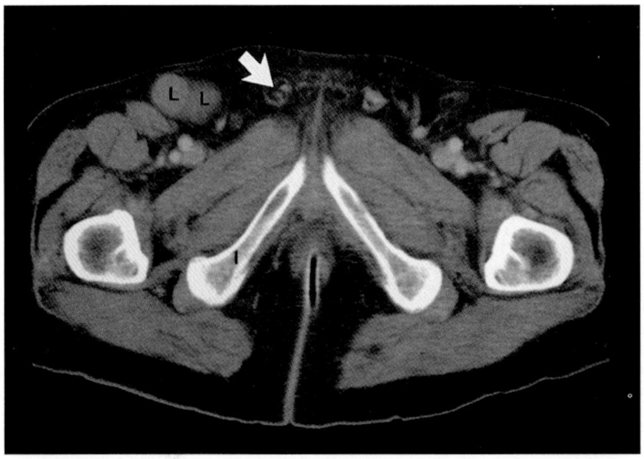

FIG. 3.27. Various normal appearance of the spermatic cord. Right spermatic cord (*arrow*) is seen as a thin-walled ring containing several dots. On the left, the cord is seen as a more homogeneous structure. An air-filled tube is seen in the distal rectum. (I, ischium; L, inguinal lymph nodes)

erally and superiorly by the transversus abdominis muscle. The **inguinal canal** is not a true canal but a space between the layers of the abdominal wall extending between the internal and external inguinal rings. It contains the vas deferens and testicular artery, vein, and lymphatics.

On CT scans, the spermatic cord is seen anterolateral to the symphysis pubis and medial to the femoral veins. It either appears as an oval mass of soft tissue density (Fig. 3.26) or as a thin-walled, ringlike structure in which the vas deferens and testicular vessels may be identified separately (Fig. 3.27). The various components of the spermatic cord can be identified within the inguinal canal, although they may not be individually differentiated.

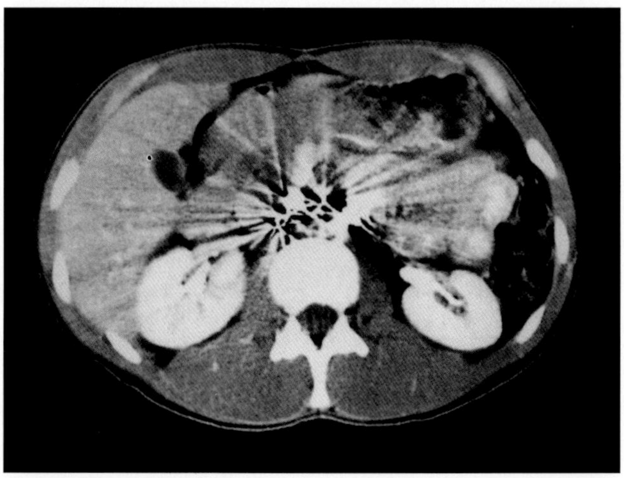

FIG. 3.28. Artifacts produced by metallic clips in a patient who had RPLND.

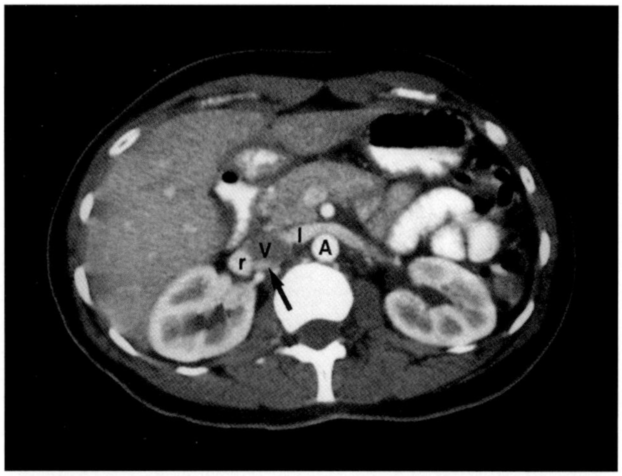

FIG. 3.29. Flow artifact within inferior vena cava (V). On ultrafast CT the inferior vena cava is seen as a lower density structure because of the inflow of nonopacified blood from the lower extremities. Note opacified blood in dependent portion of the lumen (*arrow*). (A, aorta; r, right renal vein; l, left renal vein)

Though neither the internal nor external inguinal ring may be demonstrated on CT scans, the location of the inguinal canal, including internal and external inguinal rings, can be determined by locating bony and vascular landmarks (Fig. 3.26). The external inguinal ring is just superior to the pubic ramus, and the internal inguinal ring is located approximately halfway between the sym-

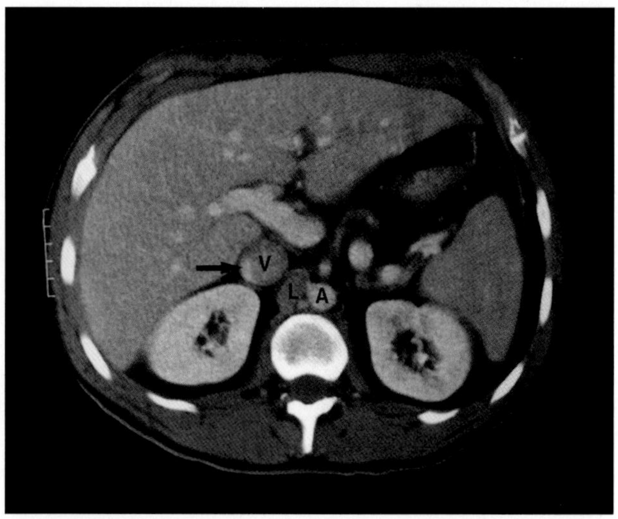

FIG. 3.30. Inferior vena cava (V) mimicking an enlarged lymph node. An enlarged crural lymph node (L) in a patient with testicular cancer is seen in the right aspect of the aorta, resembling the inferior vena cava. The inferior vena cava (v) is actually located anterolateral to this lymph node and mimics an enlarged lymph node. Opacified blood, seen in right lateral portion of the lumen (*arrow*), confirms the identification of the vessel.

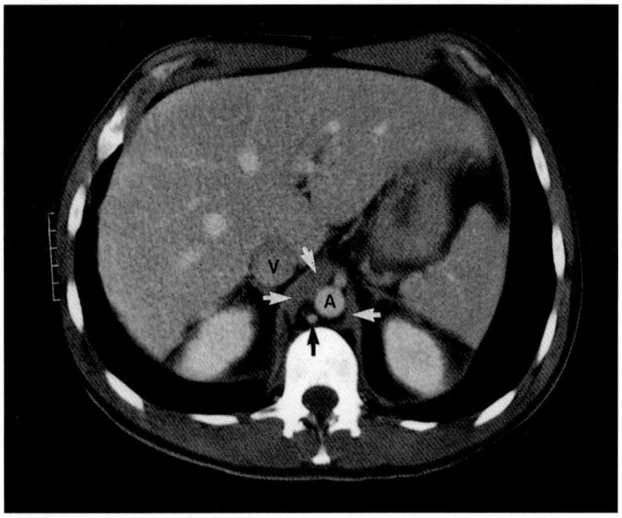

FIG. 3.31. Retrocrural lymph nodes (*white arrows*) in a patient with testicular embryonal carcinoma. The attenuation value of the nodes and adjacent crura of the diaphragm are very similar, although in this patient asymmetrical thickening of the crura is diagnostic of nodal disease. (A, aorta; V, inferior vena cava; *black arrow,* azygos vein)

physis pubis and the anterior superior iliac spine (12). Before it enters the inguinal canal, the spermatic cord lies within the subcutaneous tissue anterolateral to the symphysis pubis (Fig. 3.26). At the level of the internal inguinal ring, the vas deferens and testicular vessels diverge. The former loops behind the inferior epigastric artery and passes downward and posteriorly along the lateral pelvic wall to the seminal vesicle. The latter ascends into the abdomen. Occasionally, a segment of the vas deferens can be traced to the seminal vesicle, but spermatic vessels usually cannot be identified at this level.

ARTIFACTS

Scrotal CT images are not particularly affected by movement artifacts (from patient motion, breathing, cardiac motion, and peristalsis of the bowel), which can degrade CT images elsewhere in the body. Most commonly, artifacts encountered during the examination of the testes are caused by metallic clips in patients who have had retroperitoneal lymph node dissection (RPLND) (Fig. 3.28). Of the commercially used surgical ligation clips, tantalum clips induce the most image degradation. The impact on images progressively decreases with the use of stainless steel, titanium, and absorbable polymeric clips (13). In fact, titanium and absorbable polymeric clips produce almost no artifact (13). Other metallic foreign bodies, such as femoral prostheses, can produce similar, often more striking, artifacts. Pelvic bone can cause beam-hardening artifacts, and residual barium and the air–fluid level of bowel loops can produce streak artifacts.

Another common artifact is the flow artifact, which may mimic a thrombus in the suprarenal inferior vena cava. Laminar blood flow in the aorta and major arteries, or inflow of unopacified venous blood into inferior vena cava (Figs. 3.29 and 3.30) or portal vein can produce filling defects that may mimic intraluminal thrombi or an enlarged lymph node. Unlike true thrombi, however, such artifacts have ill-defined margins, are transient, and do not persist on delayed images.

When CT is used for evaluation of testicular cancer, it is important to be able to distinguish enlarged retrocrural lymph nodes from thickened diaphragmatic crura. As the retrocrural lymph nodes serve as a gateway of tumor spread into the thorax, even a small lymph node in this area may be of great prognostic importance. However, especially in thin subjects with little retroperitoneal fat, the retrocrural lymph nodes are often inseparable from the diaphragmatic crura on CT scans (Fig. 3.31). When it is not possible to differentiate these structures from thickened crura, MRI may be helpful.

REFERENCES

1. Robson WLM, Leung AKC, Putnins RE, Boag GS. Genital edema in children on continuous ambulatory peritoneal dialysis. *Child Nephrol Urol* 1990;10:205–210.
2. Maxwell AJ, Boggis CRM, Sambrook P. Computed tomographic peritoneography in the investigation of abdominal wall and genital swelling in patients on continuous ambulatory peritoneal dialysis. *Clin Radiol* 1990;41:100–104.
3. Berland LL. Radiation. In: Berland LL. *Practical CT: technology and techniques.* New York: Raven Press; 1987:39–43.
4. NCRP report no. 100. *Exposure of the U.S. population from diagnostic medical radiation.* Bethesda, MD: National Council on Radiation Protection and Measurements; 1989:1–72.
5. Shope TB, Gagne RM, Johnson GC. A method for describing the doses delivered by transmission x-ray computed tomography. *Med Phys* 1981;8:488–495.
6. Fearon T, Vucich J. Pediatric patient exposures from CT examinations: GE CT/T 9800 scanner. *AJR* 1985;144:805–809.
7. ICRP publication 60. 1990 recommendations of the International Commission on Radiation Protection. *Ann ICRP* 1990;21:1–77.
8. NCRP report no. 91. Recommendations on the limits for exposure to ionizing radiation. Bethesda, MD: National Council on Radiation Protection and Measurements, 1987:1–55.
9. Nishizawa K, Maruyama T, Takayama M, Okada M, Hachiya J, Furuya Y. Determinations of organ doses and effective dose equivalents from computed tomographic examination. *Br J Radiol* 1991;64:20–28.
10. Evens RG, Mettler FA. National CT use and radiation exposure: United States 1983. *AJR* 1985;144:1077–1081
11. Fearon T, Vucich J. Normalized pediatric organ-absorbed doses from CT examinations. *AJR* 1987;148:171–174.
12. Rajfer J, Tauber A, Zinner N, Naftulin E, Worthen N. The use of computerized tomography scanning to localize the impalpable testis. *J Urol* 1983;129:972–974.
13. Gross SC, Kowalski JB, Lee SH, Terry B, Honickman SJ. Surgical ligation clip artifacts on CT scans. *Radiology* 1985;156:831–832.

CHAPTER 4

Congenital Anomalies of the Testis

Congenital anomalies of the testis include anomalies of the descent (undescended testis), location (testicular ectopia), number anorchism (unilateral, bilateral), polyorchidism, and size (macro-orchidism).

UNDESCENDED TESTIS (CRYPTORCHIDISM)

A testis that lies in the normal path of testicular descent is a truly undescended testis (1). The incidence of undescended testis at birth, one of the most frequent congenital anomalies of the male, has been reported to be 3.4% for full-term infants and 30.3% for premature infants (2,3). The lower the birth weight of the infant, the greater the incidence of undescended testis. The incidence decreases as the infant grows and by 1 year of age is approximately 0.8%. Undescended testes are bilateral in approximately 10% of cases (4). Different physical and endocrine factors have been suggested for testicular descent in the scrotum, but the mechanism involved in the regulation of testicular descent is not yet fully understood. In the absence of surgical intervention when the testis is not palpated in its normal scrotal position, causes may be found to be (1) congenital absence or agenesis of the testis (3% to 5% of patients), (2) testicular ectopia (1%), (3) a retractile or migratory testis (up to 70% of patients), and (4) truly undescended testis (30% of patients).

Retractile or **migratory testes** slide back and forth between the scrotum and the external inguinal ring. Because the cremasteric reflex is most active between 2 and 7 years of age, retractile testes are common during childhood (5). This probably accounts for the inflated reported incidence of about 10% for undescended testis at 5 years of age (6). Between 25% and 33% of all boys referred to clinics because of suspected undescended testis are found to have normal but retractile testes (1).Retractile testes usually take a normal intrascrotal position at puberty and no treatment is needed.

The truly undescended testis, a condition also known as **testicular retention,** can be found at several different locations:

Intra-abdominal retention, in which the testis is found retroperitoneally between the caudal pole of the kidney and the internal inguinal ring (most commonly near the internal inguinal ring).

Inguinal (canalicular) retention, in which the testis is located between the internal and external inguinal ring.

Prescrotal retention, in which the testis lies at the top of the scrotum, below the inguinal canal and above the scrotal pouch. Because of different treatment approaches this group is further categorized into high scrotal position (this type usually necessitates orchiopexy) and midscrotal position. (Follow-up observation is advocated.)

Most commonly, the undescended testis is located just outside the external inguinal ring (in the superficial inguinal pouch) or at the neck of the scrotum. Intracanalicular and intra-abdominal locations are the second and third most frequently found. The undescended testis is palpable in about 80% of patients. Approximately 80% of nonpalpable undescended testes are located intracanalicularly, and the remaining 20% are intra-abdominal (from the renal hilum to the inguinal canal) (4). In an obese patient a relatively normal-sized testis may not be palpable. In this instance it is usually located near the external ring in the superficial inguinal pouch near the neck of the scrotum (7). An intra-abdominal testis is most commonly located near the internal inguinal ring deep to the anterior abdominal wall muscle and adjacent to the iliac vessels (7). In one large study with 295 patients, 66% of undescended testes were located distal to the external inguinal ring, 16% were in the inguinal canal, 10% were intra-abdominal, and in 3% the testis was absent (8).

Complications of Undescended Testis

Infertility, malignant degeneration, torsion, and inguinal hernia may be associated with undescended testis.

A temperature difference as small as 1.5°C to 2.0°C between the scrotum and the abdomen can inhibit spermatogenesis, and undescended testes are often associated with **infertility.** The farther the testis is from the scrotum, and the longer it remains undescended, the greater the histologic alterations (e.g., decreased size of seminiferous tubules) and the greater the likelihood of infertility (5). Infertility rates in males with bilateral undescended testes have been reported to be 40% with corrective surgery and 100% without surgery (9,10). In unilateral disease the mean fertility rate is 60% (10).

Approximately 10% of **testicular cancers** are associated with an undescended testis, and the incidence of malignant degeneration in an undescended testis has been reported to be up to 48 times as high as in the normal testis (11,12). Malignant degeneration usually occurs after puberty, even after conservative or surgical correction of the malposition (4,13). Cancer also occurs more frequently in intra-abdominal testes, where it is four times as common as in intracanalicular undescended testes (14). In patients with unilateral undescended testis, up to 20% of testicular tumors develop in the contralateral, intrascrotal testis (11). Seminomas are the most common cell type in undescended testicular tumor (5,15,16).

Torsion often occurs in undescended testes and is commonly associated with malignant degeneration. Given the increased risk of torsion of an undescended testis, an intra-abdominally twisted testis should be considered in patients presenting with acute abdominal pain and an empty ipsilateral hemiscrotum. Torsion occurs more commonly after puberty because at this time the testis tends to be larger than its mesentery. Sixty-four percent of patients with torsion of an intra-abdominal testis are reported to have associated testicular cancer (17). Torsion of a cryptorchid testis in adults is most frequently induced by an increase in volume due to a tumor.

Congenital inguinal hernias (persistent processus vaginalis peritonei) (3) are also associated with undescended testis. Inguinal hernia occurs when the narrow connection of the processus vaginalis to the abdominal cavity fails to obliterate. Testicular descent is closely related to obliteration of the processus vaginalis, and more than 90% of patients with undescended testes have hernia sacs (18).

Epididymal abnormalities, ranging from elongation of the epididymis to complete disruption of the epididymis from the testis, are found in 36% to 79% of patients with undescended testis (19,20). Epididymal abnormalities are particularly likely to occur when a patient has a patent processus vaginalis (19,20).

Congenital anomalies of the central nervous system and urinary tract are also associated with undescended testis (19–21). In one study of 144 asymptomatic boys with undescended testis (21), major urinary anomalies (including renal agenesis, ectopia, and ureteropelvic junction obstruction) were found in 5.5% of patients and minor urologic abnormalities were present in 25%.

Treatment of Undescended Testis

Because of the high incidence of complications, early treatment—including hormonal therapy, orchiopexy, and orchiectomy—is important. **Gonadotropin-releasing hormone** (GnRH) and **hCG** are currently used for hormonal therapy, but their success rate is relatively low (6% to 18% for GnRH and 14% to 50% for hCG (5). Because of the possibility of spontaneous descent, surgical intervention is usually delayed until after 1 year of age. **Orchiopexy** is usually performed in patients between 1 and 10 years of age, and **orchiectomy** is considered in patients after puberty. After 32 years of age surgical risk outweighs the risk of malignancy and surgical intervention is not undertaken (22).

Clinical Examination

On clinical examination the extrascrotal location of a testis is indicated by a hypoplastic and poorly developed empty scrotum with absent or reduced wrinkling of the scrotal skin. Testes positioned in a superficial inguinal pouch can be palpated subcutaneously. If the testis is not found in either the scrotum or the inguinal region, areas where ectopic testes may be located should be inspected and palpated.

Ultrasound in Evaluation of Undescended Testis

The primary indications for an ultrasound (US) examination in patients with undescended testis are to search for an undescended testis, to follow up patients after orchiopexy or hormone therapy for undescended testis, and to facilitate exclusion or detection and staging of a tumor arising in an undescended testis. In patients with unclear findings, a second US study is recommended to avoid a misdiagnosis of undescended testis in patients with retractile testis, since surgical intervention is required for the former, but not the latter. Sonography is also suitable for therapeutic monitoring of testicular descent in patients undergoing hormone treatment. The testicular echotexture is not affected by this therapy.

Ultrasound Appearance

When searching for an undescended testis in infants and children, it is helpful to first examine the normally descended testicle and to then search for a comparable structure on the contralateral side. The undescended testis is also oval and has a homogeneous, hypoechoic echotexture (Fig. 4.1) (23,24). It is most frequently located distal to the external inguinal ring in the subcutaneous tissue anterior to the pubic tubercle–superficial inguinal pouch (Fig. 4.1) (25). High-resolution real-time US, because of its good spatial resolution and freely selectable scanning planes (parallel to the course of the inguinal canal), is accurate in detecting a testis located between the internal inguinal ring and the scrotal neck (Fig. 4.2) (26,27). Even very small (10 mm in diameter), rudimentary testicles can be recognized if they are located in this area. Difficulty in differentiating a testicular structure from a possible inguinal hernia can be overcome by scanning during a Valsalva maneuver, while the patient is coughing, or after deliberately evoking the cremasteric reflex (by stimulating the skin on the inner side of the thigh).

The **pars infravaginalis** of the gubernaculum testis, which is hypoechoic and nodular in appearance, may mimic an atrophic testis (28). A testis can be reliably distinguished from the gubernaculum by visualization of a delicate hyperechoic intratesticular band corresponding to the mediastinum testis (Figs. 4.1 and 4.3) (28,29).

When the undescended testis is located cranial to the internal inguinal ring (intra-abdominal retention), shadowing from bowel gas and difficulty distinguishing the small testicle from other abdominal structures may produce inconclusive US findings. If the undescended testis is not found in the inguinal canal or at the base of the scrotum, the suprapubic, perineal, and femoral regions should be scanned.

In adults, US examination is performed to exclude malignancy and to locate an undescended testis if surgery is contemplated. As in children, ultrasound easily depicts testes located below the internal inguinal canal, but not those in an intra-abdominal position. An undescended testis in adults differs in its sonographic appearance from the normal, intrascrotal testis. It is small and

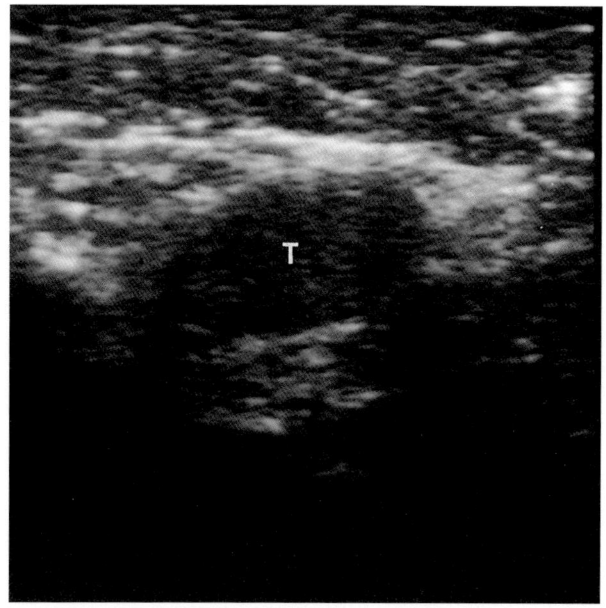

FIG. 4.2. Undescended testis (T) in intracanalicular location within the inguinal canal.

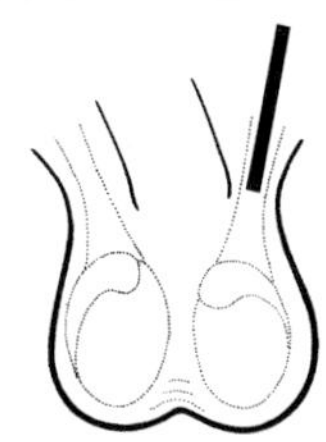

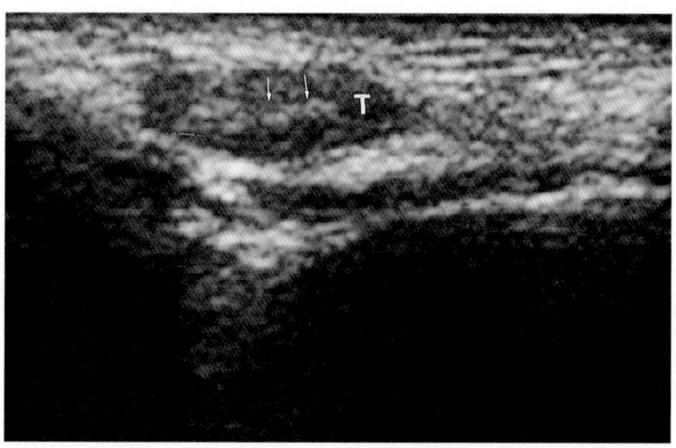

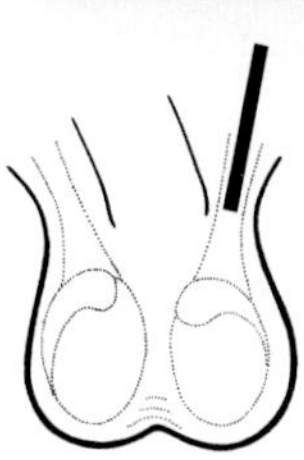

FIG. 4.1. Undescended testis (T) is located in the superficial inguinal pouch; mediastinum testis (*arrows*).

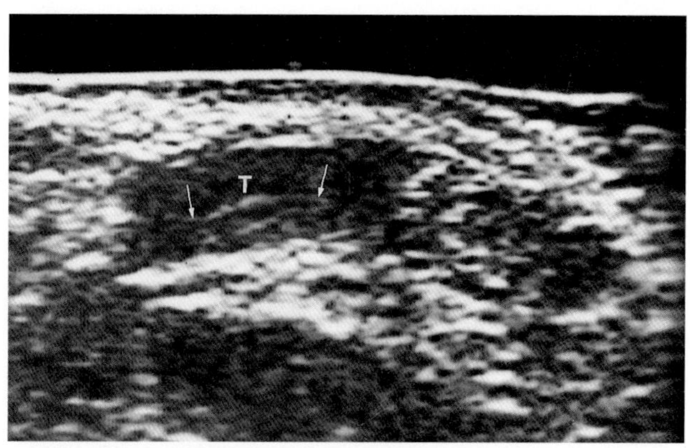

FIG. 4.3. Undescended left testis in a 2-year-old boy. The testis, located at the distal inguinal canal, has a homogeneous, hypoechoic echotexture. The mediastinum testis (*arrows*) is displayed as a thin, hyperechoic band.

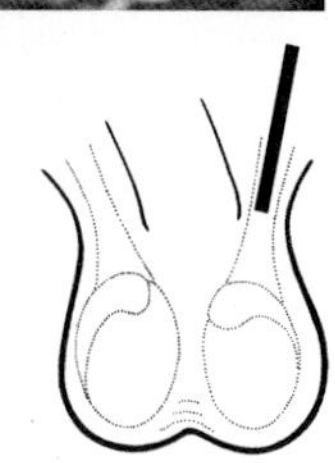

frequently hypoechoic because of damage to or incomplete development of the germinal epithelium. A testis located in the inguinal canal may be elongated rather than oval, but it retains its homogeneous echotexture. Any inhomogeneity or focal lesion within the testicular tissue suggests a testicular tumor. Examination of an undescended testis in adults may be more difficult than in children. Overlying adipose tissue is thicker, often requiring the use of a lower-frequency transducer. If a question of possible tumor in an undescended testis has not been adequately answered on US, further imaging studies preferably MRI, should be obtained.

Magnetic Resonance Imaging in Evaluation of Undescended Testis

Magnetic resonance (MR) imaging is an excellent study for demonstrating prescrotal and intracanalicular undescended testes. Intra-abdominal testes, when located close to the internal inguinal ring, can be seen lateral to the bladder or adjacent to the iliac vessels or psoas muscles. High abdominal testes, however, are difficult to demonstrate on MR.

Some changes in the routine MR protocol are necessary for evaluation of undescended testis. In infants, a head coil may be applied instead of a surface coil. Use of a pelvic multicoil may provide better resolution. Because a distended bladder can displace inguinal structures, the patient is asked to empty his bladder before the study. Using a T1-weighted sagittal localizer, transaxial T1- and T2-weighted images are obtained from the bottom of the scrotum to above the seminal vesicles. Coronal T1-weighted images can be added if the testis is found in the pelvic cavity. The examination should be extended to the lower poles of the kidneys when no testis is seen in the pelvis.

Magnetic Resonance Appearance

Magnetic resonance diagnosis of undescended testis can be made when an elliptical mass is demonstrated along the expected path of testicular descent (Fig. 4.4). When the undescended testis is in the inguinal canal, it is usually oval. In intra-abdominal locations it is more rounded (Fig. 4.5) (30). Because of its elliptical shape the whole testis is best seen on coronal plane images (Fig. 4.4). On transaxial plane images the anteroposterior dimension of the testis is usually smaller than the transverse dimension (Fig. 4.6). When it is distal to the external inguinal ring, identification of the testis is facilitated by contrast with subcutaneous fat and demonstration of the epididymis or associated fluid. The inguinal canal can be used as an anatomic landmark to locate the position of the undescended testis with a high degree of accuracy. It is also possible to distinguish an undescended testis from an inguinal lymph node on MR images (Fig. 4.4). Differentiation is made possible by the characteristic signal intensity of the testis and inner structures (i.e., the mediastinum testis) and by the typical location of the inguinal nodes (inferior to the inguinal ligament below the inguinal canal or adjacent to the femoral or iliac vessels). The signal intensity of lymph nodes may be similar to that of the testes.

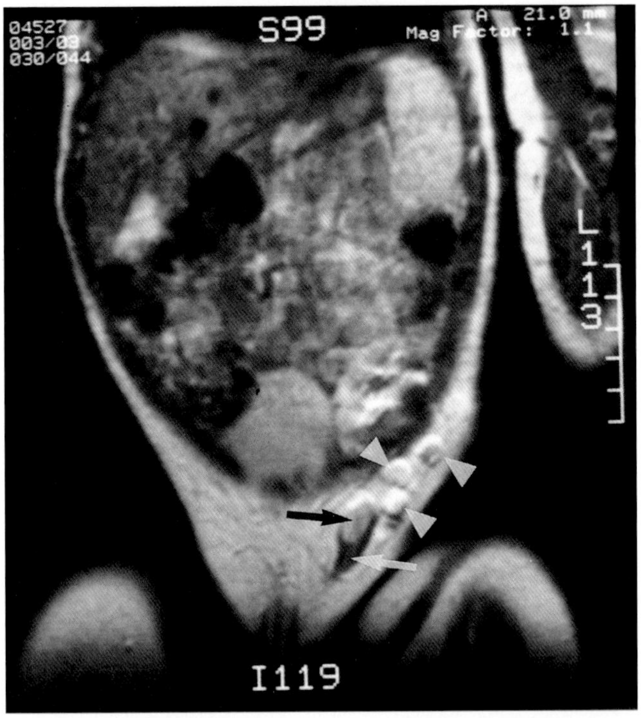

FIG. 4.4. Prescrotal location of the undescended testis. Coronal T2-weighted MR image demonstrates left undescended testis and adjacent inguinal adenopathy (*arrowheads*). The mediastinum testis (*black arrow*) is seen as a low signal intensity stripe within the testis. A gubernaculum testis (pars infravaginalis gubernaculi) (*white arrow*) is seen as a low intensity structure distal to the testis.

Although the presence or absence of the spermatic cord cannot always predict the location of an undescended testis, structures of the spermatic cord can serve as helpful landmarks. The ductus deferens and the testicular vessels can often be traced within the spermatic cord to the level of the undescended testis. The ductus is rarely present caudal to an undescended testis. However, because embryologic development of the gonads is independent of the development of the ductal structures, presence of a blind ending ductus does not always imply absence of the testis. When the undescended testis is located proximal to the external inguinal ring, an empty spermatic cord may be seen as a thin, curvilinear structure extending distally to the scrotum.

MR imaging also offers an attractive alternative to hormonal testing for the differentiation of retractile from undescended testes. In the former the volume and signal

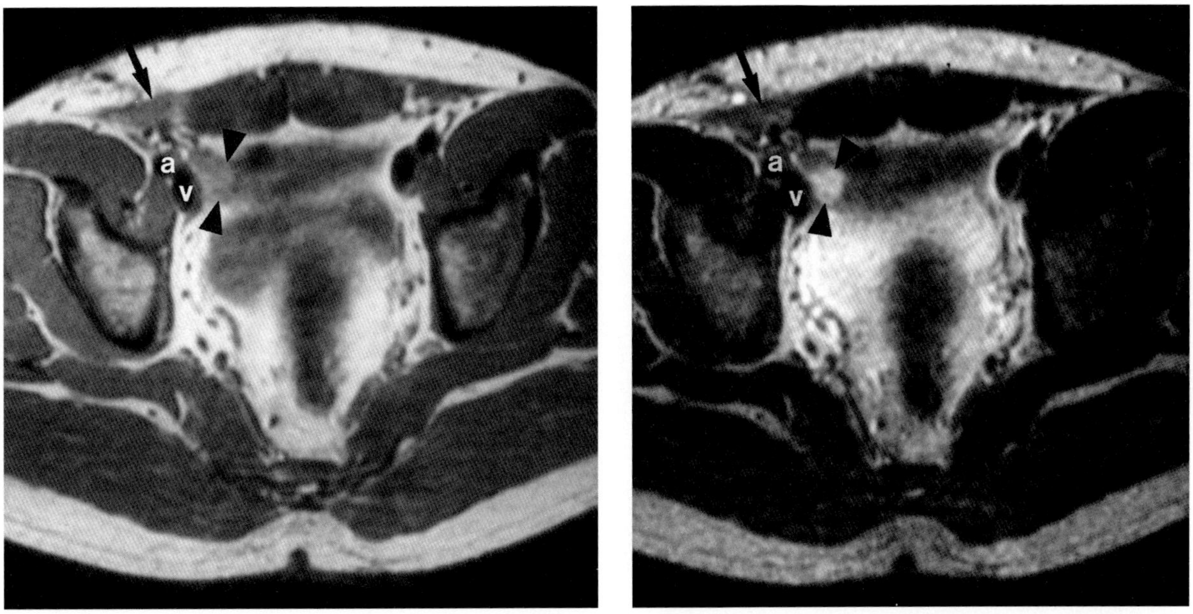

A B

FIG. 4.5. Intra-abdominal undescended testis. Transaxial **(A)** proton density, and **(B)** T2-weighted MR images. The testis (*arrowheads*) is seen medial to the iliac vessels (a and v) just outside the internal inguinal ring. The testis is round in configuration, indicating that it is outside the inguinal canal. Scar tissue (*arrow*) from previous unsuccessful surgery for localization is seen. On repeated surgery following the MR examination, the testis was found.

intensity of the testis are normal and the gubernaculum is well developed (Fig. 4.6). In an undescended testis, however, the volume of the testis may be normal or small, the gubernaculum is usually not well developed, and the signal intensity of the testis may be lower than normal on T2-weighted images.

MR imaging is also reliably able to locate remnants of **testicular regression** (i.e., regressed undescended testis composed of fibrous scar with hemosiderin deposition and calcification) (30). The diagnosis can be made when an atrophic cord is seen approaching the base of the empty scrotum. On T2-weighted images, regressed testes exhibit low signal intensity, which correlates histologically with remnant cord structures and a fibrotic nodule containing hemosiderin deposition and calcification (30).

The **pars infravaginalis gubernaculi (PIG)**, the distal bulbous termination of the gubernaculum, is always caudal to the undescended testis (Fig. 4.4). The **gubernaculum** is a cordlike structure that guides the testis during descent. It is gelatinous in early fetal life and normally atrophies after the testis descends completely (28). When the testis fails to descend to the scrotum, the gubernaculum persists as a fibrotic remnant (28). The PIG is sometimes misdiagnosed as an undescended testis on imaging studies, and differentiation between the two is essential. This is achieved on MR images by identification of the characteristic signal intensities of the testis and the gubernaculum and the presence or absence of the mediastinum testis (Fig. 4.4). Whereas the testis typically shows low signal intensity on T1-weighted images and high signal intensity on T2-weighted images, the gubernaculum demonstrates low signal intensity on both T1- and T2-weighted images. Signal intensity characteristics alone, however, are not sufficient to differentiate the gubernaculum from an atrophic undescended testis, which also demonstrates low signal intensity on T2-weighted images. Identification of the mediastinum testis, which is sometimes seen on MR images, allows a definitive diagnosis of undescended testis.

MRI also plays an important role in the detection of a tumor within an undescended testis. T2-weighted or contrast-enhanced T1-weighted images are needed for tumor depiction. (For further discussion of tumor appearance on MRI, see Chapter 5.)

Computed Tomography in Evaluation of Undescended Testis

For computed tomography (CT) evaluation of undescended testes, contiguous 5-mm sections from the inferior border of the symphysis to the anterior superior iliac spine are needed. If the testes are not visualized in the scrotal sac or inguinal regions, the examination should be extended up to the renal hilus at 10-mm intervals. When preparing children for evaluation of suspected undescended testes, ingestion of oral contrast material may be simplified by administering 500 mL of oral contrast at least 1 hour before the examination. Bolus injection of

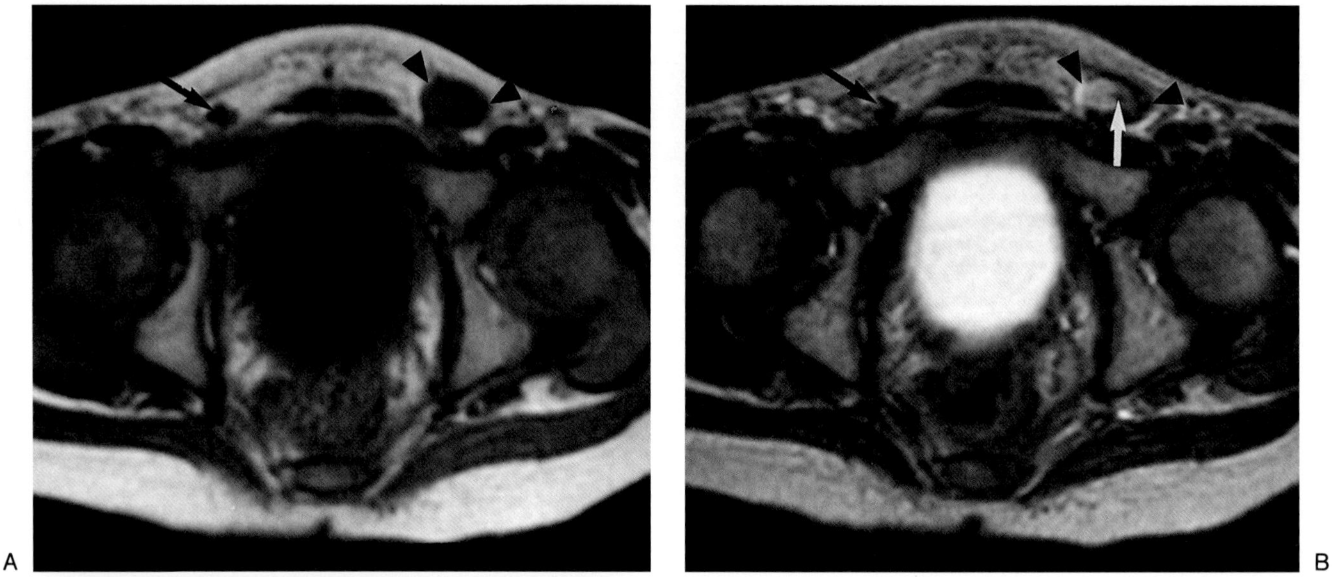

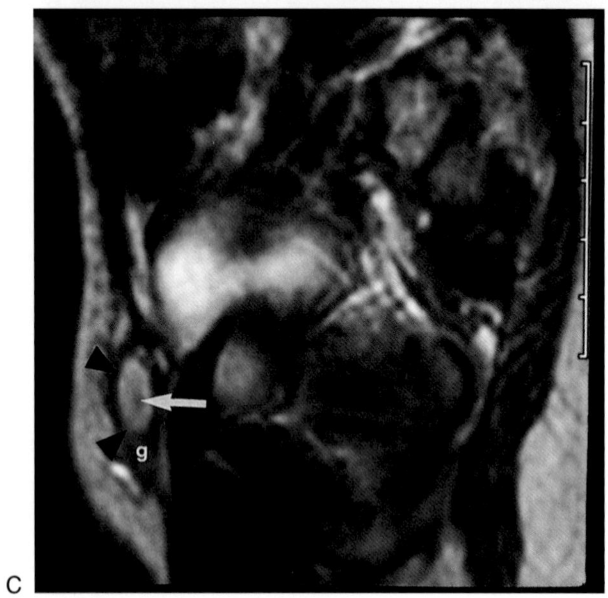

FIG. 4.6. Retractile testis just below left external inguinal ring in the superficial inguinal pouch. **(A)** Transaxial T1-weighted MR image, **(B)** transaxial T2-weighted image, and **(C)** sagittal T2-weighted MR image. Normal-sized ovoid testis (*arrowheads*). The linear low-signal-intensity mediastinum (*white arrow*) can be differentiated from the high intensity testis on the T2-weighted images. (*black arrow,* contralateral normal spermatic cord; g, gubernaculum testis).

intravenous contrast material with prompt scanning are necessary to obtain optimal vascular enhancement for the detection of undescended testes.

Computed Tomography Appearance

On CT examination, undescended testes appear as oval soft tissue masses along the expected course of testicular descent (Fig. 4.7). CT, like MRI, allows precise identification of the undescended testis in the prescrotal (Fig. 4.8), canalicular, or intra-abdominal location (Fig. 4.9). When located in the superficial inguinal pouch the undescended testes may sometimes be difficult to differentiate from inguinal lymph nodes (Fig. 4.10). Nodes are located outside the spermatic cord, inferior to the inguinal ligament (below the inguinal canal), or adjacent to the femoral or iliac vessels, deep and lateral to the inguinal canal (Figs. 4.10) (7). It is more difficult to detect intra-abdominal testes than prescrotal intracanalicular testes because the former can be confused with bowel loops, vessels, and lymph nodes (Fig. 4.11) (31). The possibility of malignant degeneration should be considered when the undescended testis is larger than 2 cm in its longest dimension (Fig. 4.12).

Scintigraphy in Evaluation of Undescended Testis

Of three case reports on the diagnosis of torsion of an undescended testicle by radionuclide scintigraphy, two cases were accurately diagnosed and one was missed (32–34). The use of pinhole and converging collimators can be helpful in visualizing torsion. A torsed redux testicle

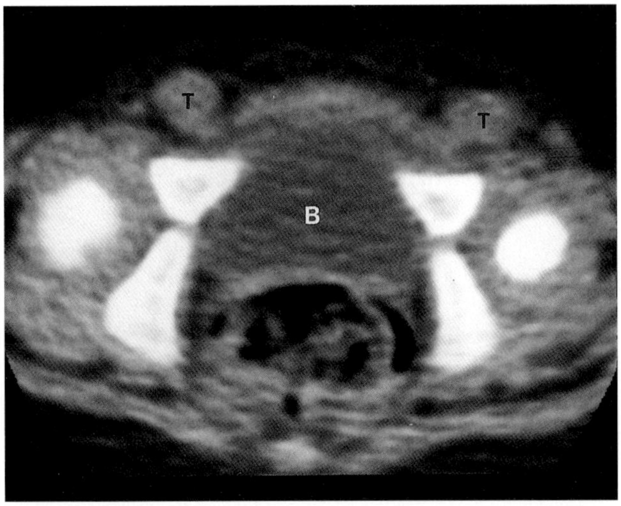

FIG. 4.7. Bilateral undescended testes (T) just below the external inguinal ring in the superficial inguinal pouch are well depicted on this noncontrast CT scan. (B, urinary bladder)

(one that retracts into the canal) has also been found by scintigraphy (33). For techniques and further discussion see Chapter 9 (32–34).

Angiography in Evaluation of Undescended Testis

For many years **testicular venography** was the most widely used diagnostic procedure (35–37). When successfully performed, it significantly reduces the need for surgical exploration. Three distinct findings have been reported in the literature: demonstration of a pampiniform plexus, demonstration of the testicular parenchyma, and demonstration of a blind-ending testicular vein. If a pampiniform plexus is demonstrated, it is most likely that a testicle is present (38). If there is a blind-ending testicular vein, it is most unlikely that a testicle is present. For a discussion of technique and further discussion see Chapter 10 (35,36).

A

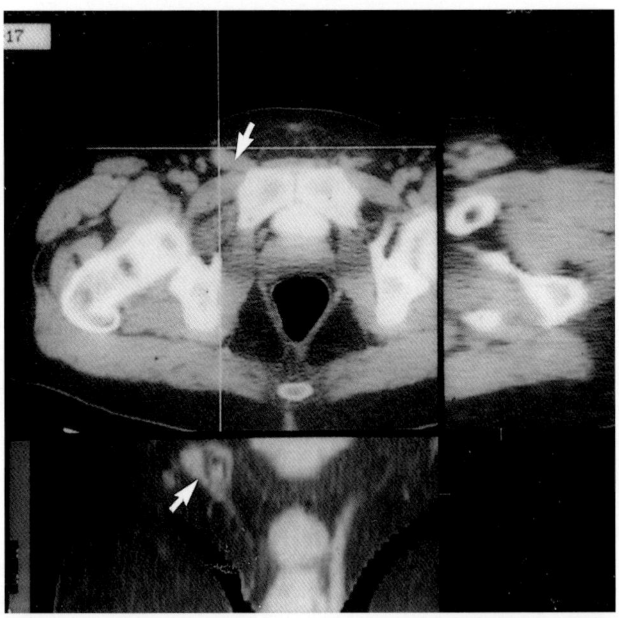

B

FIG. 4.8. Prescrotal location of the undescended testis (T) is well displayed on either **(A)** transverse or **(B)** coronal reformatted CT scan.

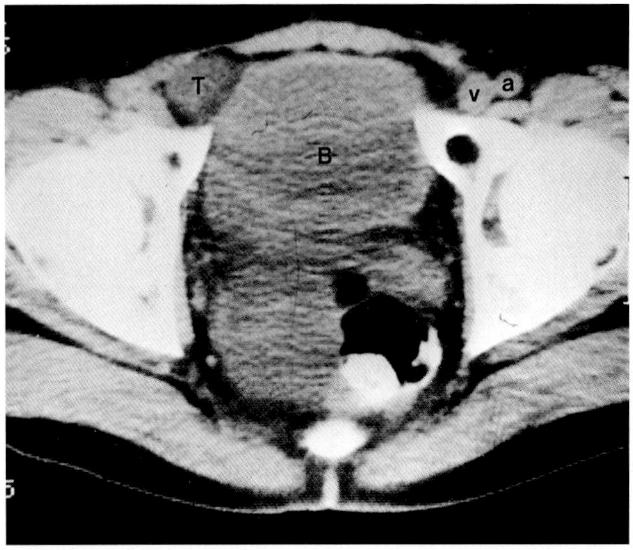

FIG. 4.9. Intra-abdominal undescended testis (T) just outside the internal inguinal ring (B, urinary bladder; a and v, femoral vessels). The orientation of the longest axis of the testis indicates that it is outside the inguinal canal. (Photo courtesy of D. Fahlenkamp, Humboldt-Universität zu Berlin.

Comparative Evaluation of Radiologic Techniques

In addition to clinical examination, ultrasound, magnetic resonance imaging (39), computed tomography

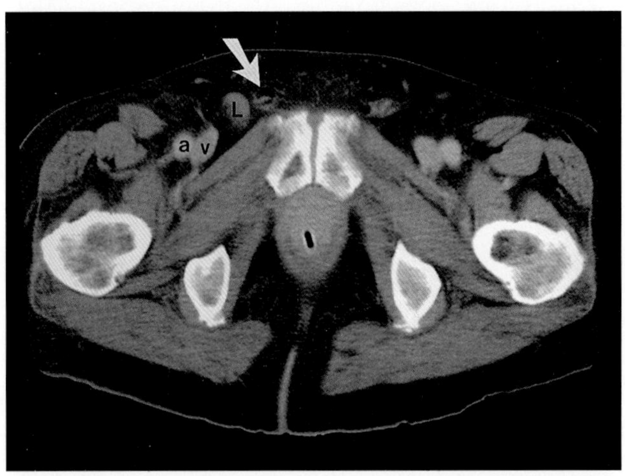

FIG. 4.10. Enlarged inguinal lymph node (L) is located below the inguinal canal and adjacent to the femoral vessels (a and v). Medial to the node, the spermatic cord is seen as a ring structure (*arrow*).

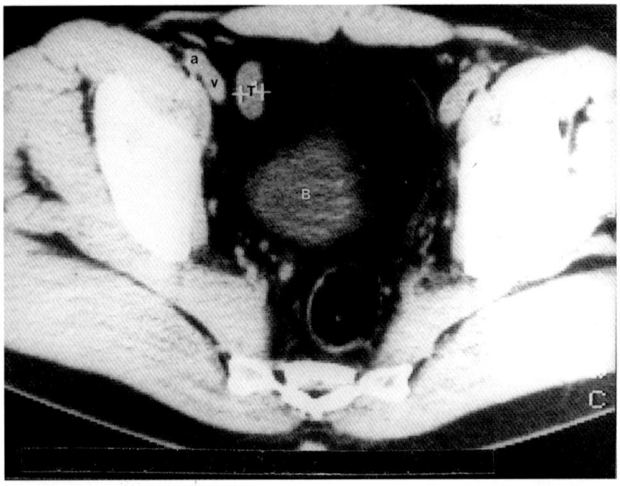

FIG. 4.11. Right intra-abdominal testis (T) is seen medial to the iliac vessels (a and v), it may be difficult to differentiate intra-abdominal testis from an unfilled bowel loop. (B, urinary bladder) (Photo courtesy of H. Derouet, Universität Homburg/ Saar.)

(22,31,40), arteriography (41), retrograde testicular venography (23,35,36), laparoscopy (42), and exploratory laparotomy can all be used in the diagnostic evaluation of undescended testes.

Ultrasound, despite a relatively smaller field of view, poor specificity, and operator dependence, is often the primary imaging modality used in the search for undescended testis.

Magnetic resonance imaging offers the advantages of noninvasiveness, excellent soft tissue contrast, a large field of view, multiplanar capability, free selection of imaging plane, and absence of ionizing radiation exposure. MRI is highly accurate (94%) in locating undescended testes, a figure comparable to CT and slightly better than US (39). Intra-abdominally located testes, however, frequently escape detection on MR examination. MRI, however, is the preferred modality when testicular tumor within an undescended testis is suspected (Fig. 4.13).

Despite poor spatial resolution, computed tomography was often used to localize undescended testes in the early 1980s. It is more expensive, however, takes longer (possibly necessitating sedation of young children), and carries a radiation risk. In addition, the lack of body fat in children limits its usefulness in the pediatric population. Additional limitations of CT include difficulty in separating the testis from the spermatic cord or from fluid, and often the inability to detect atrophic testes less than 1 cm in diameter (31). The widespread availability of US and MRI have made CT a much less frequent choice for the detection of undescended testis. It should be remembered, however, that computed tomography is as accurate as real-time sonography in the localization of testes retained in the inguinal canal, and is superior for detection of intra-abdominal testicles (40). In one study that compared CT with high-resolution US for the localization of the nonpalpable, undescended testis, the accuracy of CT and US was 96% and 91%, respectively (40). In addition, both US and MRI are limited in the ability to demonstrate intra-abdominal testes, making CT a more accurate and reliable modality in this situation (4).

Radiologic visualization of testicular vessels may be indicated when intra-abdominal retention of the testis is suspected. The most widely used angiographic procedure is retrograde, selective venography (4,23,35,36). Selective venography, however, has relatively low sensitivity and requires considerable technical skill on the part of the angiographer (4), and the radiation exposure is 5 to 10 times higher than with CT. In 30% to 40% of cases the origin of the testicular vein cannot be found or the flow of the contrast material is obstructed by the presence of valves (38). In addition, venography is an invasive procedure and may require sedation or anesthesia when performed in young children. Other major drawbacks of testicular venography are a high rate of unsuccessful procedures and the inability of the technique to distinguish cryptorchidism from testicular agenesis (since the testis is not visualized directly). As a result, testicular venography is rarely used.

Although radiologic procedures can be highly valuable and accurate, laparoscopy has become the procedure of choice for evaluating patients with impalpable testes (43). Laparoscopy is reliable in demonstrating intra-abdominal testes (Fig. 4.14) and at the same time allows mobilization of the undescended testis and orchiectomy of an atrophic or hypoplastic testis. An experienced examiner can perform a diagnostic laparoscopy in about 15 minutes and needs a total of about 30 minutes when additional endoscopic orchiectomy is performed. Laparoscopy, however, is an invasive procedure and, unless orchiectomy or orchiopexy are contemplated, imaging is

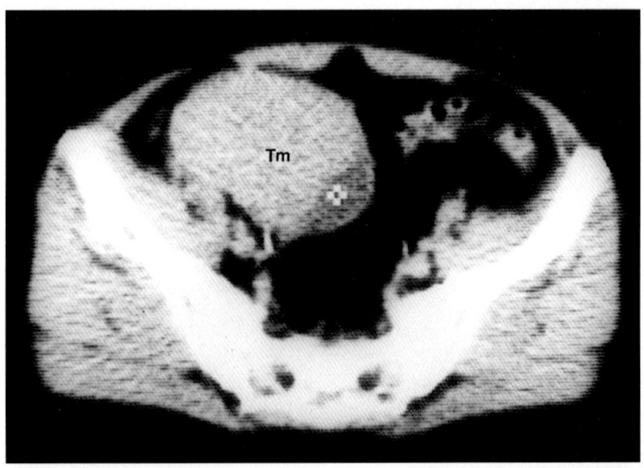

FIG. 4.12. Seminoma (Tm) arising in a right intra-abdominal undescended testis. The testis is enlarged and shows a mostly homogeneous enhancement. (From Derouet VH, Braedel HU, Ziegler M, Zwergel TH, Khorsandian CH: Computer tomographische Untersuchungen des Scrotalinhaltes, insbesondere des Hodens. *Fortschr Röntgenstr* 1988;148: 566–571.)

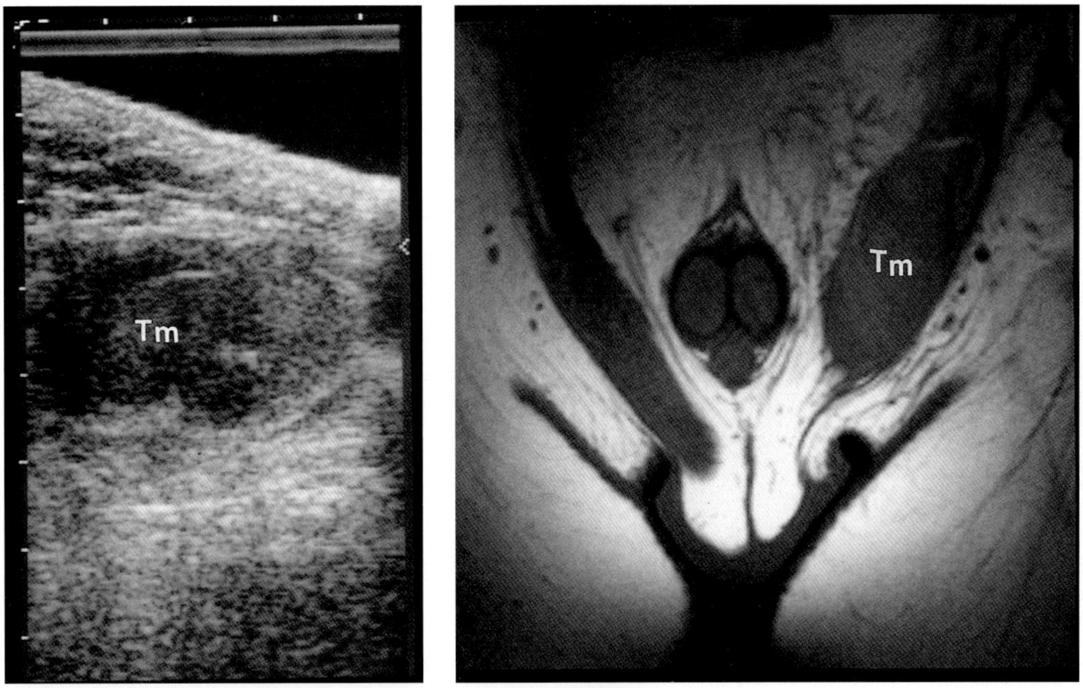

A B

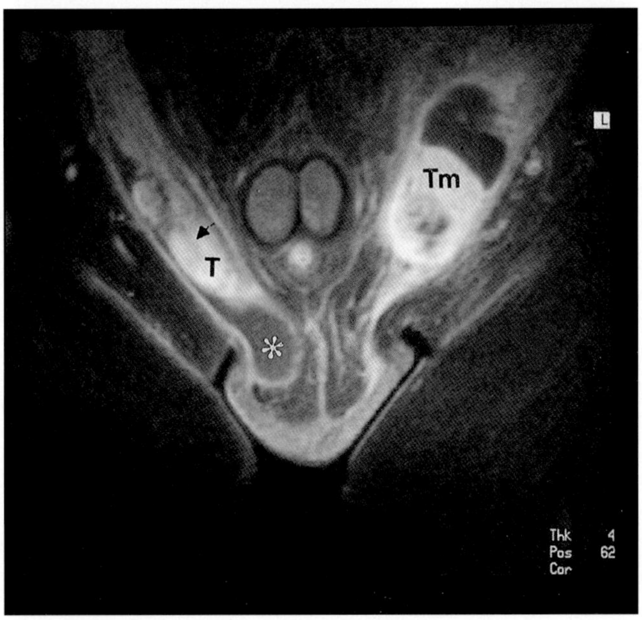

C

FIG. 4.13. Bilateral undescended testicles in a prescrotal location. Normal right testis and tumor present in the left testis: **(A)** an ultrasound scan, **(B)** noncontrast T1-weighted MR image, and **(C)** contrast-enhanced T1-weighted MR image, coronal plane of section. Ultrasound shows enlarged and inhomogeneously echogenic, undescended left testis, findings suggestive of tumor (Tm). On MRI the right undescended testis (T) with surrounding fluid in the spermatic cord (*) is well depicted on a contrast-enhanced study (Mediastinum testis [*arrowhead*]). The left undescended testis is large and demonstrates heterogeneous signal enhancement, indicating tumor involvement (Tm).

an attractive alternative. Although US is the most practical approach, because of its small field of view and operator and patient habitus dependence, it is not generally embraced. MRI is considered by many to be the single best imaging procedure for the evaluation of the undescended testis. CT is reserved for the search of intra-abdominal testis, and testicular arteriography and venography have fallen into relative disuse.

TESTICULAR ECTOPIA

Testicular ectopia is relatively rare. The most common ectopic site is the superficial inguinal pouch (a subcutaneous pocket anterolateral to the external inguinal ring). Unlike the truly undescended testis, the ectopic testis in this location cannot be manipulated into the path of testicular descent. Other sites include the perineum, the femoral canal, the suprapubic area, the penis, the diaphragm, and the opposite scrotal compartment (the least common ectopic site) (Fig. 4.15) (5,44).

ANORCHIA

Unilateral anorchia (monorchism), most common on the left side, is found in about 4% of all patients presenting with a nonpalpable testis (45). Definitive diagno-

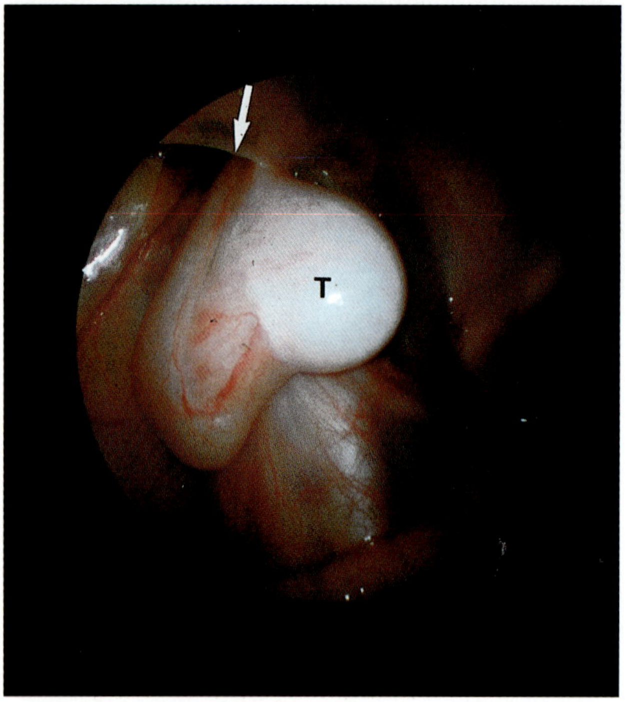

FIG. 4.14. Laparoscopic demonstration of an intra-abdominal testis (T) in a boy with right-sided cryptorchidism. Internal ring of the inguinal canal (*arrow*). (Courtesy of D. Fahlenkamp, Charité, Humboldt-Universität zu Berlin.)

sis depends on the intraoperative finding of a blind-ending, rudimentary vas deferens. Unilateral anorchia may be caused by intrauterine testicular torsion or other forms of compromised vascular supply to the testis during descent. The testis in patients with monorchism is not at increased risk of malignancy (46). Ultrasound, MRI, CT, and angiographic examinations for evaluation of unilateral absence of a testicle are the same as that described for evaluation of cryptorchidism.

Bilateral Anorchia

Complete bilateral absence of the male gonads is found in only about 0.6% to 1.0% of patients with nonpalpable testes (45). These patients are genotypically and phenotypically male and present clinically with a small, empty, and unpigmented scrotum, a micropenis, and delayed onset of puberty. Hormonal studies confirm the diagnosis. Patients with bilateral anorchia have elevated serum levels of luteinizing hormone (LH) and follicle-stimulating hormone (FSH), and do not show any response to the human chorionic gonadotropin (hCG) stimulation test (i.e., the increase in testosterone induced by hCG administration in healthy boys is absent in patients with bilateral anorchia) (22).

The hCG stimulation test, however, is not applicable after 35 years of age, because at this age the undescended testis may be too atrophied to respond to hCG administration. In addition, unilateral absence of the testis cannot be identified at present by endocrine testing.

POLYORCHIDISM

Polyorchidism (testicular duplication) is a very rare condition, and only about 80 cases have been reported in the literature to date. It is attributed to division of the gonadal primordium by peritoneal folds (47). The anomaly is more common on the left (75% of cases) and is bilateral in 5% of cases. The supernumerary testis is most commonly located in the scrotum (75%), but it can be in the inguinal canal (20%) or retroperitoneum (5%) (47). The additional testis is small and its efferent spermatic system is hypoplastic or completely absent. Polyorchidism is often associated with undescended testis (23%) or inguinal hernia (22%) (47). Because of its unstable connection to other structures, torsion of the supernumerary testis is relatively common (14%). In addition, testicular tumors may develop in the supernumerary testis (47,48).

Most patients are asymptomatic and may present with painless groin or testicular masses. On palpation, this malformation is difficult to distinguish from a tumor or a cyst. Sonographically, polyorchidism is suspected if a mass has a testislike, homogeneous echotexture, which may be iso- or hypoechoic with that of the normal testicular tissue (49–51). A single case report on MRI appearance of polyorchidism described testicular duplication with the same signal intensity of all the testicles (52). Given the rarity of this anomaly, any condition that may simulate duplicated testes (e.g., crossed testicular ectopia) should be excluded before establishing the diagnosis. Surgical exploration is usually indicated.

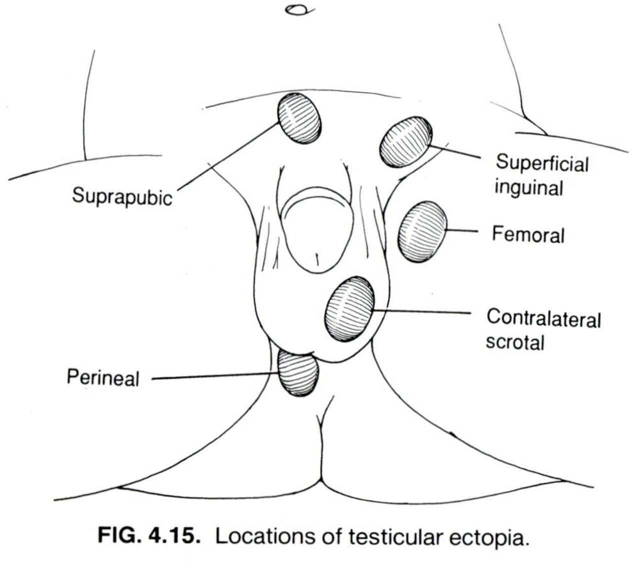

FIG. 4.15. Locations of testicular ectopia.

MACRO-ORCHIDISM

Macro-orchidism, a very rare entity, is characterized by asymptomatic, benign testicular enlargement. It is usually seen in mentally retarded patients, especially in those with a fragile X chromosome (53–56). Sporadic cases have also been reported in pubertal boys (57). The enlarged testis is smooth and symmetric, and no pathologic alteration other than larger size is detected by palpation or sonography. The echotexture in macro-orchidism is homogeneous and of medium-level intensity. The MRI or CT findings in macro-orchidism have not been reported. There is no increased risk of malignancy. It is important to differentiate this benign condition from other disorders that cause bilateral testicular enlargement. The differential diagnosis includes bilateral testicular tumors (leukemia, lymphoma, germ cell tumors, and stromal tumors), precocious puberty (either idiopathic or associated with juvenile hypothyroidism), and adrenal rests (57).

REFERENCES

1. Whitaker RH. Undescended testis: the need for a standard classification. *Br J Urol* 1992;70:1–6.
2. Scorer CG, Farrinton GH. Testis at birth and during infancy. In: Scorer CG, Farrinton GH. *Congenital deformities of the testis and epididymis.* New York: Appleton-Century-Crofts; 1971:15–27.
3. Scorer CG, Farrinton GH. *Congenital deformities of the testis and epididymis.* New York: Appleton-Century-Crofts; 1971.
4. Friedland GW, Chang P. The role of imaging in the management of the impalpable undescended testis. *AJR* 1988;151:1107–1111.
5. Rajfer J. Congenital anomalies of the testis. In: Walsh PC, Retik AB, Stamey TA, Vaughan ED, eds. *Campbell's urology,* 6th ed, vol 2. Philadelphia: WB Saunders; 1992:1543–1562.
6. Farrington GH. The position and retractability of the normal testis in childhood, with reference to the diagnosis and treatment of cryptorchidism. *J Pediatr Surg* 1968;3:53–59.
7. Wolverson MK, Jagannadharao B, Sundaram M, Riaz MA, Nalesnik WJ, Houttuin E. CT in localization of impalpable cryptorchid testes. *AJR* 1980;134:725–729.
8. Moul JW, Belman B. A review of surgical treatment of undescended testes with emphasis on anatomical position. *J Urol* 1988;140:125–128.
9. Kogan SJ. Cryptorchidism. In: Kelalis PP, King LR, Belman AB (eds.). *Clinical pediatric urology,* 3rd ed. Philadelphia: WB Saunders; 1992;1985:864–887.
10. Kogan SJ. Cryptorchidism and infertility: an overview. *Dialog Pediatr Urol* 1981;4:2–3.
11. Johnson DE, Woodhead DM, Pohl DR, Robinson JR. Cryptorchidism and testicular tumorigenesis. *Surgery* 1968;63:919–922.
12. Pinch L, Aceto T, Meyer-Bahlburg HFL. Cryptorchidism: a pediatric review. *Urol Clin North Am* 1974;1:573–592.
13. Martin DC. Germinal cell tumors of the testis after orchiopexy. *J Urol* 1979;121:422–424.
14. Campbell HE. The incidence of malignant growth of the undescended testicle: a reply and re-evaluation. *J Urol* 1959;81:663–668.
15. Mostofi FK, Price EB. Tumors of the testis. In: Mostofi FK, Price EB. *Tumors of the male genital system.* Washington, DC: Armed Forces Institute of Pathology; 1973:1–176.
16. Richie JP. Neoplasms of the testis. In: Walsh PC, Retik AB, Stamey TA, Vaughan ED, eds. *Campbell's urology,* 6th ed, vol 2. Philadelphia: WB Saunders; 1992:1222–1263.
17. Riegler HC. Torsion of intraabdominal testis: an unusual problem in diagnosis of the acute surgical abdomen. *Surg Clin North Am* 1972;52:371–374.
18. Scorer CG, Farrinton GH. Inguinal hernia and hydrocele in childhood. In: Scorer CG, Farrinton GH. *Congenital deformities of the testis and epididymis.* New York: Appleton-Century-Crofts; 1971: 157–174.
19. Koff WJ, Scaletscky R. Malformations of the epididymis in undescended testis. *J Urol* 1990;143:340–343.
20. Elder JS. Epididymal anomalies associated with hydrocele/hernia and cryptorchidism: implications regarding testicular descent. *J Urol* 1992;148:624–626.
21. Pappis CH, Argianas SA, Bousgas D, Athanasiades E. Unsuspected urological anomalies in asymptomatic cryptorchid boys. *Pediatr Radiol* 1988;18:51–53.
22. Rajfer J, Tauber A, Zinner N, Naftulin E, Worthen N. The use of computerized tomography scanning to localize the impalpable testis. *J Urol* 1983;129:972–974.
23. Diamond AB, Meng CH, Kodroff M, Goldman SM. Testicular venography in the nonpalpable testis. *AJR* 1977;129:71–75.'
24. Madrazo BL, Klugo RC, Parks JA, DiLoreto R. Ultrasonographic demonstration of undescended testis. *Radiology* 1979;133:181–183.
25. Cendron M, Huff DS, Keating MA, Snyder HM, Duckett JW. Anatomical, morphological and volumetric analysis: a review of 759 cases of testicular maldescent. *J Urol* 1993;149:570–573.
26. Hederstrom E, Forsberg L, Kullendorff CM. Ultrasonography of the undescended testis. *Acta Radiol* 1985;26:453–456.
27. Hinman F. Survey: localization and operation for nonpalpable testes. *Urology* 1987;30:193–198.
28. Rosenfield AT, Blair DN, McCarthy S, Glickman MG, Rosenfield NS, Weiss R. The pars infravaginalis gubernaculi: importance in the identification of the undescended testis. *AJR* 1989;153:775–778.
29. Johansen TE, Larmo A. Ultrasonography in undescended testes. *Acta Radiol* 1988;29:159–163.
30. Fritzsche PJ, Rifkin M, Hopkins CR, Piccoli CW. Scrotum and testes. In: Stark DD, Bradley WG. *Magnetic resonance imaging,* 2nd ed, vol 2. St Louis: Mosby–Year Book; 1992:2058–2077.
31. Lee JKT, Glazer HS. Computed tomography in the localization of the nonpalpable testis. *Urol Clin North Am* 1982;9:397–404.
32. Dravid VS, Heyman S. Torsion of an undescended testis not detected on testicular imaging. *Clin Nucl Med* 1991;16:275–277.
33. Fink-Bennett D, Uppal TK, Conway GF. Redux testis: potential pitfall in testicular imaging. *J Urol* 1979;121:821–822.
34. Ueno K, Hayashi H, Oohama K, Asano S. Missed torsion of an undescended testis detected with testicular imaging [letter]. *J Nucl Med* 1987;28:1061.
35. Amin M, Wheeler CS. Selective testicular venography in abdominal cryptorchidism. *J Urol* 1976;115:760–761.
36. Greenberg SH, Ring EJ, Oleaga J, Wein AJ. Gonadal venography for preoperative localization of nonpalpable testis in adults. *Urology* 1979;13:453–455.
37. Weiss RM, Glickman MG. Localization and management of nonpalpable undescended testes. *Surg Clin North Am* 1980;60:1253–1263.
38. Khan O, Krausz T, Williams G. Testicular venography in impalpable testis. *Eur Urol* 1993;9:341–342.
39. Fritzsche PJ, Hricak H, Kogan BA, Winkler ML, Tanagho EA. Undescended testis: value of MR imaging. *Radiology* 1987;164: 169–173.
40. Wolverson MK, Houttuin E, Heiberg E, Sundaram M, Shields JB. Comparison of computed tomography with high-resolution realtime ultrasound in the localization of the impalpable undescended testes. *Radiology* 1983;146:133–136.
41. Khademi M, Seebode JJ, Falla A. Selective spermatic arteriography for localization of an impalpable undescended testis. *Radiology* 1980;136:627–634.
42. Silber SJ, Cohen R. Laparoscopy for cryptorchidism. *J Urol* 1980;124:928–929.
43. Fahlenkamp D, Raatz D, Schönberger B. Laparoscopic diagnosis and therapy of cryptorchidism. *Urologe* 1992;31:328–332.
44. Lierse W. Testis. In: Lierse W. *Applied anatomy of the pelvis.* Berlin: Springer-Verlag; 1984:188–198.
45. Levitt SB, Kogan SJ, Engel RM, Weiss RM, Martin DC, Ehrlich RM. The impalpable testis: a rational approach to management. *J Urol* 1978;120:515–520.

46. McAlister WH, Sisler CL. Scrotal sonography in infants and children. *Curr Prob Diagnost Radiol* 1990;19(6):203–251.
47. Thum G. Polyorchidism: case report and review of literature. *J Urol* 1991;145:370–372.
48. Tulchinsky M, Eggli DF. Scintigraphy of torsion in triorchidism. *J Nucl Med* 1992;33:1854–1856.
49. Giyanani VL, McCarthy J, Venable DD, Terkeurst J, Fowler M. Ultrasound of polyorchidism: case report and literature review. *J Urol* 1987;138:863–864.
50. Goldberg RM, Chilcote W, Kay R, Bodie BH. Sonographic findings in polyorchidism. *J Clin Ultrasound* 1987;15:412–415.
51. Rifkin MD, Kurtz AB, Pasto ME, Gordberg BB. Polyorchidism diagnosed preoperatively by ultrasonography. *J Ultrasound Med* 1983;2:93–94.
52. Baker LL, Hajek PC, Burkhard TK, Mattrey RF: Polyorchidism: evaluation by MR. *AJR,* 1987;148(2):305–306.
53. Hutton L, Rankin RN, Pozsonyi J. High resolution ultrasound of macro-orchidism in mental retardation. *J Clin Ultrasound* 1985;13:19–22.
54. Nielsen KB, Tommerup N. Macroorchidism, mental retardation and the fragile X. *N Engl J Med* 1981;305:1348.
55. Ruvalcaba RHA, Myhre SA, Roosen-Runge EC, Beckwith JB. X-linked mental deficiency megalotestes syndrome. *JAMA* 1977;238:1646–1650.
56. Turner G, Daniel A, Frost M. X-linked mental retardation macro-orchidism and the Xq(27) fragile site. *J Pediatr* 1980;96:837–841.
57. Truwit CL, Jackson M, Thompson IM. Idiopathic macroorchidism. *J Clin Ultrasound* 1989;17:200–205.

CHAPTER 5

Testicular Tumors and Tumorlike Lesions

Overall, testicular cancer accounts for 1% of all cancers in men, and it is the most common malignancy among 15- to 34-year-olds (1). Fortunately, it is one of the most curable tumors, and the overall 5-year survival rate is over 90% (2). About 95% of testicular tumors are of germ cell origin. Other tumors affecting the testis include those arising from the gonadal stroma, secondary tumors from lymphoid and hematopoietic tissue, and metastatic tumors. Of the secondary tumors involving the testis, lymphoma is the most common (5% of all testicular tumors), followed by leukemia. Metastatic tumors are rare in the testis. The most common primary sites include the prostate, lung, gastrointestinal tract, skin, and kidney (2). Only 3% to 4% of testicular tumors are benign, and about 90% of these are non–germ cell tumors, such as Leydig cell tumors (1% to 3% of all testicular tumors), Sertoli cell tumors (1%), gonadoblastomas (0.5%), epidermoid cysts (1%), and adrenal rest tumors. In addition, a variety of tumorlike lesions affect the testis. Ultrasound (US) is the most commonly used modality for evaluation of testicular tumors, but no imaging modality can provide a histologic diagnosis.

TESTICULAR CANCER

Approximately 6,600 new cases of testicular cancer are reported every year, and it is estimated that about 350 deaths are related to this disease annually in the United States (3). The annual incidence in the United States is 2.4 to 2.92 per 100,000 male inhabitants. A worldwide increase in testicular cancer has been observed over the last 40 years (4). The majority (90% to 95%) of testicular tumors are malignant germ cell tumors. Common histologic types include seminomas (35%), embryonal carcinomas (20%), teratomas (5%), choriocarcinomas (<1%), teratocarcinomas (a combination of teratoma and embryonal carcinoma) (25%), and other combined tumors (15%) (5). Seminomas occur most commonly in men 35 to 39 years of age and are rare before 10 or after 60 years of age (6). Most nonseminomatous germ cell tumors (NSGCT) occur between the ages of 25 and 35, but pure teratomas and yolk sac tumors (endodermal sinus tumors or infantile-type embryonal cell cancers) most commonly occur in childhood. Malignant lymphomas are the most common testicular tumors in patients over 50 years of age. Undescended testis is associated with testicular cancer in 10% of patients, and about half of bilateral tumors are associated with unilateral or bilateral undescended testes.

New diagnostic techniques and combination chemotherapy protocols have resulted in earlier diagnoses and have considerably improved the prognosis for testicular cancer (7). The overall survival rate has increased from 50% to 95% within the last decade (8).

Clinical Presentation

The most common symptom of testicular cancer is a lump or painless swelling of the testis. Scrotal pain, if present, is usually dull or heavy in nature. Approximately 27% of patients complain of scrotal pain, confirming that the presence of pain does not exclude the diagnosis of testicular cancer. In approximately 10% of patients, testicular cancer is associated with acute pain, usually caused by hemorrhage or infarction, mimicking torsion or epididymitis. Some patients report a feeling of heaviness in the affected hemiscrotum. About two thirds of all patients report awareness of a testicular mass for up to 3 months before seeking medical advice (9). In patients with seminomas, the delay in presentation may be even longer (10). Tumor involving the epididymis or spermatic cord occurs in 10% to 15% of patients (1), and 20% to 40% of patients have metastatic disease at the time of diagnosis. In approximately 10% of patients presenting symptoms—such as back pain (most common), supraclavicular lymphadenopathy, respiratory symptoms, central nervous system symptoms, bone pain, and lower leg swelling—are related to metastatic disease (6).

In another 10% of cases, reactive hydrocele is associated with testicular tumor and may preclude correct diagnosis of the coexisting tumor. Gynecomastia occurs in 5% of patients with germ cell tumors and in 30% to 50% of patients with Sertoli and Leydig cell tumors (2).

Testicular cancer occurs more commonly on the right side than on the left, and tumors are bilateral in approximately 2% to 3% of cases. Histologically, most bilateral tumors are seminomas. On physical examination, seminomas, which are usually diffuse, can be palpated as painless, rubbery enlargements. Teratomas and embryonal cell carcinomas, on the other hand, may be recognized as irregular nodular masses on palpation (11).

Several **tumor markers** are closely related to the tumor burden of testicular cancer and are useful for detection, staging, and monitoring response to treatment. **Alpha-fetoprotein (AFP), human chorionic gonadotropin (hCG),** and **lactic acid dehydrogenase (LDH)** are the most commonly used markers. Elevation of tumor markers varies, depending on the various cell types of testicular tumor (Table 5.1). AFP is elevated to varying degrees in many NSGCTs, but it is never elevated in pure seminoma or choriocarcinoma. Similarly, hCG is commonly elevated in most NSGCTs, including choriocarcinoma, and is elevated in about 7% of seminomas. Even in advanced stages, however, approximately 10% of patients with NSGCTs have negative AFP and hCG. Despite a high false-positive rate, LDH can be used as an indicator of tumor burden in NSGCT or advanced seminoma.

Germ Cell Tumors (Seminomas and Nonseminomatous Germ Cell Tumors)

Germ cell testicular tumors are either seminomas or nonseminomatous germ cell tumors. Seminomas are divided into three histologic subtypes—"classic" or typical seminoma (82% to 85%), anaplastic seminoma (5% to 10%), and spermatocytic seminoma (2% to 12%) (6). Nonseminomatous tumors include embryonal cell carcinoma, teratoma, choriocarcinoma, and any combination of these tumors.

TABLE 5.1. *Incidence of tumor marker elevation in testis cancer*

Histology	hCG (%)	AFP (%)
Seminoma	7	0
Embryonal carcinoma	60	70
Teratoma	25	38
Teratocarcinoma	57	64
Choriocarcinoma	100	0

From Tanagho EA, McAninch JW, eds. *Smith's general urology,* 13th ed. Norwalk, CT: Appleton & Lange; 1992:416.
AFP, alpha-fetoprotein; hCG, human chorionic gonadotropin.

Anaplastic seminomas are the most aggressive with the least favorable prognosis. Spermatocytic seminomas, which most commonly occur in elderly men, rarely metastasize and frequently have a favorable outcome. Compared with pure seminomas, nonseminomatous tumors more often metastasize and usually have a less favorable prognosis. Mixed seminomatous and nonseminomatous germ cell tumors behave and are treated like nonseminomatous tumors. Although the precise etiology of germ cell tumors is not known, predisposing factors include a history of cryptorchidism (12) and a previous testicular tumor on the contralateral side (13). Additional possible risk factors include testicular atrophy, mumps orchitis, a positive family history of testicular tumors, and testicular microlithiasis (14–19). The most important risk from a clinical perspective is that of malignant transformation of the remaining testis in patients having undergone unilateral orchiectomy for a testicular tumor. Contralateral testicular intraepithelial neoplasia (TIN) (see later) is histologically demonstrated in 4% to 7% of all patients with germ cell tumors. Of these, 50% develop a malignant tumor within 5 years (20). TIN cannot be diagnosed clinically, but a random biopsy of the contralateral testicle will identify those patients with a high risk of developing a second testicular tumor (20). A second tumor may develop in the contralateral testicle even after a very long interval, and patients require prolonged surveillance with regular follow-up and instruction in scrotal self-examination.

There are a number of systems for the classification of germ cell tumors based on different theories of histogenesis. The theory of **common germ cell origin,** originally proposed by Friedman and Moore (21), was modified first by Dixon and Moore (22) and later by Mostofi (23). This theory postulates that all germ cell tumors arise from a single precursor lesion, namely, testicular intraepithelial neoplasia (TIN) (20,24). This precursor may differentiate into seminomatous (except spermatocytic seminoma) or nonseminomatous tumors, which, in accordance with the biologic potential of germ cells, may histologically resemble different abortive stages of human embryogenesis (20,25). The WHO classification of testicular tumors (Table 5.2) (26) reflects this theory of common histogenesis, and identifies six different histologic patterns that occur either alone or, more frequently, in any combination. The British nomenclature according to Pugh (27), which was used frequently in the past, is based on an outdated dualistic germ cell tumor theory.

About 10% of all patients with germ cell tumors present with symptoms related to metastatic disease. An intrascrotal tumor can be diagnosed in two-thirds. The other one third may have a true extragonadal germ cell

TABLE 5.2. *WHO classification of testicular tumors*

1. Germ cell tumors
   1.1. Tumors of one histologic type
      1.1.1. Seminoma
      2. Spermatocytic seminoma
      3. Embryonal carcinoma
      4. Yolk sac tumor
      5. Polyembryoma
      6. Choriocarcinoma
      7. Teratoma
         Mature
         Immature
         With malignant transformation
   1.2. Tumors of more than one histologic type
      1.2.1. Teratocarcinoma (embryonal carcinoma + teratoma)
      2. Choriocarcinoma and any other types
      3. Other combinations
2. Sex cord/stromal tumors
   2.1. Well-differentiated forms
      2.1.1. Leydig cell tumor
      2. Sertoli cell tumor
      3. Granulosa cell tumor
   2.2. Mixed forms
   2.3. Incompletely differentiated forms
3. Tumors containing both germ cell and sex cord/stromal elements
   3.1. Gonadoblastoma
   3.2. Others
4. Miscellaneous tumors
   4.1. Carcinoid
   4.2. Others
5. Lymphoid and hematopoietic tumors
6. Secondary tumors (metastases)
7. Tumors of collecting ducts, rete, epididymis, spermatic cord, capsule, supporting structures, and appendices
8. Tumorlike lesions
   8.1. Epidermal (epidermoid) cyst
   8.2. Dermoid cyst
   8.3. Others

tumor, malignancy of an intra-abdominal testicle, or a so-called **burned-out testicular tumor** (19). In these "burned-out" tumors, immunologic or vascular processes (exactly which are not yet fully understood) have caused the primary tumor to regress while metastatic spread continues (19). Metastatic spread from a burned-out testicular tumor may be mistaken for a **primary extragonadal germ cell tumor**. The latter, however, which accounts for 3% to 5% of primary germ cell tumors, occurs in midline structures, such as the mediastinum, retroperitoneum, pineal gland, prostate, or thymus (11,28). These tumors tend to be aggressive and often present in the advanced stages of disease with early metastases. Because a primary tumor in the testis cannot be effectively treated by chemotherapy (the testis is believed to be a "sanctuary organ") (29–31), the major aim of diagnostic imaging is to exclude testicular tumor in patients with presumed primary extragonadal tumor (e.g., in retroperitoneum) (32). If an occult or "burned-out" tumor is found, patients can be referred for unilateral orchiectomy and will be spared a random bilateral testicular biopsy.

Tumors of the Gonadal Stroma (Leydig Cell Tumors, Sertoli Cell Tumors, and Gonadoblastomas)

The most frequent nongerminal neoplasms are **Leydig cell tumors** (representing 2% to 3% of all testicular tumors). Bilateral involvement is seen in 5% to 9% of patients and is often associated with an adrenogenital syndrome. Leydig cell tumors are most common in children between 5 and 10 years of age and in adults between 30 and 35 years of age. Only 5% to 10% of Leydig cell tumors are malignant, and these generally occur during the sixth and seventh decades of life (33). Endocrine symptoms—caused by elevation of estrogen, androgen, progesterone, and corticosteroid concentrations in plasma (34,35)—are found in 30% to 40% of patients. In adults, unilateral or bilateral gynecomastia may develop months before testicular enlargement becomes apparent. In children the production of androgen and estrogen may induce precocious puberty (36). Leydig cell tumors are usually small and tend to grow slowly. Except in cases of malignant degeneration, the prognosis is good. Orchiectomy is the therapy of choice.

Rare tumors of the gonadal stroma include Sertoli cell tumors, granulosa cell tumors, androblastomas, and tumors of the supporting connective tissue (e.g., adenocarcinoma of the rete testis). **Sertoli cell tumors**, which account for about 1% of testicular tumors, are malignant in approximately 10% of cases. Patients may present with gynecomastia or endocrinopathy, but this is uncommon (37–38). **Gonadoblastoma,** a rare mixed tumor accounting for 0.5% of testicular tumors, contains both germ cell and stromal elements and is seen almost exclusively in association with gonadal dysgenesis (39). Patients have intersex problems and present with abnormalities of the gonads and external genitalia. Most of the patients are phenotypically female with XY, XO, or XO/XY chromosome patterns (39).

Lymphoid/Hematopoietic Tumors

Lymphoid and hematopoietic tumors represent a separate group in the WHO classification of intrascrotal tumors (Table 5.2). **Lymphoma** is the most common testicular tumor in men over 60 years of age. The testis may be the initial site of manifestation, or it may be the site of secondary invasion in the presence of systemic disease. It is the most common secondary testicular tumor, accounting for approximately 5% of metastatic disease. Simultaneous or successive involvement of both testicles

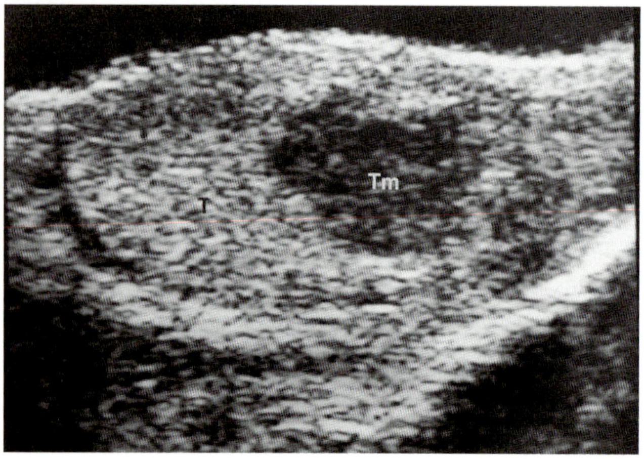

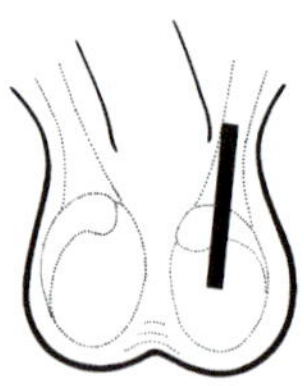

FIG. 5.1. A small, hypoechoic, intratesticular tumor (Tm) in a 32-year-old patient. Histologic examination showed the tumor to be a seminoma. (T, testis)

is not uncommon (approximately 50% of cases), and there is a relatively high incidence of tumor recurrence in the testis in patients having undergone chemotherapy for leukemia or malignant lymphoma (40). There is one report of a case of AIDS presenting as a primary testicular lymphoma (41). Testicular lymphomas are commonly associated with hemorrhage and necrosis.

Leukemic infiltration of the testis is most commonly seen in children, and the testis is the most common site of relapse of acute leukemia (42,43). Bilateral disease is found in approximately half of the patients. Testicular irradiation combined with adjuvant chemotherapy is currently used for treatment of patients with leukemic infiltration.

Metastatic Tumors of the Testis

Intrascrotal metastases secondary to malignant tumors of other organs are uncommon. When they do occur, they are usually found in older patients (more than 50 years of age) and are associated with primaries in advanced stages. Carcinoma of the prostate, lung, and kidney, as well as malignant melanoma, are the most frequent neoplasms that metastasize to the scrotum (44). All intrascrotal structures are usually affected. The clinical picture is dominated by the advanced primary cancer.

Differential Diagnosis of Testicular Cancer

Since the treatment for a testicular cancer is radical orchiectomy, differentiation of tumors from other testicular lesions is of primary importance (6,11,45). Because the clinical presentation, physical examination, and laboratory findings for different testicular diseases overlap, testicular cancer is often misdiagnosed and treated as tor-

A

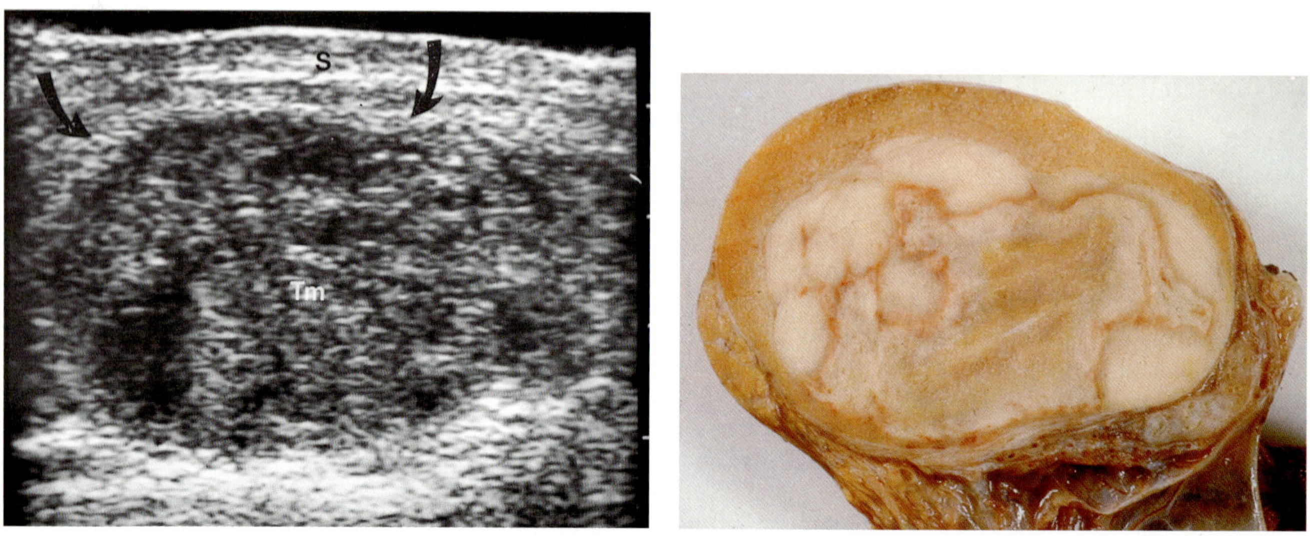

B

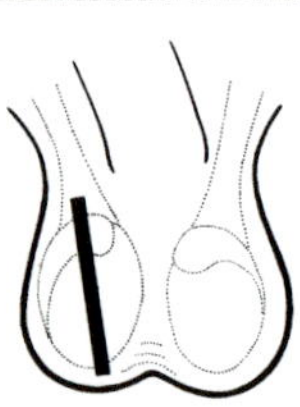

FIG. 5.2. Seminoma in a 22-year-old patient. **(A)** Sonogram demonstrates a large, inhomogeneous echotexture testicular tumor (Tm) with a thin rim of normal testicular parenchyma (*curved arrows*). (S, scrotal skin) **(B)** Surgical specimen.

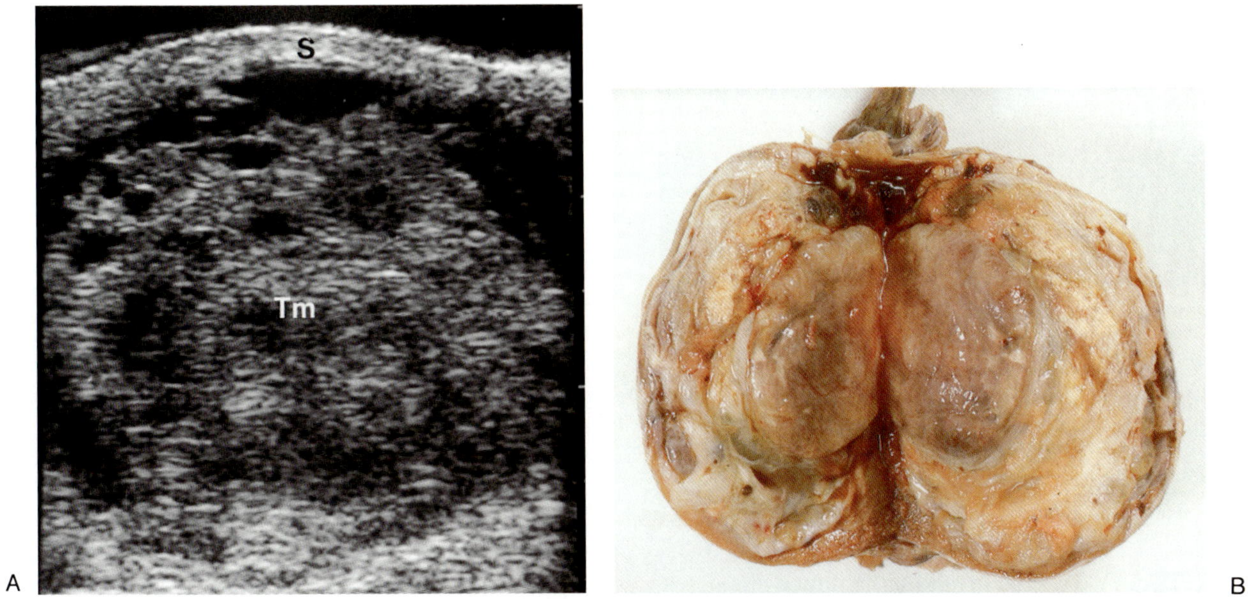

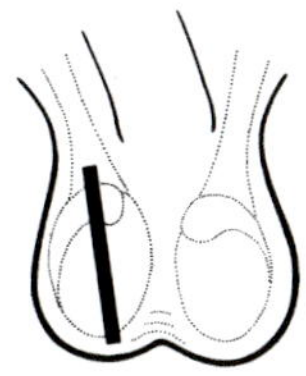

FIG. 5.3. Mixed tumor, with elements of embryonal carcinoma, choriocarcinoma, and teratoma in a 32-year-old patient. **(A)** Sonogram showing a large, inhomogeneous tumor (Tm) with solid and cystic areas infiltrating the entire testis. (S, scrotal skin) **(B)** Surgical specimen.

sion, epididymitis, or epididymo-orchitis, resulting in delay in appropriate treatment (11). Any suspicions for an intratesticular mass, either on palpation or on imaging, should be considered a neoplasm until proven otherwise (6,11). Often a combination of findings—from the history, palpation, and imaging—is necessary to arrive at a definite diagnosis. Surgical exploration is indicated in all cases where malignancy cannot be ruled out. Percutaneous biopsy of a testicular lesion is not commonly performed, since it may promote local metastatic spread (28).

Ultrasound in Evaluation of Testicular Cancer

Sonography is the most commonly used modality to evaluate the testis. It is very sensitive for detection of intratesticular lesions, clearly differentiating testicular from paratesticular tissue and allowing direct visualization of suspicious lesions discovered by palpation (46,47). It is not possible, however, to differentiate benign from malignant tumors or tumor from inflammatory lesions using sonographic criteria alone (47–52). Given the high incidence of malignancy in the testis, any intratesticular solid lesion should be suspected of being malignant and requires surgical exploration. Ultrasound is indicated for testicular tumor evaluation in the following cases:

- To confirm or rule out the presence of a tumor if findings on palpation are inconclusive
- To corroborate the diagnosis of tumor by direct visualization in patients presenting with testicular enlargement as the primary clinical symptom
- To search for an underlying testicular tumor in the presence of a hydrocele or epididymitis
- To follow patients with testicular microlithiasis to exclude development of tumor
- To search for an occult testicular tumor in patients presenting with metastatic disease and an unknown primary
- To eliminate anxiety in carcinophobic patients (a rare indication)

Ultrasound Appearance. The homogeneous echotexture of normal testicular tissue provides an excellent background for detection of intratesticular lesions. Small tumors are displayed as focal lesions (Fig. 5.1); larger tumors may leave only a thin rim of testicular tissue with normal, medium-level echogenicity (Fig. 5.2); and extensive tumors may infiltrate the entire testis (Fig. 5.3).

Tumor borders may be either smooth (Fig. 5.4) or irregular (Fig. 5.5). Although most primary germ cell tumors are solitary lesions (Fig. 5.4), mixed tumors (made up of two or more cell types) and seminomas may be multicentric (Figs. 5.5 and 5.6). If the tumor does not extend beyond the testis, the testis usually retains its oval

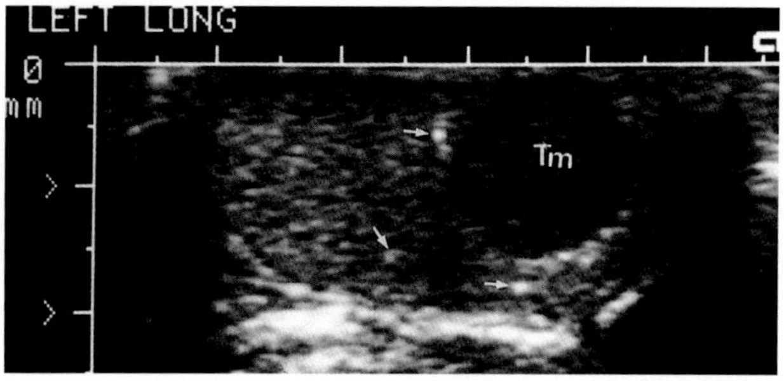

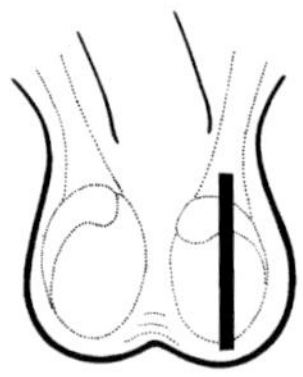

FIG. 5.4. Seminoma in a 28-year-old patient. The tumor (Tm) shows homogeneous hypoechoic echotexture and a sharp (smooth) interface toward normal testicular parenchyma. Also present is microlithiasis (*arrows*).

shape (Fig. 5.7). Tumors invading the tunica albuginea, the epididymis, or other extratesticular structure, however, partly or completely distort the contour of the testicle (Fig. 5.8). Most testicular tumors are hypoechoic, but they are sometimes seen as hyper- or mixed echogenic lesions (53). Cystic areas within a tumor correspond to necrosis, hemorrhage, or cysts (Fig. 5.9). Hemorrhage and necrosis are more common in advanced disease than in small lesions.

Color-coded Doppler sonography (CCDS) provides additional information in tumor vascularity. Tumor vascularity may be increased or decreased, and sometimes prominent venous flow is present (Fig. 5.8). Tumor vascularity correlates with the size of the tumor (although it has no relation to tumor histology). Larger tumors tend to be hypervascular, and smaller ones are more likely to be hypovascular. In one study of 28 patients with testicular tumors, 95% of tumors larger than 1.6 cm were hypervascular (Fig. 5.6), and 86% of tumors smaller than 1.6 cm were hypovascular (54). It should be noted that this correlation has no clinical significance, and hypervascularity within tumors cannot be differentiated from the US appearance of focal or diffuse orchitis (54,55). CCDS is also helpful in detecting diffuse infiltrative lesions, such as lymphoma or leukemia, which are often hypervascular and may be readily depicted. These lesions cannot, however, be differentiated from inflammatory processes. In general, the lack of specificity prevents CCDS from providing significant additional information to gray-scale imaging.

Ultrasound Appearance of Seminoma. Most seminomas (70% in one study [53]) have a homogeneous hypoechoic echotexture consistent with the regular surface of the surgical specimen (Figs. 5.4 and 5.7). Heterogeneous areas in a seminoma most often result from hemorrhage (Fig. 5.10) or regressive changes like necrosis (Fig. 5.2), which may also produce cystlike spaces (53,56,57). TIN, which consists of atypical cells, is not seen sonographically and can only be identified by histologic evaluation.

Ultrasound Appearance of Nonseminomatous Tumors. NSGCTs and mixed malignant germ cell tumors of the testis (e.g., embryonal carcinoma, choriocarcinoma, and teratoma) typically show an inhomogeneous echotexture (53) (see Figs. 5.3 and 5.9). Hemorrhage and necrosis are common in these tumors, partly accounting for their heterogeneity. Embryonal cell carcinomas tend to invade the tunica albuginea, demonstrating a bulge in the testicular contour (Fig. 5.8). Cystic spaces are primarily seen in teratomas (Fig. 5.9), and despite more frequent demonstration of the once rarely detected simple cyst, any intratesticular cystic structure should be evaluated for malignancy. (See also the discussion of seminiferous tubular ectasia of the rete testis, p. 82.) Dense echogenic foci within a tumor result from scarring, calcification, ossification, or cartilage formation (56) and are present in 35% of all nonseminomatous tumors (53) (Fig. 5.11).

Ultrasound Appearance of Occult and "Burned-Out" Testicular Tumor. Ultrasonography plays an important role in evaluating patients with clinically occult testicular tumors (58). Sonographically, occult testicular tumors resemble clinically manifest tumors and are visualized as small, well-defined, hypoechoic masses with an occa-

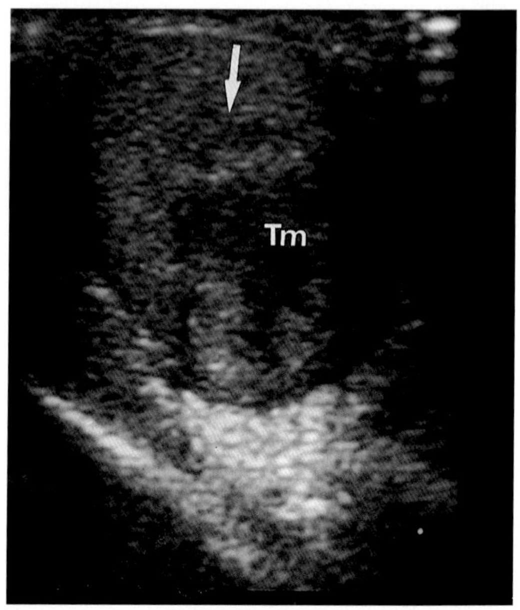

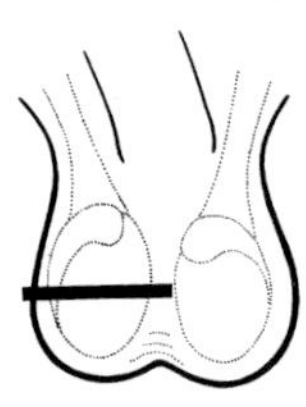

FIG. 5.5. Anaplastic multifocal seminoma in a 25-year-old patient. The large tumor (Tm) is hypoechoic and has a sharp but irregular margin toward the normal parenchyma. Smaller lesion (*arrow*) is seen anteriorly.

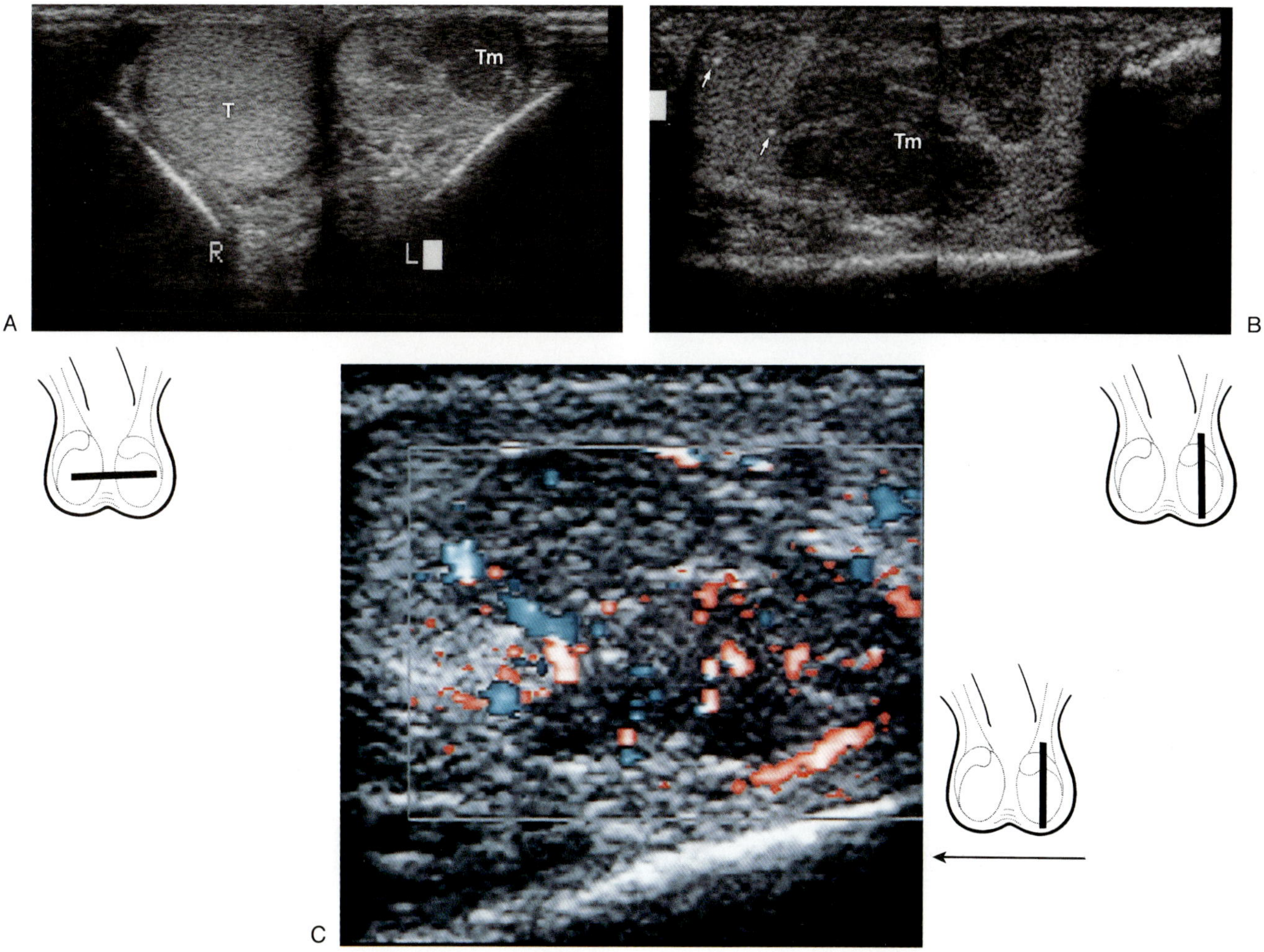

FIG. 5.6. Left testicular seminoma in a 24-year-old patient. **(A)** Transverse and **(B)** longitudinal gray-scale sonogram showing lobulated hypoechoic mass (Tm) in left testis. The tumor is multicentric and additional small foci are seen in the left testis. Also present are tiny echogenic foci (*arrows*) indicating testicular microlithiasis. (T, right testis) **(C)** Longitudinal color-coded-duplex sonogram demonstrating heterogeneous tumor vascularity.

sionally inhomogeneous echotexture. Scrotal ultrasound is used to search for an occult testicular neoplasm in patients (especially those 20 to 40 years of age) presenting with retroperitoneal metastases from an unknown primary. Small (3- to 5-mm) nonpalpable lesions can be detected by ultrasound. Ultrasound is also indicated in cases of suspected extragonadal germ cell tumor or in patients presenting with gynecomastia or other symptoms of endocrinopathy (28,32,59–61).

In **burned-out testicular tumors** a scar is found at the site of the original lesion, frequently appearing as a dense echogenic focus (Fig. 5.12) (58). Larger, homogeneous fibrotic structures may be hypoechoic and suggest a viable tumor (62). Occasionally, there may be some residual tumor tissue as well as histologic evidence of atypical spermatogonia consistent with TIN (63,64).

Ultrasound Appearance of Lymphoid/Hematopoietic Tumors. The sonographic appearance of leukemic infiltration or malignant lymphoma of the testis is nonspecific. The testes are usually enlarged, and areas of tumor invasion appear hypoechoic compared to the normal testicular tissue (Fig. 5.13). Testicular involvement may be either diffuse or focal (47,65–68). Intratesticular manifestations are frequently bilateral. Typical striations of echolucency radiating from a hypoechoic mediastinum testis represent intratesticular lymphatic infiltration and have been described in patients with testicular lymphoma (66). Relapse of lymphoproliferative disease with testicular localization is likely in patients with known systemic disease or in those who have been treated for such disorders previously. The effect of chemotherapy on the testis is limited, and intratesticular

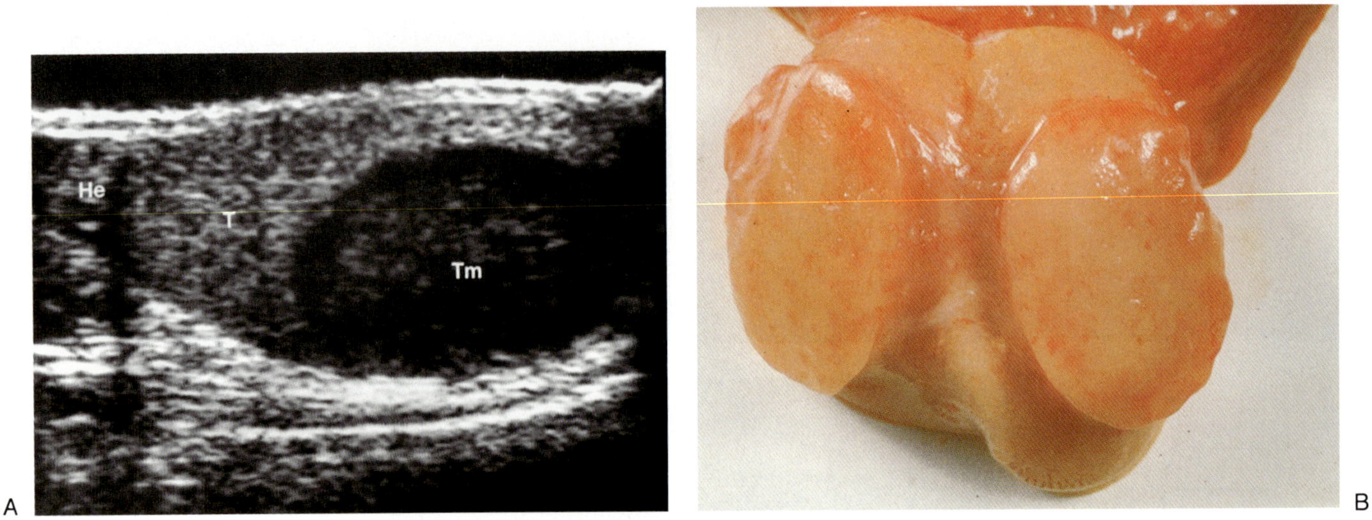

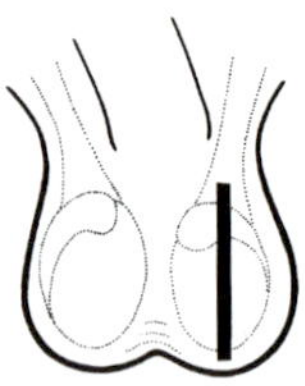

FIG. 5.7. Seminoma in a 32-year-old patient. **(A)** Sonogram showing a smoothly demarcated, hypoechoic testicular tumor (Tm). The testis is enlarged but remains oval in configuration. (He, head of the epididymis; T, normal testis) **(B)** Surgical specimen.

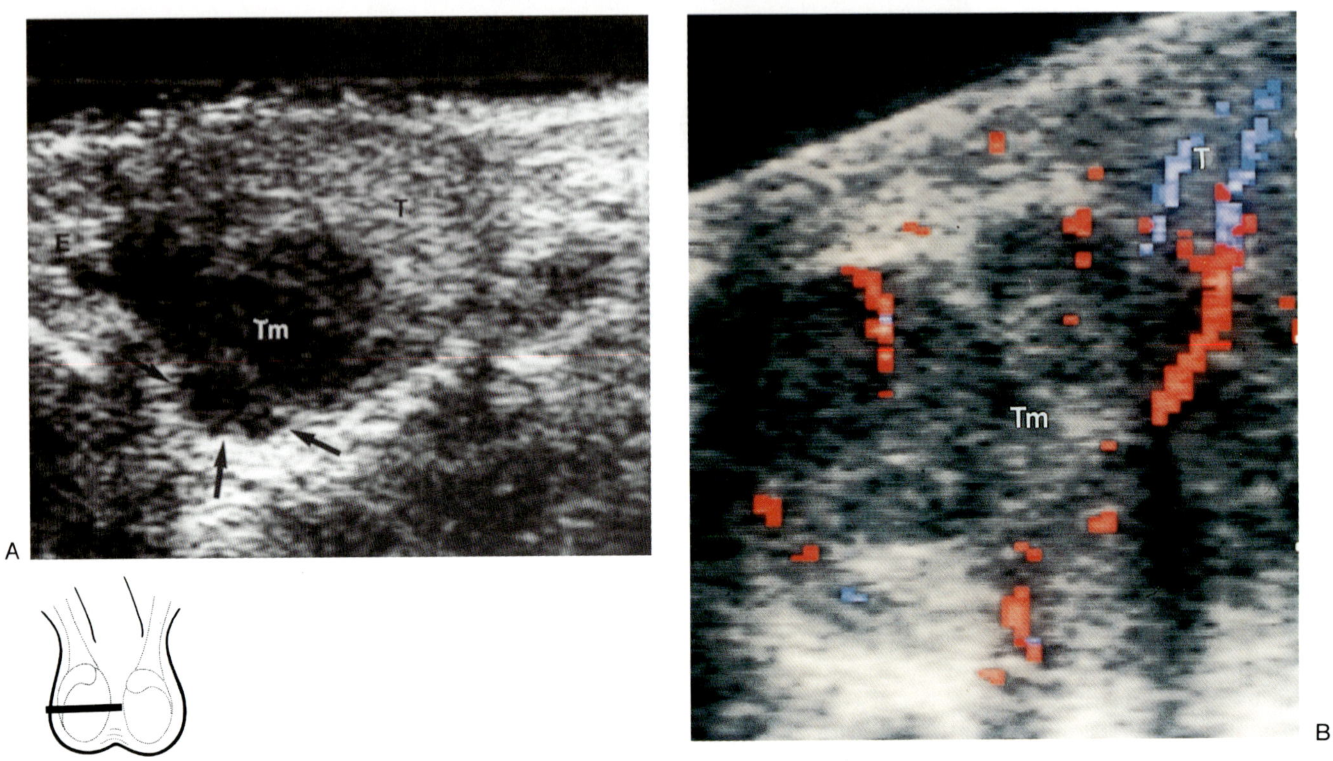

FIG. 5.8. Embryonal cell carcinoma in a 30-year-old patient, stage pT2 N1 M0. **(A)** Transverse scan showing a hypoechoic mass (Tm) extending beyond the tunica albuginea (*arrows*) and invading the epididymis (E). (T, remaining testicular parenchyma) **(B)** Color-coded Doppler demonstrates increased vascularity at the periphery of the tumor.

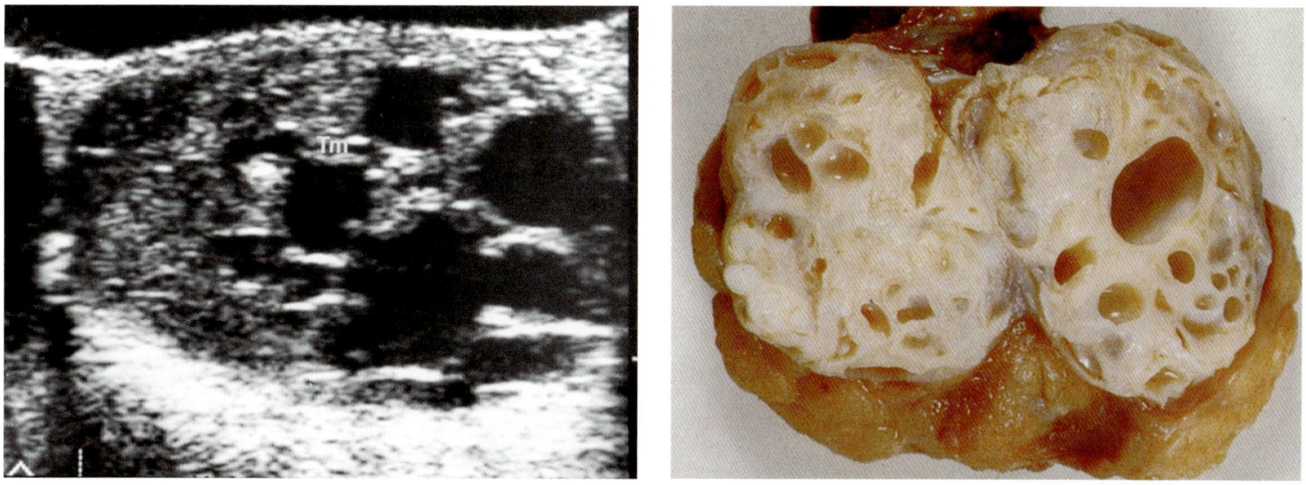

A B

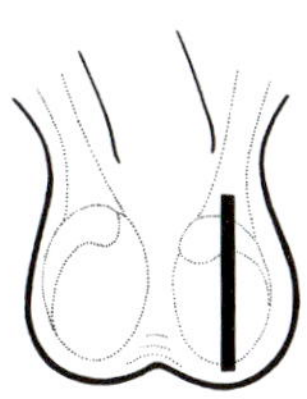

FIG. 5.9. A mature teratoma with cysts and elements of seminoma in a 24-year-old patient. **(A)** Sonogram. The testis is enlarged, and the tumor demonstrates solid (Tm) and cystic features. **(B)** Surgical specimen.

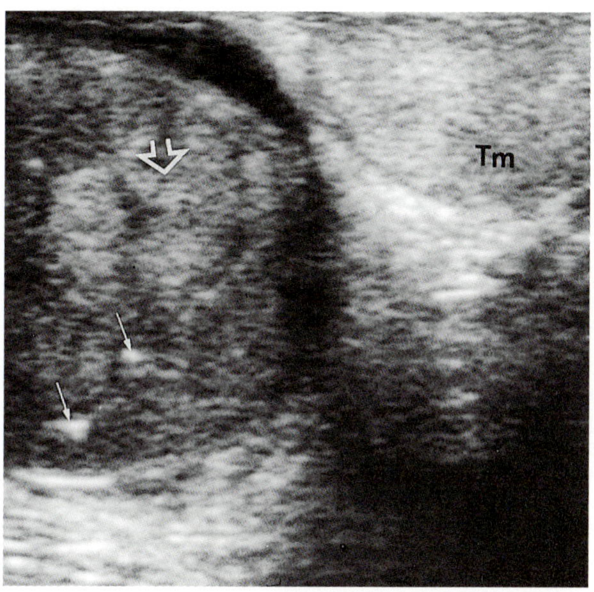

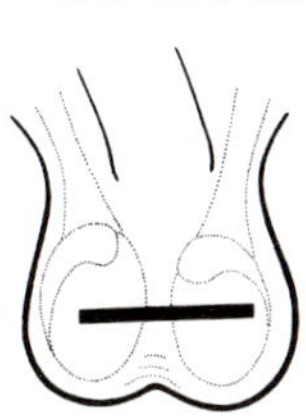

FIG. 5.10. Bilateral seminomas in a 29-year-old patient. The right testis is markedly enlarged. It demonstrates heterogeneous hypo- and hyperechoic (*open arrow*) echotexture. Also seen is testicular microlithiasis (*arrows*). The tumor (Tm) in the left testis is hypoechoic and has irregular shape.

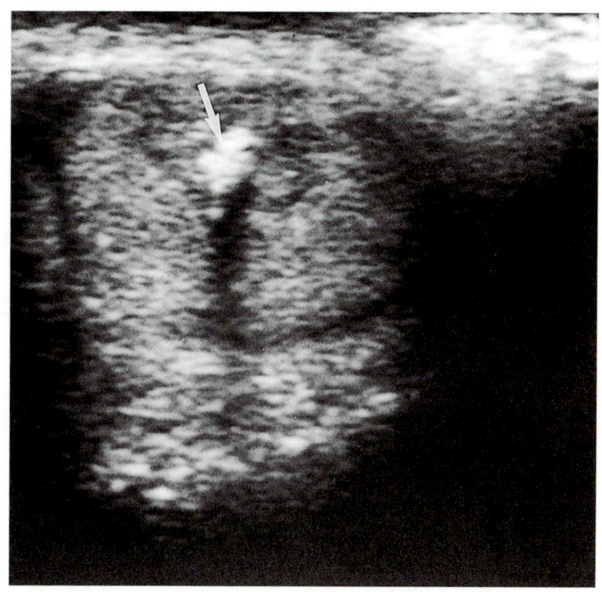

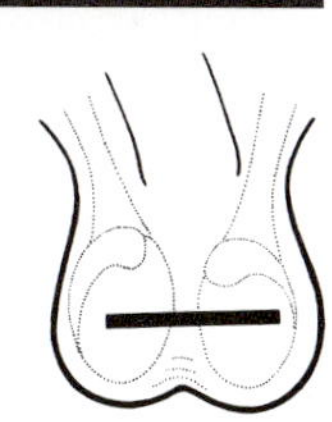

FIG. 5.11. Teratoma in a 26-year-old patient. The tumor is hypoechoic with a central area of calcification (*arrow*).

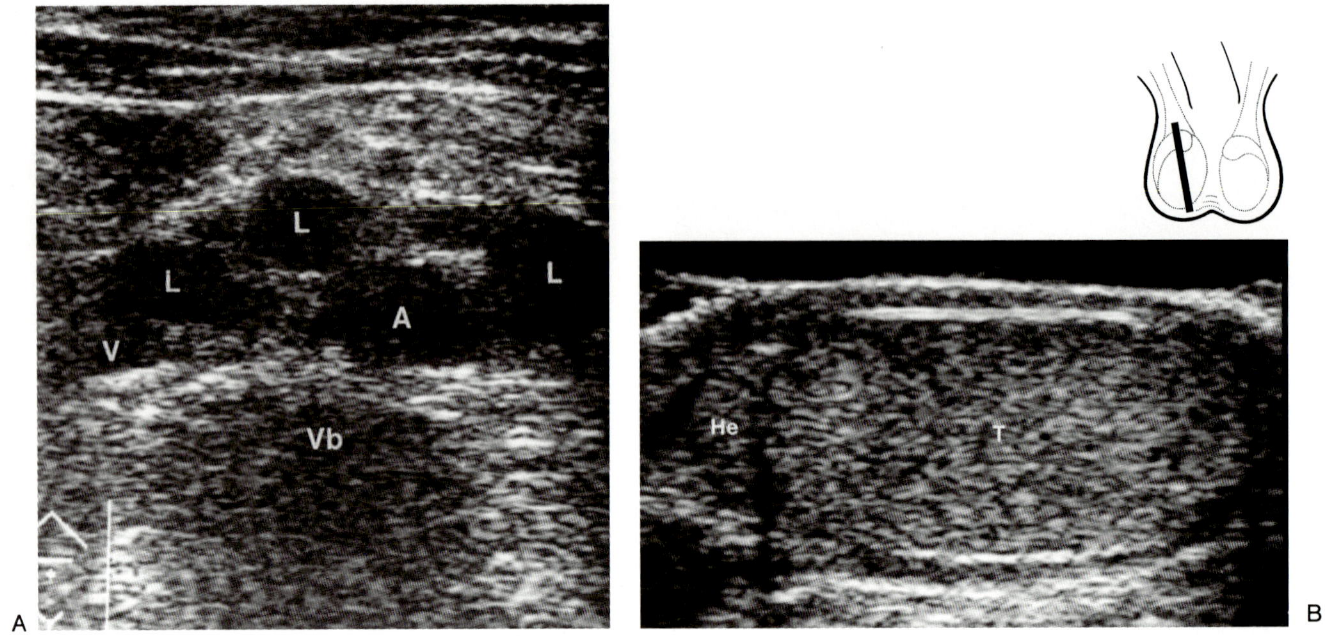

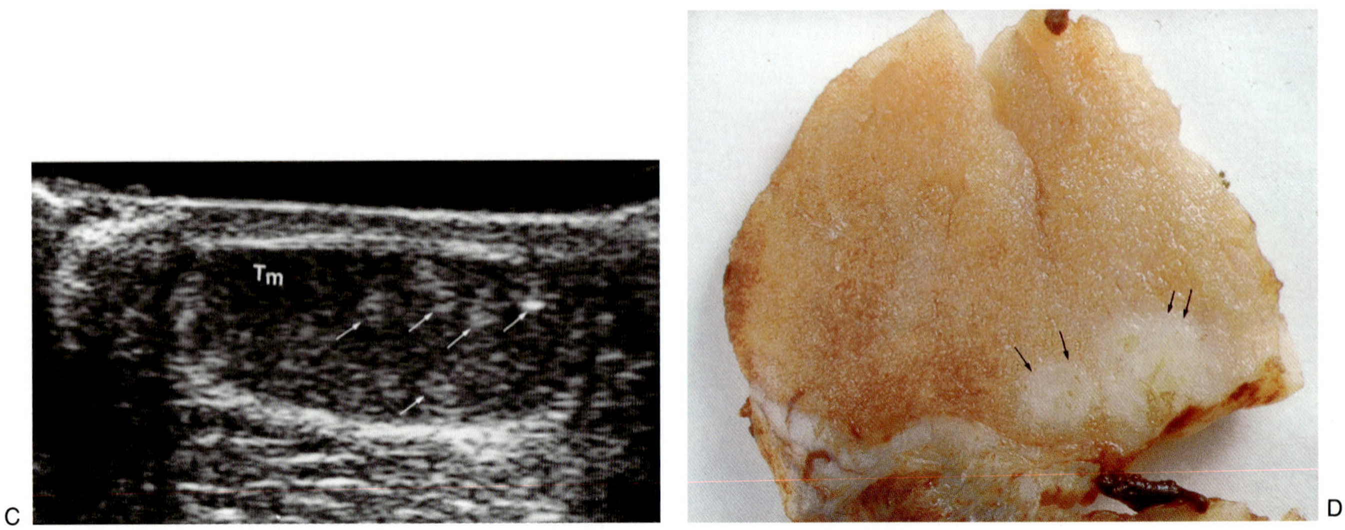

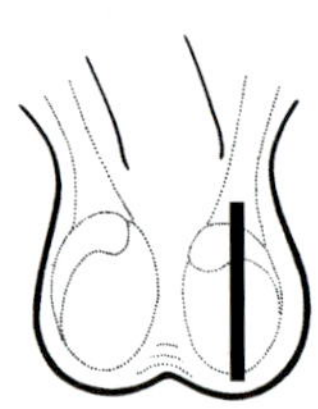

FIG. 5.12. Extensive retroperitoneal lymphadenopathy in a 28-year-old patient with normal palpatory findings in both testes. **(A)** Transverse abdominal sonogram. (A, aorta; V, inferior vena cava; Vb, vertebral body; L, retroperitoneal lymphadenopathy) **(B)** Normal sonographic appearance of the right testis (T). (He, head of the epididymis) **(C)** Small foci of echo-dense alterations (*arrows*) in the left testis that histologically proved to be focal intratesticular scars and isolated seminoma cells consistent with a burned-out testicular tumor. Ill-defined hypoechoic area anteriorly (Tm) corresponds to the largest scar seen on **(D)** surgical specimen (*arrows* demonstrate a scarlike lesion).

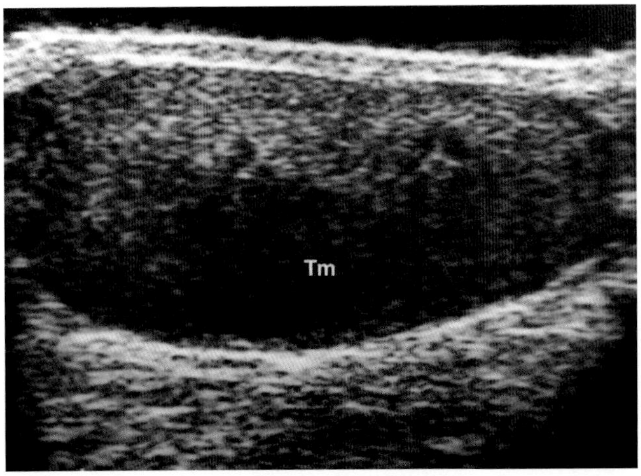

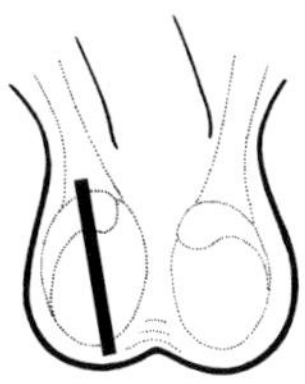

FIG. 5.13. Acute lymphoblastic leukemia in a 35-year-old patient. On clinical examination, the testis felt indurated. Ultrasound scan shows a poorly demarcated, hypoechoic area (Tm) in the testis consistent with the underlying disease.

recurrence can be seen even after complete bone marrow remission (68,69). Ultrasonography can detect these lesions, even when no abnormal findings are present on palpation (69), but the sensitivity of ultrasound is not sufficiently reliable for making therapeutic decisions.

Ultrasound Appearance of Stromal Tumors. Most Leydig cell tumors are sonographically visualized as smoothly demarcated, intratesticular masses with a homogeneous hypoechoic appearance (Fig. 5.14) (61,70). There are no sonographic features to distinguish Leydig cell tumors from malignant germ cell tumors, although the former tend to be smaller and more circumscribed than malignant neoplasms (Fig. 5.14). The tentative diagnosis of a Leydig cell tumor can be made in the presence of gynecomastia (71).

Ultrasound Appearance of Secondary Testicular Tumors. The sonographic characteristics in metastatic disease resemble those of primary testicular cancer (i.e., well-circumscribed hypoechoic masses with variable heterogeneity). The lesions may be multiple and bilateral.

Ultrasound in Differential Diagnosis of Testicular Cancer

Sonographic findings are not specific enough to distinguish benign testicular tumors and tumorlike lesions, such as epidermoid cyst and aberrant adrenal tissue, from primary germ cell tumors (47,57), nor is it possible to identify testicular tumors on the basis of their perfusion characteristics (54). Ultrasound can be useful in differentiating testicular tumors from some forms of orchitis (53,72,73). Sonographically, orchitis (p. 98) (similar to tumor) is characterized by echo-poor, focal, or diffuse intratesticular lesions, but the associated findings of scrotal wall thickening, hydrocele, and enlarged epididymis reinforced the diagnosis of an inflammatory disease. Granulomatous and chronic fibrotic inflammations, however, present as firm masses, often without associated findings and masquerade as tumors. Although color-coded duplex sonography (CCDS) may be helpful in making some distinctions, it cannot provide definitive information for differentiating structural disorders of the testis from testicular tumor or focal orchitis, since both testicular tumors and orchitis may be associated with either increased or decreased blood flow (54). Other etiology that sonographically may mimic testicular tumor is testicular atrophy. Atrophic testis is hypoechoic, and the abnormality can be localized or diffuse (Fig. 5.15). It often can be differentiated from testicular neoplasm by preserved vascular anatomy, by demonstration of normal mediastinum testis, and on the basis of clinical findings. Size of the testis is not always a helpful finding of differentiation; as in localized atrophy the testis size may be normal. Furthermore, cancer can coexist in small testis. The sonographic characteristics of intratesticular hematoma (p. 119) or abscess (p. 98) may also resemble those of tumor with a very low echogenicity. The correct

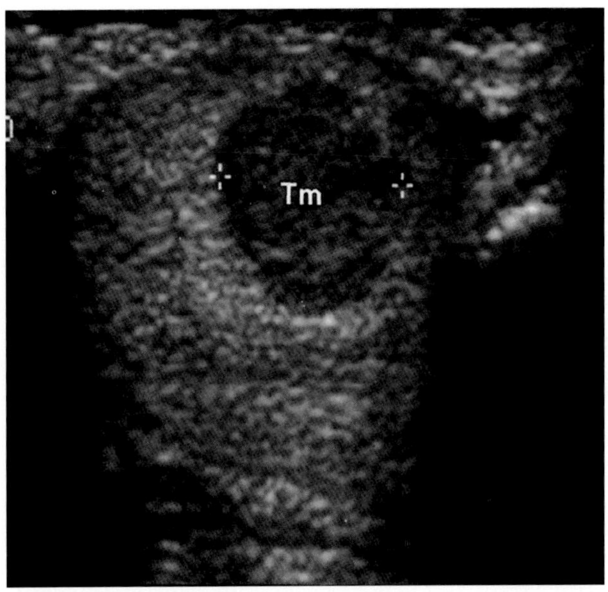

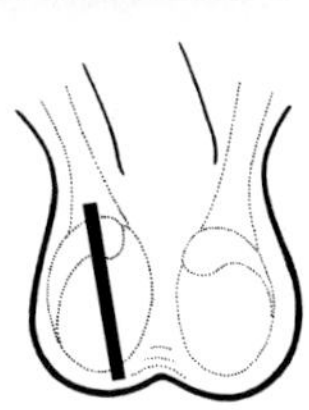

FIG. 5.14. Leydig cell tumor in a 32-year-old patient. The tumor (Tm) is hypoechoic and sharply marginated. Sonographically, it cannot be differentiated from a malignant neoplasm.

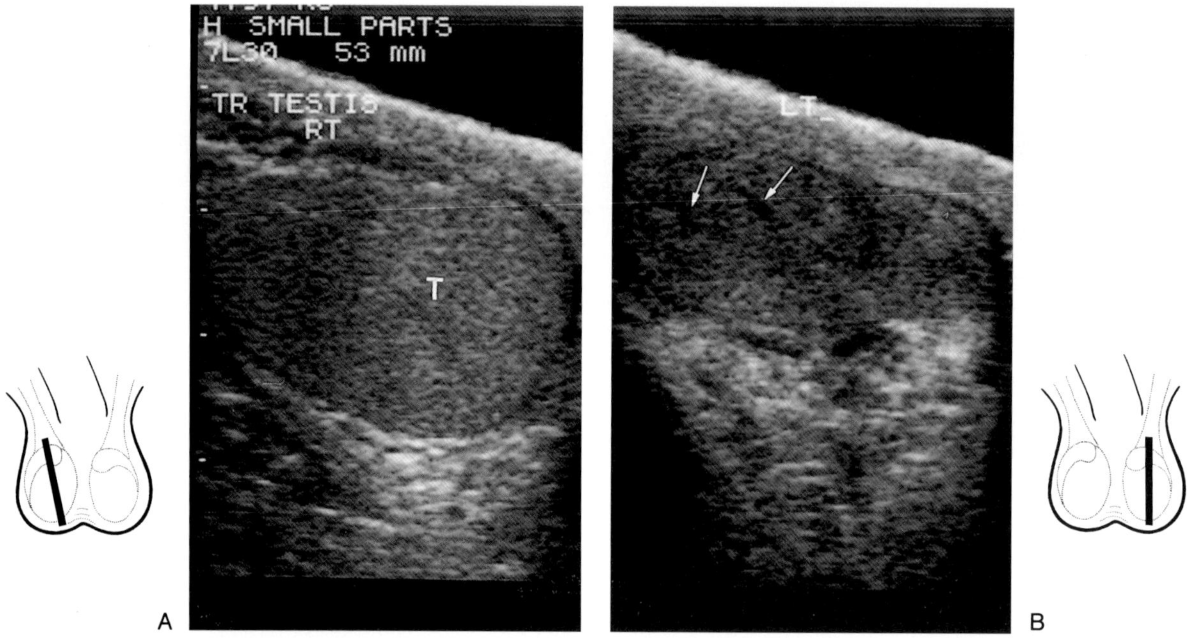

FIG. 5.15. Testicular atrophy. **A)** The right testis (T) is normal. **B)** The left testis is small, with heterogeneous but predominantly hypoechoic echotexture. Undisplaced vessels (*arrows*) are a helpful finding that this does not represent testicular tumor.

diagnosis is suggested by history and clinical data, but the patient should be followed closely to assure resolution (see Chapter 6, Scrotal Trauma). Other conditions to be considered in the differential diagnosis of testicular tumor are testicular infarction (p. 125), small testicular cyst (Fig. 5.16), and epidermoid cyst. In addition, it is important to differentiate small, firm fibrotic plaques of the tunica albuginea from a subcapsular tumor. A regressed or burned-out tumor should be considered if a small, echo-dense scar in the testis is seen on ultrasonography. Evaluation of the retroperitoneal lymph nodes is mandatory in such cases.

Magnetic Resonance Imaging in Evaluation of Testicular Cancer

Although MRI has a high sensitivity rate for detection of primary testicular tumors, findings are variable and rarely specific for tumor type (70). Most commonly, testicular tumors demonstrate a signal intensity similar to the normal testis on T1-weighted images. On T2-weighted images they are mostly hypointense to the normal testis and may be either homogeneous or heterogeneous signal intensity (Figs. 5.17 and. 5.18). Occasionally, they demonstrate a signal intensity similar to the normal testis on T2-weighted images (70) (Fig. 5.19). On gadolinium chelates contrast-enhanced T1-weighted MR images when dynamic scans are used, the tumor enhancement is seen earlier than the adjacent normal testicular tissue. Tumor enhancement is often greater than normal testicular tissue (Fig. 5.20) (74). In general, noncontrast T1- and T2-weighted images are essential for tumor detection (70). Contrast-enhanced T1-weighted images should be obtained if lesion detection or characterization needs reinforcement (70). It has been suggested that signal intensity and degree of heterogeneity

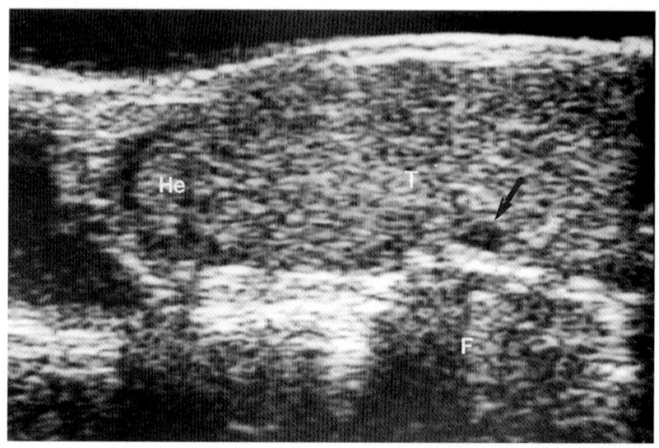

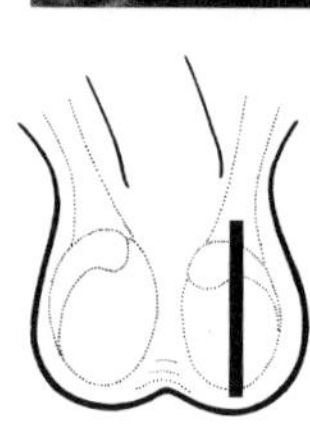

FIG. 5.16. A small (3 mm in diameter) testicular cyst in a 42-year-old patient. Although there is smooth demarcation of the lesion (*arrow*) without distortion of adjacent testicular parenchyma (T), there are questionable internal echoes, making it difficult to differentiate a simple cyst from a small cancer. Indentation of the testis was made by the palpating finger (F). (He, head of the epididymis)

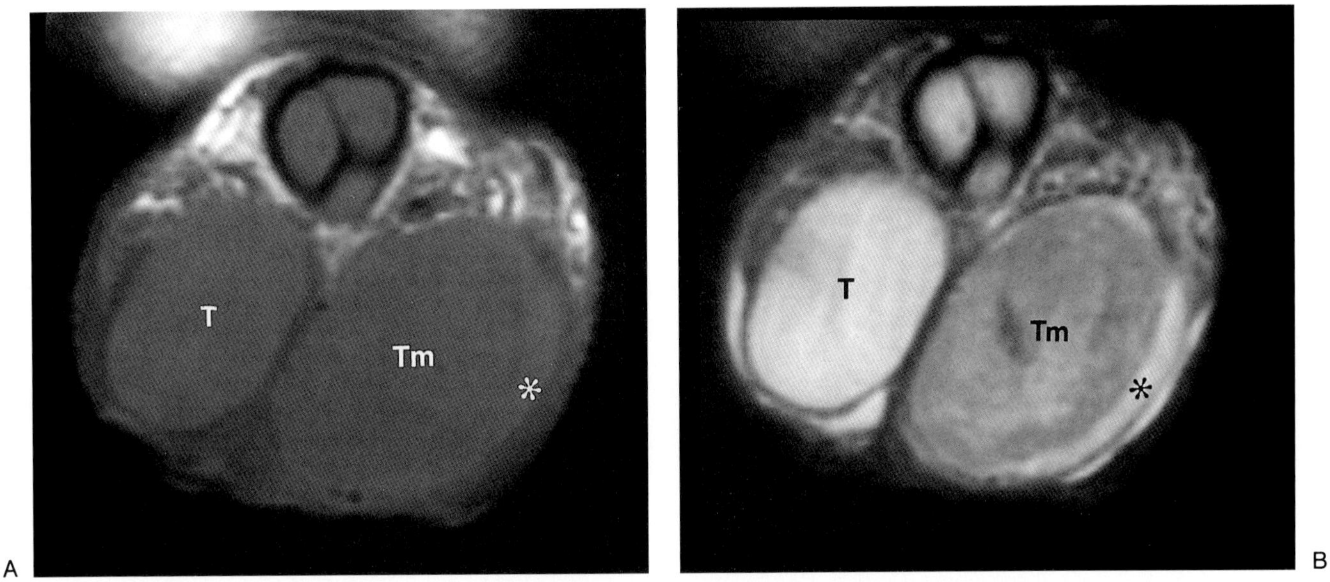

FIG. 5.17. Left testicular seminoma. **(A)** Coronal T1- and **(B)** T2-weighted images. The left testis is enlarged and almost completely replaced with tumor (Tm). On the T1-weighted image, the tumor is hypointense as compared with the normal right testis (T) or the remaining left testicular tissue (*). The tumor (Tm) is hypointense as compared with the normal testis on the T2-weighted image.

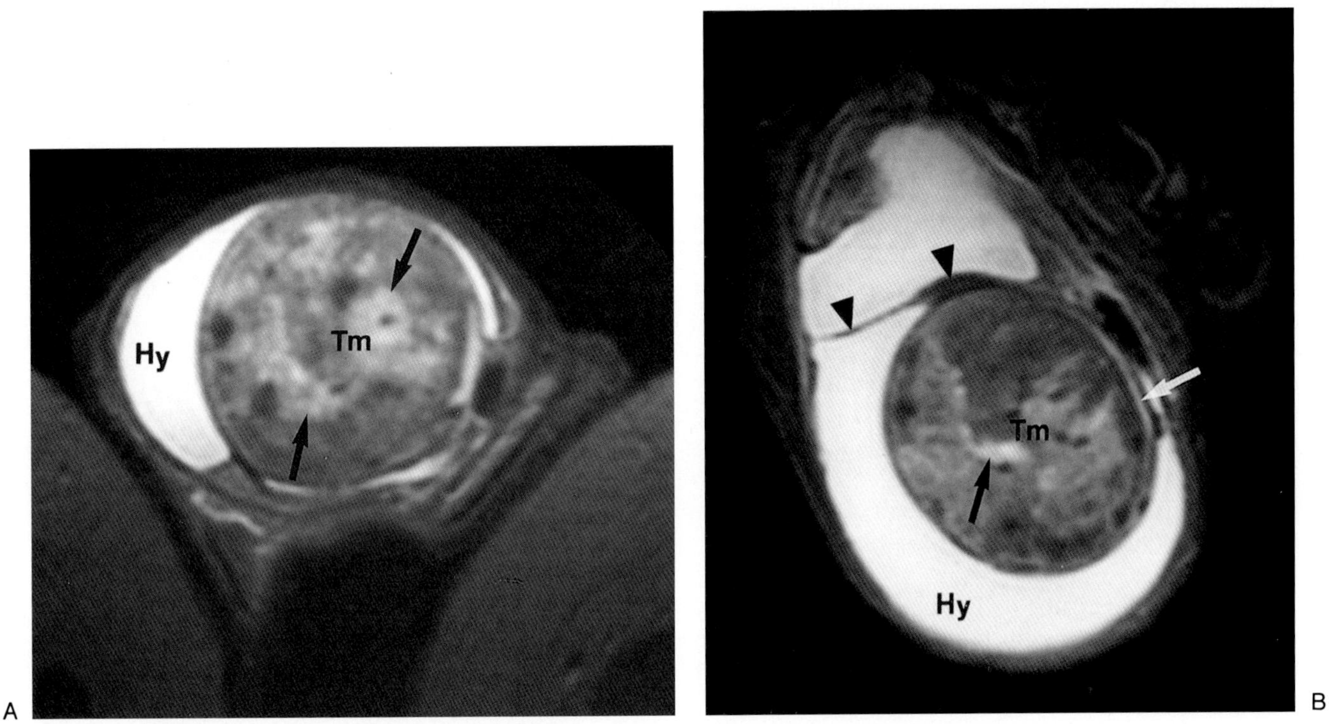

FIG. 5.18. Left testicular seminoma. **(A)** Transaxial and **(B)** coronal T2-weighted images. A large, heterogeneous-signal-intensity testicular tumor (Tm) replaces almost all the testicular tissue. A hydrocele (Hy) with intervening fibrous septum (*arrowheads*) is also seen (*white arrow*, a thin rim of the remaining testicular tissue).

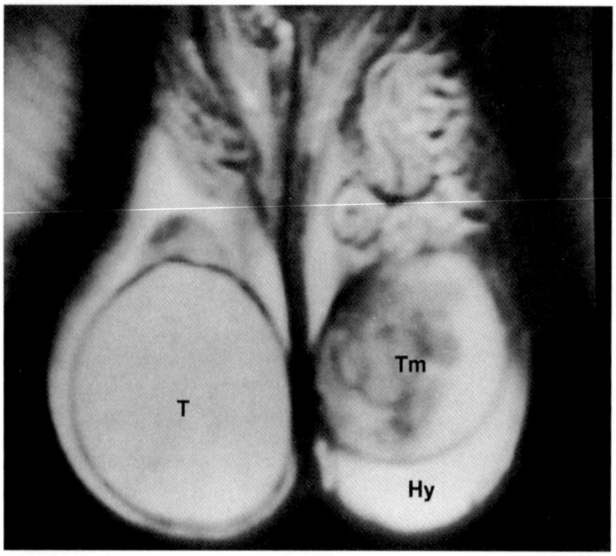

FIG. 5.19. Embryonal cell carcinoma. Coronal T2-weighted image. The tumor (Tm) demonstrates heterogeneous signal intensity that is only slightly lower than that of the adjacent testis. Tumor has a lobulated appearance. (Hy, hydrocele; T, normal right testis)

may correlate with specific tumor histology (75). **Seminomas** are typically isointense with the normal testis on T1-weighted images, and homogeneous and hypointense on T2-weighted images (Fig. 5.17). On the other hand, **nonseminomatous tumors** are often heterogeneous and demonstrate higher signal intensity (isointense or slightly hyperintense to normal testis) on T2-weighted images (Fig. 5.19). A dark outer margin sometimes detected on T2-weighted images correlates with a fibrous tumor capsule on histologic examination. Marked heterogeneity of signal intensity in NSGCT is thought to be due to hemorrhage (especially in embryonal cell carcinomas (76)), fibrosis, or calcification (77). Exceptions to these characteristic findings are not uncommon. Seminomas sometimes demonstrate medium to high signal intensity on T1-weighted images and heterogeneous high signal intensity on T2-weighted images (Fig. 5.18). On histologic examination the areas of high signal intensity were shown to be hemorrhages within a pure seminoma (78).

Stromal tumors, such as Leydig and Sertoli cell tumors, are well circumscribed and resemble seminomas in signal intensity (homogeneous and isointense on T1-weighted images and markedly hypointense on T2-weighted images). When these tumors are malignant (10% of cases), they may have hemorrhage and necrosis, in which case they mimic the MR appearance of nonseminomatous tumors (75). In general, the MR appearance of benign tumors is similar to that of testicular cancer, preventing distinction between them (78).

Signal intensity of **secondary testicular tumors** is similar to that of primary tumors, most commonly low signal intensity on T2-weighted images. **Lymphomas** and **leukemias** are usually diffuse and infiltrative (Fig. 5.21).

Magnetic Resonance Imaging in Differential Diagnosis

In the evaluation of an intratesticular mass, MR imaging is a problem-solving modality when US findings are inconclusive. It has higher specificity than US in

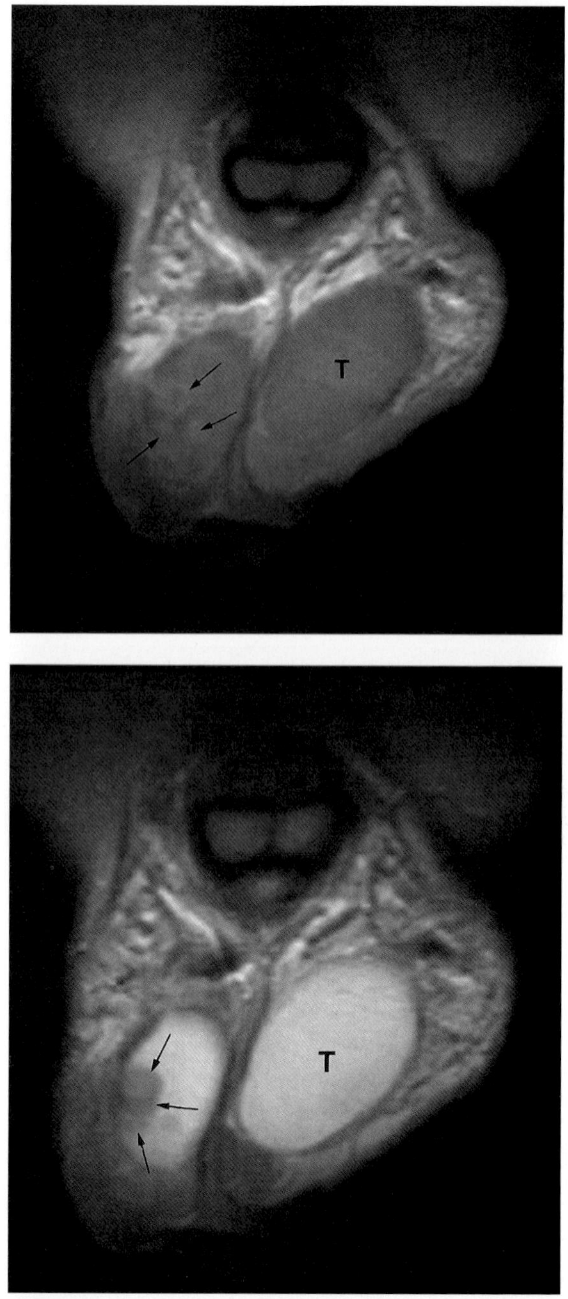

FIG. 5.20. Seminoma. Coronal plane **(A)** T2-weighted image, **(B)** Gd-DTPA enhanced T1-weighted image. A tumor (*arrows*) is present in the small, atrophic right testis. It demonstrates low signal intensity on T2-weighted images and shows greater enhancement than adjacent testicular tissue on postcontrast scans. Normal left testis (T).

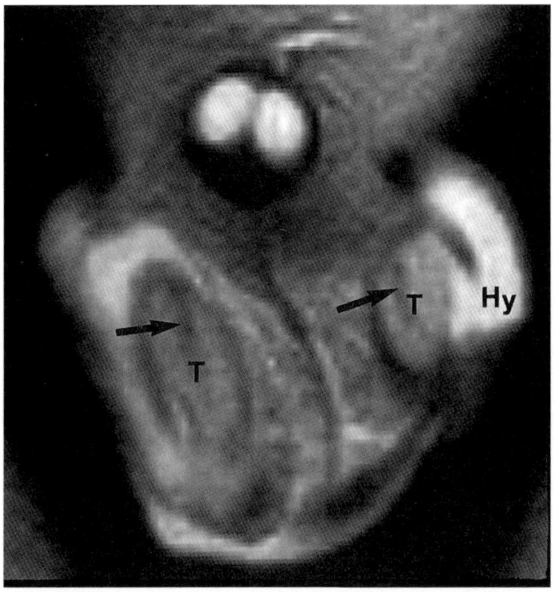

FIG. 5.21. Lymphocytic leukemia involving both testes. Coronal T2-weighted image shows hypointense testes (T) due to diffuse leukemic infiltration. (Hy, hydrocele; *arrows*, mediastinum testis)

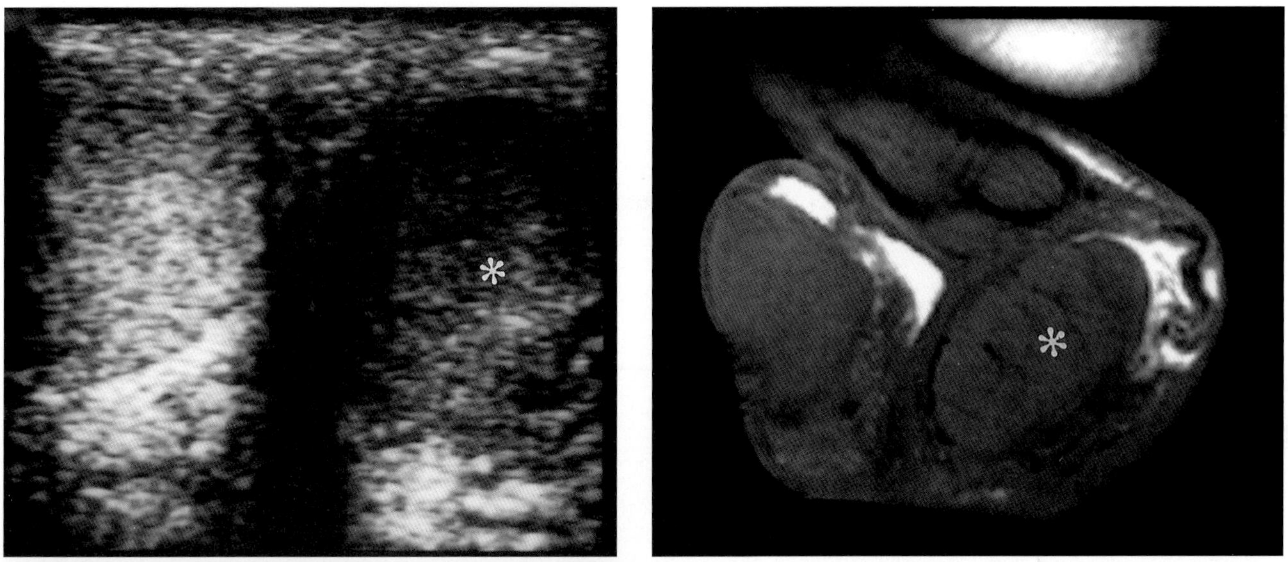

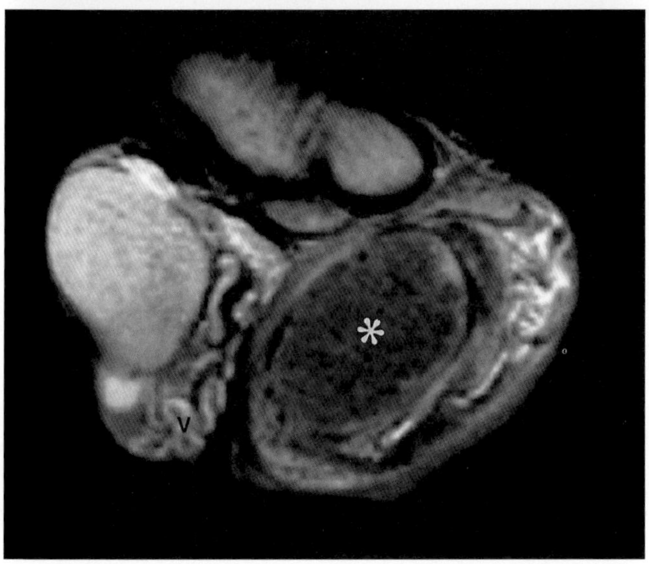

FIG. 5.22. Granulomatous orchitis (*) misdiagnosed as tumor on both **(A)** US and MRI, **(B)** T1-weighted and **(C)** T2-weighted images. The abnormal area (*) demonstrates homogeneous hypoechoic echotexture on sonogram and low signal intensity indistinguishable from cancer on T2-weighted MR image. Varicocele (v) on the right.

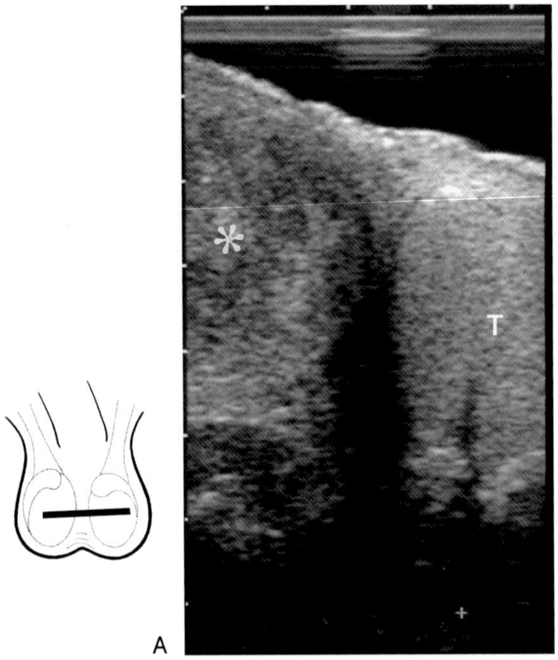

A

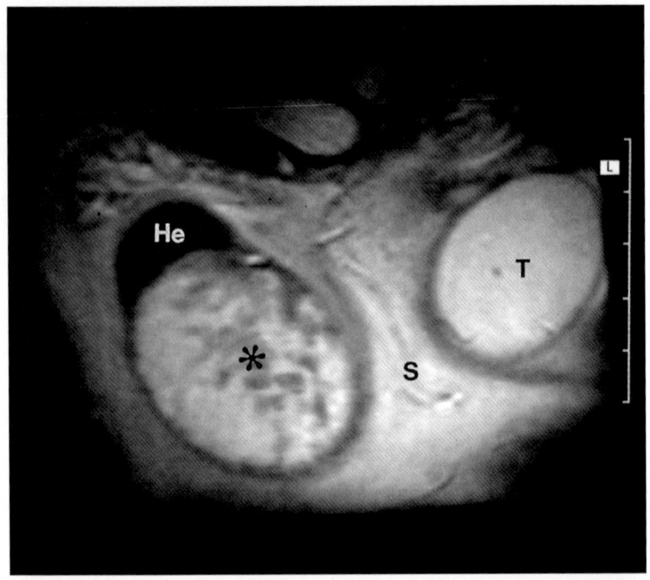

B

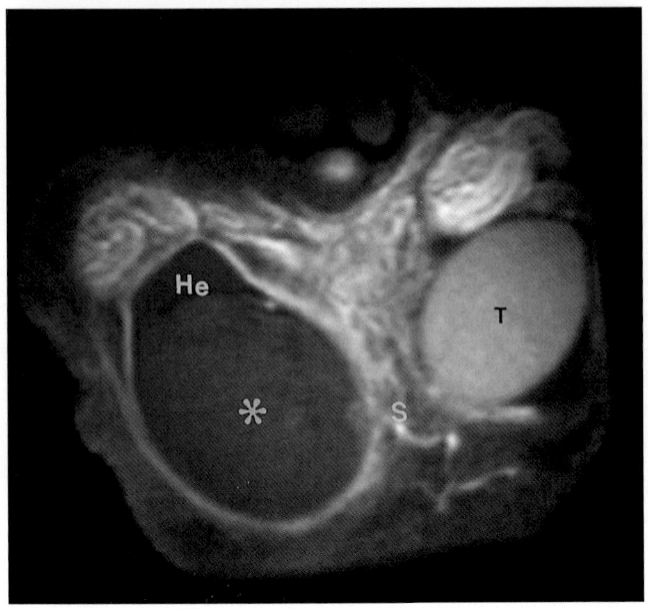

C

FIG. 5.23. Chronic testicular torsion (>48 hours) in a 42-year-old patient. **(A)** Ultrasound and coronal MRI, **(B)** T2-weighted image, and **(C)** contrast-enhanced T1-weighted image. On sonogram, the right testis is enlarged, heterogeneous, and predominantly hypoechoic. On the T2-weighted image, the right testis demonstrates low-signal-intensity foci, but no mass lesion is seen. Contrast-enhanced study shows lack of enhancement and reinforces the diagnosis of extensive testicular infarction. (T, normal left testis; He, hematocele; S, edematous scrotal septum)

differentiating orchitis from testicular tumor (78,79). In addition to the indirect findings also used by US (e.g., thickening of the scrotal skin, enlarged epididymis, and hydrocele), orchitis usually demonstrates high signal intensity on T2-weighted images; but homogeneous or heterogeneous hypointensity on T_2-weighted images can be seen as well. (Tumors most commonly demonstrate low signal intensity.) Granulomatous orchitis, however, represents a problem on MRI as well (Fig. 5.22). MRI can also be helpful in the diagnosis of testicular infarcts, especially when contrast-enhanced studies are used (Fig. 5.23). Infarcts will demonstrate lack of enhancement, whereas tumor enhancement is similar or higher than normal testis. Similarly, in the diagnosis of hematoma (Fig. 5.24) and other intratesticular pathology, such as testicular cysts, better tissue contrast of MRI justifies its use as a problem-solving approach.

Computed Tomography in Evaluation of Testicular Cancer

Although CT examination is not presently used for evaluation of primary testicular cancer (it is usually used for staging and follow-up), certain histologic types of testicular cancers show typical CT findings (80). **Seminomas** tend to show a homogeneous high attenuation value (Fig. 5.25). **Teratomas** are usually inhomogeneous and

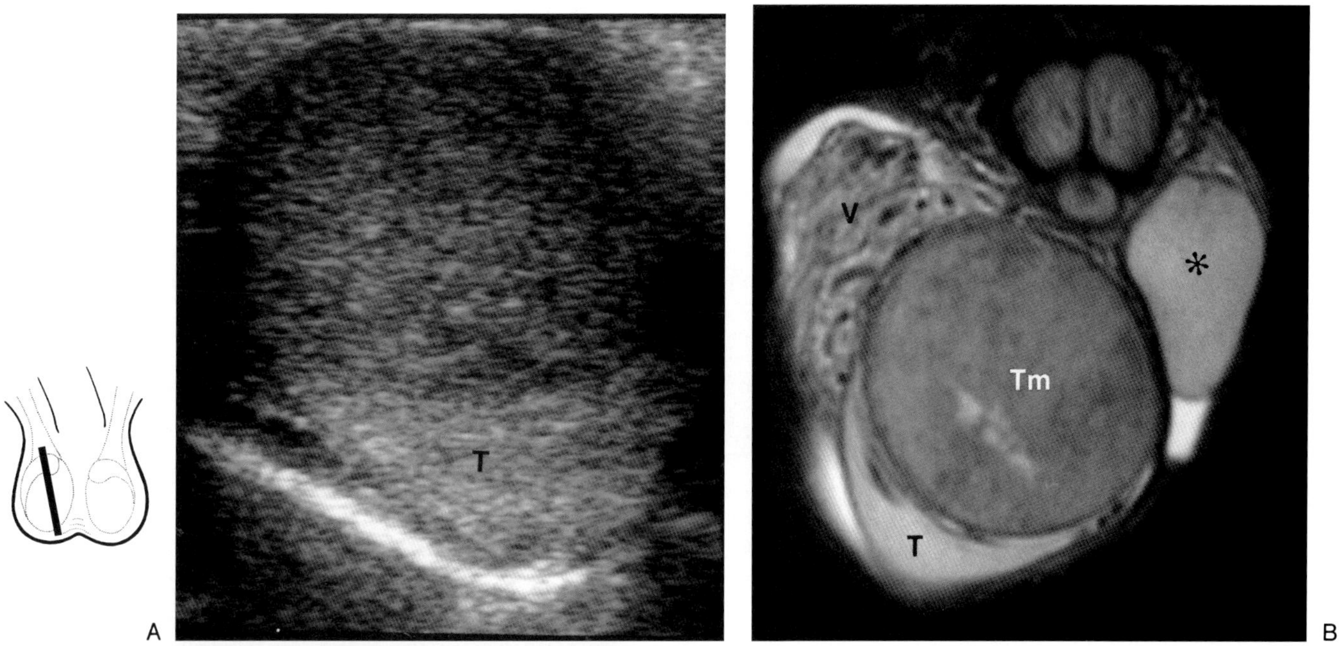

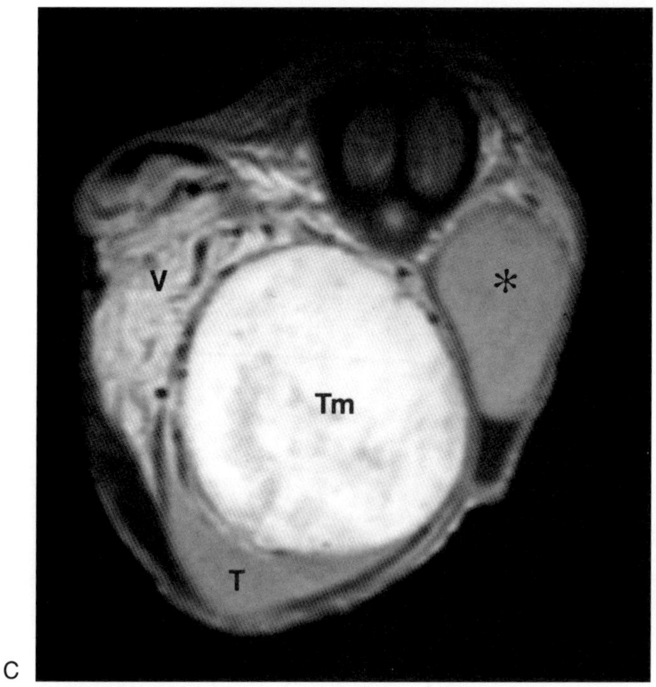

FIG. 5.24. Seminoma in a 15-year-old boy seen 2 weeks after trauma. **(A)** Sonogram, **(B)** T2-weighted MR image, **(C)** contrast-enhanced T1-weighted image. Anterior to the right testis (T) is a large mass misdiagnosed as hematoma on US. The mass (Tm) demonstrates low signal intensity on T2-weighted image and marked enhancement on postcontrast study, findings that unequivocally indicate tumor on MRI study. (v, varicoceles; *, left testis)

typically contain low-density areas (Fig. 5.26). The presence of fat leads to a diagnosis of **lipoma** or **liposarcoma** (Fig. 5.27). Unfortunately, none of these findings is specific for testicular tumors.

Computed Tomography in Differential Diagnosis

Computed tomography is not recommended for the detection or characterization of testicular lesions. Although a finding of fatty tissue or intratesticular calcifications assist in specific diagnosis of testicular tumors, diffuse infiltrative diseases, such as granulomatous orchitis (Fig. 5.28), may demonstrate similar CT findings.

Staging, Treatment, and Follow-up of Testicular Cancer

Staging

Correct clinical staging is critical for optimal therapeutic choices. Unfortunately, understaging is quite common. Approximately 15% of stage IIA testicular cancers are understaged clinically as stage I disease (11,81). A va-

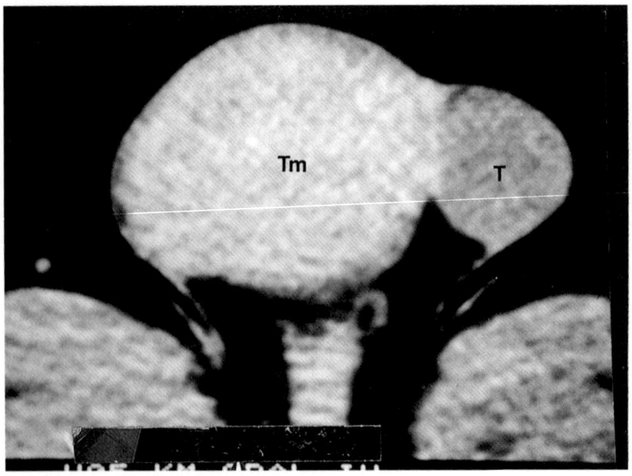

FIG. 5.25. Seminoma of the right testis (Tm). Compared with the normal left testis (T), the right testis is markedly enlarged and shows homogeneous enhancement. (Photo courtesy of H. Derouet, Universität Homburg/Saar.)

riety of systems has been proposed for staging testicular tumors, although none has gained widespread acceptance. Most are modifications of the original staging system proposed by Boden and Gibb (Fig. 5.29). One of the most commonly used clinical staging systems is summarized in Table 5.3 (6,11). The TNM system (Table 5.4), proposed by the American Joint Committee on Staging and End Results Reporting, is a pathologic staging system similar to that used for staging tumors in other parts of the body (81). In evaluating patients with testicular

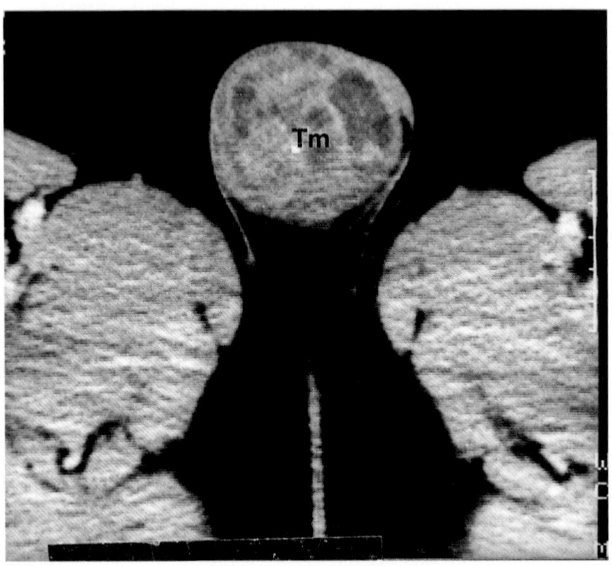

FIG. 5.26. Teratoma of the right testis. The scrotum is enlarged. The testicular tissue is replaced with a heterogeneous mass that contains multiple foci of low density. (From Derouet H, Braedel HU, Ziegler M, Zwergel TH, Khorsandian CH: Computertomographische Untersuchungen des Skrotalinhaltes, insbesondere des Hodens. *Fortschr Röntgenstr* 1988;148:566–571.)

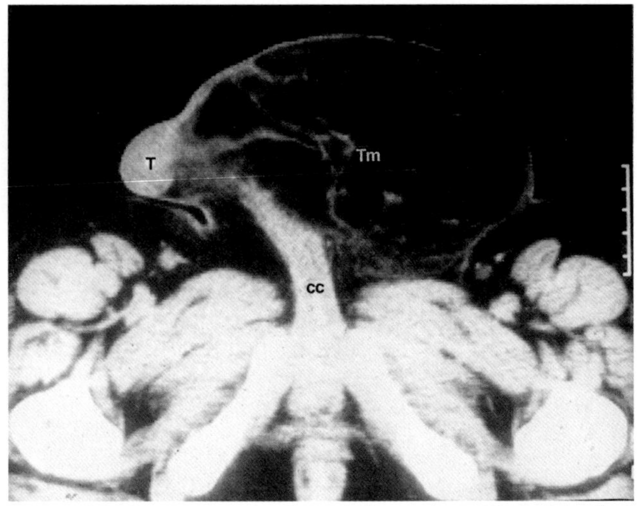

FIG. 5.27. Liposarcoma of the left scrotum (Tm). A typical fatty mass enlarging the left scrotum and invading the scrotal skin and the corpora cavernosa (cc). Normal right testis (T). (From Derouet VH, Braedel HU, Ziegler M, Zwergel TH, Khorsandian CH: Computertomographische Untersuchungen des Skrotalinhaltes, insbesondere des Hodens. *Fortschr Röntgenstr* 1988;148:566–571.)

tumors, staging of the primary tumor (T-stage; Fig. 5.30) is of minor importance because all suspected testicular tumors are evaluated surgically. Preoperative T-staging of testicular tumors, however, is relevant only if there is involvement of the scrotal skin or if there is tumor extension high into the spermatic cord and inguinal canal. Involvement of the scrotal skin necessitates hemiscrotectomy, and tumor extension in the inguinal canal requires an extended surgical approach. The TNM classification has not gained wide acceptance among clinicians. There

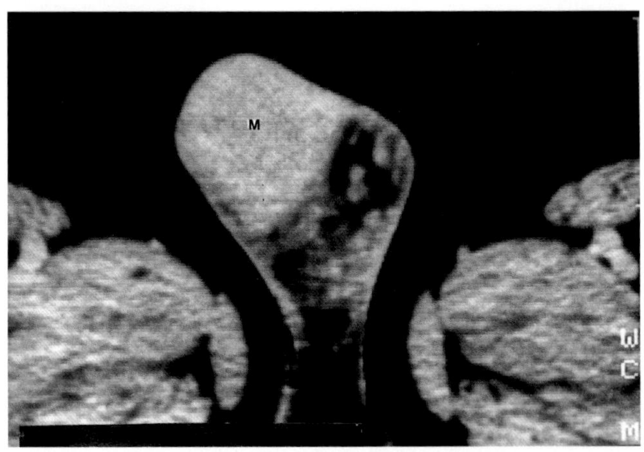

FIG. 5.28. Granulomatous orchitis of the right testis. An inflammatory mass (M) shows homogeneous enhancement, resembling the CT appearance of seminoma. (From Derouet H, Braedel HU, Ziegler M, Zwergel TH, Khorsandian CH. Computertomographische Untersuchungen des Skrotalinhaltes, insbesondere des Hodens. *Fortschr Röntgenstr* 1988;148:566–571.)

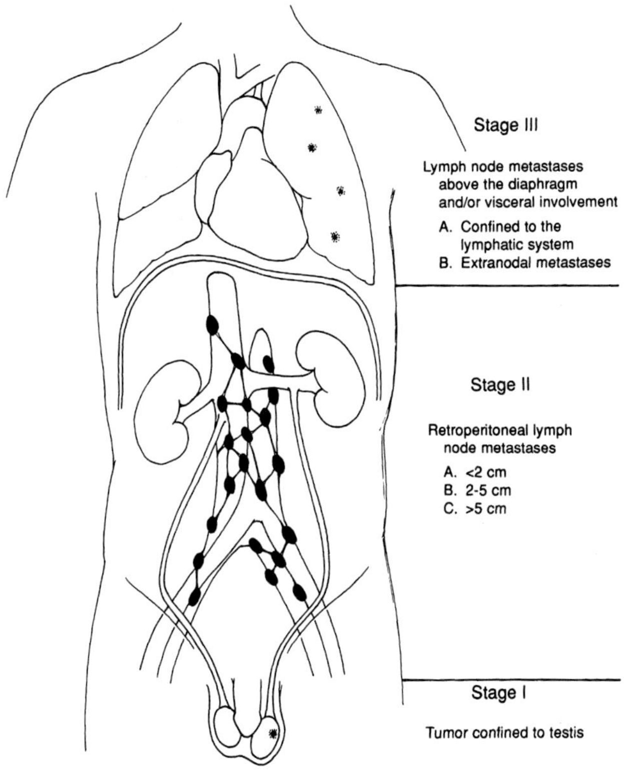

FIG. 5.29. Clinical staging of testicular tumors. (Staging system of Royal Marsden Hospital.)

is no grading system for classifying germ cell tumors according to the degree of morphologic differentiation of the tumor cells.

The **metastatic potential** of a testicular tumor is primarily determined by its histologic type, the local extent of the primary tumor, and the presence or absence of lymphatic and blood vessel invasion (82,83). Metastases are present at the time of diagnosis in 20% to 25% of pure seminomas, and in more than 40% of nonseminomatous tumors (11). With the exception of choriocarcinoma, which shows early hematogenous spread, most germ cell tumors spread via the lymphatics. Lymphatic drainage from the testis usually follows its vascular supply and is directed toward primary drainage sites, "sentential nodes" of the para-aortic chain (Fig. 5.31) (6,11,84,85). Lymphatic spread is generally orderly, with the right testis draining mainly to the aortocaval region below the level of the right renal hilum (Fig. 5.31), and subsequently to the precaval, preaortic, paracaval, right common iliac, and right external iliac lymph nodes. The primary drainage site of the left testis is the left para-aortic area (Fig. 5.31), just below the level of left renal vein. Spread then extends to the preaortic, left common iliac, and left external iliac lymph nodes. Occasionally, the testes drain to the regional nodes of the internal, external, and common iliac nodes along the epididymal and cremasteric arteries. Testicular cancer may also spread to the cisterna chyli, thoracic duct, and supraclavicular lymph nodes (usually on the left side). Midline crossover of metastatic tumors occurs in 15% to 20% of cases (more commonly from right to left) (6,11,86). In most cases metastases first occur in the ipsilateral lymph node regions. When no ipsilateral metastatic lesion is found, the incidence of contralateral involvement is very low (86).

Tumor invasion of the epididymis or spermatic cord may cause lymph node enlargement in distal external iliac and obturator chains. The inguinal nodes are not considered regional nodes of the testis, but tumor invasion of these nodes can occur in patients with extensive involvement of the scrotum (Fig. 5.31), with massive retroperitoneal disease, or with prior scrotal or inguinal surgery (87). The inguinal nodes can also be involved by

TABLE 5.3. *Clinical staging of testicular tumors (proposed by the Royal Marsden Hospital)*

Stage I (or A)	Tumor confined to the testis
Stage II (or B)	Tumor metastatic to the lymph nodes below the diaphragm
IIA (B1)	Retroperitoneal lymph node enlargement less than 2 cm (5 cm[a])
IIB (B2)	Retroperitoneal lymph node enlargement greater than 2 cm (5 cm[a]), but less than 5 cm (10 cm[a])
IIC (B3)	Retroperitoneal lymph node enlargement greater than 5 cm (10 cm[a])
Stage III (C)	Tumor metastatic to lymph nodes above the diaphragm or viscera
IIIA	Confined to the lymphatic system
IIIB (IV)	Extranodal metastases

[a] Memorial Sloan-Kettering Cancer Center.

TABLE 5.4. *TNM staging**

T: Primary tumor
- TX: Primary tumor cannot be assessed
- T0: No evidence of primary tumor
- T1: Tumor limited to testis, including rete testis
- T2: Tumor invades beyond tunica albuginea or into epididymis
- T3: Tumor invades spermatic cord
- T4: Tumor invades scrotum

N: Regional lymph nodes
- NX: Regional lymph nodes cannot be assessed
- N0: No regional lymph node metastasis
- N1: Metastasis in a single lymph node, 2 cm or less in greatest dimension
- N2: Metastasis in a single lymph node, more than 2 cm but not more than 5 cm in greatest dimension, or multiple lymph nodes, none more than 5 cm in greatest dimension
- N3: Metastasis in a lymph node, more than 5 cm in greatest dimension

M: Distant metastasis
- MX: Distant metastasis cannot be assessed
- M0: No distant metastasis
- M1: Distant metastasis present

* AJC: American Joint Committee on Staging and End Results Reporting (1986).

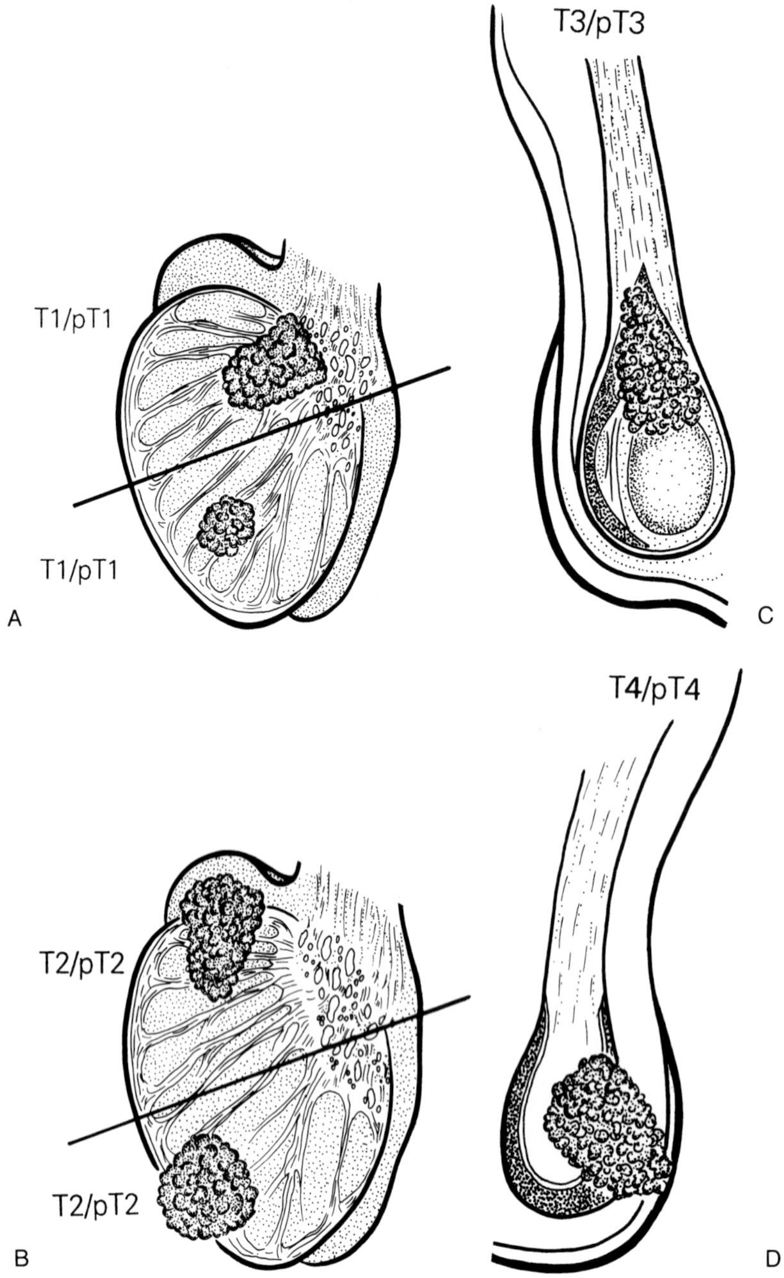

FIG. 5.30. T-stages of testicular tumors (UICC, 1987). **(A)** Stage T1 tumor confined to the testis or infiltration of the rete testis. **(B)** Stage T2 tumor infiltration of the tunica albuginea or epididymis. **(C)** Stage T3 tumor infiltration of the spermatic cord. **(D)** Stage T4 tumor infiltration of the scrotal wall.

retrograde spread from the iliac nodes. In extensive retroperitoneal disease, the iliac and inguinal nodes may be involved in a retrograde fashion and/or the suprahilar retrocrural nodes may be affected, eventually involving the posterior mediastinum. When metastatic disease is extensive, unusual patterns of tumor drainage (such as involvement of the mesenteric nodes by retrograde filling due to lymphatic obstruction) or hematogenous metastases to the viscera can occur. At this stage, most patients have also developed hematogenous organ metastases.

Primary hematogenous metastases occur in about 10% of cases. They are often seen in patients with choriocarcinoma or in more advanced stages of other types of tumor. It is unclear whether elements of choriocarcinoma in a mixed tumor result in a significantly poorer prognosis (88). The lung, liver, brain, kidney, gastrointestinal tract, bone, adrenal glands, peritoneum, and spleen may be involved (in order of decreasing frequency) (89). Choriocarcinoma often metastasizes to unusual sites such as the spleen (2).

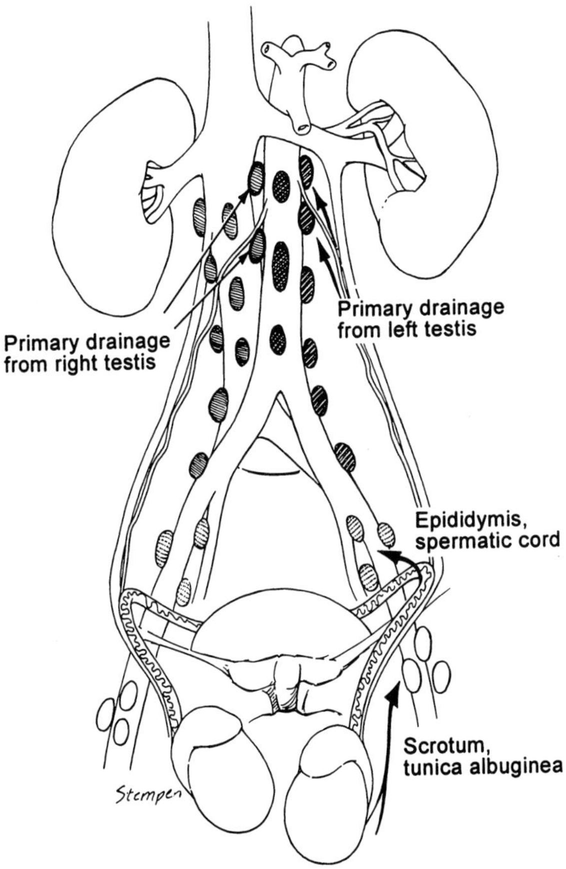

FIG. 5.31. Lymphatic drainage of the testis. The right and left testes drain to different locations as illustrated. There is some overlap between the two sides (mostly to the preaortic and interaortocaval nodes). Testicular cancer usually metastasizes along the testicular vessels and reaches the primary drainage sites ("sentinel nodes") outlined in bold. Then it tends to spread sideways and also distally to the iliac nodes. Sometimes it extends up to the thorax or supraclavicular lymph nodes via the suprahilar lymph nodes. Tumor invasion of the epididymis or spermatic cord may cause lymph node enlargement in the distal external iliac and obturator chains, and invasion of the tunica albuginea with scrotal involvement may produce inguinal lymphadenopathy.

The histology of metastatic lesions may differ from that of the primary tumor in the testis. Seminomas may metastasize as NSGCTs, and NSGCTs may metastasize as pure seminomas. Mixed germ cell tumors may metastasize as pure seminomas or as NSGCTs, such as teratoma.

Various imaging modalities are used as an adjunct to clinical staging. Testicular metastases tend to cause enlargement of the involved nodes, and all imaging techniques use nodal enlargement as the basis for identification of affected nodes. Abdominal sonography, CT, and MRI can all be used to evaluate metastatic involvement of the retroperitoneum and the abdominal organs (90). Computed tomography is considered the single best modality for the evaluation of the retroperitoneum and is often used as a primary approach. False-negative results, however, can be encountered in as many as 20% of patients, and a tailored approach with close clinical correlation remains essential (91). A chest X-ray in two planes is generally sufficient to screen for metastatic disease. If, however, an abdominal CT demonstrates retroperitoneal tumor spread, or if there is no decrease in tumor markers following unilateral orchiectomy or RPLND, potential metastatic involvement of the mediastinum and other regions needs to be evaluated by thoracic CT, cranial CT, or MRI as well as by skeletal scintigraphy.

Treatment

Germ cell tumors are initially treated by radical orchiectomy, followed by either surveillance, irradiation, chemotherapy, or retroperitoneal lymph node dissection (RPLND), depending on the type and stage of the tumor (Table 5.5) (2,6,11). Seminomas, which are radiosensitive, are usually treated by postorchiectomy radiation therapy. Chemotherapy and surgery other than orchiectomy (i.e., RPLND) are utilized only in advanced disease

TABLE 5.5. *Current treatment options for testis cancer*

Stage	Seminoma	NSGCT
Stage I	Surveillance, irradiation	Surveillance, modified RPLND[a]
Stage IIA	Irradiation, chemotherapy	RPLND, chemotherapy
Stage IIB–C	Chemotherapy	Chemotherapy (±RPLND[b])
Stage III	Chemotherapy	Chemotherapy (±RPLND[b])

[a] Modified retroperitoneal lymph node dissection (RPLND)—to preserve ejaculation function, the RPLND is modified to include the primary landing sites of the disease.

[b] RPLND is often performed following chemotherapy in patients with advanced nonseminomatous germ cell tumors if tumor markers have returned to normal.

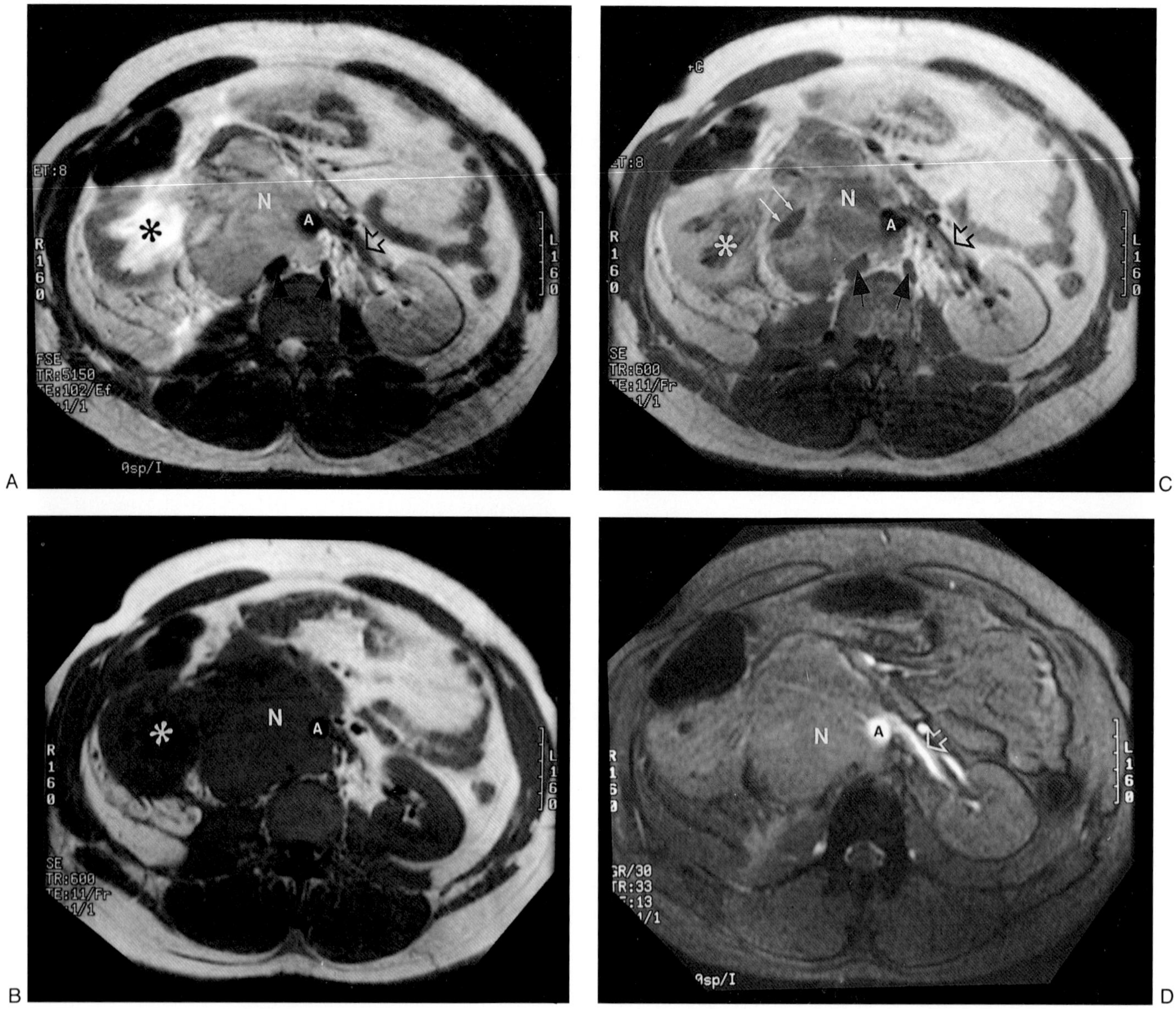

FIG. 5.32. Metastatic lymphadenopathy in a patient with testicular cancer. **(A)** T1-weighted image, **(B)** T2-weighted image, **(C)** contrast-enhanced T1-weighted image, **(D)** GRE image. The contrast between the nodes (N) and adjacent vessels (A, aorta) and fat is best seen on T1-weighted images. On contrast-enhanced image, heterogeneous enhancement and the area of necrosis (*small white arrow*) are seen. GRE indicates obstruction of the inferior vena cava, while the aorta and the left renal vessels (*open arrowhead*) are clearly seen. The right kidney is hydronephrotic (*). (*Black arrows,* the crus of the diaphragm).

or for residual disease after irradiation. Serum tumor markers are not very helpful in staging seminomas (Table 5.1) (2).

Nonseminomatous and mixed germ cell tumors (including histologically proven seminomas with elevated serum tumor markers) are usually treated by orchiectomy followed by lymphadenectomy (with or without chemotherapy). Serum tumor markers play an important role in diagnosis and follow-up in patients with NSGCT. Either hCG or AFP is elevated in approximately 90% of patients with advanced NSGCTs (86), and in patients with choriocarcinoma hCG is always elevated but AFP is normal (Table 5.1). However, since serum levels of hCG and AFP are normal in 30% of patients with NSGCTs, treatment decisions should not be based on negative tumor markers alone and the information should be correlated with imaging findings.

Most patients with nonseminomatous tumors are evaluated with **diagnostic RPLND** during surgery. It is used for staging and treatment of patients with early dis-

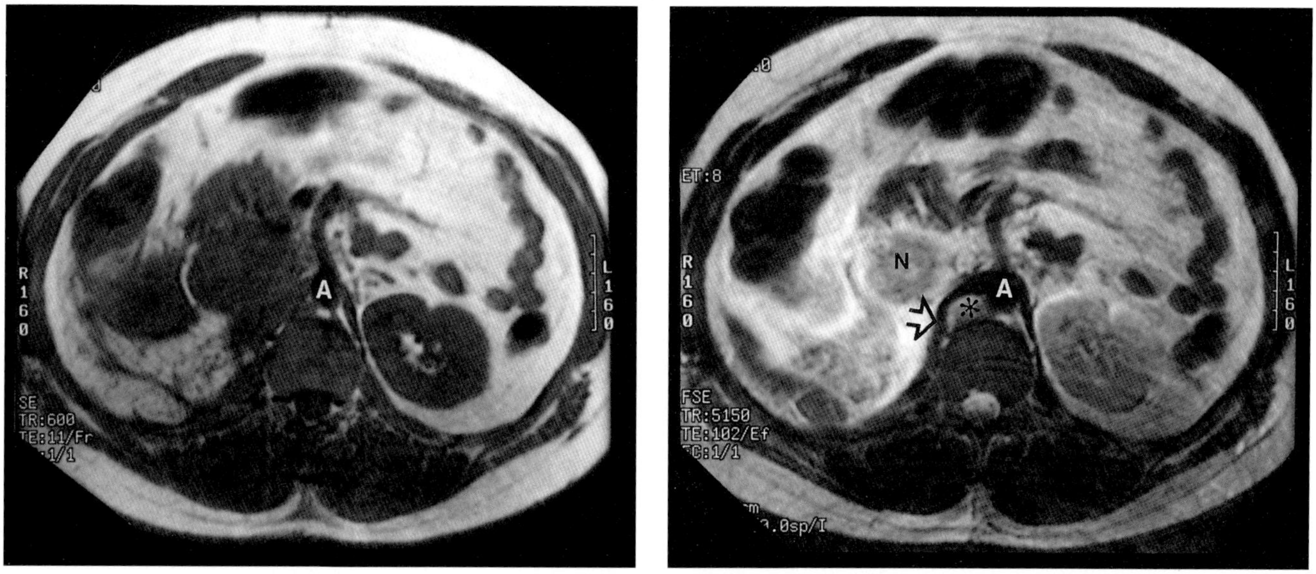

A B

FIG. 5.33. Metastatic retrocrural adenopathy. **(A)** T1-weighted and **(B)** T2-weighted images. Retrocrural nodes (*), the crus of the diaphragm (*arrow*), and retroperitoneal nodes (N) demonstrate similar signal intensity on the T1-weighted image, but it is clearly differentiated on the T2-weighted image. (A, Aorta)

ease (stages 1 and 2A) (Table 5.5). If histologic evaluation during surgery does not demonstrate lymph node metastases in the ipsilateral lymphatic drainage system, a modified RPLND, without systematic removal of all retroperitoneal lymph nodes, may be performed (9,92,93). RPLND is also performed in patients with more advanced disease (stages 2B–C and 3) if, after chemotherapy, tumor markers return to normal but a residual mass is found on CT (Table 5.5).

Tumor Recurrence

Patients with testicular cancer should be carefully followed after treatment. With the exception of seminomas, germ cell tumors tend to grow very fast. Recurrence of seminomas is most common from 2 to 10 years after initial treatment. NSGCT recurrences are most common within the first 8 to 10 months (2). Physical examination, chest radiography, and serum marker assays should be performed periodically (e.g., monthly during the first year, every 2 months during the second year, and every 6 months thereafter) (11). CT examinations should be performed at 3-month intervals for the first year and then yearly for at least the next 3 years (94). Any interval changes seen on follow-up CT examination should be carefully evaluated and correlated with serum tumor markers. Percutaneous fine-needle biopsy or even surgical reexploration may be necessary to obtain tissue confirmation.

In about 60% of cases recurrence of testicular cancer is at the initial metastatic site. Occasionally (26% of cases), however, testicular cancer recurs in both the initial and a new site (6,11,95). Both serum markers and CT examination are usually positive in testicular cancer recurrence. However, in 18% of patients CT alone is positive, and in 8% serum markers alone are positive (95). After chemotherapy, serum markers usually return to normal and on CT scans the metastatic lesions are reduced in size or disappear. Persistently elevated levels of serum markers suggest failure of treatment or presence of residual disease. A persistent elevation of marker levels after orchiectomy indicates stage II or III disease, and a persistent elevation after RPLND suggests stage III disease (96).

Residual masses are observed in 24% to 60% of cases after chemotherapy (97). In patients with NSGCTs, histologic evaluation of residual masses reveals either scar or necrosis (40% of cases), teratoma (40% of cases), or carcinoma (20% of cases) (2,98). In patients with pure seminoma, the presence of teratoma or carcinoma in residual masses is uncommon, and histology of the residual mass is more likely to reveal fibrosis and scar (90% of cases). This fibrotic scar is often diffuse and densely adherent to the great vessels. Patients with a primary testicular teratoma are at high risk of new or residual teratoma and/or carcinoma in the retroperitoneum (98). In a study done by Donohue et al. (99), 78% of patients with teratomatous elements in the primary tumor had either teratoma or carcinoma in the RPLND specimens despite having a greater than 90% decrease in tumor volume in the retroperitoneum after chemotherapy. In patients without teratomatous elements in the original tumor who had a greater than 90% decrease in the volume of retroperitoneal masses, however, none had teratoma or active cancer at RPLND (99).

Ultrasound in Staging and Follow-up of Testicular Cancer

Evaluation of the local tumor stage (T-staging) by ultrasonography is unreliable because the procedure frequently fails to demonstrate slight infiltration of the rete testis (T1), tunica albuginea (T2), or epididymis (T2) (100). In cases of large tumors, the examination should be extended to include the spermatic cord up to the internal inguinal ring, and tumor adhesion to the scrotal skin should be checked. In both cases the finding will impact the surgical approach.

Staging of testicular tumors relies heavily on the involvement of retroperitoneal lymph nodes, which, as discussed, are nearly always the initial site of metastatic involvement. The aorta, the inferior vena cava, and the iliac vessels serve as lines of orientation in the sonographic search for lymph node metastases. Any constant, nodular, solid mass is suggestive of metastatic involvement. Under favorable examination conditions, sonography can detect metastatic lymph nodes as small as 10 to 15 mm in diameter. They have a hypoechoic texture that is either homogeneous or heterogeneous and may contain cystic spaces (see Fig. 5.12). Sonography, however, is not used as a definitive staging approach.

Magnetic Resonance Imaging in Staging and Follow-up of Testicular Cancer

On T2-weighted images, testicular tumors commonly demonstrate low signal intensity that is similar to that of the tunica albuginea and the mediastinum testis, making it difficult to assess tumor extension into the tunica. While tumor extension into the spermatic cord can be depicted, concomitant inflammation or edema lowers the specificity of MR imaging findings.

In staging and follow-up of retroperitoneal lymphadenopathy, MR accuracy is comparable to that of CT (101). On T1-weighted images the nodes demonstrate medium signal intensity, rendering an excellent contrast among vessels, nodes, and retroperitoneal fat (Fig. 5.32). On T2-weighted images the nodes usually demonstrate increase in signal intensity (Fig. 5.32), rendering excellent contrast as compared with the low-signal-intensity muscle (including crus of the diaphragm) (Fig. 5.33). The signal intensity of the nodes is often homogeneous, but large nodes will demonstrate heterogeneous signal intensity. Involved lymph nodes demonstrate various degrees of enhancement following gadolinium chelates injection (Fig. 5.32). MR is helpful when vascular invasion or thrombosis is suspected. In those patients addition of gradient recalled echo (GRE) is essential (Fig. 5.32).

Like CT (see later), MR imaging can be used for follow-up after irradiation or chemotherapy (Fig. 5.34). The differentiation between residual teratoma and fibrosis can be attempted on MRI. Mature fibrosis demonstrates low signal intensity on both T1- and T2-weighted MR images, whereas residual or recurrent tumor demonstrates higher signal intensity. Unfortunately, fibrosis after cancer treatment varies from solid to cystic and is often accompanied by an inflammatory reaction, which makes reliable differentiation impossible.

Computed Tomography Staging of Testicular Cancer

Staging and follow-up in patients with testicular cancer is the primary indication for CT. When used in com-

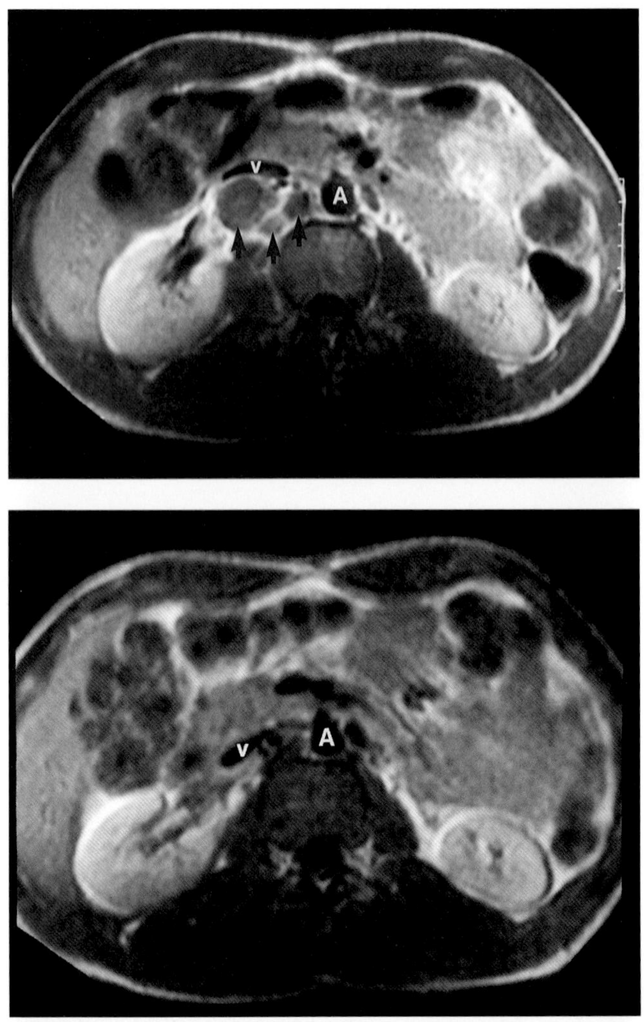

A

B

FIG. 5.34. Postchemotherapy follow-up in a patient with testicular cancer. Contrast-enhanced T1-weighted images **(A)** before and **(B)** after chemotherapy. Large retrocaval lymph nodes demonstrate low and heterogeneous enhancement and are no longer seen after treatment. (A, aorta; V, inferior vena cava)

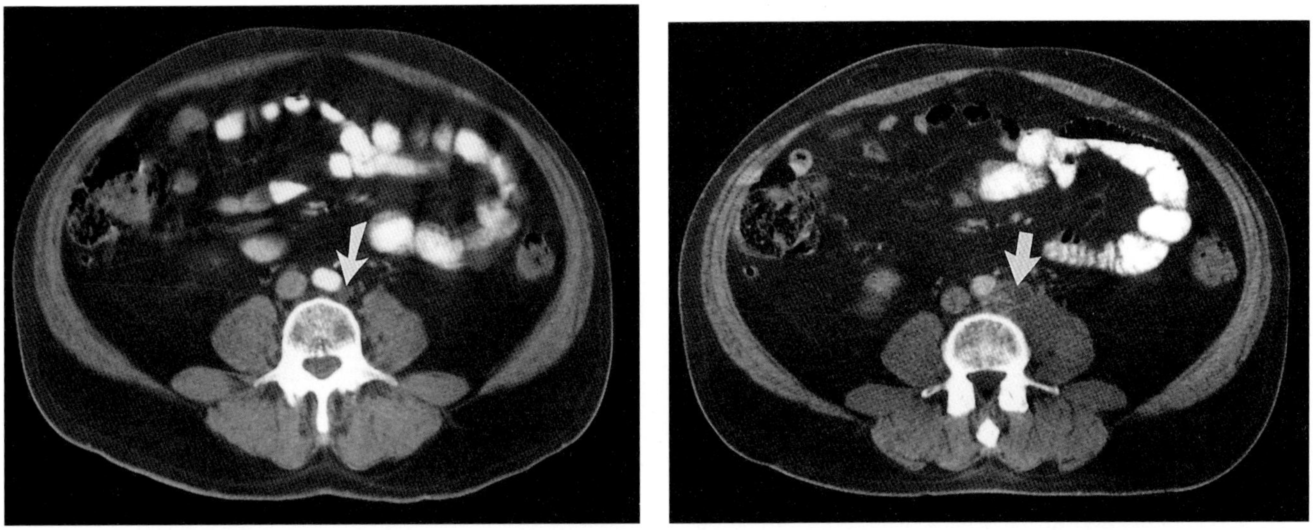

A B

FIG. 5.35. Metastatic left para-aortic lymph node (teratoma) in patient with left testicular mixed germ cell tumor who underwent surveillance. A small (9-mm) lymph node (*arrow*) in left para-aortic area on initial CT scan **(A)** has markedly enlarged on a follow-up CT scan, 6 months later **(B)**. Any lymph nodes in the typical draining sites for testicular cancer should be found suspicious for metastasis and carefully correlated with clinical course and tumor markers.

bination with radioimmunoassay of AFP, hCG, and LDH, CT staging accuracy approaches 80% to 90% (86). Although normal-sized lymph nodes may contain microscopic metastatic foci, on CT examination abdominal lymph nodes less than 1.0 cm are usually not considered abnormal (96). In patients with testicular cancer, however, even lymph nodes of less than 1.0 cm in diameter should be considered suspicious if they are located in a typical testicular tumor drainage area (e.g., the aortocaval area for right-side tumors, and the preaortic and left para-aortic areas for left-side tumors) (Fig. 5.35). The lymphatic drainage from the right-side tumor most commonly includes the aortocaval area (Fig. 5.36); lymphatic drainage from the left-side tumor often includes the left para-aortic area (Fig. 5.37). In extensive disease, retrocrural and mediastinal nodes will be involved (Fig. 5.38). Retrocrural nodes are usually considered enlarged if they are greater than 6 mm (102). Inguinal lymphadenopathy can be involved by retrograde spread or secondary to the invasion of the scrotum (Fig. 5.39).

The CT appearance of metastatic lymph nodes varies, depending on the histology and the extent of disease. Me-

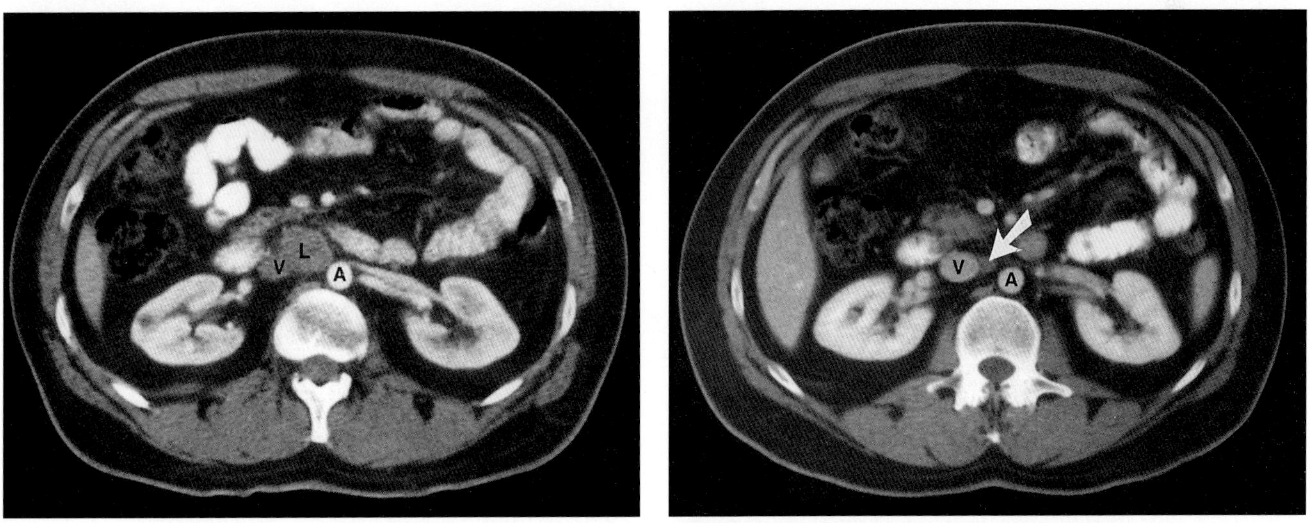

A B

FIG. 5.36. Metastatic interaortocaval node (L) in patient with right testicular seminoma **(A)** before and **(B)** after chemotherapy. This is the most common location of right-side testicular cancer drainage. After chemotherapy, the node has shrunken but a small residual mass (*arrow*) remains. (A, aorta; V, inferior vena cava)

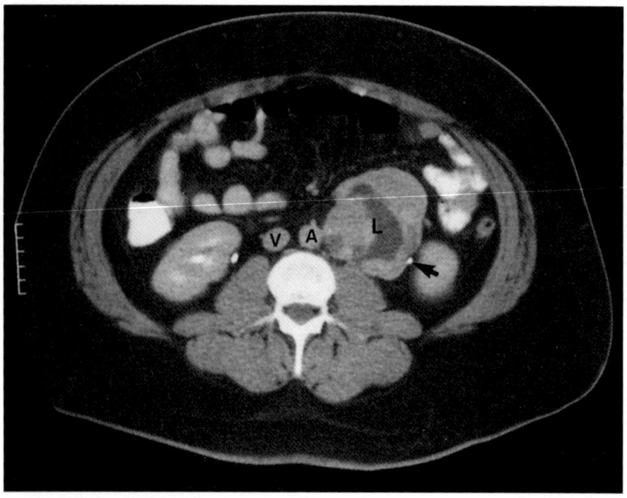

FIG. 5.37. Metastatic left para-aortic lymph node (L) in patient with left testicular teratoma. This is the most common site of lymph node metastasis from a left testicular cancer. (A, aorta; V, inferior vena cava; *arrow*, displaced left ureter)

tastases from seminomas and pure embryonal carcinomas usually show increased density on CT examination (greater than 30 HU) (Fig. 5.36), and teratomas and mixed germ cell tumors containing teratomatous elements tend to demonstrate lower attenuation (less than 30 HU) (Figs. 5.38 and 5.40) (100). However, even seminomas and embryonal carcinomas, especially when bulky, may contain low-density areas caused by tumor necrosis (Fig. 5.41). In one study retroperitoneal metastatic lymph nodes showed low density (10 to 30 HU) in 48% of the patients (103). CT is useful not only for the evaluation of the retroperitoneum, but for that of intraperitoneal (Fig. 5.42) and liver/spleen metastasis.

Computed tomography, especially in combination with serum tumor markers, is also a reliable method for evaluation of the effects of therapy and for detection of cancer recurrence following irradiation or chemotherapy. It can also serve as a method of surveillance for stage I seminomas and NSGCTs after primary orchiectomy

A

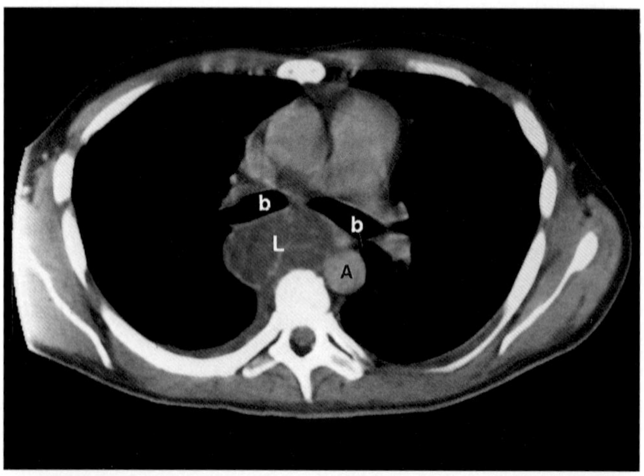

B

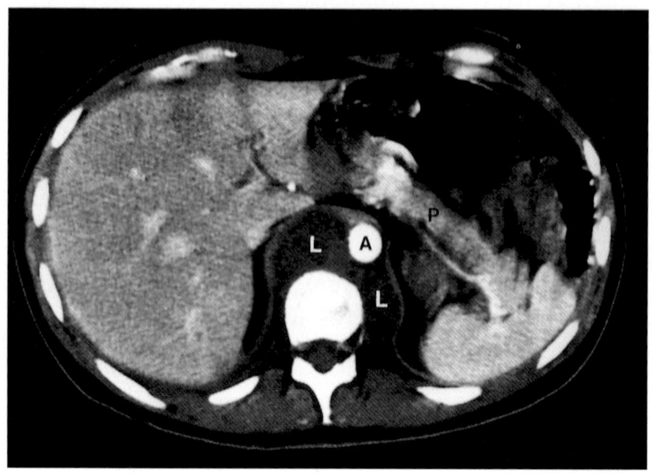

C

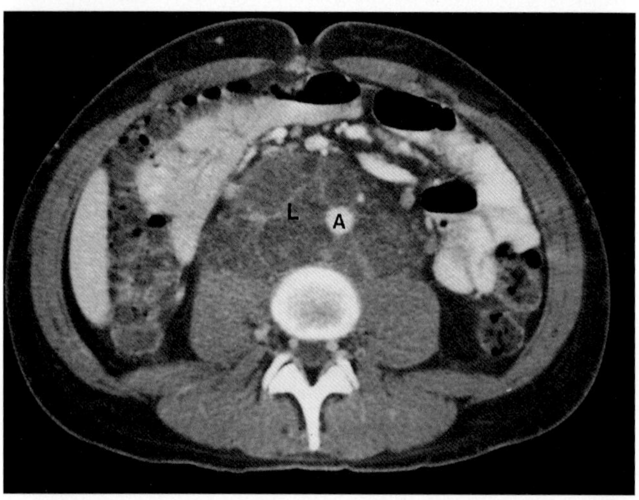

FIG. 5.38. Extensive metastatic teratoma in patient with right testicular mixed germ cell tumor (teratoma, embryonal carcinoma, and seminoma). **(A)** Subcarinal, **(B)** retrocrural, and **(C)** para-aortic and paracaval lymph nodes (L). Note the typical low density of metastatic nodes and the continuity of retrocrural metastases to the subcarinal region suggesting direct extension of the tumor into the mediastinum. Because of different window settings, the densities of the nodes in different sections look different. (A, aorta; b, main bronchus; P, pancreas)

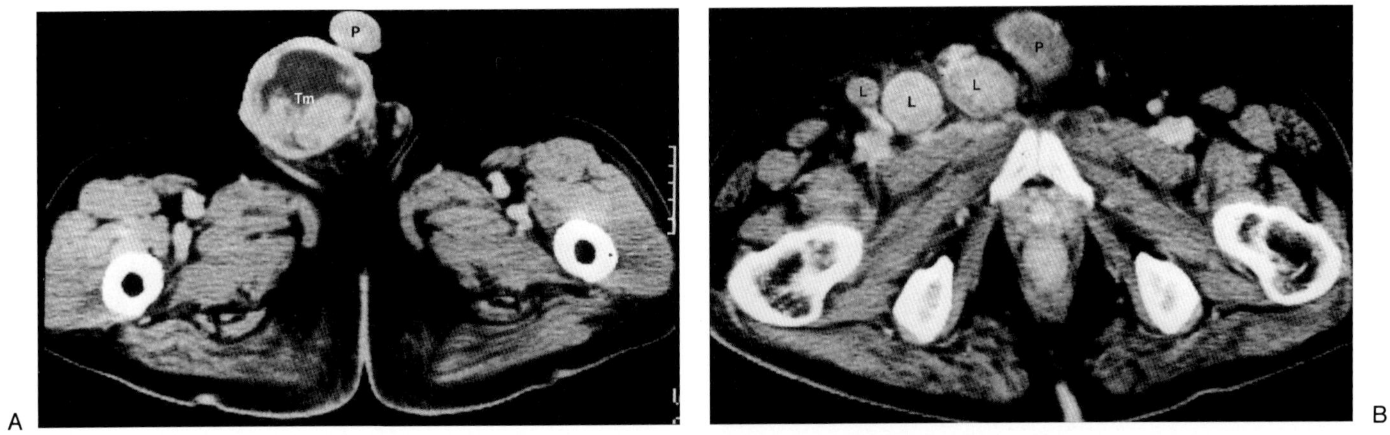

FIG. 5.39. Teratoma of the right testis. **(A)** Primary tumor (Tm), and **(B)** inguinal lymph node metastases (L). Inguinal lymphadenopathy is probably from direct invasion of the scrotal wall. (P, penis)

(104,105). Posttreatment CT changes are sometimes difficult to interpret, and presence or absence of malignancy in a residual mass cannot be predicted by CT morphologic findings or attenuation value measurements (96,106). A decrease in CT attenuation value as well as in the size and number of enlarged nodes may indicate a favorable response, even though small foci of residual malignancy cannot be ruled out (Fig. 5.36). However, a posttreatment decrease in CT attenuation may also be caused by tumor necrosis and presence of lipid-laden macrophages or by tumor evolution to teratoma (96). In addition, residual fibrotic masses may persist after successful treatment, making CT differentiation between posttreatment fibrosis or necrosis and residual or recurrent tumor difficult, especially in patients treated with cisplastin-containing chemotherapy regimens (Fig. 5.43). The incidence of fibrosis is particularly high in patients with seminoma, and in this case, residual cancer is suspected only when the mass is large (>3 cm) and well circumscribed (107).

Comparative Imaging Evaluation

Of the currently available radiologic studies, US serves as the primary modality for detection of testicular tumors and CT is most commonly recommended for staging (evaluation of metastases in the retroperitoneum, lung, and mediastinum). Magnetic resonance imaging is considered a "problem-solving" modality after US for the primary tumor detection, and after CT for cancer staging and follow-up.

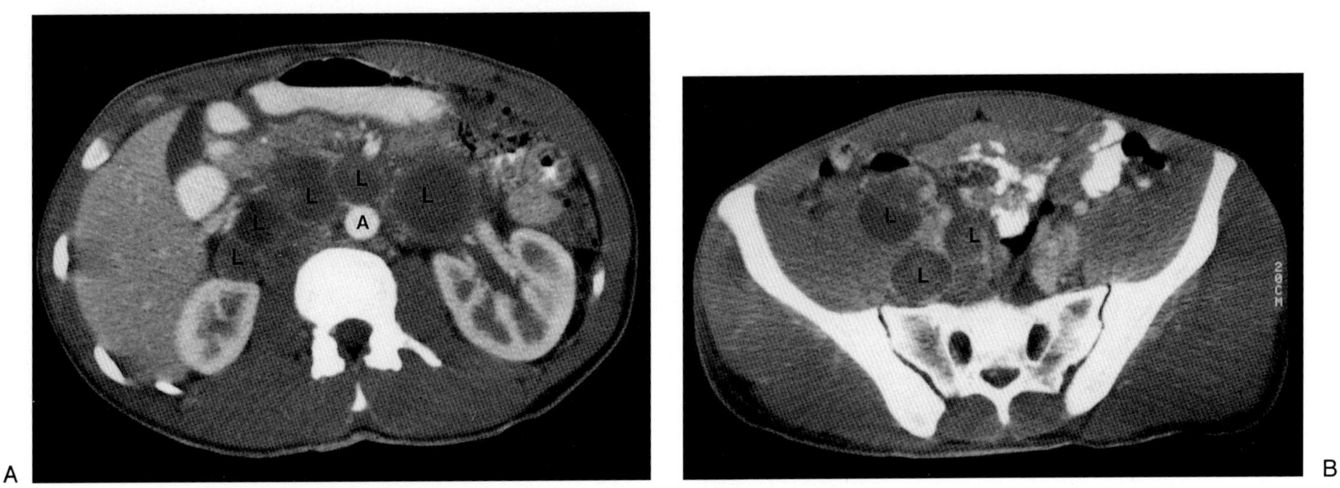

FIG. 5.40. Extensive metastatic lymph nodes (L) from right testicular mixed germ cell tumor can be seen in the retroperitoneum **(A)** and in the pelvis. **(B)** Note the low density of enlarged lymph nodes with rim enhancement. (A, aorta)

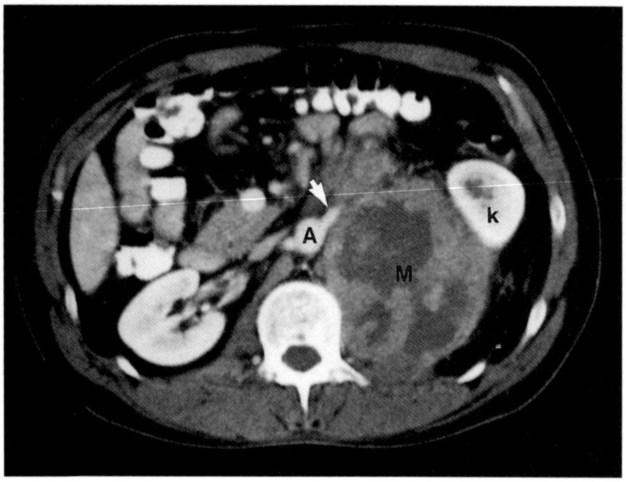

FIG. 5.41. Left paraspinal metastasis (M) in a patient with testicular embryonal carcinoma. The metastatic mass is inseparable from left psoas muscle, displacing the left kidney (k) anterolaterally. Note irregular low density within the mass. (*arrow*, left renal artery; A, aorta)

Tumor Detection

Ultrasound is a highly sensitive imaging modality for the detection of an intratesticular lesion. In most patients, US study is the only imaging needed before treatment. However, when US findings are equivocal, US scan is technically suboptimal, or when there is a discrepancy between clinical and US findings, MRI should be performed. Magnetic resonance imaging is superior to US in diffuse infiltrative disease and in extensive bilateral disease. For patients who have undergone unilateral orchiectomy, US evaluation of the remaining testis is difficult, since comparison with a normal testis is not possible. Because up to 6% of patients with testicular seminoma have bilateral disease, US is insufficient in this situation and MRI is preferred.

Staging and Follow-up

For local staging of testicular tumors despite excellent tissue contrast, MRI is no more accurate than US. The figures for both modalities are disappointingly low—63% for MRI and 45% for US (100). MRI is not very helpful in locoregional staging of testicular cancer. Accuracy rates for the detection of metastatic lymph nodes by CT (59% to 89%), MRI (62% to 92%), and lymphangiography (69% to 92%) are comparable (94,101,108). Lymphangiography is slightly more accurate overall, has a similar sensitivity rate, and has a slightly higher specificity (108). False-negative rates for lymphangiography are reported to be 10% to 25%, and those for CT are 29% to 34%. False-positive rates for lymphangiography are 5% to 10% (97,108). Although lymphangiography is slightly more accurate (especially for nonenlarged nodes), visualization of lymph nodes in the upper part of the retroperitoneum and near the renal hilum ("sentinel nodes") is limited. In addition, lymphangiographic contrast material may cause lymphoid hyperplasia and fibrosis of lymph nodes, rendering subsequent RPLND difficult. With CT it is possible not only to visualize mesenteric and renal hilar nodes, but to evaluate other organs, such as the liver, kidneys, and lungs. Although a combination of CT and lymphangiography increases both sensitivity and overall accuracy for detecting lymph node metastasis, a combined approach does not contribute to an essential improvement in the assessment of malignant retroperitoneal nodes (108). It is generally agreed, there-

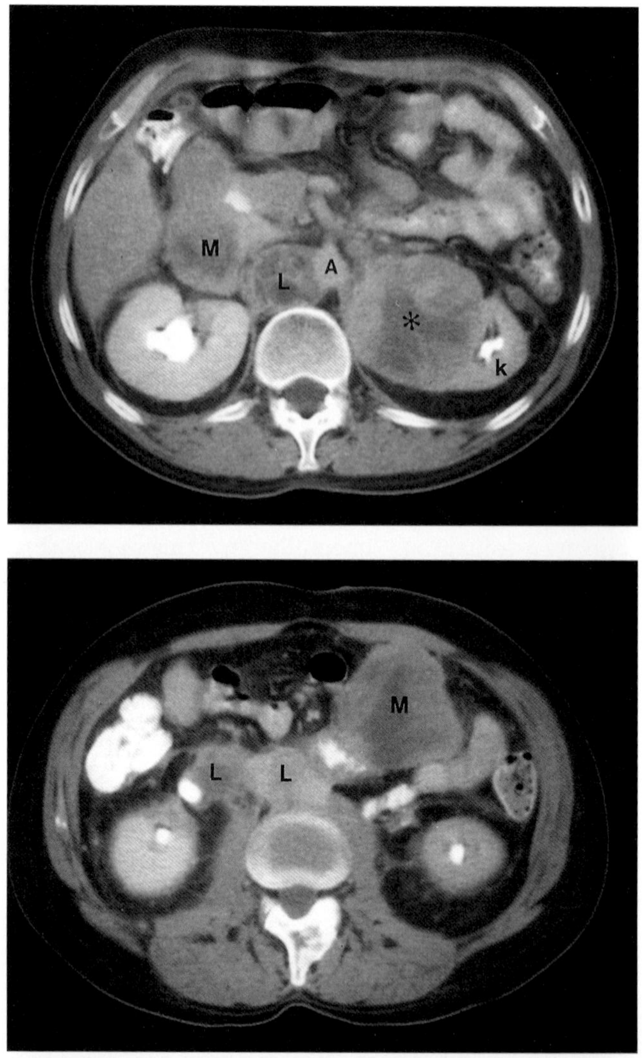

A

B

FIG. 5.42. CT scans at the level of the celiac axis **(A)** and the lower pole of left kidney **(B)** showing extensive intra- and retroperitoneal metastatic testicular cancer. Extensive lymph node metastases (L) are seen in para-aortic and paracaval area. Similar density masses (M) are seen intraperitoneally and retroperitoneally medial to the left renal hilum (*). (A, aorta; k, displaced left kidney)

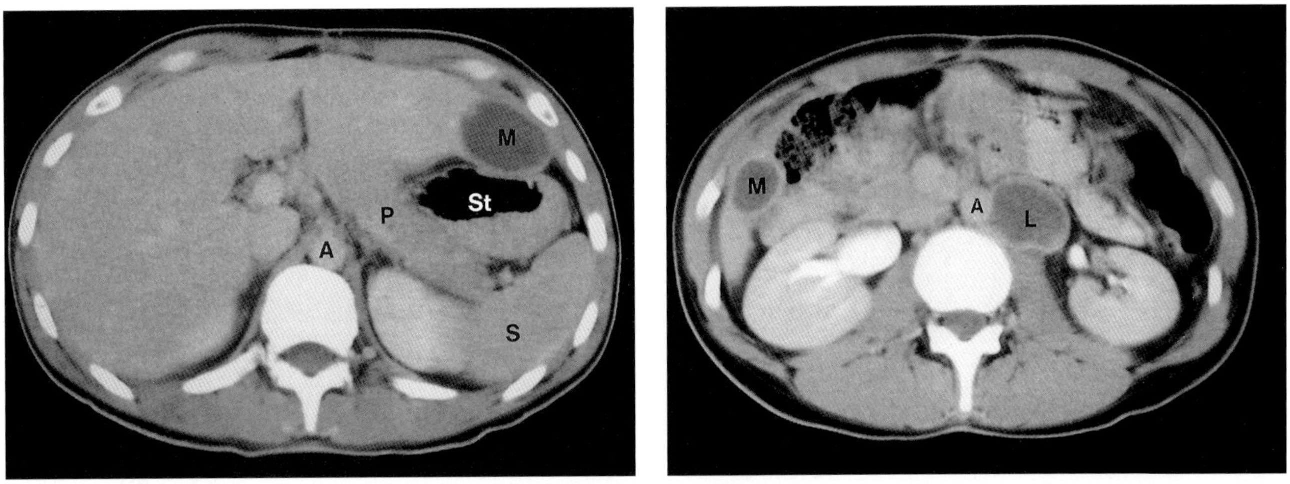

A B

FIG. 5.43. Postchemotherapy necrosis and fibrosis of left para-aortic lymph node (L) and liver metastases (M) in a patient with testicular seminoma. CT sections through **(A)** the body of the pancreas (P) and **(B)** the right renal hilum. A necrotic node and hepatic metastases in both the right and left tips of the liver are seen as round, low-density structures with rim enhancement. At surgery, no viable tumor cell was found within the masses. (A, aorta; S, spleen; St, stomach)

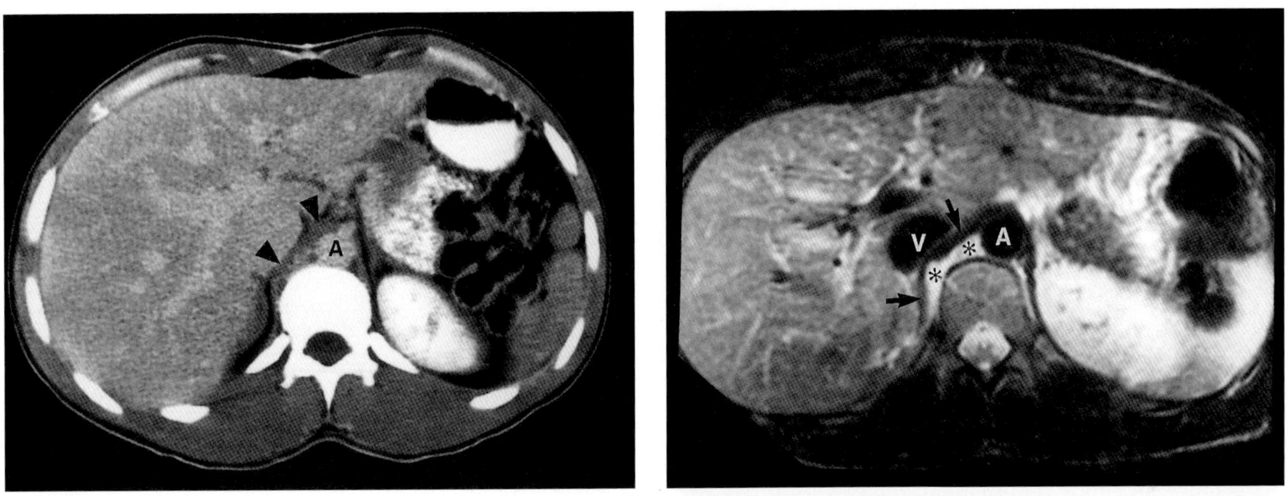

A B

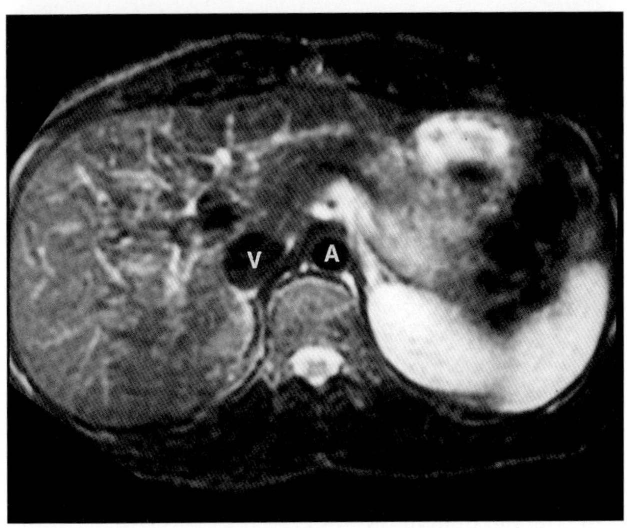

C

FIG. 5.44. Retrocrural metastatic lymphadenopathy in a patient with testicular cancer. **(A)** CT scan, **(B)** T2-weighted MR image performed 10 days after CT scan, and **(C)** T2-weighted image performed after chemotherapy (3 months after image B). On the CT scan the right crus (*arrowheads*) is thickened and nodular as compared to the contralateral side. Paucity of retroperitoneal fat, however, makes it difficult to identify retrocrural nodes separately from crura. On MR images the retrocrural nodes (*) demonstrate high signal intensity in contrast to the low-signal-intensity crura (*arrows*). The nodes have resolved after chemotherapy. (A, aorta; V, inferior vena cava)

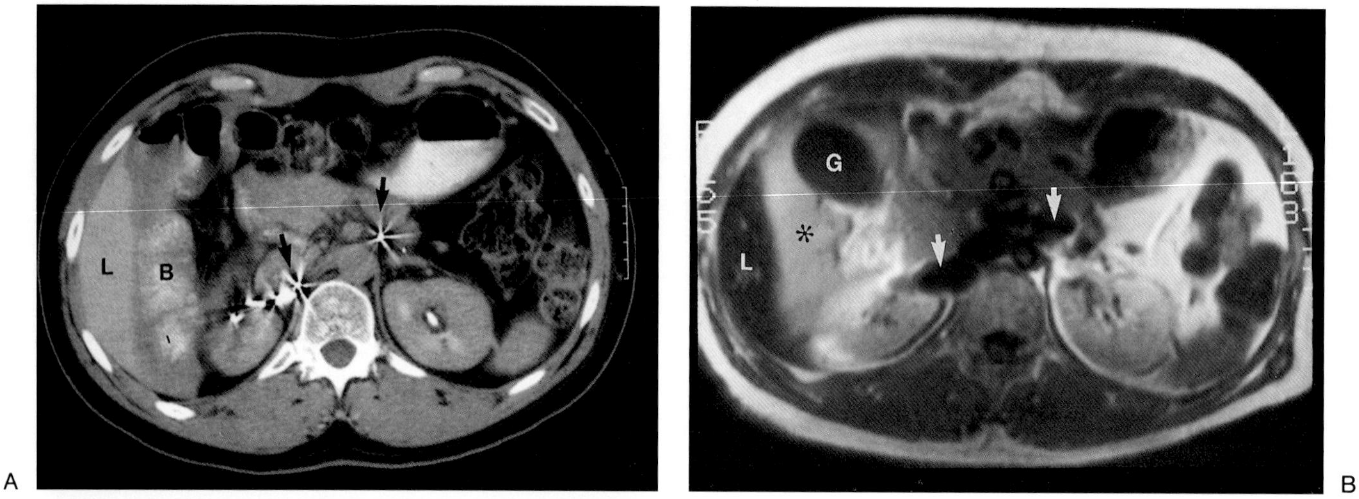

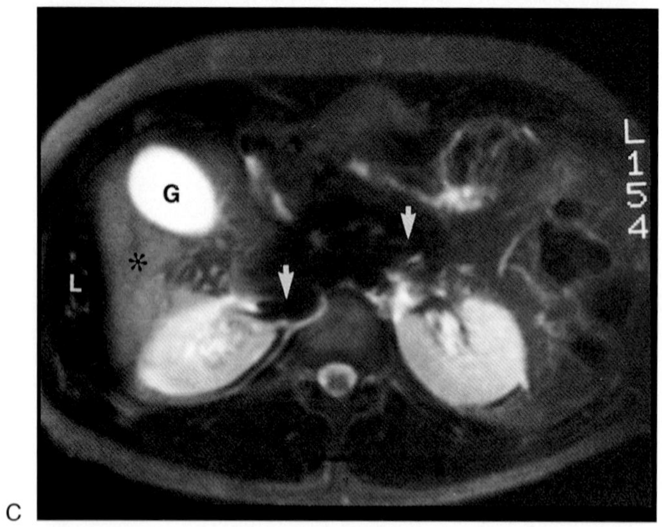

FIG. 5.45. Fluid-filled bowel (well seen on CT scan) mimics subhepatic metastases on MR images (*asterisk*). **(A)** CT scan; **(B)** contrast-enhanced, T1-weighted MR image; and **(C)** T2-weighted image. (*arrows*, surgical clips; B, contrast-filled small bowel loops; G, gallbladder; L, liver)

fore, that CT should be considered the primary modality for staging and that lymphangiography should be performed only when a technically adequate CT study fails to show enlarged retroperitoneal nodes in the presence of elevated tumor markers. As a problem-solving modality, MRI is by many preferred to lymphangiography. In staging and follow-up of patients with testicular cancer, MRI is as accurate as CT in evaluating retroperitoneal lymphadenopathy (101). Futhermore, MRI is better than CT for evaluation of retrocrural lymph nodes in a thin subject where paucity of retroperitoneal fat makes it difficult to differentiate lymph nodes from diaphragm or adjacent vessels (Fig. 5.44). MR imaging is also superior to CT for follow-up of patients with previous lymph node dissection, since there is little image degradation by surgical clips (see Section B of Chapter 3). MRI is recommended in patients in whom iodinated contrast media are contraindicated. Evaluation of intraperitoneal disease, however, can be difficult on MRI because postsurgical adhesions and unopacified bowel loops can mimic metastatic disease (Figs. 5.45 and 5.46). Even when all available diagnostic methods are used, understaging rates may still reach 10% to 20%.

BENIGN TESTICULAR TUMORS AND TUMORLIKE LESIONS

About 4% of all intrascrotal tumors are benign (21,23). In addition, a variety of benign tumorlike lesions affect the testis.

Cystic Testicular Lesions

Simple Testicular Cysts

Simple testicular cysts, which used to be regarded as rare, are being detected more frequently since the introduction of scrotal ultrasound (109–111). They present a particular diagnostic dilemma because testicular neoplasms may also contain cystic spaces and these must be reliably distinguished from simple cysts (110). Because

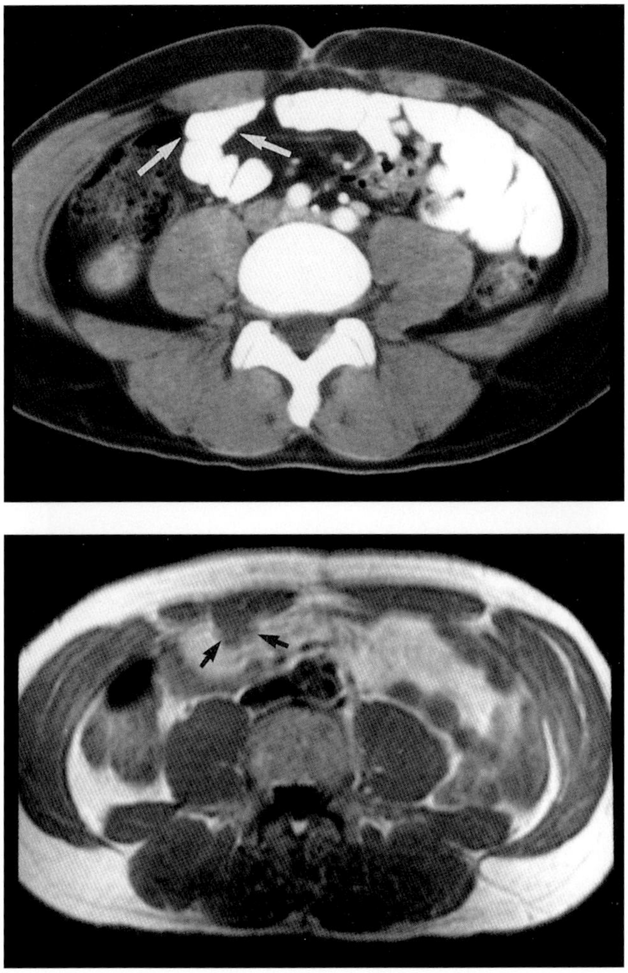

A

B

FIG. 5.46. Adhesion of small bowel loop mimicking intraperitoneal metastasis. **(A)** CT scan and **(B)** contrast-enhanced T1-weighted image. On the MR image a round, medium-intensity lesion (*black arrows*) is seen in the right anterior part of the abdominal cavity, inseparable from the anterior abdominal wall. On CT, however, the lesion corresponds to a small bowel loop (*white arrows*).

the majority of testicular masses are malignant and because benign testicular lesions may coexist with testicular cancer, simple cysts of the testis used to be treated by orchiectomy. With technologic improvements in ultrasonography, however, testicular cysts are now more easily recognized and, because of their benign nature, can be treated by conservative organ-preserving surgery (112,113). With small cysts, for which organ-preserving excision is difficult, a strategy of surveillance can be adopted in asymptomatic patients (112,113).

Two types of simple, benign cysts can be identified—cysts of the tunica albuginea and intratesticular cysts.

Tunica albuginea cysts are typically very small and are palpated as firm masses of pinhead size. They cannot be distinguished from small subcapsular tumors by palpation alone. The incidence of these cysts has been reported to increase with age (114). Patients may be asymptomatic or may present with pain and swelling (114). Several theories have been proposed to explain the pathogenesis of tunica albuginea cysts, the most plausible being that they are an anomalous efferent ductule or postinflammatory cystic dilatation of individual ductules (115–117).

As they are not associated with induration and escape detection by palpation, most simple **intratesticular cysts** are discovered incidentally. Simple cysts of the testis are most frequently solitary, and even the larger ones are rarely palpated because of their flaccid consistency. They are typically located near the mediastinum testis (110). Histologic studies show that simple intratesticular cysts originate from the rete testis. They may contain spermatozoa in the cystic fluid and are frequently associated with spermatoceles, suggesting communication with the testicular tubular system (118). Both dysgenic predisposition and alterations caused by inflammatory processes or trauma are also possible causes.

Cystic Dysplasia of the Testis

Cystic dysplasia of the testis, a rare congenital malformation, is characterized by cystic changes (predominantly in the mediastinum testis) and usually involves the rete testis and adjacent seminiferous tubules. Typically, it occurs in combination with ipsilateral renal agenesis or dysplasia of both kidneys. It is usually diagnosed in childhood (119,120) and may be due to a congenital defect of connection between the rete testis and efferent ductules (119). The lesion may extend into the testicular parenchyma, with testicular enlargement and atrophy of the remaining parenchyma (120). No malignant transformation has been reported.

Epidermoid Cysts

Epidermoid cysts, the most frequent benign lesion of the testis, represent less than 1% of all testicular tumors. Although not included in the WHO classification, epidermoid cysts are believed to be of germ cell origin and may represent monodermal teratoma (121). Palpation reveals a painless, firm, and isolated lump in the testis. Epidermoid cysts are almost always unilateral (122). They form cystic cavities lined by stratified squamous epithelium. Histologic examination reveals horny lamellae (desquamated keratinized epithelium) but no dermal adnexal structures such as sebaceous glands or hair follicles. Unlike testicular teratoma, carcinoma in situ is not found in the seminiferous tubules adjacent to an epidermoid cyst. Clinical findings do not permit differentiation between epidermoid cysts and malignant tumors, and a surgical procedure is necessary to make the diagnosis. In the case of an epidermoid cyst, however, since the testis can be preserved (123–126), a tentative diagnosis based on imaging findings can provide important information, possibly sparing the patient an orchiectomy (121,127). No local recurrence or metastasis has been reported after enucleation or orchiectomy (121).

Dermoid Cysts

Dermoid cysts differ from epidermoid cysts in that they contain dermal adnexa and are difficult to distinguish from mature teratoma as defined in the WHO classification. Malignancy is the most important differential diagnosis. A mature teratoma occurring before puberty is regarded as a benign lesion, since only nonmetastasizing cases have been described to date. The leading symptom, as in all other testicular tumors, is painless enlargement of the testicle. In children, however, this may occasionally be associated with local inflammation and must be differentiated from testicular torsion or epididymis.

Ultrasound in Evaluation of Testicular Cysts

Reliable distinction of benign cysts from malignant tumors is of primary importance. The correct diagnosis can nearly always be made on the basis of palpation in combination with ultrasound. All testicular tumors are of higher consistency than normal testicular tissue and can therefore be palpated as a mass if they are large enough. Sonographically, cystic portions of malignant neoplasms are seen as multiple cysts disseminated within a solid tumor.

On ultrasound, simple cysts of the tunica albuginea, which are palpable, are demonstrated as small, marginally located and sharply demarcated, often multilocular, cystic spaces in the area of the palpated mass. There is no structural disturbance of the adjacent testicular parenchyma (Fig. 5.47), and there should be no suspicion about solid portions.

In contrast, a simple intratesticular cyst is never discovered as a palpable mass. It is discovered incidentally on sonography frequently in the area of the mediastinum testis. In the majority of cases, it is a solitary lesion, but multiple cysts can also be present (Fig. 5.48) (110,111). Difficulties in interpretation may arise when very small lesions in the center of the testis are found on sonography. These are not accessible to palpation and may represent either a cyst of the rete testis or a small cystic teratoma.

Epidermoid cysts cannot be distinguished from tumors by palpation, but sonographically they are seen as hypoechoic, well-circumscribed round or oval lesions in the testis. They may actually have a cystlike appearance in some instances, showing a markedly hyperechoic margin but with additional internal echoes (110,122,

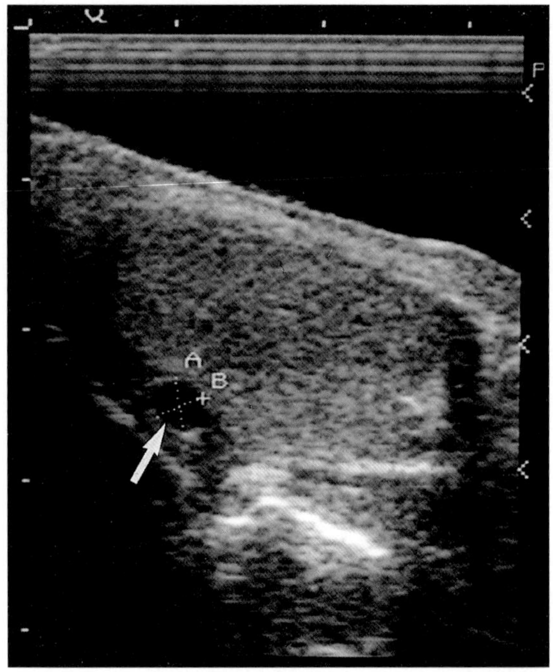

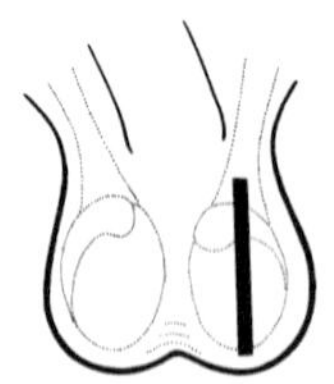

FIG. 5.47. Cyst of the tunica albuginea in a 42-year-old man presenting with a small firm mass on self-examination. Longitudinal sonogram demonstrates small cyst (*arrow*) of the tunica albuginea.

128,129,130) (Fig. 5.49). Ultrasonographic findings in epidermoid cysts are variable and nonspecific and various unusual appearances have been reported, including a mass with a "target appearance" (a central hyperechoic area surrounded by a echolucent rim) (122), an "onion appearance" (alternating rings of hyper- and hypoechogenicity) (129), an echogenic mass with dense acoustic shadowing (due to calcification) (130), and a well-circumscribed solid mass with a hyperechoic rim (131). Epidermoid cysts are differentiated from simple cysts by associated internal echoes.

Magnetic Resonance Imaging in Evaluation of Testicular Cysts

Testicular cysts, like cysts elsewhere in the body, are usually seen as sharply marginated lesions with the characteristic signal intensity of fluid (low on T1-weighted images, high on T2-weighted images, and demonstrating lack of enhancement on contrast-enhanced T1-weighted images) (Fig. 5.50). Their relationship to the mediastinum testis is demonstrated (Fig. 5.50). The signal intensity characteristics of epidermoid cysts resemble those of simple cysts, but often they can demonstrate high signal intensity on T_1-weighted image due to higher protein content. Furthermore, epidermoid cysts may be differ-

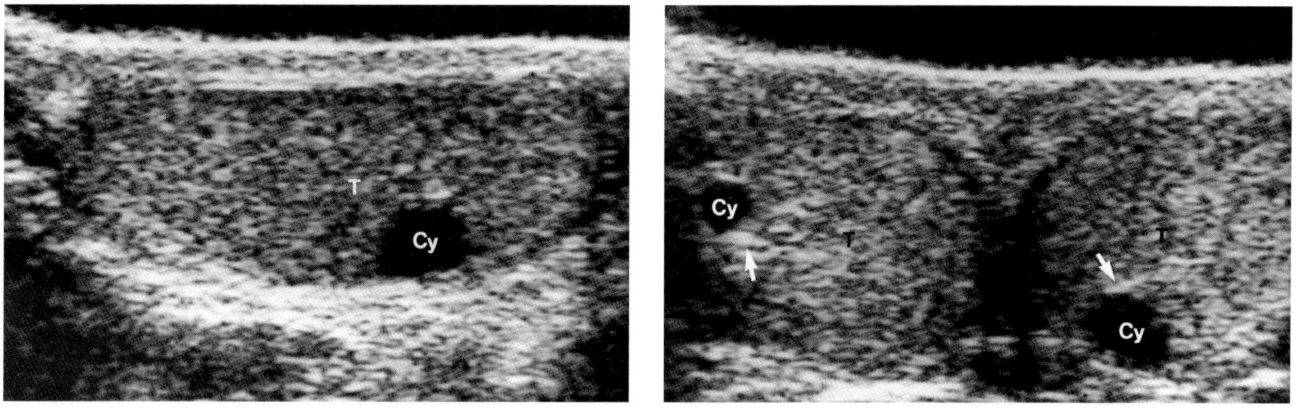

A B

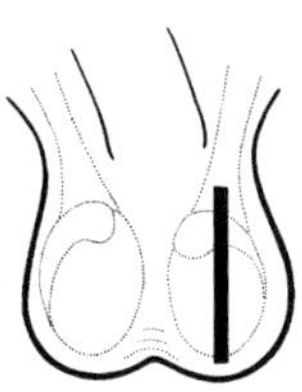

FIG. 5.48. Bilateral simple cysts (confirmed by surgery) in a 45-year-old patient with normal clinical examination. **(A)** Longitudinal scan of the left testis. **(B)** Transverse scan of both testes demonstrating a smoothly demarcated cysts (Cy) adjacent to the mediastinum testis. (T, testes; *arrows*, mediastinum testis)

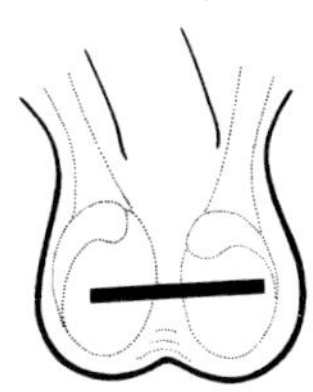

entiated from the latter by demonstration of a low-signal-intensity outer-rim capsule (Fig. 5.51). The use of contrast media helps in confirming the cystic nature of the lesion.

Computed Tomography Evaluation of Testicular Cysts

CT depiction of testicular cysts is incidental. Simple testicular cysts are seen as well-defined cystic lesions of low attenuation value (near water density). The CT findings of epidermoid cysts have not been reported.

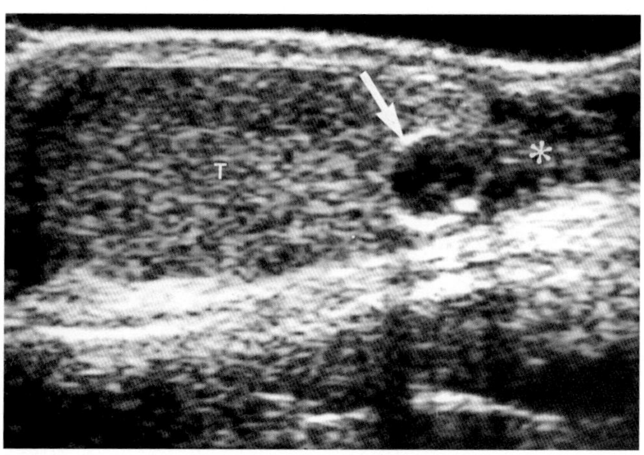

FIG. 5.49. Epidermoid cyst in a 20-year-old patient. Sonogram shows "cystlike" focal intratesticular mass (*arrow*) in the lower pole of the testis. The lesion, however, has hyperechoic margin and internal echoes. (T, normal testicular tissue; *, tail of the epididymis)

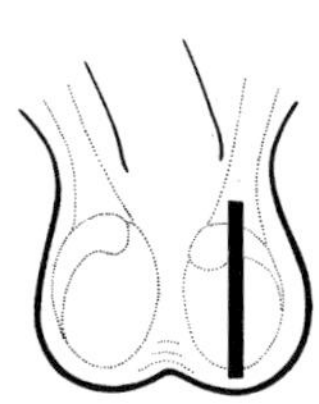

Miscellaneous Benign Tumors

Testicular gummas, a tertiary manifestation of syphilis, are rare and develop 2 to 5 years after the initial infection. Clinical symptoms resemble those of malignant testicular tumors. Patients have a positive syphilis test.

Other benign lesions—such as fibroma, angioma, neurofibroma, leiomyoma, and fibrous pseudotumors—of the testis are rare. Aberrant splenic and adrenal tissue (so-called **adrenal rest tumors**) have also been found in the testis. The pathogenesis of aberrant adrenal tissue is not fully understood, but may be related to the common embryologic origin of the adrenal gland and gonads (see Chapter 1). It occurs in about 8% of patients with congenital adrenal hyperplasia. Histologically, these lesions are difficult to differentiate from Leydig cell tumors (132). Although it is unclear whether adrenal rest tumors represent true neoplasms or hyperplasia, they present as bilateral testicular tumors with associated congenital adrenal hyperplasia and elevated serum levels of adrenocorticotropic hormone (ACTH). Patients with this tumor can be treated by corticosteroids (133). Aberrant adrenal tissue produces echo-poor foci near the mediastinum testis, commonly on both sides (134). Imaging findings on either US or MRI are indistinguishable from other benign or malignant testicular tumors.

Adenomatoid tumors, which usually occur in the epididymis, may also be found within the testis. They have been reported to represent up to 5% of all testicular tumors. They arise from the tunica albuginea and are therefore always found in the periphery of the testicle. These benign histologic entities cannot be differentiated from testicular malignancies on clinical grounds or imaging findings (135,136). On ultrasound scans they are

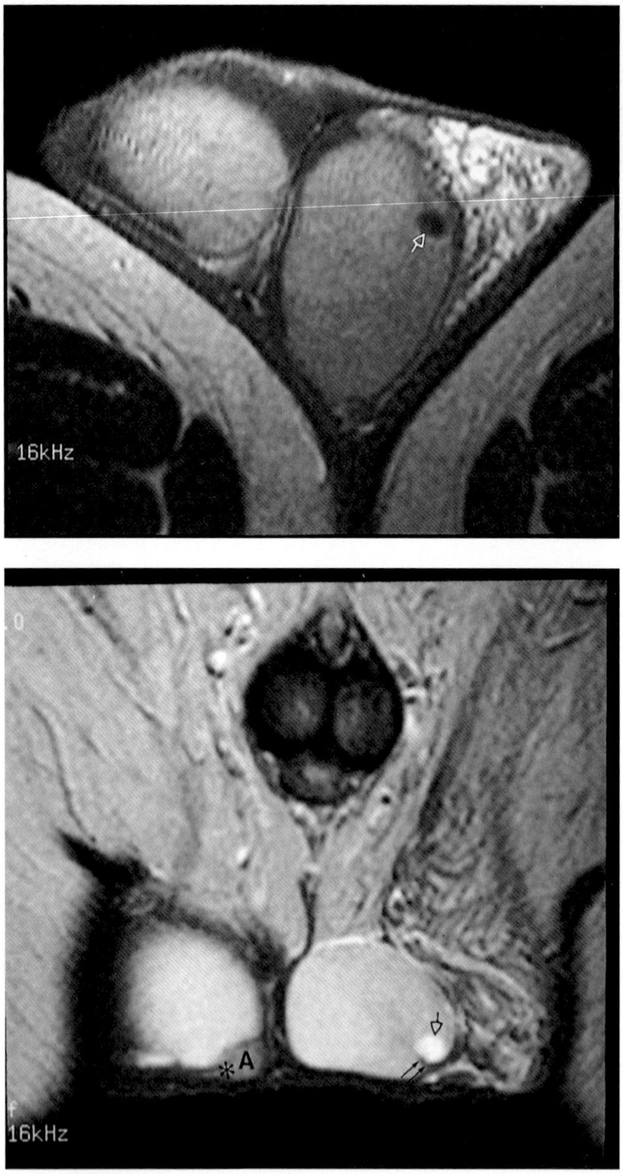

A

B

FIG. 5.50. Solitary testicular cyst of the left testis and adenomatoid tumor of the right epididymis. **(A)** Contrast-enhanced T1-weighted and **(B)** T2-weighted images. Testicular cyst (*open arrowhead*) demonstrates characteristic low signal intensity on T1-weighted image and increase in signal intensity on the T2-weighted image. The cyst is adjacent to the mediastinum testis (*arrows*). Adenomatoid (A) tumor in the right epididymis (*).

most commonly seen as oval-shaped masses on the surface of the testis. The echogenicity varies, but they are predominantly homogeneous and hyperechoic. The solid nature of the lesion helps differentiate them from cysts of the tunica albuginea, but not from other solid testicular neoplasms.

Seminiferous Tubular Ectasia of the Rete Testis

Seminiferous tubular ectasia of the rete testis is a benign condition, often bilateral, which usually occurs in elderly men. It is commonly associated with epididymal abnormalities (i.e., spermatoceles, epididymal cysts, or epididymitis) (137,138) and shares a common location (i.e., within the mediastinum testis) with cystic dysplasia of the testis and testicular cysts (139). Obstruction caused by trauma or inflammation is thought to be a causative factor in seminiferous tubular ectasia and testicular cysts (137).

Ultrasound in Evaluation of Seminiferous Tubular Ectasia of Rete Testis

Ultrasound reveals numerous small, tubular or round cystic structures within the mediastinum testis. This is a characteristic finding that, in combination with its typical location, makes it easy to identify and differentiate from other entities (Fig. 5.52). On relatively rare occasions, the differential diagnosis may include cystadenoma of the epididymis, adenocarcinoma of the rete testis, non-Hodgkin's lymphoma, and secondary dilatation of the rete testis resulting from testicular tumor (138,140).

MR in Evaluation of Seminiferous Tubular Ectasia of Rete Testis

On T1-weighted images, tubular ectasia of rete testis is depicted as a low-signal-intensity serpiginous tubular cystic structure in the vicinity of the mediastinum testis. It demonstrates signal intensity similar or higher than testis on T2-weighted images and lack of enhancement on postcontrast study. Associated spermatocele is depicted as well (139).

Computed Tomography in Evaluation of Seminiferous Tubular Ectasia of Rete Testis

Computed tomographic appearance of seminiferous tubular ectasia has not been reported.

Fibrosis of the Tunica Albuginea

Small fibrotic foci of the tunica albuginea may develop secondary to inflammation or trauma. They are palpated as small, circumscribed, firm masses. Clinically, these fibrotic foci cannot be distinguished from subcapsular tumors.

Ultrasound in Evaluation of Fibrosis of the Tunica Albuginea

The diagnosis of fibrosis of the tunica albuginea is facilitated by ultrasonography, which should be performed in conjunction with physical examination. Although cir-

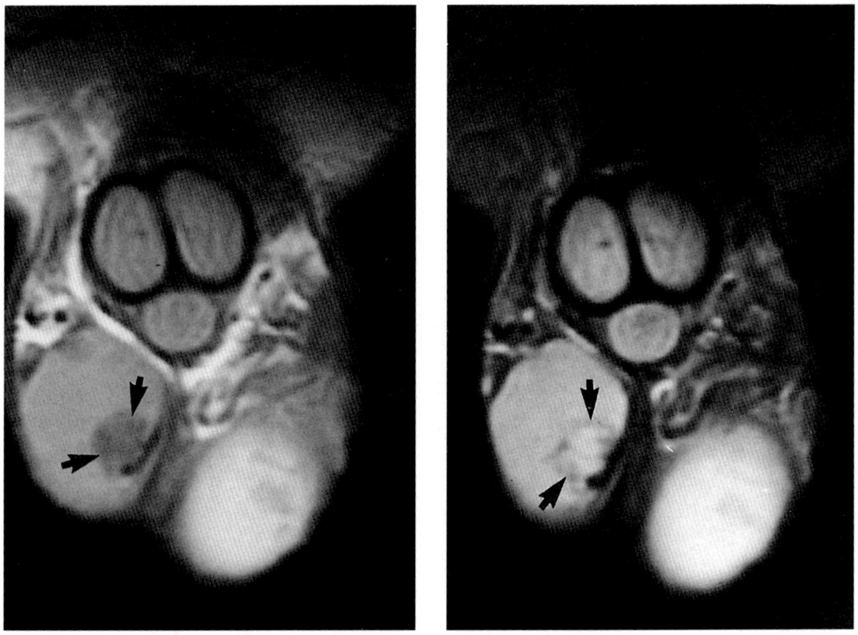

A,B

FIG. 5.51. Epidermoid cyst, right testis. **(A)** Proton density and **(B)** T2-weighted images. Although the signal intensity of the lesion is characteristic for a cyst (*arrows*), the margin is irregular and its thick low-signal-intensity band is seen medially.

cumscribed fibrosis of the tunica albuginea may be seen as slight focal thickening, sonography usually fails to demonstrate any abnormalities, and the diagnosis is suggested when the homogeneous echotexture of the subcapsular testicular tissue is preserved. Intratesticular structural disturbances around the palpable lesion, however, indicate a neoplasm.

Plaquelike calcifications of the tunica albuginea are also palpated as circumscribed, firm lesions. In this case, however, ultrasonography reveals a hyperechoic plaque in the calcified area of the tunica albuginea, typically associated with acoustic shadowing (Fig. 5.53). Additional scanning of the testis from the opposite side facilitates evaluation of the testicular tissue behind the calcified area to rule out a focal tumorous lesion.

MR and CT in Evaluation of Fibrosis of the Tunica Albuginea

Neither MRI nor CT findings of fibrosis of tunica albuginea have been reported. Calcified plaque of the tunica albuginea is easily demonstrated by CT.

Echo-Dense Intratesticular Alterations

Echo-dense structural disorders within the testis are unusual. They may occur singly or multiply, and most frequently correspond to small focal scars or calcifications. **Intratesticular calcifications** may represent an incidental finding of no clinical relevance (calcifications outside the testis are not uncommon and are usually benign), or they may, especially when multiple and tiny, be associated with testicular cancer (see below, under testicular microlithiasis). Whenever an echo-dense intratesticular focus is demonstrated by ultrasound, it is important to exclude tumorous processes. When interpreting these scans, ultrasonographic artifacts—caused by air bubbles within the water path, sonographer's fingers beneath the scrotal sac, or bowel-filled scrotal hernia—

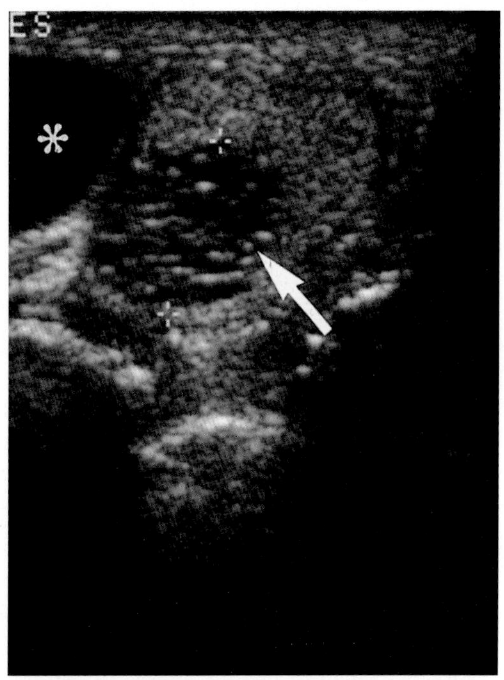

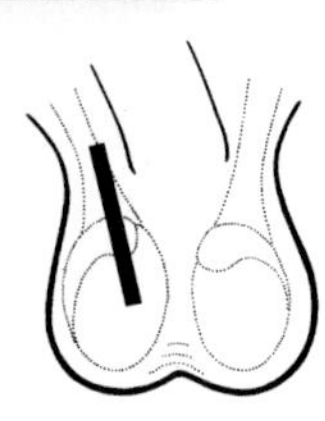

FIG. 5.52. Tubular ectasia of the rete testis. Sonogram demonstrates tubular cystic structures (*arrow*) in the vicinity of the mediastinum testis. Spermatocele (*).

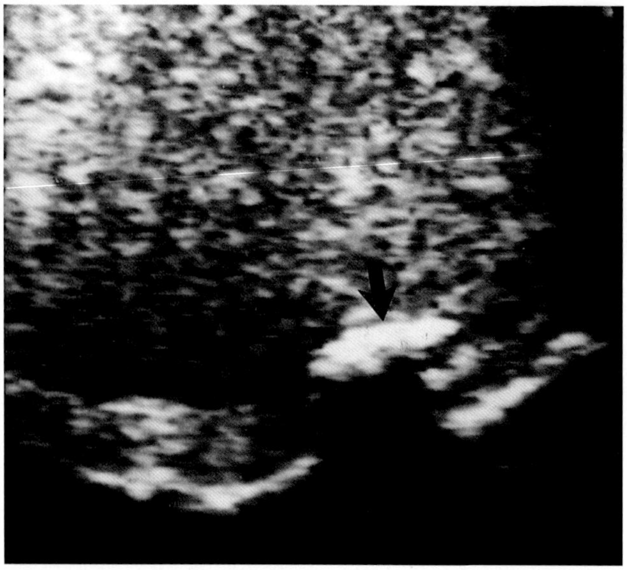

FIG. 5.53. Calcification of the tunica albuginea seen as an echogenic focus with posterior acoustic shadowing (*arrow*). Testicular parenchyma is normal.

should first be excluded. Dense echogenic scars, calcifications, or cartilaginous structures may indicate nonseminomatous germ cell tumors (141) or a burned-out testicular tumor. Testicular tumor should be excluded by careful palpation. A burned-out testicular tumor can be excluded after the examination of the retroperitoneal lymph nodes is negative.

Clues from the patient's history may also be useful for the further differentiation of echo-dense intratesticular lesions. Scarring or calcification can occur after orchiopexy or trauma, or may be secondary to tuberculous epididymo-orchitis or granulomatous orchitis (142,143). Small foci of disseminated testicular scars are sometimes also observed in patients who have undergone systemic chemotherapy.

It is not always possible to find an explanation for echo-dense changes in testicular tissue. Sometimes an idiopathic structural disorder must be assumed. However, this assumption can only be made after the possibility of a testicular tumor has been excluded, and even then US follow-up study should be recommended.

Testicular Microlithiasis

Histologically, testicular microliths represent calcified concretions within the lumina of the seminiferous tubules (144). Although the pathogenesis of testicular microlithiasis is not well known, associated disorders include cryptorchidism, testicular tumor, Klinefelter's syndrome, male pseudohermaphroditism, and infertility (17,144). To date there is no answer to the question of whether testicular microlithiasis is directly related to development of testicular cancer. A high coincidence between microlithiasis and tumor (24 out of 61 reported cases, or 39%), however, has been reported in the literature (16,17). In evaluation of patients with testicular microlithiasis, additional attention should be paid to the possible presence of a testicular tumor. Patients should be instructed in testicular self-examination and short-interval (annual) follow-up is recommended.

Ultrasound in Evaluation of Testicular Microlithiasis

Scrotal ultrasonography reveals tiny (1 to 2 mm in diameter), disseminated echogenic foci throughout the testis (Fig. 5.54) (16,17,144,145). They usually involve both testes but may be unilateral. The microliths are very tiny and, therefore, usually show no acoustic shadowing.

Magnetic Resonance Imaging in Evaluation of Testicular Microlithiasis

On T1-weighted MR images, small, scattered, low-signal-intensity foci can be detected (Fig. 5.55). On T2-weighted images the small foci of microlithiasis may not be detected, especially when image resolution is degraded by poor signal-to-noise level (Fig. 5.55)

Computed Tomography in Evaluation of Testicular Microlithiasis

Although punctate calcifications can be demonstrated, the CT findings of testicular microlithiasis are not established.

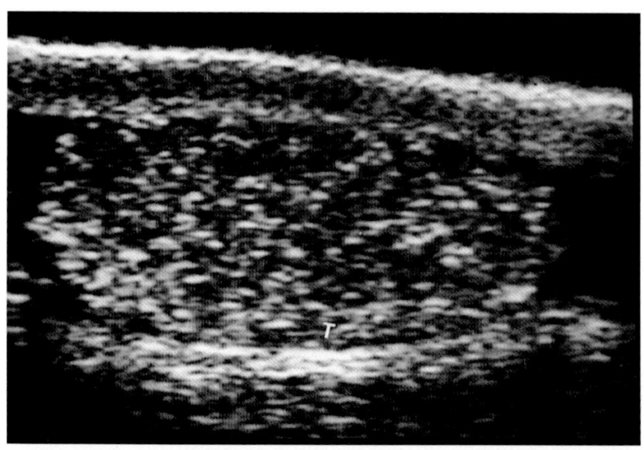

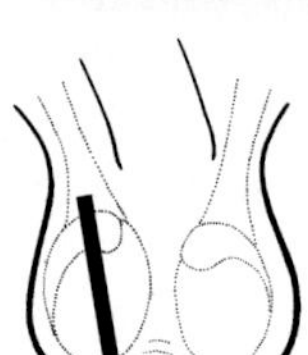

FIG. 5.54. Testicular microlithiasis demonstrating disseminated echogenic foci throughout the testicular parenchyma (T) in this 26-year-old patient with a normal clinical examination.

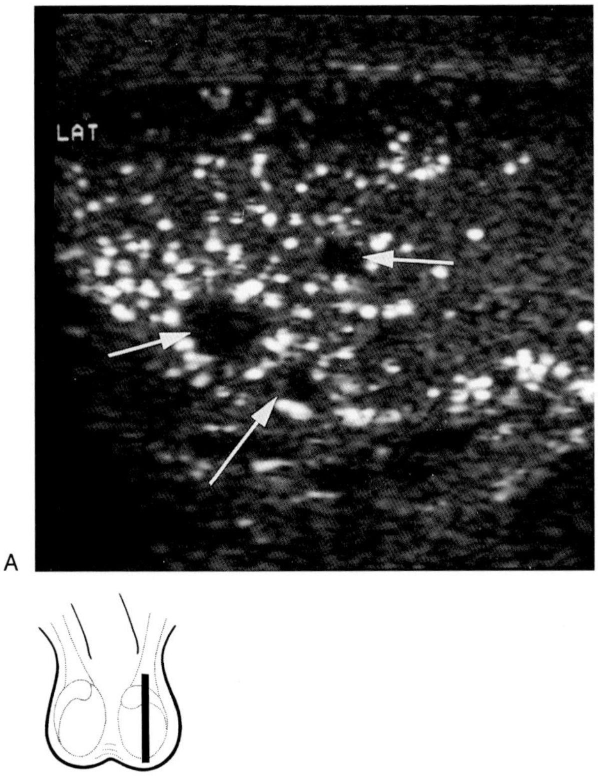

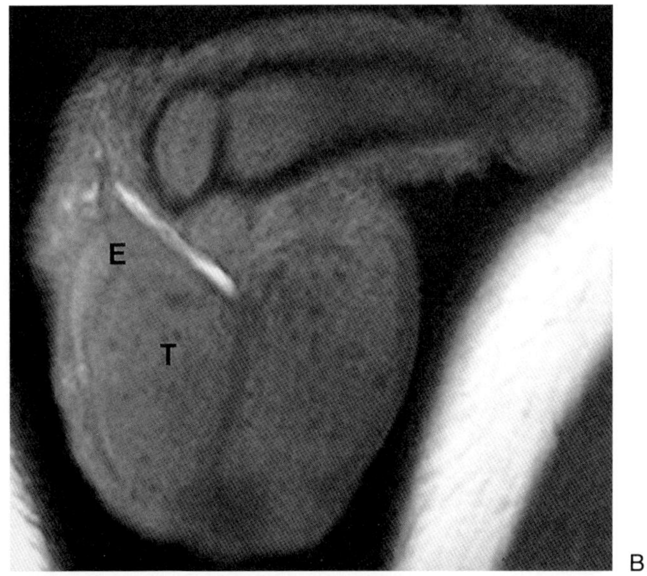

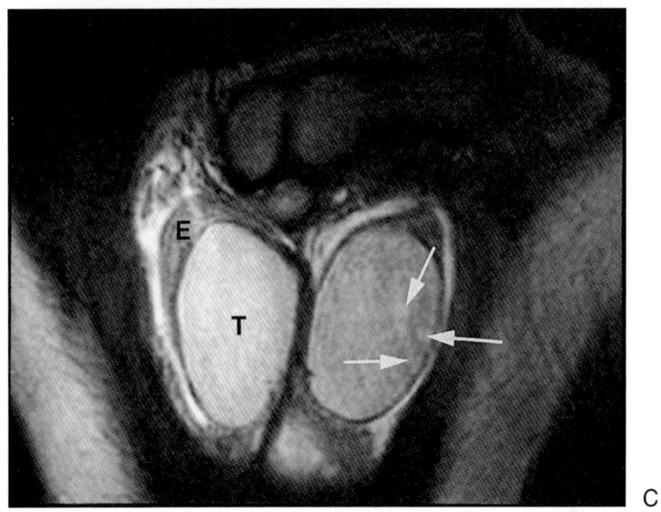

FIG 5.55. Testicular microlithiasis in a 34-year-old patient. **(A)** Longitudinal ultrasonogram showing three hypoechoic lesions (*white arrows*) and multiple disseminated echogenic dots throughout left testis. **(B)** Coronal T1-weighted and **(C)** T2-weighted MR images. Multiple disseminated foci demonstrate low signal intensity on T1-weighted image and are not seen on T2-weighted image. High signal intensity foci (*arrows*) corresponded to hypoechoic lesions on US. At surgery, however, no tumor was present. Epididymis (E). Normal right testis (T).

Comparative Evaluation

In the evaluation of benign tumors and tumorlike conditions of the testis, US is the primary imaging approach. Only in rare cases when US diagnosis of simple cyst (which requires no surgical intervention) needs reinforcement, is MRI study warranted. Solid benign tumors cannot be differentiated from malignant neoplasms on either US or MR.

Testicular Tumors in Children

Testicular tumors are rare in children, accounting for only about 1% of pediatric malignant neoplasms. Approximately 3.5% of all testicular tumors occur in children, with a peak incidence in the second year of life. In contrast to adults, in whom the incidence of primary germ cell tumors is approximately 95%, germinal tumors constitute only 60% to 75% of testicular tumors occurring during childhood (50,146). Most testicular neoplasms in children are malignant, with benign tumors occurring about one fourth of the time (146). The most frequent malignancies are yolk sac tumors (approximately 50% of all childhood testicular tumors), followed by teratoma and secondary manifestations of lymphoma and leukemia. Seminomas are rarely seen in children. They do not develop before the onset of spermatogenesis and are regarded as postpubertal tumors. Benign testicular tumors are primarily Leydig cell and Sertoli cell tumors. Rhabdomyosarcoma is the most frequent childhood tumor of the spermatic cord.

Clinical Presentation

Testicular tumors in children typically present with an asymptomatic, firm swelling of the scrotal contents

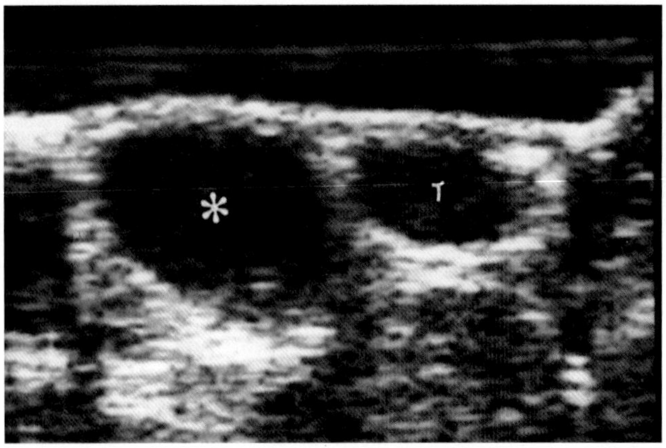

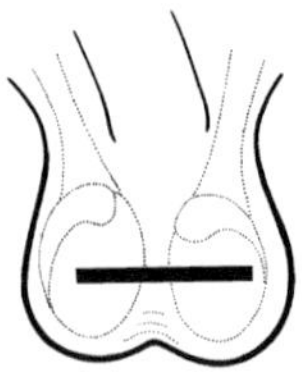

FIG. 5.56. Acute lymphoblastic leukemia and scrotal swelling on the right in a 10-year-old boy. The right testis (*) is enlarged and hypoechoic consistent with leukemic infiltration. The left testis (T) is of normal size and shows the age-appropriate hypoechogenicity. However, leukemic infiltration of the left testis cannot be ruled out.

(147). **Yolk sac tumors**, the most frequent testicular neoplasm in children, occur more frequently in younger children than do teratomas and are seen primarily during the first 2 years of life. Yolk sac tumor is characterized by slow growth, and testicular swelling often persists for some time before seeking medical help. Metastatic spread is primarily hematogenous (e.g., pulmonary metastases). Most children with yolk sac tumors have elevated levels of AFP, whereas those with teratomas do not.

Leydig cell tumors are most frequent around the fifth year of life. If they are testosterone producing, the clinical picture may be dominated by secondary alterations, such as rapid growth, bone age greater than chronologic, a deep voice, premature growth of the penis, and development of pubic hair. The cornerstones of diagnosis of a Leydig cell tumor are precocious puberty, testicular mass, and elevated urinary excretion of 17-ketosteroids. Gynecomastia may also be present.

Sertoli cell tumors are the second most frequent benign tumors in children. They have a peak incidence during the first 6 months of life and are generally not associated with endocrine disorders.

Gonadoblastoma most commonly occurs in infants and children under 2 years of age. These children present with intersex problems, usually without endocrinopathy (50).

The most common neoplasms causing secondary testicular manifestations in children are **lymphoma** and **leukemia. Metastatic tumors** of the testis are relatively rare in children. When they are found, the most common primary tumors include Wilms' tumor, neuroblastoma, his-

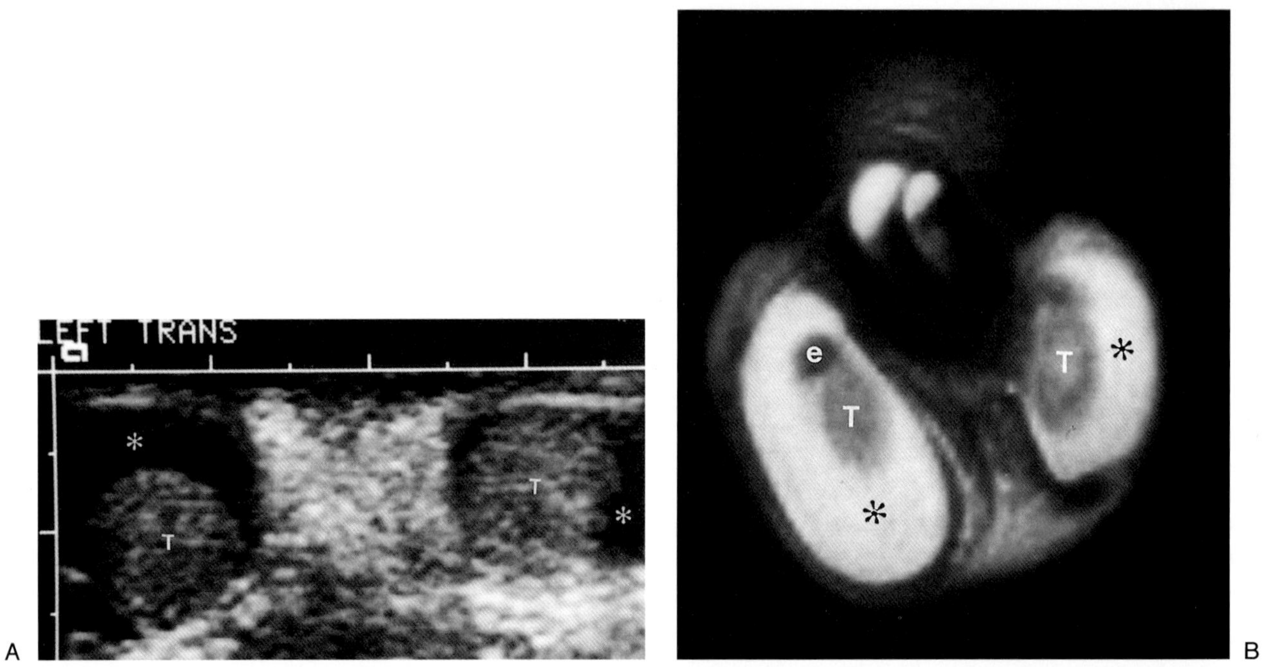

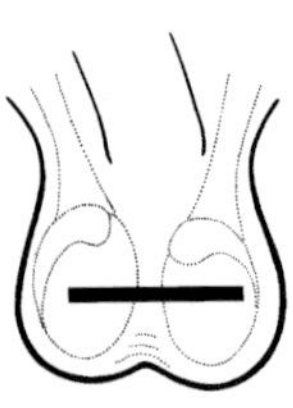

FIG. 5.57. Lymphocytic leukemia involving both testes. **(A)** Sonogram and **(B)** T2-weighted MR image. Both testes (T) are of normal size and echogenicity for the child's age. On MRI, however, the diffuse low signal intensity of both testicles is consistent with a clinical diagnosis of leukemic infiltration. (e, head of the epididymis; *, hydrocele)

tiocytosis X, retinoblastoma, and rhabdomyosarcoma (50,148).

Ultrasound in Evaluation of Pediatric Testicular Tumors

Although transillumination can distinguish a hydrocele from a large solitary mass, ultrasound is the most suitable procedure for the direct demonstration of an intratesticular tumor. The sonographic characteristics (hypoechoic, commonly inhomogeneous, focal or diffuse intratesticular alterations) are the same as those described for testicular tumors in adults (Fig. 5.56). However, two factors make ultrasound evaluation more difficult in children. First, the prepubertal testis is normally of lower echogenicity, and visualization of small tumors, which may not stand out against the hypoechoic background of the normal testicular tissue, is more difficult. Comparison with the normal contralateral testis is, however, helpful in overcoming this difficulty. Second, problems may arise from the small size of the organ and its mobility, especially in young infants. Despite these drawbacks ultrasound has an important role in distinguishing a solid mass from a hydrocele and an intratesticular lesion from a paratesticular one (148). It is also useful in differentiating testicular tumor from other testicular disorder (e.g., epididymitis, inguinal hernia, torsion).

In the evaluation of lymphoma and leukemic infiltration, demonstration of a hypoechoic lesion or enlargement of the testis is suggestive of this diagnosis (66). The leukemic infiltration is often bilateral. Ultrasound is insensitive for diffusely infiltrative testicular lesions, especially when the size of the testis is normal or both testes are involved (Fig. 5.57) (149). These lesions are better shown by MR imaging (100).

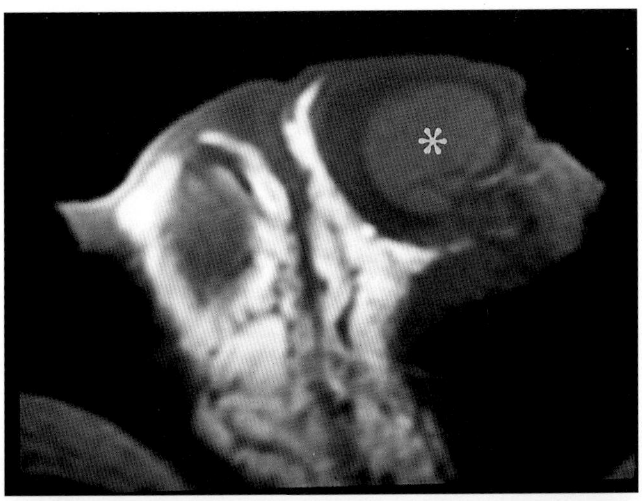

A

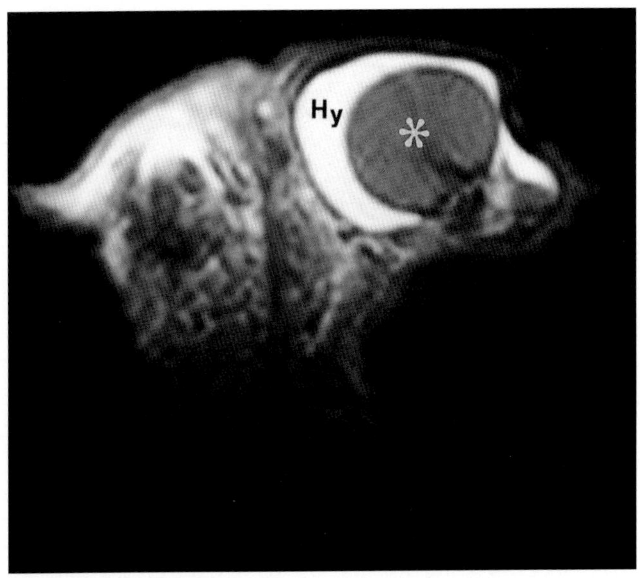

B

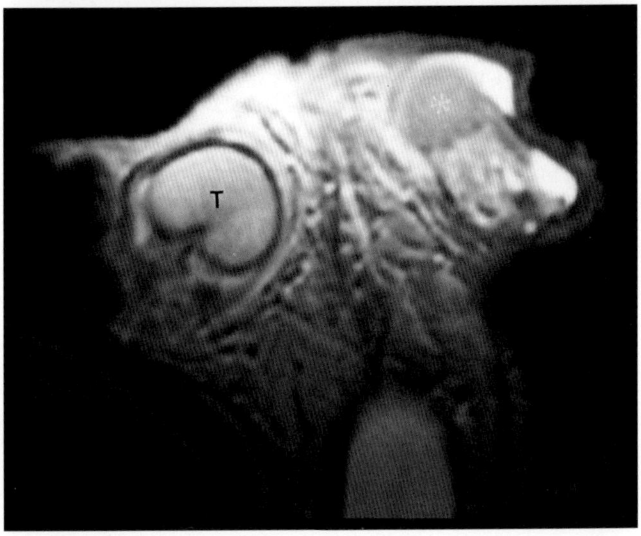

C

FIG. 5.58. Leydig cell hypertrophy of the left testis (proven by biopsy) in this 7-year-old boy with pubertas precox. US was normal. **(A)** T1-weighted and **(B)** T2-weighted images at the same level, and **(C)** T2-weighted image 1.5 cm cranially (superiorly). The right (T) and the left (*) testes are of similar size. The left testis demonstrates diffuse decrease in signal intensity. The right testis is normal. The MRI finding warranted surgical evaluation. (Hy, hydrocele)

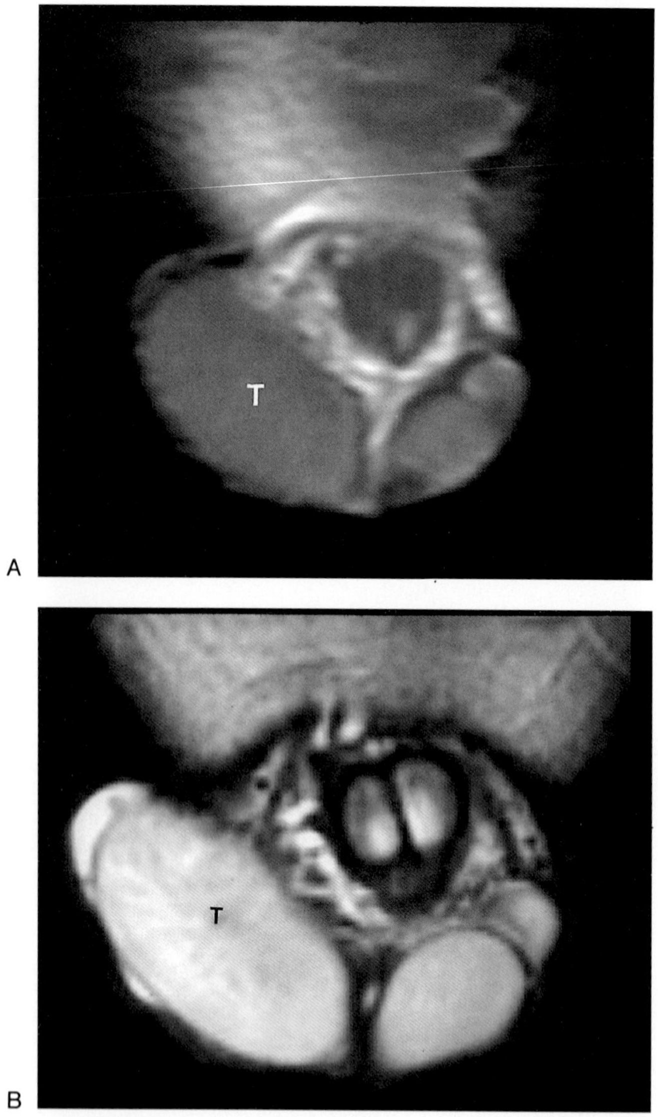

FIG. 5.59. Normal but uneven testis size in a 9-year-old boy. On physical examination, testis size was asymmetrical but consistency was normal. Ultrasound showed no abnormalities. Because of the parents' anxiety and the child's carcinophobia, MRI study was done. **(A)** T1-weighted and **(B)** T2-weighted images demonstrated an enlarged but normal-signal-intensity right testis (T), reinforcing the impression of normal variant of discordant testicular size.

Magnetic Resonance Imaging in Evaluation of Pediatric Testicular Tumors

On MRI the sensitivity and imaging findings for the pediatric testicular tumors are similar to those in adults. Prepubertal testis demonstrates high signal intensity on T2-weighted images serving as an excellent backup for the low-signal-intensity tumorous infiltration (Fig. 5.58). Localized as well as diffuse tumors are well depicted (Fig. 5.57). Although they are highly sensitive, the MRI findings are nonspecific, limiting the differentiation between benign and malignant intratesticular disease (Figs. 5.57 and 5.58).

Computed Tomography in Evaluation of Pediatric Testicular Tumors

Computed tomography is not recommended for the evaluation of intratesticular tumors, and CT findings have not been well established.

Comparative Evaluation of Pediatric Testicular Tumors

Sonography remains the primary approach in the evaluation of pediatric testicular tumors (148). The sonographic evaluation of the prepubertal testis, however, is more difficult than that in the adult, and testicular involvement in the pediatric population is often infiltrative and/or bilateral. Whenever there is a discrepancy between sonographic findings and clinical impression (Fig. 5.57), MRI study should be obtained. Better tissue contrast of MRI and an objective standard of reference for testicular signal intensity result in superior depiction of intratesticular pathology. This also applies to the cases where tumor due to an asymmetrical size of the testis needs to be excluded (Fig 5.59). CT plays no role in the evaluation of pediatric testicular disease.

REFERENCES

1. Silverberg E. Cancer in young adults (ages 15 to 34). *CA* 1982;32:32–42.
2. Presti JC, Herr HW. Genital tumors. In: Tanagho EA, McAninch JW. *Smith's general urology,* 13th ed. Norwalk, CT: Appleton & Lange; 1992:413–425.
3. American Cancer Society. *Cancer facts and figures—1993.* American Cancer Society, Atlanta, Georgia, 1993.
4. Pottern LM, Goedert JJ. Epidemiology of testicular cancer. In: Javadpour N, ed. *Principles and management of testicular cancer.* New York: Thieme; 1986:108–119.
5. Mostofi FK. Proceedings: Testicular tumors. epidemiologic, etiologic, and pathologic features. *Cancer* 1973;32:1186–1201.
6. Richie JP. Neoplasms of the testis. In: Walsh PC, Retik AB, Stamey TA, Vaughan ED, eds. *Campbell's urology,* 6th ed, vol 2. Philadelphia: WB Saunders; 1992:1222–1263.
7. Motzer RJ, Bosl GJ, Geller NL, et al. Advanced seminoma: the role of chemotherapy and adjunctive surgery. *Ann Int Med* 1988;108:513–518.
8. Einhorn LH. Treatment strategies of testicular cancer in the United States. *Int J Androl* 1987;10:399–405.
9. Weissbach L, Boedefeld EA. Localization of solitary and multiple metastases in stage II nonseminomatous testis tumor as basis for a modified staging lymph node dissection in stage I. *J Urol* 1987;138:77–82.
10. Dieckmann KP, Becker T, Bauer HW. Testicular tumors: Presentation and role of diagnostic delay. *Urol Int* 1987;42:241–247.
11. Einhorn LH, Crawford ED, Shipley WU, Loehrer RJ, Williams SD. Cancer of the testes. In: De Vita VT, Hellman S, Rosenberg SA. *Cancer: principles and practice of oncology,* 3rd ed, vol 1. Philadelphia: JB Lippincott; 1989:1071–1098.
12. Kuber W. Testicular tumor and cryptorchidism. *Eur Urol* 1982;8:280–283.

13. Dieckmann KP, Boeckmann W, Brosig W, Jonas D, Bauer HW. Bilateral testicular germ-cell tumors. Report of nine cases and a review of the literature. *Cancer* 1986;57:1254–1258.
14. Depue RH, Pike MC, Henderson BE. Estrogen exposure during gestation and risk of testicular cancer. *J Nat Cancer Inst* 1983;71: 1151–1155.
15. Dieckmann KP, Becker T, Jonas D, Bauer HW. Inheritance and testicular cancer. Arguments based on a report of three cases and a review of the literature. *Oncology* 1987;44:367–377.
16. Patel MD, Olcott EW, Kerschmann RL, Callen PW, Gooding GAW. Sonographically detected testicular microlithiasis and testicular carcinoma. *J Clin Ultrasound* 1993;21:447–452.
17. Höbarth K, Susani M, Szabo N, Kratzik C. Incidence of testicular microlithiasis. *Urology* 1992;40:464–467.
18. von der Maase H, Rorth M, Walblom-Jorgensen S, et al. Carcinoma in situ of contralateral testis in patients with testicular germ-cell cancer: study of 27 cases in 500 patients. *Br Med J Clin Res Ed* 1986;293:1398–1401.
19. Bernini G, Sgro M, Bartolommei A, et al. Retroperitoneal seminoma secondary to "burned out" testicular tumor in an acromegalic patient. *Eur J Surg Oncol* 1992;18:191–194.
20. Skakkebaek NE, Berthelsen JG, Giwercman A, Muller J. Carcinoma in situ of the testis: possible origin from gonocytes and precursor of all types of germ cell tumours except spermatocytoma. *Int J Androl* 1987;10:19–28.
21. Friedman NB, Moore RA. Tumors of the testis: a report on 922 cases. *Milit Surg* 1946;99:573–593.
22. Dixon FJ, Moore RA. Testicular tumors: a clinicopathological study. *Cancer* 1953;6:427–454.
23. Mostofi FK. Testicular tumors: epidemiologic, etiologic, and pathological features. *Cancer* 1973;32:1186–1201.
24. Loy V, Dieckmann KP. Carcinoma in situ of the testis: intratubular germ cell neoplasia or testicular intraepithelial neoplasia? *Hum Pathol* 1990;21:457–458.
25. Jacobsen GK. Histogenetic considerations concerning germ-cell tumours. Morphological and immunohistochemical comparative investigation of the human embryo and testicular germ cell tumours. *Virchows Arch Pathol Anat Histopathol* 1986;408:509–525.
26. Mostofi FK. Histological typing of testis tumours. International histological classification of tumours. No. 16. World Health Organization, Geneva 1977:15–36.
27. Pugh RCB. *Pathology of the testis*. Oxford: Blackwell, 1976.
28. Weaver DJ, Havey AD, Weinstein SH, Tully RJ. Nonpalpable occult testis tumor. *Urology* 1989;34:218–220.
29. Fowler JE, Whitmore WF. Intratesticular germ cell tumors: observations on the effect of chemotherapy. *J Urol* 1981;126:412–414.
30. Greist A, Einhorn LH, Williams SD, Donohue JP, Rowland RG. Pathologic findings at orchiectomy following chemotherapy for disseminated testicular cancer. *J Clin Oncol* 1984;2:1025–1029.
31. Snow BW, Rowland RG, Donohue JP, Einhorn LH, Williams SD. Review of delayed orchiectomy in patients with disseminated testis tumors. *J Urol* 1983;129:522–523.
32. Shawker TH, Javadpour N, O'Leary T, Shapiro E, Krudy AG. Ultrasonographic detection of "burned-out" primary testicular germ cell tumors in clinically normal testes. *J Ultrasound Med* 1983;2:477–479.
33. van der Hem KG, Boven E, van Hennik MB, Pinedo HM. Malignant Leydig cell tumor of the testis in complete remission on o, p'-dichlorodiphenyl-dichloroethane. *J Urol* 1992;148:1256–1259.
34. Düe W, Dieckmann KP, Loy V, Stein H. Immunohistological determination of oestrogen receptor, progesterone receptor, and intermediate filaments in Leydig cell tumours, Leydig cell hyperplasia, and normal Leydig cells of the human testis. *J Pathol* 1989;157:225–234.
35. Gabrilove JL, Nicolis GL, Mitty HA, Sohval AR. Feminizing interstitial cell tumor of the testis: personal observations and a review of the literature. *Cancer* 1975;35:1184–1202.
36. Kaufman E, Akiya F, Foucar E, Grambort F, Cartwright KC: Virilization due to Leydig cell tumor diagnosis by magnetic resonance imaging. case management report. *Clin Pediatr* 1990;29: 414–417.
37. Gabrilove JL, Freiberg EK, Leiter E, Nicolis GL. Feminizing and non-feminizing Sertoli cell tumors. *J Urol* 1980;124:757–767.
38. Sharma S, Seam RK, Kapoor HL. Malignant Sertoli cell tumor of the testis in a child. *J Surg Oncol* 1990;44:129–131.
39. Cortez JC, Kaplan GW. Gonadal stromal tumors, gonadoblastomas, epidermoid cysts, and secondary tumors of the testis in children. *Urol Clin North Am* 1993;20:15–26.
40. Hsueh C, Gonzalez-Crussi F, Murphy SB. Testicular angiocentric lymphoma of postthymic T-cell type in a child with T-cell acute lymphoblastic leukemia in remission. *Cancer* 1993;72:1801–1805.
41. Armenakas NA, Schevchuk MM, Brodherson M, Fracchia JA. AIDS presenting as primary testicular lymphoma. *Urology* 1992;40:162–164.
42. Ritzen EM. Testicular relapse of acute lymphoblastic leukemia (ALL). *J Reprod Immunol* 1990;18:117–121.
43. Musmanno MC, White JM. Scrotal ultrasonography as adjunct to testis biopsy in leukemia. *Urology* 1990;35:239–241.
44. Dieckmann KP, Düe W, Loy V. Intrascrotal metastasis of renal cell carcinoma. Case reports and review of the literature. *Eur Urol* 1988;15:297–301.
45. Kromann-Andersen B, Hansen LB, Larsen PN, et al. Clinical versus ultrasonographic evaluation of scrotal disorders. *Br J Urol* 1988;61:350–353.
46. Benson CB. The role of ultrasound in diagnosis and staging of testicular cancer. *Semin Urology* 1988;6:189–202.
47. Fournier GR, Laing FC, Jeffrey RB, McAninch JW. High resolution scrotal ultrasonography: a highly sensitive but nonspecific diagnostic technique. *J Urol* 1985;134:490–493.
48. Benson CB, Doubilet PM, Richie JP. Sonography of the male genital tract. *AJR* 1989;153:705–713.
49. Kratzik C, Hainz A, Kuber W, et al. Sonographic appearance of benign intratesticular lesions. *Eur Urol* 1988;15:196–199.
50. Rifkin MD, Kurtz AB, Pasto ME, Goldberg BB. Diagnostic capabilities of high-resolution scrotal ultrasonography: prospective evaluation. *J Ultrasound Med* 1985;4:13–19.
51. Snyder HM, D'Angio GJ, Evans AE, Raney RB. Pediatric oncology. In: Walsh PC, Retik AB, Stamey TA, Vaughan ED, eds. *Campbell's urology*, 6th ed. Philadelphia: WB Saunders; 1992: 1967–2014.
52. McAlister WH, Sisler CL. Scrotal sonography in infants and children. Current problems in diagnostic radiology, vol 19, no 6. St Louis: Mosby–Year Book; 1990.
53. Schwerk WB, Schwerk WN, Rodeck G. Testicular tumors: prospective analysis of real-time US patterns and abdominal staging. *Radiology* 1987;164:369–374.
54. Horstman WG, Melson GL, Middleton WD, Andriole GL. Testicular tumors: findings with color Doppler US. *Radiology* 1992;185:733–737.
55. Mitchell DG. Color doppler imaging: principles, limitations, and artifacts. *Radiology* 1990;177:1–10.
56. Grantham JG, Charboneau JW, James EM, et al. Testicular neoplasms: 29 tumors studied by high-resolution US. *Radiology* 1985;157:775–780.
57. Hricak H, Filly RA. Sonography of the scrotum. *Invest Radiol* 1983;18:112–121.
58. Bockrath JM, Schaeffer AJ, Kies MS, Neiman HL. Ultrasound identification of impalpable testicle tumor. *J Urol* 1983;130:355–356.
59. Bohle A, Studer UE, Sonntag RW, Scheidegger JR. Primary or secondary extragonadal germ cell tumors? *J Urol* 1986;135:939–943.
60. Glazer HS, Lee JK, Melson GL, McClennan BL. Sonographic detection of occult testicular neoplasms. *AJR* 1982;138:673–675.
61. Hendry WS, Garvie WH, Ah-See AK, Bayliss AP. Ultrasonic detection of occult testicular neoplasms in patients with gynaecomastia. *Br J Radiol* 1984;57:571–572.
62. Gross GW, Rohner TJ, Lombard JS, Abrams CS. Metastatic seminoma with regression of testicular primary: ultrasonographic detection. *J Urol* 1986;136:1086–1088.
63. Daugaard G, von der Maase H, Olsen J, Rorth M, Skakkebaek NE. Carcinoma in situ testis in patients with assumed extragonadal germ-cell tumours. *Lancet II* 1987;2(8558):528–530.
64. Trias I, Algaba F, Hocsman H. Intratubular germ cell tumor. Re-

lation with "burned-out" tumor and testicular germinal neoplasia. *Eur Urol* 1991;19:81–84.
65. Portalez D, Song MY, Marty MH, Joffre F. Ultrasonographic patterns of testicular non-Hodgkin's lymphoma: a report of five cases. *Eur J Radiol* 1982;2:222–225.
66. Tweed CS, Peck RJ. A sonographic appearance of testicular lymphoma. *Clin Radiol* 1991;43:341–342.
67. Phillips G, Kumari-Subaiya S, Sawitsky A. Ultrasonic evaluation of the scrotum in lymphoproliferative disease. *J Ultrasound Med* 1987;6:169–175.
68. Lupetin AR, King W, Rich P, Lederman RB. Ultrasound diagnosis of testicular leukemia. *Radiology* 1983;146:171–172.
69. Rayor RA, Scheible W, Brock WA, Leopold GR. High resolution ultrasonography in the diagnosis of testicular relapse in patients with acute lymphoblastic leukemia. *J Urol* 1982;128:602–603.
70. Hricak H. The testis. In: Hricak H, Carrington BM. *MRI of the pelvis: a text atlas*. London: Martin Dunitz; 1991:343–381.
71. Emory TH, Charboneau JW, Randall RV, Scheithauer BW, Grantham JG. Occult testicular interstitial-cell tumor in a patient with gynecomastia: ultrasonic detection. *Radiology* 1984;151: 474.
72. Baker WC, Bishai MB, DeVere White RW. Misleading testicular masses. *Urology* 1988;31:111–113.
73. Rifkin MD, Kurtz AB, Pasto ME, et al. The sonographic diagnosis of focal and diffuse infiltrating intrascrotal lesions. *Urol Radiol* 1984;6:20–26.
74. Kaiser WA, Reinges M, Miersch WD, Reiser MF, Hahn D. Dynamic MR imaging of benign and malignant lesions in testes. Presented at the 79th Scientific Assembly and Annual Meeting of the Radiological Society of North America, Chicago, 1993.
75. Johnson JO, Mattrey RF, Phillipson J. Differentiation of seminomatous from nonseminomatous testicular tumors with MR imaging. *AJR* 1990;154:539–543.
76. Cramer BM, Schlegel EA, Thueroff JW. MR imaging in the differential diagnosis of scrotal and testicular disease. *Radiographics* 1991;11:9–21.
77. Lorigan JG, Shirkhoda A, Dexeus FH. CT and MR imaging of malignant germ cell tumor of the undescended testis. *Urol Radiol* 1989;11:113–117.
78. Mattrey R, Trambert M. MR imaging of the scrotum and testis. In: Edelman RR, Hesselink JR, eds. *Clinical magnetic resonance imaging*. Philadelphia: WB Saunders; 1990:952–979.
79. Baker LL, Hajek PC, Burkhard TK, et al. MR imaging of the scrotum: pathologic conditions. *Radiology* 1987;163: 92–98.
80. Derouet VH, Braedel HU, Ziegler M, Zwergel Th, Khorsandian Ch. Computertomographische Untersuchungen des Scrotalinhaltes, insbesondere des Hodens. Fortschr. *Röentgenstr* 1988; 148:566–571.
81. International Union Against Cancer (UICC). *TNM atlas: illustrated guide to the TNM/pTNM—classification of malignant tumors*, 3rd ed. Berlin: Springer-Verlag, 1989.
82. Fung CY, Kalish LA, Brodsky GL, Richie JP, Garnick MB. Stage I nonseminomatous germ-cell testicular tumor: prediction of metastatic potential by primary histopathology. *J Clin Oncol* 1988;6:1467–1473.
83. Hoeltl W, Kosak D, Pont J, et al. Testicular cancer: prognostic implications of vascular invasion. *J Urol* 1987;137:683–685.
84. Johnson DE. Clinical staging. In: Donohue JP. *Testis tumors*. Baltimore: Williams & Wilkins; 1983:131–144.
85. Richter E, Feyerabend T. Pelvic and inguinal region. In: Richter E, Feyerabend T. *Normal lymph node topography: CT atlas*. Berlin: Springer-Verlag, 1991:113–147.
86. Heiken JP, Balfe DM, McClennan BL. Testicular tumors: oncologic imaging and diagnosis. *Int J Radiation Oncol Biol Phys* 1984;10:275–287.
87. Stein M, Steiner M, Suprun H, Robinson E. Inguinal lymph node metastases from testicular tumor. *J Urol* 1985;134:144–145.
88. Ramon Y, Cajal S, Pinango L, Barat A, Moldenhauer F, Olivia H. Metastatic pure choriocarcinoma of the testis in an elderly man. *J Urol* 1987;137:516–519.
89. Johnson DE, Appelt G, Samuels ML, Luna M. Metastases from testicular carcinoma: study of 78 autopsied cases. *Urology* 1976;8:234–239.
90. Poskitt KJ, Cooperberg PL, Sullivan LD. Sonography and CT in staging nonseminomatous testicular tumors. *AJR* 1985;144:939–944.
91. Samuelsson L, Forsberg L, Olsson AM. Accuracy of radiological staging procedures in non-seminomatous testis cancer compared with findings from surgical exploration and histopathological studies of extirpated tissue. *Br J Radiol* 1986;59:131–134.
92. Javadpour N. Overview of testicular cancer. In: Javadpour N, ed. *Principles and management of testicular cancer*. New York: Thieme; 1986:1–12.
93. Richie JP. Clinical stage I testicular cancer: the role of modified retroperitoneal lymphadenectomy. *J Urol* 1990;144:1160–1163.
94. Scoutt LM, McCarthy SM, Moss AA. Computed tomography and magnetic resonance imaging of the pelvis. In: Moss AA, Gamsu G, Genant HK. *Computed tomography of the body with magnetic resonance imaging*, 2nd ed, vol 3. Philadelphia: WB Saunders; 1992:1183–1265.
95. Stomper PC, Socinski MA, Kaplan WD, Garnick MB. Failure patterns of nonseminomatous testicular germ cell tumors: radiographic analysis of 51 cases. *Radiology* 1988;167:641–646.
96. Heiken JP. Tumors of the testis and testicular adnexa. In: Pollack HM. *Clinical urography: an atlas and textbook of urological imaging*, vol 2. Philadelphia: WB Saunders; 1990:1414–1441.
97. Coscojuela P, Llauger J, Pérez C, Germá J, Castañer E. The growing teratoma syndrome: radiologic findings in four cases. *Eur J Radiol* 1991;12:138–140.
98. Sagalowsky AI, Ewalt DH, Molberg K, Peters PC. Predictors of residual mass histology after chemotherapy for advanced testis cancer. *Urology* 1990;35:537–542.
99. Donohue JP, Rowland RG, Kopecky K, et al. Correlation of computed tomographic changes and histological findings in 80 patients having radical retroperitoneal lymph node dissection after chemotherapy for testis cancer. *J Urol* 1987;137:1176–1179.
100. Thurnher S, Hricak H, Carroll PR, Pobiel RS, Filly RA. Imaging the testis: comparison between MR imaging and US. *Radiology* 1988;167: 631–636.
101. Ellis JH, Bies JR, Kopecky KK, Klatte EC, Rowland RG, Donohue JP. Comparison of NMR and CT imaging in the evaluation of metastatic retroperitoneal lymphadenopathy from testicular carcinoma. *JCAT* 1984;8:709–719.
102. Crawford ED, Mettler FA, Duncan PR. Retrocrural lymphadenopathy in testicular cancer. *J Urol* 1984;131:343–345.
103. Husband JE, Peckham MJ, MacDonald JS. The role of abdominal computed tomography in the management of testicular tumors. *Comput Tomogr* 1980;4:1–16.
104. Crawford SM, Rustin GJS, Begent RHJ, Newlands ES, Bagshawe KD. Safety of surveillance in the management of stage I anaplastic germ cell tumors of the testis. *Br J of Urol* 1988;61:250–253.
105. Charig MJ, Hindley AC, Lloyd K, Golding SJ. 'Watch policy' in patients with suspected stage I testicular seminoma: CT as a sole staging and surveillance technique. *Clin Radiol* 1990;42:40–41.
106. Scatarige JC, Fishman EK, Kuhajda FP, Taylor GA, Sigelman SS. Low attenuation nodal metastases in testicular carcinoma. *JCAT* 1983;7:682–687.
107. Stanton GF, Bosl GJ, Whitmore WF Jr, et al. VAB-6 as initial treatment of patients with advanced seminoma. *J Clin Oncol* 1985;3:336–339.
108. Tesoro-Tess JD, Pizzocaro G, Zanoni F, Musumeci R. Lymphangiography and computed tomography in testicular carcinoma: how accurate in early stage disease? *J Urol* 1985;133:967–970.
109. Leung ML, Gooding GAW, Williams RD: high-resolution sonography of scrotal contents in asymptomatic subjects. *AJR* 1984;143:161–164.
110. Hamm B, Fobbe F, Loy V. Testicular cysts: differentiation with US and clinical findings. *Radiology* 1988;168:19–23.
111. Gooding GA, Leonhardt W, Stein R. Testicular cysts: US findings. *Radiology* 1987;163:537–538.
112. Altadonna V, Snyder HM, Rosenberg HK, Duckett JW. Simple cysts of the testis in children: preoperative diagnosis by ultrasound and excision with testicular preservation. *J Urol* 1988;140: 1505–1507.
113. Dmochowski RR, Rudy DC, Weitzner S, Corriere JN. Simple cyst of the testis. *J Urol* 1989;142:1078–1081.

114. Tammela TL, Karttunen TJ, Mattila SI, Mäkäräinen HP, Hellström PA, Kontturi MJ. Cysts of the tunica albuginea—more common testicular masses than previously thought? *Br J Urol* 1991;68:280–284.
115. Redman JF, Rountree GA. Bilateral cysts of tunica albuginea of testes. *Urology* 1988;32:259–261.
116. Mancilla-Jimenez R, Matsuda GT. Cysts of the tunica albuginea. Report of 4 cases and review of the literature. *J Urol* 1975;114:730–733.
117. Mennemeyer RP, Mason JT. Non-neoplastic cystic lesions of the tunica albuginea: an electron microscopic and clinical study of 2 cases. *J Urol* 1979;121:373–375.
118. Yalowitz BR, Eble JN, Wilks DC. Spermatozoa-containing simple cysts of the rete testis. *J Urol* 1989;142:1572–1573.
119. Cho CS, Kosek J. Cystic dysplasia of the testis: sonographic and pathologic findings. *Radiology* 1985;156:777–778.
120. Nistal M, Regadera J, Paniagua R. Cystic dysplasia of the testis. Light and electron microscopic study of three cases. *Arch Pathol Lab Med* 1984;108:579–583.
121. Reinberg Y, Manivel JC, Llerena J, Niehans G, Fraley EE. Epidermoid cyst (monodermal teratoma) of the testis. *Br J Urol* 1990;66:648–651.
122. Maxwell AJ, Mamtora H. Sonographic appearance of epidermoid cyst of the testis. *J Clin Ultrasound* 1990;18:188–190.
123. Berger Y, Srinivas V, Hajdu SI, Herr HW. Epidermoid cysts of the testis: role of conservative surgery. *J Urol* 1985;134:962–963.
124. Malek RS, Rosen JS, Farrow GM. Epidermoid cyst of the testis: a critical analysis. *Br J Urol* 1986;58:55–59.
125. Schlecker BA, Siegel A, Weiss J,Wein AJ . Epidermoid cyst of the testis: a surgical approach for testicular preservation. *J Urol* 1985;133:610–611.
126. Goldstein AM, Mendez R, Vargas A, Terry R. Epidermoid cysts of testis. *Urology* 1980;15:186–189.
127. Kaasinen E, Taavitsainen M, Lehtonen T. Epidermoid cyst of the testis. Case report with a review of the literature. *Eur Urol* 1988;15:141–143.
128. Poster RB, Spirt BA, Tamsen A, Surya BV. Complex tunica albuginea cyst simulating an intratesticular lesion. *Urol Radiol* 1991;13:129–132.
129. Malvica RP. Epidermoid cyst of the testicle: an unusual sonographic finding. *AJR* 1993;160:1047–1048.
130. Meiches MD, Nurenberg P. Sonographic appearance of a calcified simple epidermoid cyst of the testis. *J Clin Ultrasound* 1991;19:498–500.
131. Cohen EL, Mandel E, Goodman JD, Carr L, Feigin G, Dikman S. Epidermoid cyst of the testicle. Ultrasonographic characteristics. *Urology* 1984;24:79–81.
132. Cunnah D, Perry L, Dacie JA, et al. Bilateral testicular tumors in congenital adrenal hyperplasia: a continuing diagnostic and therapeutic dilemma. *Clin Endocrinol* 1989;30:141–147.
133. Kirkland RT, Kirkland JL, Keenan BS, Bongiovanni AM, Rosenberg HS, Clayton GW. Bilateral testicular tumors in congenital adrenal hyperplasia. *J Clin Endocrinol Metab* 1977;44:369–378.
134. Seidenwurm D, Smathers RL, Kan P, Hoffman A. Intratesticular adrenal rests diagnosed by ultrasound. *Radiology* 1985;155:479–481.
135. Friedrichs R, Rbben H, Lutzeyer W. Differential diagnosis and therapy of rare testicular tumors. *Eur Urol* 1986;12:217–223.
136. Petersen RO. *Urologic pathology*. Philadelphia: JB Lippincott; 1986.
137. Weingarten BJ, Kellman GM, Middleton WD, Gross ML. Tubular ectasia within the mediastinum testis. *J Ultrasound Med* 1992;11:349–353.
138. Brown DL, Benson CB, Doherty FJ, et al. Cystic testicular mass caused by dilated rete testis: sonographic findings in 31 cases. *AJR* 1992;158:1257–1259.
139. Tartar VM, Trambert MA, Balsara ZN, Mattrey RF. Tubular ectasia of the testicle: sonographic and MR imaging appearance. *AJR* 1993;160:539–542.
140. Thomas RD, Dewbury KC. Ultrasound appearances of the rete testis. *Clin Radiol* 1993;47:121–124.
141. Martin B, Tubiana JM. Significance of scrotal calcifications detected by sonography. *J Clin Ultrasound* 1988;16:545–552.
142. Mullins TL, Sant GR, Ucci AA, Doherty FJ. Testicular microlithiasis occurring in postorchiopexy testis. *Urology* 1986;27:144–146.
143. Vick CW, Bird KI, Rosenfield AT, Viscomi GN, Taylor KJ. Scrotal masses with a uniformly hyperechoic pattern. *Radiology* 1983;148:209–211.
144. Janzen DL, Mathieson JR, Marsh JI, et al. Testicular microlithiasis: sonographic and clinical features. *AJR* 1992;158:1057–1060.
145. Jaramillo D, Perez-Atayde A, Teele RL. Sonography of testicular microlithiasis. *Urol Radiol* 1989;11:55–57.
146. Weissbach L, Altwein JE, Stiens R. Germinal testicular tumors in childhood. Report of observations and literature review. *Eur Urol* 1984;10:73–85.
147. Barth RA, Teele RL, Colodny A, Retik A, Bauer S. Asymptomatic scrotal masses in children. *Radiology* 1984;152:65–68.
148. Kratzik C, Kuber W, Donner G, Lunglmayr G, Frick J, Schmoller HJ. Impact of sonography on diagnosis of scrotal diseases: a multicenter study. *Eur Urol* 1988;14:270–275.
149. Klein EA, Kay R, Norris DG, George CR, Richmond B. Noninvasive testicular screening in childhood leukemia. *J Urol* 1986;136:864–866.

CHAPTER 6

The Acute Scrotum

Acute scrotum is a broad term encompassing clinical conditions characterized by the sudden onset of scrotal symptoms—particularly pain, swelling, and reddening—that may occur alone or in any combination. From a clinical point of view, it is essential to differentiate, as early as possible, conditions (such as testicular torsion or rupture) that require immediate surgery from those (such as epididymitis) that are adequately treated by antibiotic therapy.

Physical examination of the acute scrotum is limited by swelling or pain. Clinical history (e.g., trauma) may play a crucial role in identifying the causes of acute scrotal abnormalities. Various imaging modalities can also be used to facilitate the notoriously difficult identification of the underlying cause in acute scrotum, but surgery should not be delayed if findings are equivocal. One of the common causes of an acute scrotum is testicular torsion, a condition that requires prompt surgical intervention (detorsion) to prevent necrosis.

The following guidelines are considered golden rules for evaluating patients with acute, nontraumatic scrotal abnormalities:

1. Testicular torsion is the most common cause of acute scrotum in children.
2. In patients presenting with acute scrotal symptoms, swelling and/or pain must be considered indicative of testicular torsion until proven otherwise. It is important to remember that trauma does not exclude the possibility of torsion.
3. The extent of testicular damage is determined mainly by the degree of torsion and, to a lesser extent, by its duration. In severe ischemia the germinal epithelium is irreversibly damaged after only 2 hours.
4. Undescended testicles undergo torsion 13 times more frequently than those in the scrotum.
5. Extravaginal torsion is most common in neonates and infants, and intravaginal torsion is most common just before and during puberty. Appendiceal torsion is most common in school-age children.
6. Testicular pain may radiate to the abdomen, and the diagnostic evaluation of infants and children with acute abdominal symptoms must always include the scrotum.
7. In torsion, pain occurs before swelling. In inflammatory processes, however, swelling is the leading symptom.
8. Testicular tumors may also mimic an acute scrotum, especially if a patient "suddenly" discovers a scrotal swelling or painful mass.

The major causes of an acute scrotum are (in descending order of incidence):

- Acute inflammation (e.g., epididymitis, orchitis, abscess)
- Testicular torsion
- Torsion of the appendix epididymis or testis
- Trauma
- Incarcerated inguinal hernia
- Testicular tumor
- Testicular vasculitis, infarction

Other less common scrotal and abdominoscrotal disorders that may also present with the characteristics of an acute scrotum include idiopathic scrotal edema, thrombophlebitis of the pampiniform plexus, necrosis of the intrascrotal fatty tissue, meconium periorchitis, and appendicitis in a hernial sac. These are, however, rare conditions. The following discussion focuses on the diagnostic considerations of acute inflammation and infection, testicular and appendiceal torsion, and trauma. In the miscellaneous grouping the discussion addresses meconium periorchitis, vasculitis and testicular infarcts, and necrosis of the intrascrotal fatty tissue. Incarcerated inguinal hernia is discussed in Chapter 8, and testicular tumors are discussed in Chapter 5.

A. Inflammation and Infection

EPIDIDYMITIS AND ORCHITIS

Of all pathologic processes involving the epididymis, epididymitis is the most common cause of the acutely swollen and painful scrotum in adult men. Epididymitis can often be diagnosed on the basis of the clinical findings and urine analysis. Imaging may be used to (1) determine the extent of the inflammatory process, especially with regard to possible involvement of the testis (epididymo-orchitis); (2) confirm the diagnosis of inflammatory process in a patient with poor or no response to antibiotic treatment; (3) exclude abscess formation; and (4) follow up patients with complicated disease. Acute epididymitis is defined as a pathologic condition of inflammation, pain, and swelling of the epididymis of less than 6 weeks' duration (1). Chronic epididymitis, on the other hand, represents irreversible end-stage epididymitis, characterized by long-standing pain in the epididymis and testis, usually without swelling (1).

Acute nonspecific epididymitis is almost always caused by descending, intracanalicular spread of pathogens in patients with prostatitis, urethritis, or other urinary tract infections. Lymphogenous or hematogenous spread from a bacterial focus is rare. In children and older men the disease is most frequently caused by nonsexually transmitted organisms, including *E. coli, Proteus*, enterococci, *Pseudomonas aeruginosa*, and (less often) staphylococci. Structural urologic abnormalities most likely play a role in such cases (2). In young men (under 35 years of age), sexually transmitted organisms such as gonococci (*N. gonorrhoeae*), chlamydia (*C. trachomatis*), and mycoplasma (*M. hominis*) are most often found (3,4). Rarely, epididymitis is caused by systemic disease, such as **tuberculosis**, *Cryptococcus*, and *Brucella*. Coexistent **orchitis** is found in up to 20% of patients with epididymitis. Isolated orchitis is rare except when caused by a viral infection such as mumps. **Mumps orchitis**, the most common form of infectious orchitis, occurs in postpubertal males, usually associated with parotitis. **Idiopathic granulomatous orchitis**—nonspecific (apparently noninfectious) inflammation of the testis—occurs in middle-aged and older men, and clinically often mimics testicular tumor. Inflammation usually begins in the tail of the epididymis and may spread to the rest of the epididymis and into the testis.

Chronic epididymitis must be differentiated from epididymal tumors, epididymal tuberculosis, and spermatocele. It is also necessary to exclude testicular tumor from the diagnosis.

Clinical Presentation

Acute Epididymitis

The patient with acute inflammation of the epididymis presents with pain, fever, and progressive swelling of the scrotal contents accompanied by erythema and scrotal edema. Severe scrotal pain develops abruptly and may radiate to the ipsilateral groin and flank area. Dysuria, pyuria, fever, and other signs and symptoms of urethritis or prostatitis often accompany epididymitis (5). On physical examination early in the course, the epididymis can be palpated as an enlarged, indurated, tender structure. A few hours after the onset of symptoms, it is palpated as one enlarged mass not separable from the testis (4). The spermatic cord is usually swollen and tender. Chronic pain, infarction, abscess or gangrene formation, infertility and testicular atrophy may complicate acute epididymitis (6). Pyocele may also occur and is usually associated with pyogenic testicular abscess.

It is often difficult to differentiate acute epididymitis from torsion of the spermatic cord or testicular tumor on a clinical basis. Since a diagnostic delay in patients with testicular torsion may hamper salvage of a testis, accurate diagnosis is very important. Unfortunately, misdiagnosis is common, especially in men under 35 years of age, in whom both epididymitis and torsion are common. After this age, torsion occurs infrequently, whereas epididymitis is common. Since epididymitis is rare in prepubertal boys, torsion is the prime diagnostic consideration of the cause of an acute scrotal pain in children.

Clinically, scrotal pain associated with epididymitis is usually relieved when the scrotum is elevated over the symphysis (**Prehn's sign**) (4). This may help in clinically differentiating between epididymitis and torsion of the spermatic cord, in which scrotal pain is aggravated with this maneuver. The presence of urethritis and swelling confined to the distal epididymis further helps a clinical diagnosis of epididymitis. However, in 15% of patients,

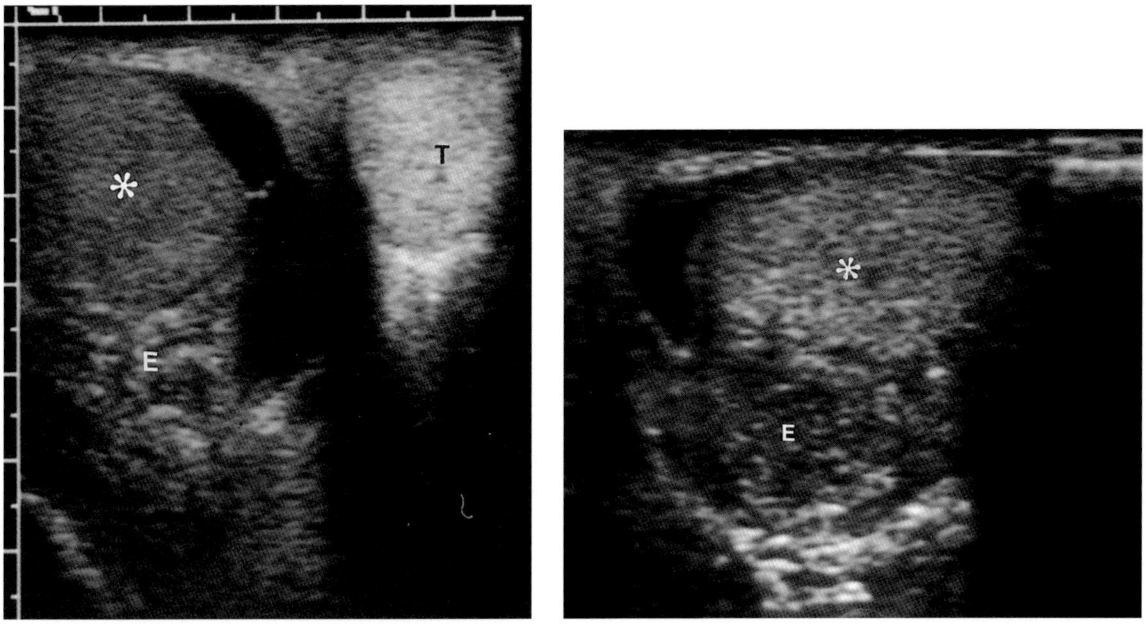

A B

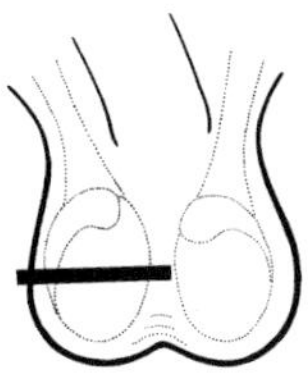

FIG. 6.1. Acute epididymo-orchitis in a 29-year-old patient. **(A)** Transverse and **(B)** longitudinal scans demonstrate markedly enlarged and hypoechoic body of the epididymis (E). The right testis (*) is also enlarged and uniformly hypoechoic. The left testis (T) is normal.

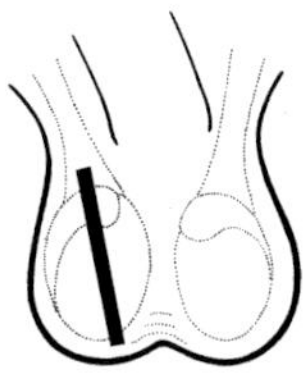

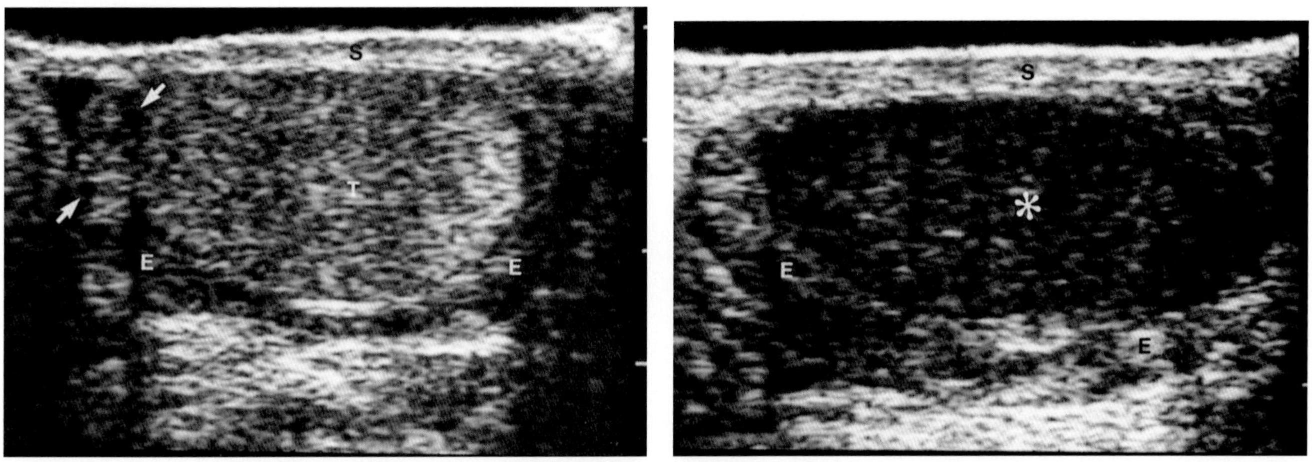

A B

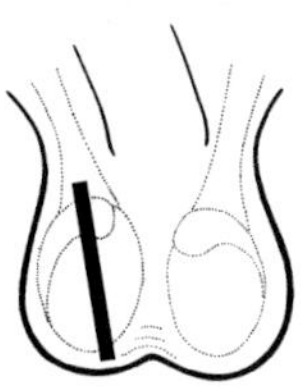

FIG. 6.2. Orchitis secondary to epididymitis in a 56-year-old patient. Longitudinal sonogram of **(A)** the right and **(B)** left scrotum. Compared with the normal right testis (T) and epididymis (E), epididymo-orchitis on the left is associated with enlargement and heterogeneous echogenicity of the epididymis (E) and generalized, homogeneous hypoechogenicity of the testis (*). (S, scrotal skin; *arrows*, small epididymal cysts)

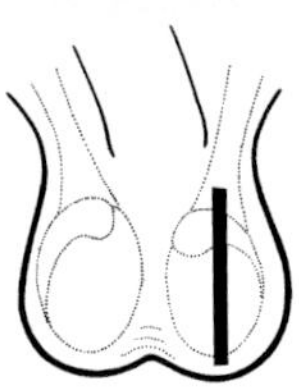

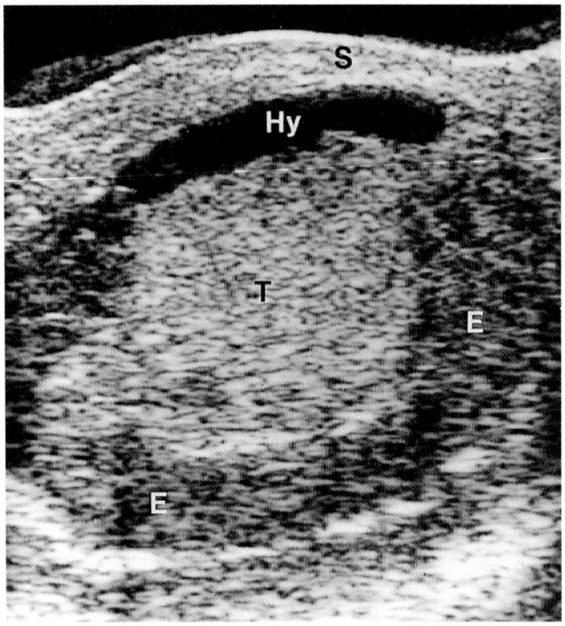

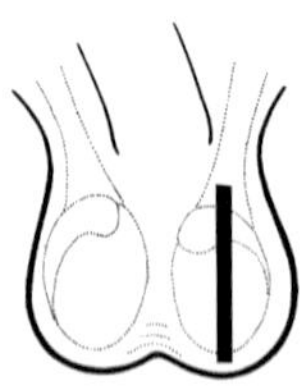

FIG. 6.3. Acute epididymitis in a 55-year-old patient. The entire left epididymis is enlarged (E) and demonstrates diffusely hypoechoic coarse and inhomogeneous echo pattern. (Hy, hydrocele; S, moderate edema of the scrotal skin) The testis (T) retains its normal echotexture.

early torsion also presents with localized swelling of the epididymis, compromising clinical differentiation between the two entities (7).

Indirect signs of inflammation—reactive hydrocele and thickening of the scrotal skin—are seen in most cases (8). Hydrocele is a nonspecific finding, however, since it may be present without inflammation or in association with torsion or tumor. Edematous and inflammatory thickening of the scrotal skin may be helpful in differentiating an acute inflammatory condition from a tumorous lesion. It is important to remember, however, that scrotal skin thickening may also occur in testicular torsion and that it may be absent in chronic inflammation.

Epididymitis should be treated promptly with antimicrobial drugs. If adequately treated, acute epididymitis may resolve completely without any sequelae. If untreated, an inflammatory tumorous conglomeration develops, precluding differentiation of the testis and epididymis on palpation. Epididymitis may then evolve into an orchitis and/or **epididymal** or **scrotal abscess**. When an abscess is large enough, it is palpated as a fluctuation. Although severe infection often results in abscess, spread of the infectious process into the testis (**epididymo-orchitis**) is not as common. Tenderness and swelling of the spermatic cord are not uncommon, and a reactive hydrocele often develops. Laboratory tests generally demonstrate pronounced leukocytosis, bacteriuria, and leukocyturia. Eventually, untreated disease develops into chronic epididymitis.

Chronic Epididymitis

Chronic epididymitis is characterized by persistent or recurrent dragging pain in the scrotal area. On palpation, the epididymis is moderately tender and indurated and can be differentiated from the testis. Most patients present with a history of recurrent urinary tract infection.

Sperm granuloma, a subtype of chronic, nonspecific epididymitis, is a granulomatous inflammation that de-

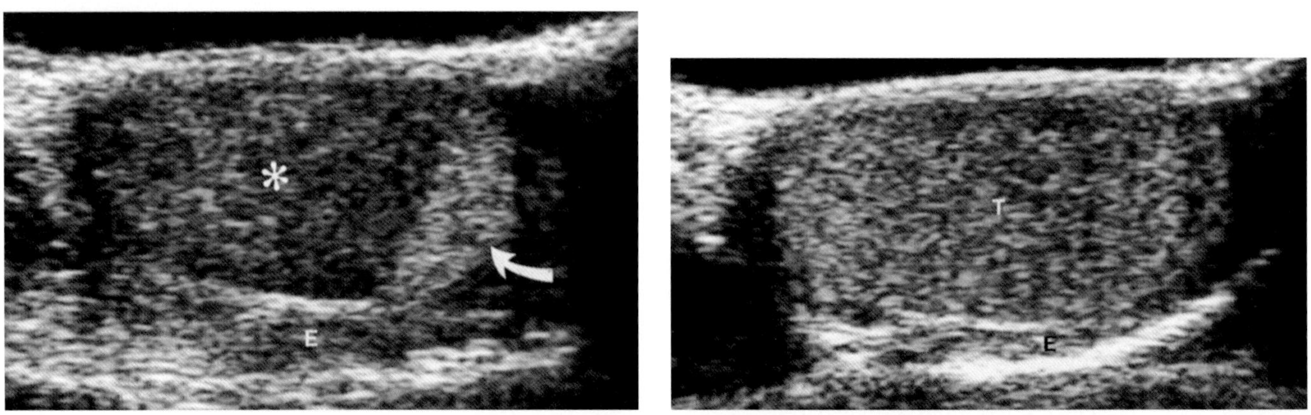

A B

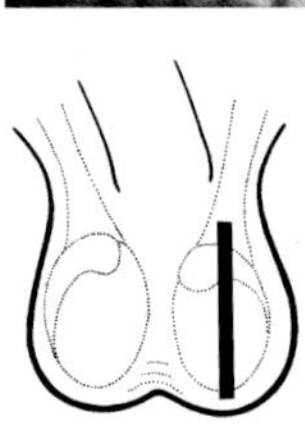

FIG. 6.4. Epididymo-orchitis in a 24-year-old patient. **(A)** A sonogram taken during the acute stage of inflammation shows enlarged epididymis (E) and focal homogeneously decreased echogenicity (*) of the upper and middle portion of the testis with normal echotexture (*arrow*) in the lower pole. **(B)** Follow-up sonogram 1 month later shows normal appearance of the testis (T) and epididymis (E) after an uncomplicated clinical course.

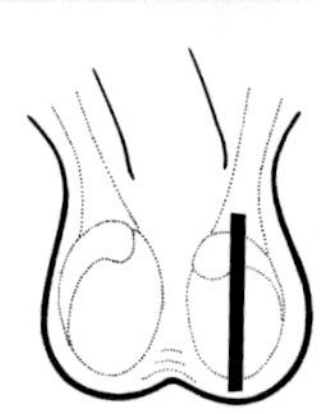

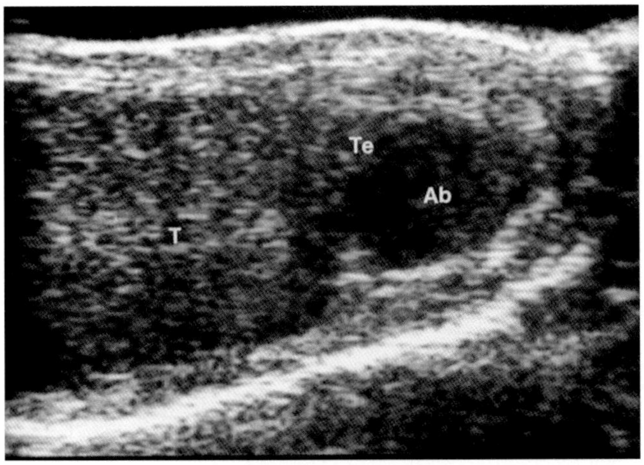

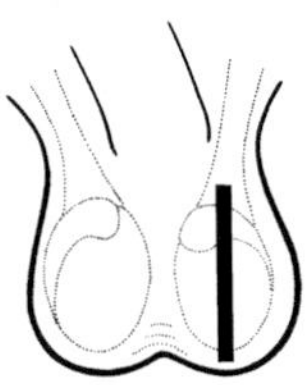

FIG. 6.5. Epididymal abscess subsequent to epididymitis in a 59-year-old patient. A circumscribed hypoechoic lesion (Ab) is seen in the enlarged tail of the epididymis (Te). The adjacent lower pole of the testis (T) retains its normal echotexture.

velops around interstitial sperm extravasated from damaged tubules. A sperm granuloma commonly presents as a roundish mass, which does not transilluminate. It most commonly occurs in the epididymal head.

Chronic inflammatory or granulomatous lesions of the epididymis may also occur as a reaction to prolonged obstruction of the efferent sperm ducts following vasectomy (9). They may or may not be associated with pain or other symptoms and are often palpated in the tail and body of the epididymis.

Treatment of chronic epididymitis includes management of underlying urinary tract infection or prostatitis and antimicrobial agents in case of acute exacerbation. In the later stages of the disease, surgery may be necessary (10).

Ultrasound in the Evaluation of Inflammation

During the **acute stage** the epididymis is markedly enlarged and may reach a transverse diameter of up to 30 mm (Fig. 6.1). Depending on the extent of the inflammatory process, either the entire organ is enlarged or swelling is confined to the tail area (Figs. 6.2 and 6.3). Although the testis and epididymis cannot be palpated separately, differentiation should be possible on ultrasound.

The acutely inflamed epididymis usually has an inhomogeneous texture with a coarse distribution of echoes (Figs. 6.2 and 6.3). Compared with the normal testis, the echogenicity of the epididymis is typically reduced (Figs. 6.1 and 6.3), but it may occasionally be increased (Fig. 6.2) (possibly because of small epididymal hemorrhages) (10–13). Successful therapy leads to a reduction in size, and in most cases, the epididymis will regain its normal shape, size, and echogenicity (Fig. 6.4). Abnormal ultra-

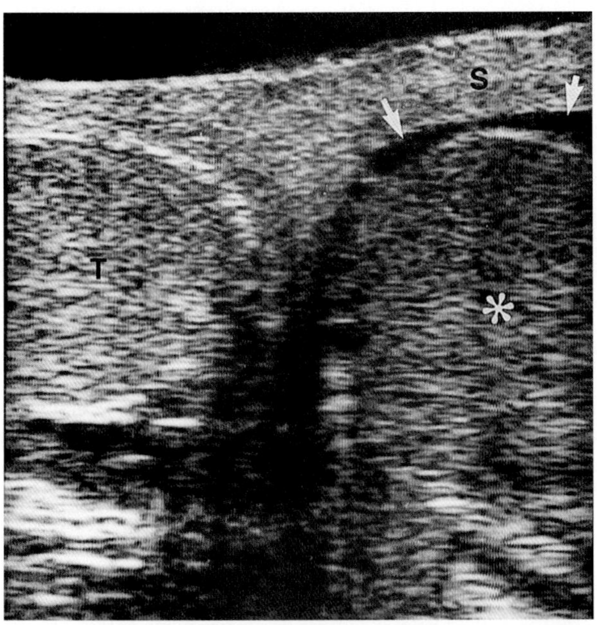

A

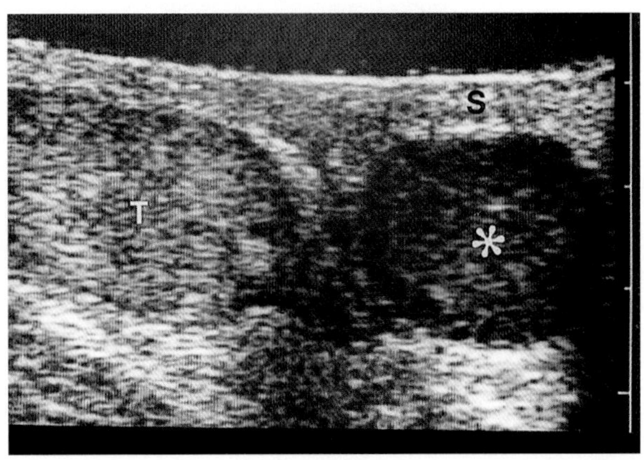

B

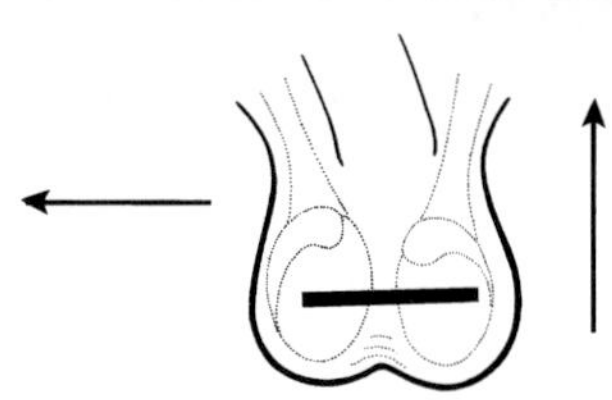

FIG. 6.6. Severe epididymo-orchitis with subsequent atrophy of the affected testis in a 61-year-old patient. Transverse plane of section **(A)** at the time of diagnosis and **(B)** 6 months later. Initially, the left testis (*) is enlarged and hypoechoic; the scrotal skin (S) is thickened. Hydrocele (*arrows*). The right testis (T) is normal. On a follow-up study the left testis (*) is small and hypoechoic, indicating atrophy.

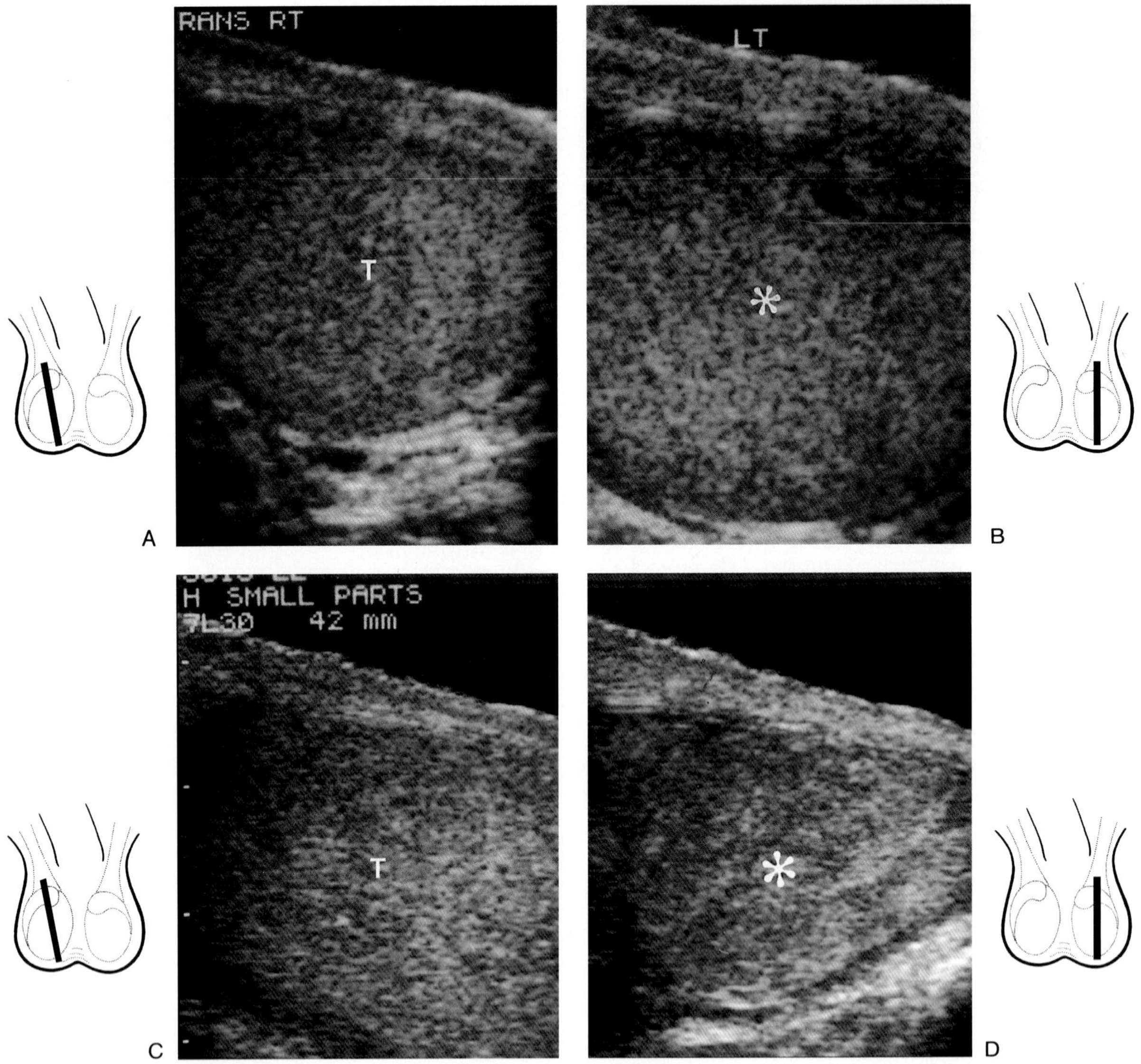

FIG. 6.7. Acute epididymo-orchitis with subsequent testicular atrophy in a 35-year-old man. **(A** and **B)** Sonogram at the time of initial diagnosis and **(C** and **D)** 3 months later. The right testis (T) is normal. The left testis (*) is initially enlarged but of normal echogenicity. On follow-up examination the left testis (*) demonstrates decrease in size and echogenicity, indicating atrophy. Clinical symptoms subsided after 2 weeks of initial study.

sound findings, however, often persist 2 to 3 weeks after the clinical symptoms have subsided.

Sonography is extremely valuable in demonstrating the complications of epididymitis, such as abscess formation or epididymo-orchitis (13). An **abscess** is visualized as a circumscribed, hypoechoic lesion within the enlarged epididymis (Fig. 6.5). Very rarely, an abscess with small gas inclusions produces a heterogeneous pattern with hyperechoic punctate echoes. The diagnosis of **epididymo-orchitis** is suggested by the sonographic demonstration of focally or diffusely decreased echogenicity in the testis (Figs. 6.2 and 6.4). The involved areas of the testis most commonly demonstrate a homogeneous decreased echotexture (Fig. 6.4). Diffuse reduction of testicular echogenicity and marked testicular swelling during the early phase of epididymitis indicate a poor prognosis (14). A sequel to such orchitis may be testicular atrophy (Figs. 6.6 and 6.7). Pronounced inflammatory swelling of the epididymis can impede testicular blood supply, resulting in focal or diffuse infarction of the testis (15,16). In severe orchitis the testis is hypoechoic, but its echotexture is heterogeneous, and an early abscess formation can be overlooked (Fig. 6.8). Such patients require sonographic follow-up, although patients with uncomplicated epididymitis do not. Patients who do not respond to therapy should also undergo an ultrasound

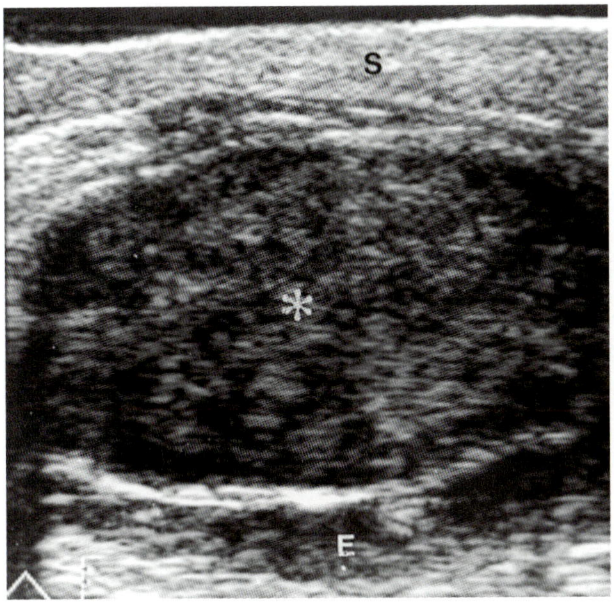

A

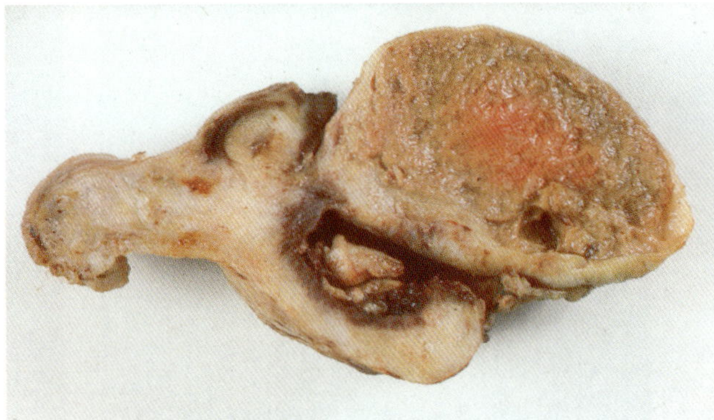

B

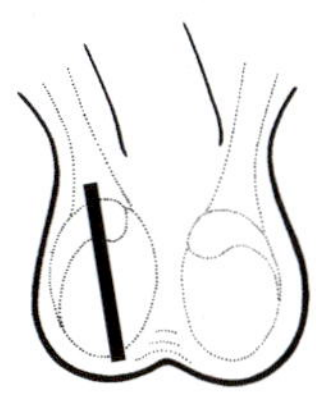

FIG. 6.8. Extensive orchitis with abscess formation in a 46-year-old patient. **(A)** Ultrasound scan showing an enlarged and hypoechoic testis (*). The testicular echotexture is coarse and inhomogeneous, but no definite abscess is seen. Secondary signs of inflammation include enlargement of the epididymis (E) and edema of the scrotal skin (S). **(B)** Surgical specimen revealed severe necrotizing and diffuse abscess-forming orchitis.

examination to identify possible abscess formation (Figs. 6.8 and 6.9) or to detect an underlying testicular tumor. Any heterogeneous intratesticular area that corresponds to a clinically palpated firm mass (as opposed to a fluctuant abscess) should be treated as a tumor until proven otherwise by surgical exploration.

Color-coded duplex sonography (CCDS) can be helpful in differentiating epididymitis from torsion. Whereas blood flow in the testis and epididymis is typically reduced or absent in patients with torsion, flow to the testis and paratesticular tissue is increased (producing hypervascularity) in patients with epididymitis (Fig. 6.10) (17–19). In addition, abscess formation in extensive epididymitis is characterized by a hypovascular center with a tissue rim of increased vascularization (Fig. 6.11), making an early diagnosis possible. In the differentiation between orchitis and tumor, however, CCDS findings are not helpful, as various flow patterns can be seen with either condition.

Ultrasonographic findings in **chronic epididymitis** are nonspecific, and the diagnosis is usually established on the basis of clinical findings, after exclusion of other disorders. The diffuse, chronic-inflammatory alterations of the epididymis are barely detectable on ultrasound; the only change that may be seen is moderate enlargement of the organ (Fig. 6.12).

Among the specific forms of epididymitis, **tuberculous involvement of the epididymis** is of particular importance. Its diagnosis, however, is based primarily on the clinical presentation, laboratory findings, and bacteriologic tests, not imaging studies (20). Sonographically, the characteristics of tuberculous epididymitis are the same as those seen in nonspecific epididymitis. The inflammatory process sometimes extends to the testis. When present, caseating necrosis is visualized as abscesslike focal lesions with markedly reduced echogenicity.

Sarcoidosis of the epididymis is a rare disease. The diagnosis is based on the overall clinical presentation, since the circumscribed, hypoechoic granulomatous lesions resemble the sonographic appearance of a sperm granuloma or a tumor of the epididymis (21).

Sperm granulomas present a diagnostic dilemma. They resemble epididymal tumors in that they present on ultrasound as circumscribed, well-demarcated, hypoechoic intraepididymal lesions (22). A history of previous inflammation, trauma, or surgery (e.g., vasectomy) may suggest the correct diagnosis in these cases.

After vasectomy, up to 45% of men exhibit morphologic changes in the epididymis. These include epididymal enlargement, cystic lesions, and inhomogeneous echotexture (23).

MR in the Evaluation of Inflammation

In **acute epididymitis** the epididymis is enlarged and demonstrates a heterogeneous and most commonly high

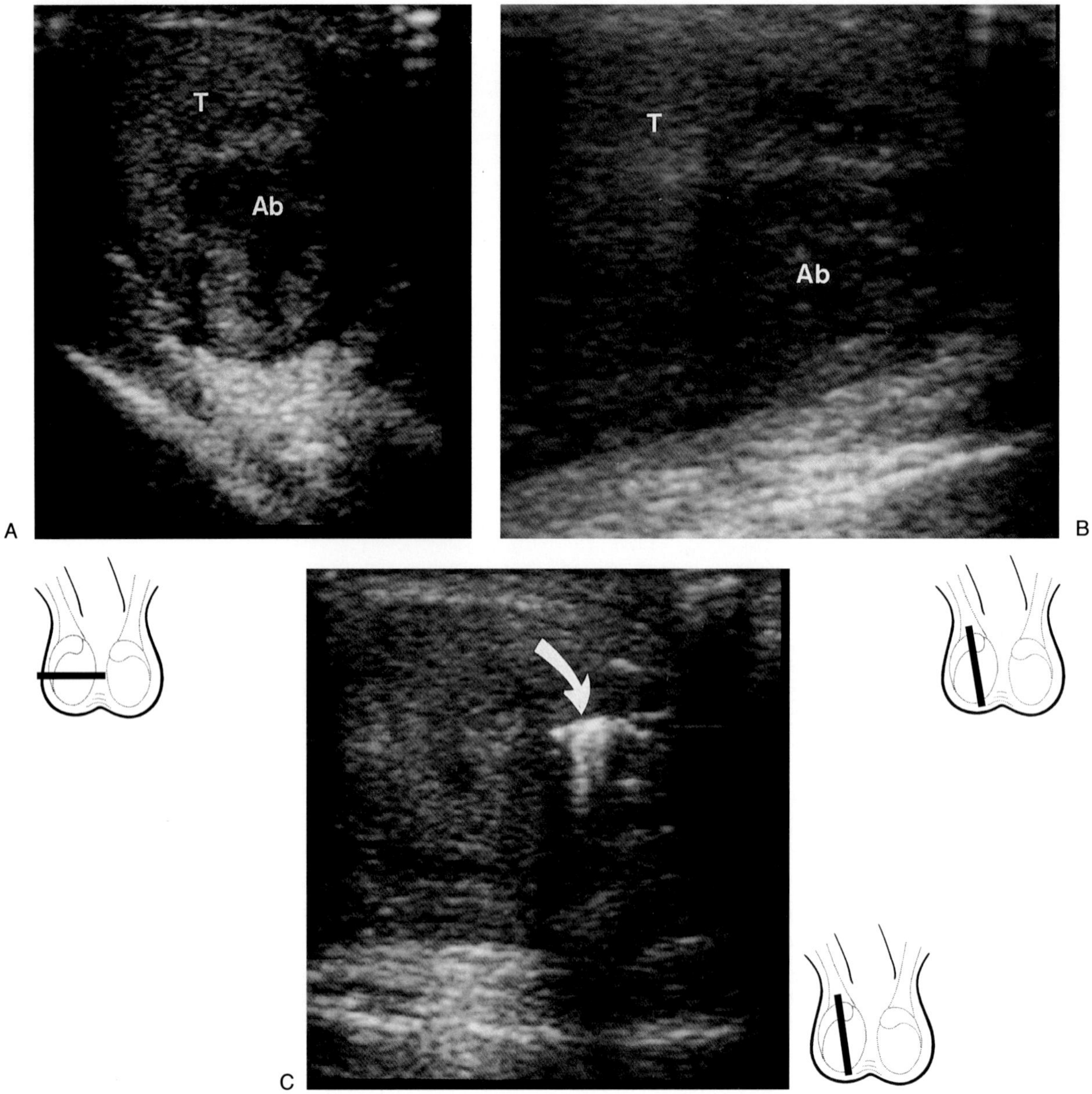

FIG. 6.9. Serial scans in a 27-year-old HIV-positive patient with severe epididymo-orchitis. **(A)** Sonogram at the time of initial diagnosis; **(B)** 2 weeks later, patient had poor response to medical treatment; and **(C)** 1 month later, clinically, patient had no response to antibiotic therapy. Initially, irregular hypoechoic focus (Ab) is seen in the testis (T). Two weeks later, the involved area of the testis has enlarged and demonstrates heterogeneous but predominantly hypoechoic echotexture (Ab). No liquified portion, indicating an abscess, is seen. One month later, air (*curved arrow*) within the abscess is identified. Necrotizing orchitis was present at surgery.

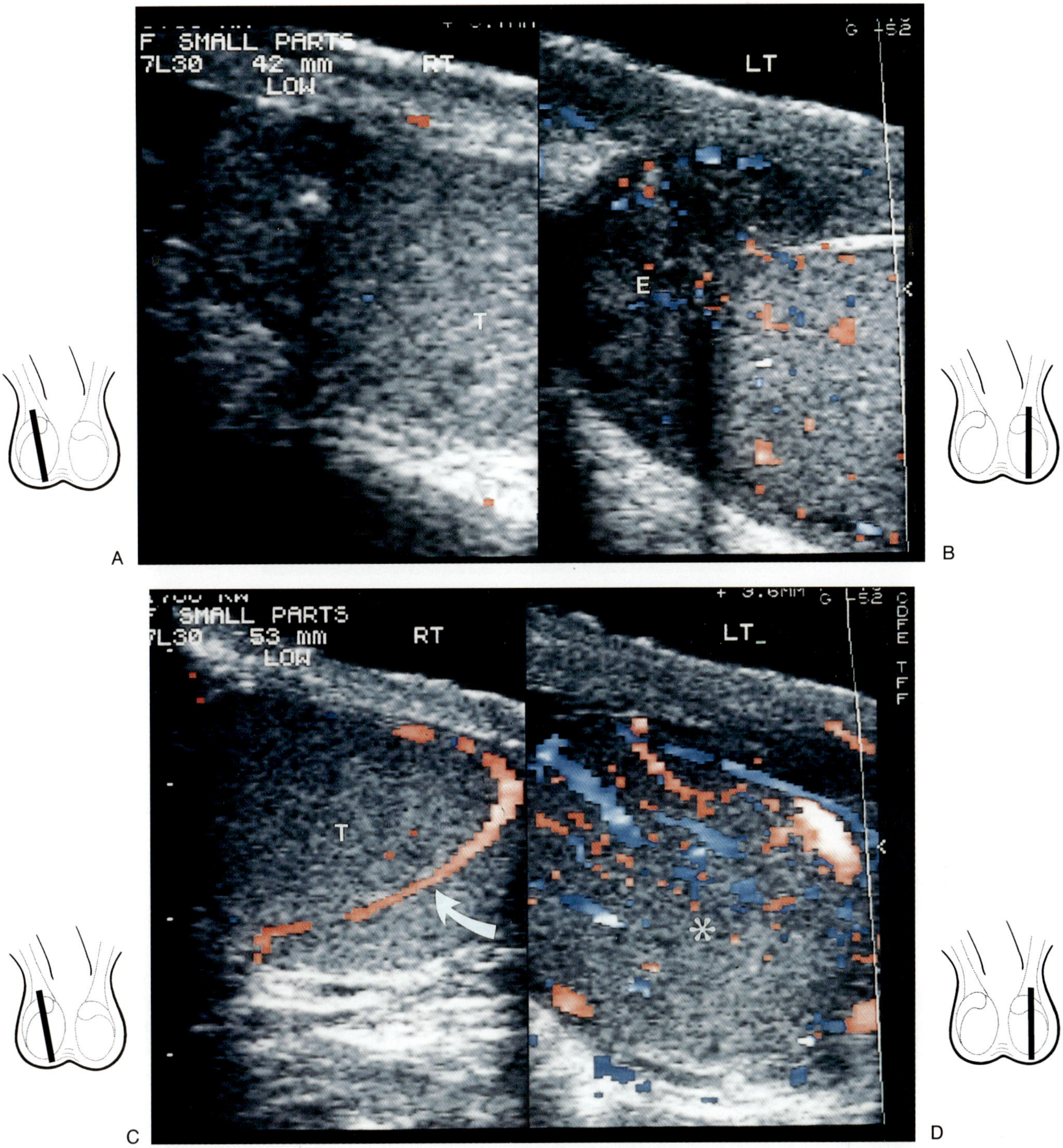

FIG. 6.10. Color-coded duplex sonogram in a 38-year-old patient with acute epididymo-orchitis. Longitudinal scans of **(A)** right and **(B)** left epididymal heads and **(C)** right and **(D)** left testes. The left head of the epididymis (E) is enlarged and hypoechoic. The left testis (*) is enlarged, but the echogenicity is normal and is symmetrical as compared with the right testis (T). The left testis (*), however, shows markedly increased vascularity. Capsular artery (*arrow*) in the right testis.

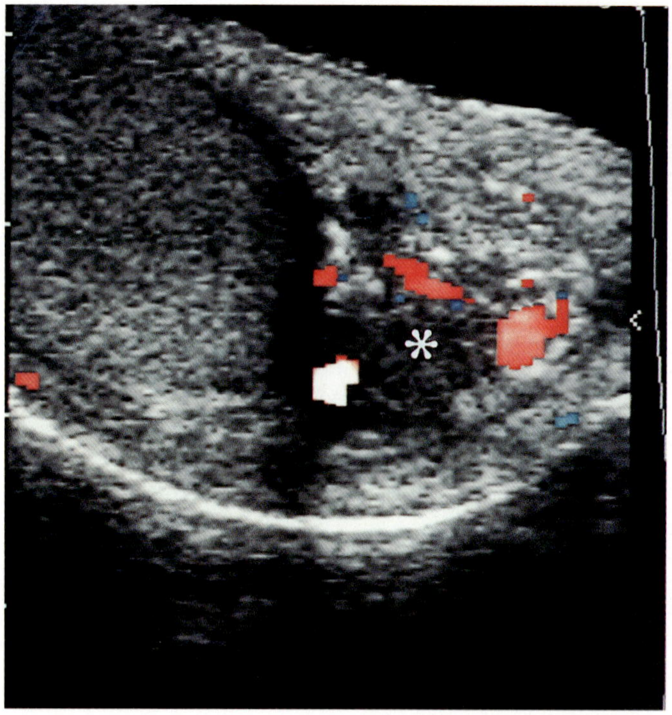

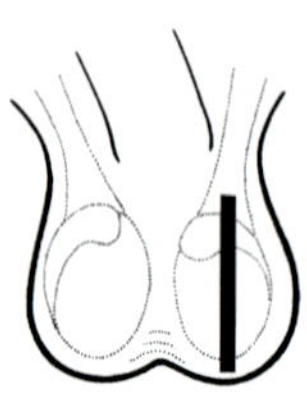

FIG. 6.11. Abscess in the tail of the epididymis in a 39-year-old patient with a 3-week history of epididymitis. Color-coded Doppler sonogram shows enlarged tail of the epididymis with localized, hypoechoic, hypovascular focus (*) surrounded by a rim of increased vascularity. Surgically proven abscess was suspected because of CCDS finding.

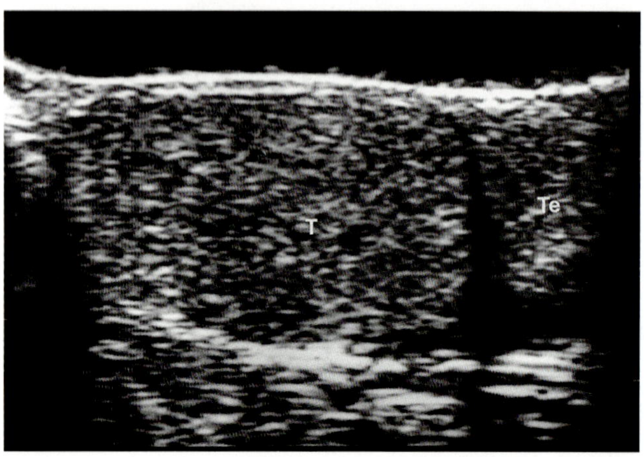

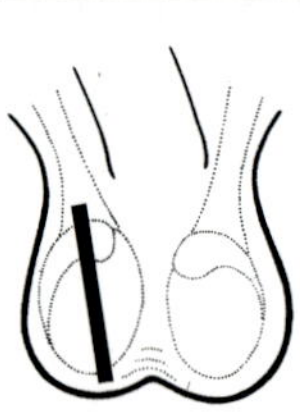

FIG. 6.12. Chronic epididymitis in a 53-year-old patient with intermittent, moderate pain and status history of recurrent epididymitis. The sonogram shows a moderately enlarged but homogeneous epididymal tail (Te) with otherwise normal intrascrotal findings. (T, testis)

signal intensity (Fig 6.13) on T2-weighted images (24). Findings of enlarged but low-signal-intensity epididymis on T2-weighted images have also been reported (Fig. 6.14). Hemorrhage may complicate acute epididymitis (especially when severe), producing varying signal intensity on T1- (Fig. 6.13) and T2-weighted images. The spermatic cord is often thickened. On T1-weighted images the inflammatory infiltration and multiple engorged vessels with signal void (reflecting hypervascularity) can be detected (Fig. 6.15). This latter finding is not usually seen in patients with torsion, assisting in MR differentiation between acute epididymitis and torsion. Reactive hydrocele with associated thickening of the scrotal skin and inguinal lymphadenopathy are also frequently seen in a patient with epididymitis. Acute epididymitis demonstrates marked enhancement on postcontrast T1-weighted images (Figs. 6.16 and 6.17).

In **chronic epididymitis** the epididymis is enlarged and demonstrates low signal intensity.

Associated **orchitis**, if present, on T2-weighted images

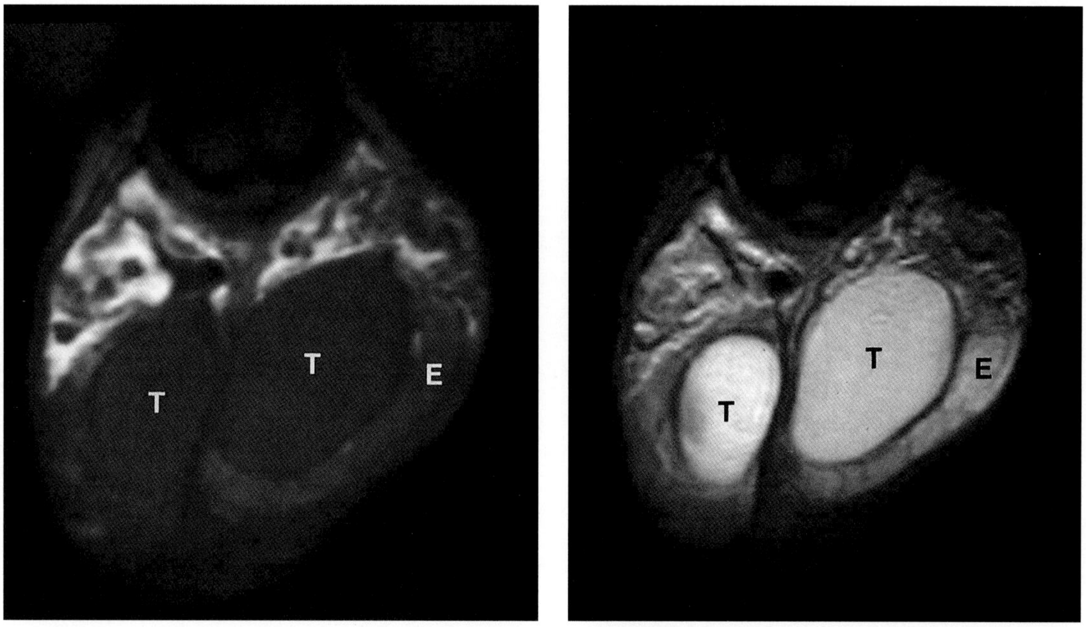

FIG. 6.13. Epididymitis in a 44-year-old man with an acute onset of scrotal pain, swelling, and erythema. **(A)** Coronal T1-weighted and **(B)** T2-weighted MR images. The left epididymis (E) is enlarged and demonstrates slightly increased signal intensity on the T1-weighted image and high signal intensity (similar to the adjacent testis) on the T2-weighted image. (T, testis)

appears as a homogeneous or heterogeneous hypointense lesion within the normal-sized or enlarged testis (Fig. 6.14). Compared with testicular tumors, orchitis usually does not produce a mass effect. On the contrast-enhanced T1-weighted image, orchitis will demonstrate

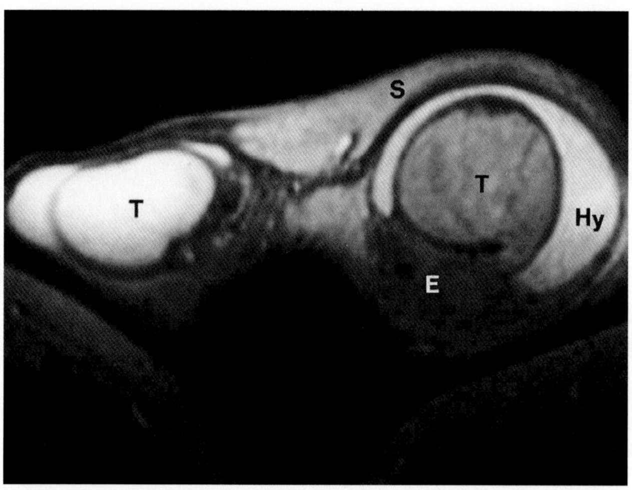

FIG. 6.14. Acute epididymo-orchitis in a 35-year-old man. Transaxial T2-weighted image shows enlarged left epididymis (E) of markedly low signal intensity. The left testis (T) demonstrates lower signal intensity than the contralateral right testis (T). Reactive hydrocele (Hy) and scrotal skin thickening (S) are also present.

different patterns of enhancement. In ischemic orchitis (e.g., seen with marked swelling of the epididymis and subsequent impediment of testicular blood supply), the involved testis is morphologically normal but shows less enhancement than the normal testis (Fig. 6.16). In acute inflammatory orchitis enhancement of the involved testis is much greater than normal (Fig. 6.17).

On noncontrast and contrast-enhanced MR images, **idiopathic granulomatous orchitis** presents as a tumor mass indistinguishable from cancer (see Chapter 5).

Pseudotumor of the Tunica Albuginea

Following epididymitis, fibrotic thickening of the tunica albuginea is common and is sometimes so marked that it cannot be clinically distinguished from testicular cancer (25). On MR scans the thickened tunica can be identified by its typical low signal intensity on both T1- and T2-weighted images.

Nuclear Scintigraphy in the Evaluation of Inflammation

In epididymitis, flow studies show augmented flow through the cord and hyperemia to the area of the epididymis. The activity may extend inferiorly and involve the testis. An associated reactive hydrocele with a semi-

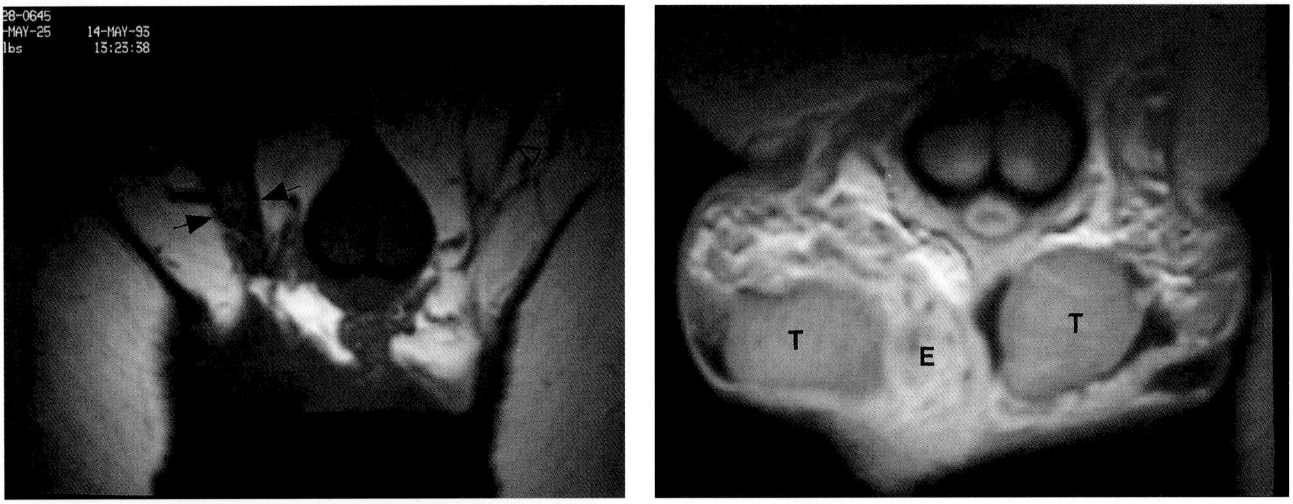

A C

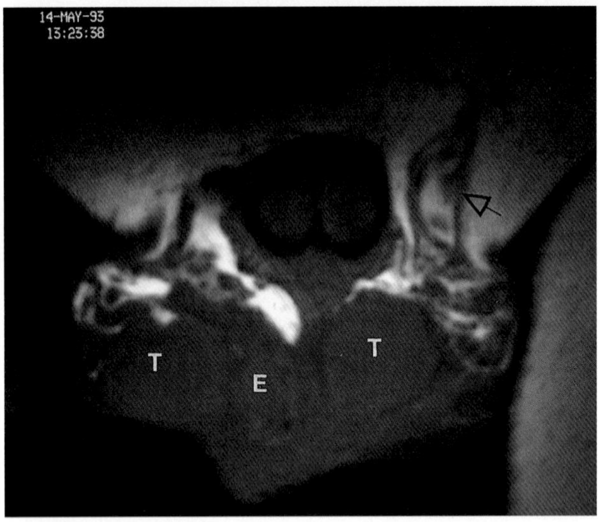

B

FIG. 6.15. Acute epididymitis with involvement of the spermatic cord in a 25-year-old man. Coronal plane of section. **(A)** and **(B)** are two consecutive sections of T1-weighted images, and **(C)** is contrast-enhanced T1-weighted image (at the same anatomic location as that in **[B]**). The right epididymis (E) is enlarged and shows marked enhancement on postcontrast study. Both testes (T) show normal size and echogenicity. The right spermatic cord (*solid arrows*) demonstrates diffuse medium signal intensity (indicating inflammation), and fat is detected within the normal left spermatic cord (*open arrow*).

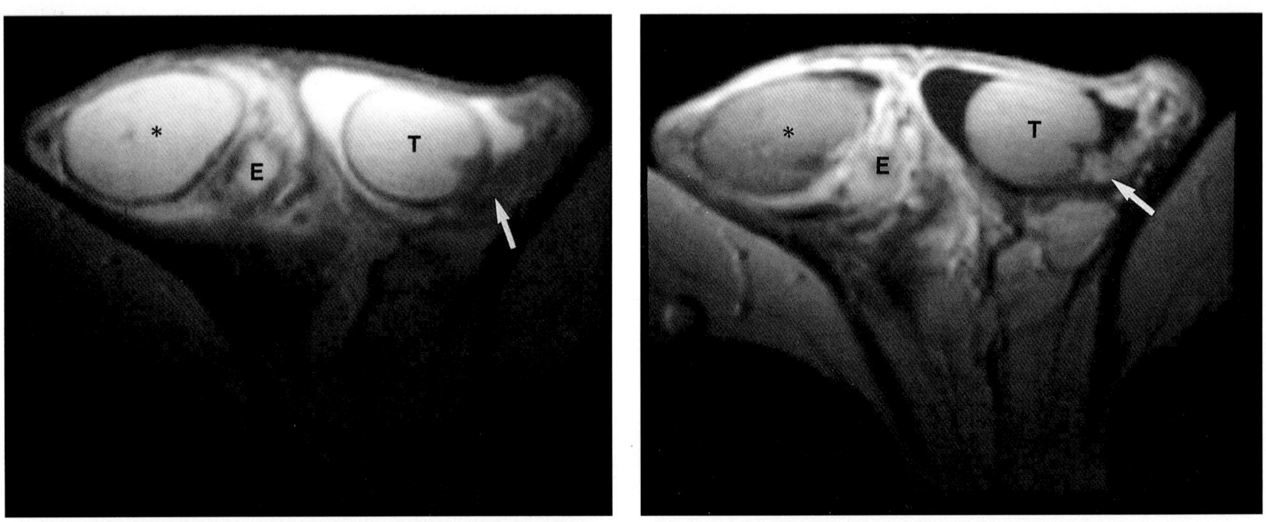

A B

FIG. 6.16. Acute epididymo-orchitis in a 27-year-old man. Transaxial **(A)** T2-weighted and **(B)** contrast-enhanced T1-weighted MR images. Compared with the contralateral side, the right epididymis (E) is enlarged and demonstrates high signal intensity on the T2-weighted scan and enhancement on postcontrast study. A normal size and signal intensity left epididymis (*arrow*). The right testis (*) is enlarged and of normal signal intensity on the T2-weighted image. On the contrast-enhanced T1-weighted image, the right testis (T), however, demonstrates less enhancement than the left testis (T), indicating an early ischemic orchitis.

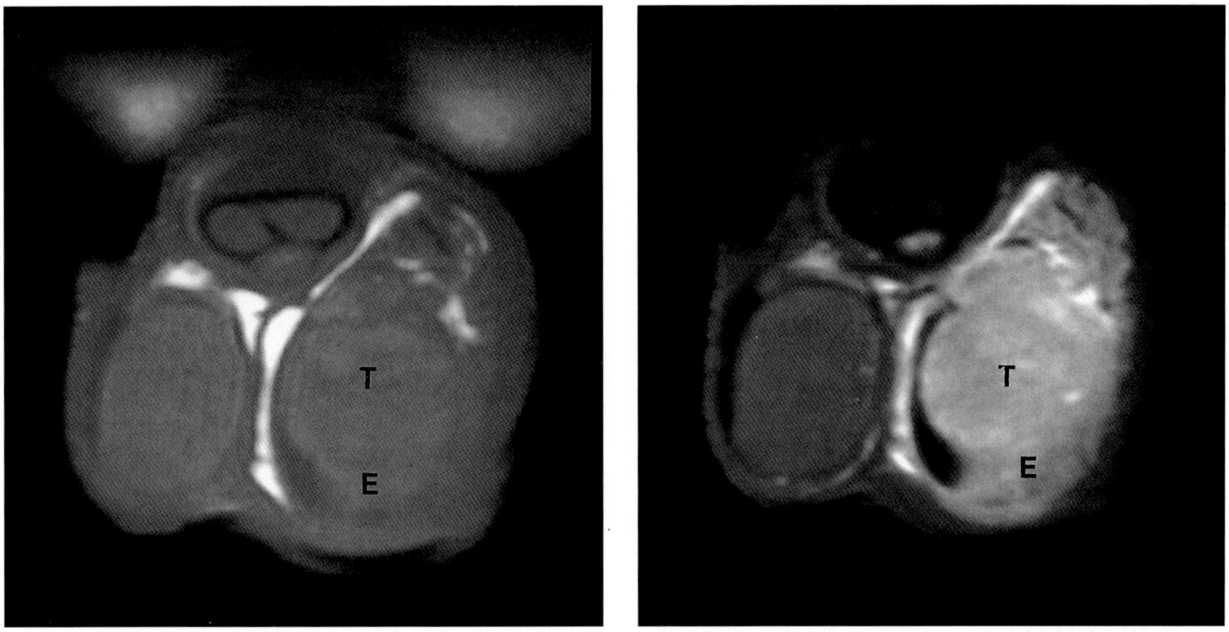

A B

FIG. 6.17. Epididymo-orchitis. Coronal plane of section. **(A)** Noncontrast and **(B)** contrast-enhanced T1-weighted images. The left epididymis (E) and testis (T) are enlarged and demonstrate marked enhancement on postcontrast study. The right testis is normal.

lunar shape is generally present (14,26,27). When large enough, the hydrocele may mimic a torsed testicle (27,28). In addition to orchitis, abscess formation may develop, in which case the scan pattern shows a "cold" defect. Testicular infarction, related to compression of the cord by inflammation, may also complicate epididymitis (14,29,30). A detailed discussion of nuclear medicine techniques and findings in epididymitis can be found in Chapter 9.

Comparative Evaluation

Imaging is necessary for the diagnosis of epididymitis and orchitis when the findings from clinical history and physical examination are insufficient or when a patient does not respond to antibiotic therapy. US is usually the initial study, and although it is highly accurate for evaluation of acute epididymitis, it can be insufficient for distinguishing orchitis from testicular tumor. MR examination can be performed when US findings are limited or equivocal or when differentiation of associated orchitis is needed, but differentiation between tumor and orchitis may remain an obstacle with MR as well.

REFERENCES

1. Berger RE. Sexually transmitted diseases. In: Walsh PC, Retik AB, Stamey TA, Vaughan ED, eds. *Campbell's urology*, 6th ed, vol 1. Philadelphia: WB Saunders; 1992: 823–846.
2. Rajfer J. Congenital anomalies of the testis. In: Walsh PC, Retik AB, Stamey TA, Vaughan ED, eds. *Campbell's urology*, 6th ed, vol 2. Philadelphia: WB Saunders; 1992:1543–1562.
3. Doble A, Taylor-Robinson D, Thomas BJ, Jalil N, Harris JR, Witherow RO. Acute epididymitis: a microbiological and ultrasonographic study. *Br J Urol* 1989;63:90–94
4. Meares EM, Jr. Nonspecific infections of the genitourinary tract. In: Tanagho EA, McAninch JW, eds. *Smith's general urology,* 13th ed. Norwalk, CT: Appleton & Lange; 1992:195–239.
5. Ward JP. Epididymo-Orchitis. In: Whitfield HN, Hendry WF, eds. *Textbook of genitourinary surgery*. Edinburgh: Churchill Livingstone; 1985:567–578.
6. Gartman E. Epididymitis: reappraisal *Am J Surg* 1961:101–756.
7. Del Villar RG, Ireland GW, Cass AS. Early exploration in acute testicular conditions. *J Urol* 1972;108:887–888.
8. Trambert MA, Mattrey RF, Levine D, Berthoty DP. Subacute scrotal pain: evaluation of torsion versus epididymis with MR imaging. *Radiology* 1990;175:53–56.
9. Selikowitz SM, Schned AR. A late postvasectomy syndrome. *J Urol* 1985;134:494–497.
10. Benson CB, Doubilet PM, Richie JP. Sonography of the male genital tract. *AJR* 1989;153:705–713.
11. Krone KD, Carroll BA. Scrotal ultrasound. *Radiol Clin North Am* 1985;23:121–139.
12. Rifkin MD. Scrotal ultrasound. *Urol Radiol* 1987;9:119–126.
13. Rifkin MD, Kurtz AB, Goldberg BB. Epididymis examined by ultrasound. *Radiology* 1984;151:187–190.
14. Desai KM, Gingell JC, Haworth JM. Fate of the testis following epididymitis: a clinical and ultrasound study. *J Roy Soc Med* 1986;79: 515–519.
15. Bird K, Rosenfield AT. Testicular infarction secondary to acute inflammatory disease: demonstration by B-scan ultrasound. *Radiology* 1984;152:785–788.
16. Vordermark JS, Favila MQ. Testicular necrosis: a preventable complication of epididymitis. *J Urol* 1982;128:1322–1324.
17. Ralls PW, Jensen MC, Lee KP, Mayekawa DS, Johnson MB, Halls JM. Color Doppler sonography in acute epididymitis and orchitis. *J Clin Ultrasound* 1990;18:383–386.
18. Horstman WG, Middleton WD, Melson GL. Scrotal inflammatory disease: color Doppler US findings. *Radiology* 1991;179:55–59.

19. Horstman WG, Middleton WD, Melson GL, Siegel BA. Color Doppler US of the scrotum. *Radiographics* 1991;11:941–957.
20. Heaton ND, Hogan B, Michell M, Thompson P, Yates-Bell AJ. Tuberculous epididymo-orchitis: clinical and ultrasound observations. *Br J Urol* 1989;64:305–309.
21. Forte MD, Brant WE. Ultrasonographic detection of epididymal sarcoidosis. *J Clin Ultrasound* 1988;16:191–194.
22. Ramanathan K, Yaghoobian J, Pinck RL. Sperm granuloma. *J Clin Ultrasound* 1986;14:155–156.
23. Jarvis LJ, Dubbins PA. Changes in the epididymis after vasectomy: sonographic findings. *AJR* 1989;152:531–534.
24. Baker LL, Hajek PC, Burkhard TK, et al. MR imaging of the scrotum: pathologic conditions. *Radiology* 1987;163:92–98.
25. Cramer BM, Schlegel EA, Thueroff JW. MR imaging in the differential diagnosis of scrotal and testicular disease. *Radiographics* 1991;11:9–21.
26. Abu-Sleiman R, Ho JE, Gregory JG. Scrotal scanning: present value and limits of interpretation. *Urology* 1979;13:326–330.
27. Chen DC, Holder LE, Melloul M. Radionuclide scrotal imaging: further experience with 210 patients. Part 1: Anatomy, pathophysiology, and methods. *J Nucl Med* 1983;24:735–742.
28. Dunn EK, Macchia RJ, Chauhan PS, Laungani GB, Solomon NA. Scintiscan for acute intrascrotal conditions. *Clin Nucl Med* 1986;11:381–388.
29. Eisner DJ, Goldman SM, Petronis J, Millmond SH. Bilateral testicular infarction caused by epididymitis. *AJR* 1991;157:517–519.
30. Vieras F. Evolution of acute epididymitis to testicular infarction. Scintigraphic demonstration. *Clin Nucl Med* 1986;11:158–160.

B. Torsion

TESTICULAR (SPERMATIC CORD) TORSION

Testicular torsion is defined as "rotation of the testis on the longitudinal axis of the spermatic cord." When the spermatic cord torses, venous drainage is initially blocked, resulting in edema and hemorrhage. Since the arterial supply of the testicle (the testicular, deferential, and cremasteric arteries) divides in the spermatic cord and there is no significant collateral circulation with the scrotal blood supply (the internal and external pudendal arteries) (1–3), arterial flow in early torsion is impaired and hemorrhagic necrosis of the entire gonad follows. Testicular torsion is considered a surgical emergency, as delay in intervention may result in irreversible damage to the testis. Specific types of testicular torsion include traumatic torsion, torsion of the undescended testicle, habitually recurrent torsion (intermittent, transient torsion with spontaneous untwisting), and prenatal, intrauterine torsion (asymptomatic).

Based on the site of twisting, torsion is classified as **extravaginal** (supravaginal), **intravaginal**, and **mesorchial** (Fig. 6.18) (1,4).

Extravaginal torsion is a rare type of torsion found almost exclusively in newborns. The torsion occurs outside the tunica vaginalis when the testis and gubernaculum are not fixed and are free to rotate within the scrotum (Fig. 6.18) (5,6). It is thought that this type of torsion occurs in utero and often at birth is present as a mass in the groin (7). The testicle is almost always necrotic.

Intravaginal torsion occurs within the tunica vaginalis. A variety of predisposing factors has been implicated, including (1) a long and narrow mesorchium **(mesorchial torsion)**; (2) absence of or defective fixation by the gubernaculum; and (3) an entwined cremasteric muscle (8,9). Normally, the testis and the epididymis adhere closely to one another and are connected to the posterolateral aspect of the scrotum by a broad and short mesorchium, so that the testis cannot rotate. An abnormally narrow mesenteric attachment (mesorchium) from the cord to the testis and the epididymis allows the testis to rotate freely and predisposes to torsion (9). Two additional structures fix the testis to the scrotum—the gubernaculum, which fixes the testis to the floor of the scrotum, and the parietal peritoneum of the tunica vaginalis, which covers the epididymis (10). Sometimes the testis is almost completely covered by the tunica vaginalis except for a thin stalk. This so-called **bell-clapper deformity** often occurs bilaterally and predisposes to intravaginal testicular torsion. This deformity occurs in a contralateral testis in approximately 85% of patients with unilateral anorchism (11). Intravaginal torsion usually affects boys after puberty, when the gubernaculum is fixed and the testis and epididymis rotate intravaginally.

Torsion is not uncommon, and the risk of developing torsion of the testis or its appendage by the age of 25 has been reported to be as high as 1 out of 160 (12). Anatomic abnormalities such as the greater mobility associated with an undescended testicle, retractile testis, or abnormal mesorchial attachment increase the likelihood of

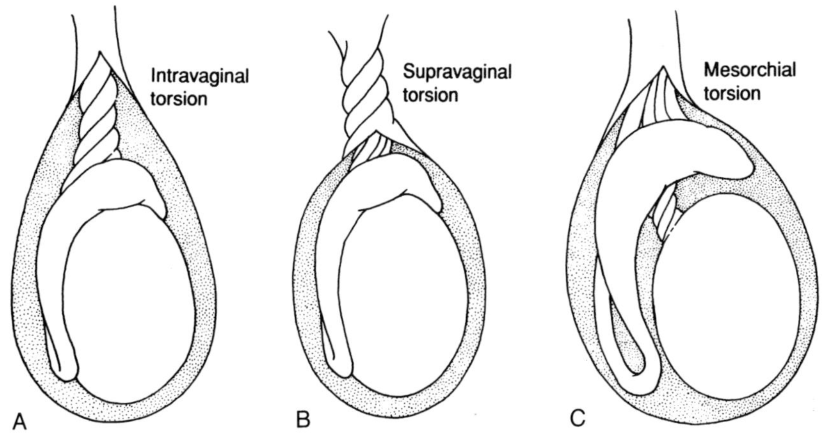

FIG. 6.18. Types of testicular torsion: **(A)** Intravaginal, **(B)** supravaginal, and **(C)** mesorchial.

torsion. Other contributing factors include abrupt rotational movements of the body, sudden exertion, or blunt trauma. Bilateral torsion has been reported in approximately 2% of cases (13). In one study of 395 boys 17 years of age or younger, torsion of the testis and appendix testis was the cause of acute scrotal pain in 38% and 24% of cases, respectively. Epididymitis or orchitis accounted for another 31% (14).

Clinical Presentation

Approximately two thirds of cases of torsion occur in adolescent males (between 12 and 18 years old) (12). The incidence slowly decreases with increasing age (9). Too much emphasis should not be placed on the patient's age, however, because the three most common disorders causing acute scrotal symptoms (testicular torsion, appendiceal torsion, and epididymo-orchitis) may occur at any age (Fig. 6.19).

The cardinal symptom of testicular torsion is sudden scrotal pain followed by swelling, which may occur in an otherwise completely healthy patient. The pain may initially be dragging and progress rapidly, or it may strike abruptly, with full intensity, accompanied by nausea, vomiting, and symptoms of shock (15). Body temperature is usually normal and urinalysis is clear (16). In one third to one half of cases there have been previous episodes of scrotal pain (5). In infants the symptoms may be absent or nonspecific (e.g., irritability, restlessness, and lack of appetite) (9) and may be associated only with redness and swelling of the scrotum. In about 40% of cases the pain radiates to the ipsilateral inguinal region or to the lower abdomen. As a result, testicular torsion in infants may be mistaken for appendicitis. Some patients report onset of pain at night or in the morning.

On physical examination the scrotum is asymmetrically swollen and tender, and the epididymis may be palpated anterior to the testis. The scrotum is usually reddened, although this sign may be absent in early stages of the disease, and there may be pitting of the skin at the base of the scrotum (**Ger's sign**). The affected testicle has a high and horizontal lie (**Brunzel's sign**) (15), and, in contradistinction to epididymitis, elevation of the testis does not relieve pain (**negative Prehn's sign**). The cremasteric reflex on the affected side is absent. Early in the course, normal urinary sediments and absence of fever and leukocytosis are important criteria for differentiating torsion from acute epididymitis.

Differentiation of torsion from epididymitis is problematic in up to 50% of cases (17), although epididymitis is rare before puberty. Clinical findings of fever, urethral discharge, and pyuria or bacteriuria support the diagnosis of epididymitis. Other diagnostic considerations

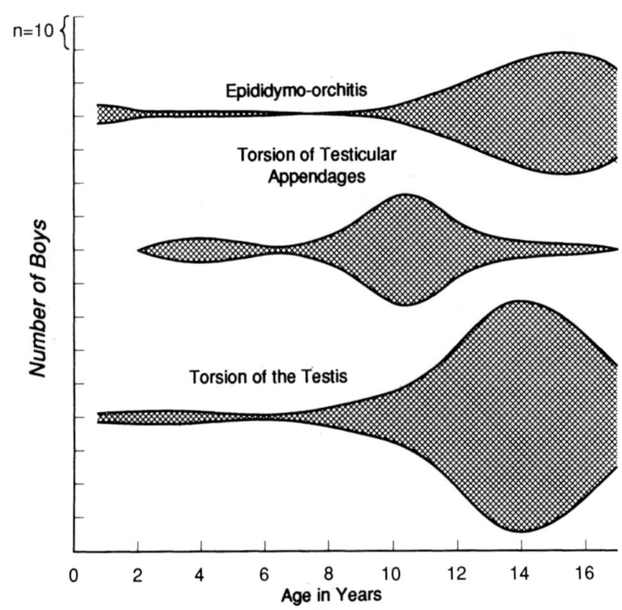

FIG. 6.19. Age distribution for testicular torsion, appendiceal torsion, and epididymo-orchitis in children, not including neonates. (From Knight PJ, Vassy LE. The diagnosis and treatment of the acute scrotum in children and adolescents. *Ann Surg* 1984;200:664–673.)

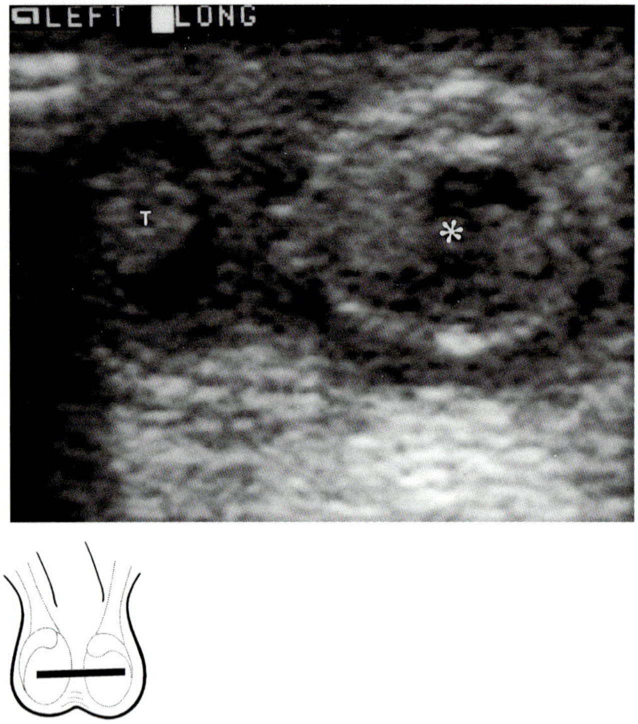

A

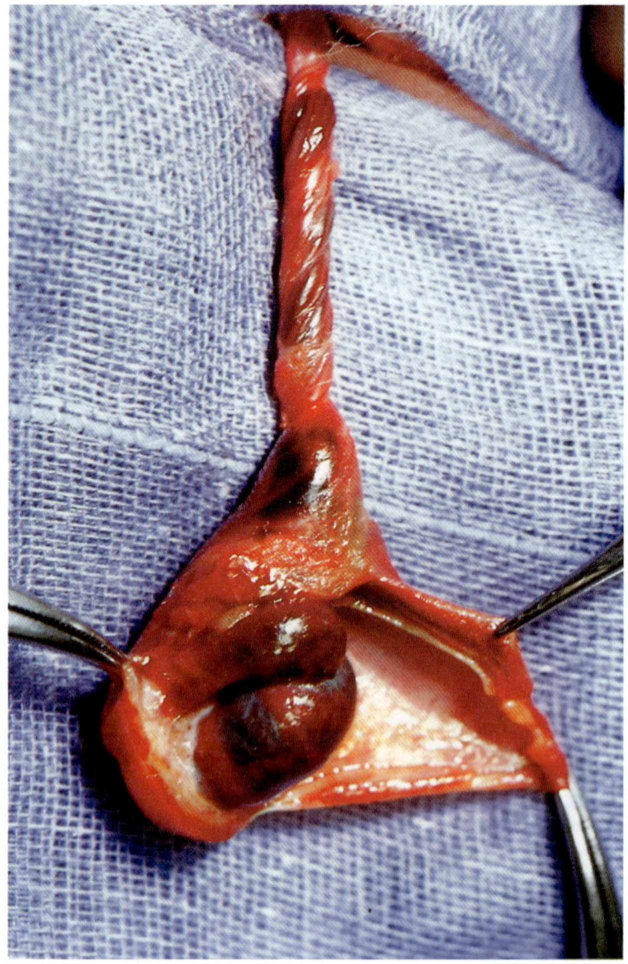

B

FIG. 6.20. Supravaginal testicular torsion in a 4-day-old newborn. **(A)** Transverse sonogram and **(B)** intraoperative view. The left testis (*) is markedly enlarged and demonstrates heterogeneous echogenicity and peripheral echogenic rim. Normal right testis (T).

include strangulated hernia, hematocele, hydrocele, testicular tumor, and idiopathic scrotal edema (16). Abnormal seminal features and reduced fertility have been reported in patients following unilateral testicular torsion, even after successful corrective surgery (18). Histologic abnormalities are found in the contralateral testis in up to 60% of cases. Those are thought to be caused by immune mechanisms (18).

The time interval between the onset of symptoms and operative reduction is critical for testicular salvage. The first 7 hours is considered the early phase of testicular torsion. From 7 to 24 hours is the middle phase. The late phase, or "missed torsion," occurs after 24 hours. The salvage rate is almost 100% when surgery is done within 3 hours. If it is delayed for more than 24 hours from the onset of symptoms, however, virtually all testicular function is lost (5,19).

If the testis is viable, treatment includes manual and surgical detorsion and bilateral orchiopexy. Prophylactic fixation of the contralateral testis is needed, since in more than 50% of cases of intravaginal torsion there is a similar defect in the contralateral testis. If surgery, including contralateral orchiopexy, is performed within 4 to 6 hours of the onset of symptoms, the prognosis is usually good (16). For late or missed torsion, surgical removal of the testis with contralateral orchiopexy is performed. Surgery is not necessary for extravaginal torsion, unless pyogenic infection occurs, because the lesion is usually found too late to salvage the testis. The nonsurgical approach to extravaginal torsion is, however, controversial.

Ultrasound in the Evaluation of Torsion

The sonographic appearance of testicular torsion is nonspecific (20–24), and diagnostic information from gray-scale ultrasound is limited. Ultrasound examination of the scrotum should include duplex sonography study. Even when both types of sonographic examinations are performed, the value of sonography is mainly to exclude the diagnosis of torsion by (1) providing a rapid overview of intrascrotal morphology (which is nearly impossible to obtain by palpation) and (2) excluding other causes of acute scrotal abnormalities, such as inflammatory disease, a tumor, or an incarcerated inguinal hernia.

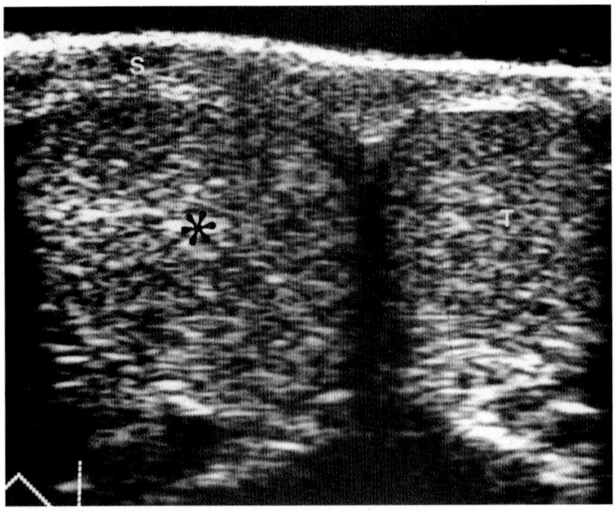

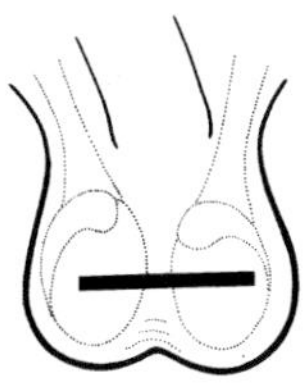

FIG. 6.21. Acute torsion of the right testis in a 16-year-old. Transverse sonogram. The right testis (*) is enlarged but of normal echogenicity. There is associated thickening of the scrotal skin (S). The left testis (T) is normal.

An **extravaginal torsion** is seen in the newborn. Sonographically, the torsed testis is round and enlarged, and frequently hydrocele and skin thickening are found (25). Heterogeneous parenchymal echoes and peripheral echogenic rims (with or without an outermost, circumferential hypoechoic region) are common US findings (Fig. 6.20) (25,26). Because this type of torsion occurs in utero, at the time of clinical examination, the testis is usually infarcted and necrotic. US is therefore very sensitive in depicting testicular abnormality, and sonography is valuable in differentiating an extravaginal torsion from other causes of scrotal enlargement in a newborn (e.g., hernia, tumor, hydrocele).

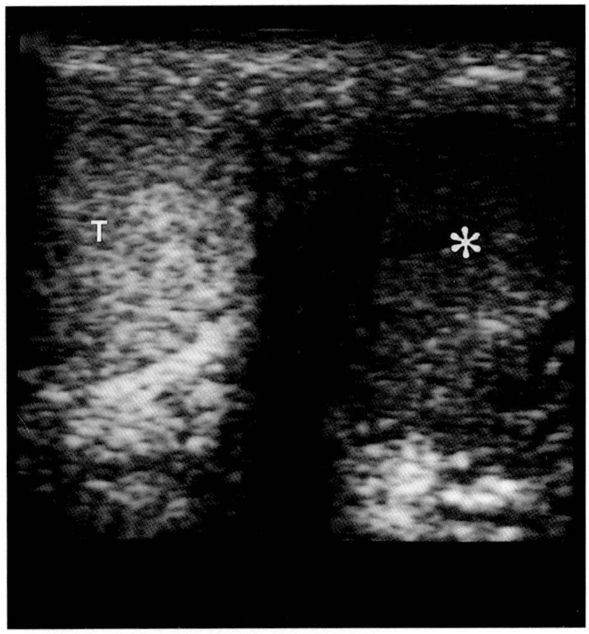

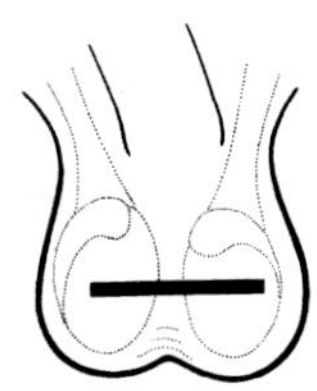

FIG. 6.22. Acute torsion of the left testis in a 14-year-old. Transverse sonogram. The left testis (*) and epididymis are enlarged and of markedly reduced echogenicity. Normal right testis (T).

In the **intravaginal torsion**, the sonographic findings are less reliable. The testis and the epididymis may appear normal, or the spectrum of sonographic findings can be seen. Torsed testis may be enlarged with normal (Fig. 6.21) or decreased (Fig. 6.22) echogenicity. Hypoechoic changes within the testis may be focal or diffused and may demonstrate homogeneous (Fig. 6.22) or heterogeneous echotexture (Fig. 6.23). The decrease in the testicular echogenicity is difficult to evaluate in children be-

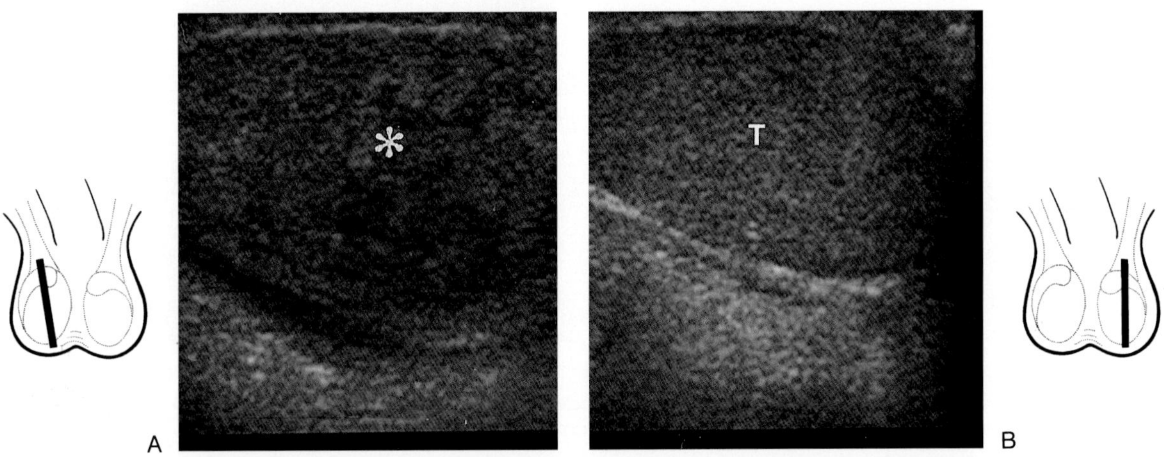

FIG. 6.23. Acute torsion of the right testis in a 22-year-old. The right testis (*) is enlarged, hypoechoic, and of heterogeneous echotexture. Normal left testis (T). Longitudinal sonogram **(A)** right testis; **(B)** left testis.

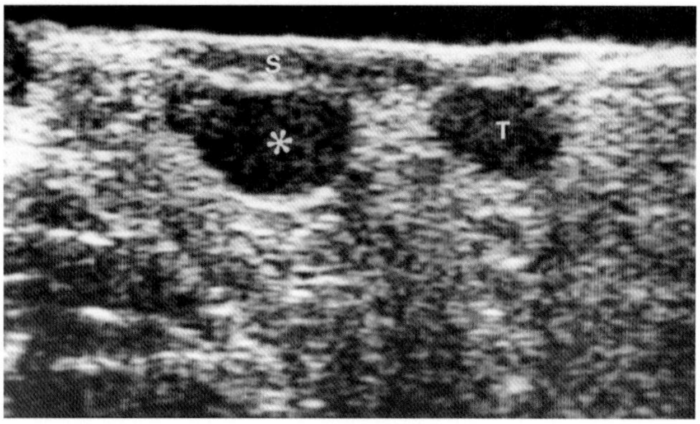

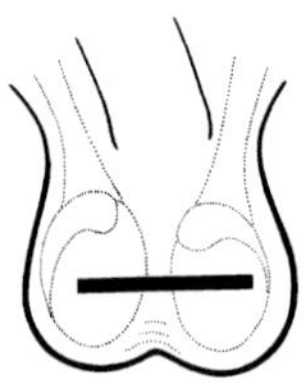

FIG. 6.24. Early phase of torsion of the right testis in a 5-year-old boy. Transverse sonogram. The right testis (*) is enlarged and there is edema of the scrotal skin (S). Note the low echogenicity of the normal left testis (T).

cause of the low echogenicity of the normal prepubertal testis (Fig. 6.24). Changes in the epididymis include enlargement and decreased echogenicity. Edema of the scrotal skin and reactive hydrocele are other findings seen in torsion (27,28). These changes, however, may not always be present in acute testicular torsion (Fig. 6.25), and when present, they are often too general to establish the diagnosis. (Similar ultrasound findings may also be present in the early stage of epididymo-orchitis.)

In the **late phase of testicular torsion**, the sonographic appearance is characterized by tissue necrosis and parenchymal hemorrhages. The echogenicity of the testis is markedly reduced, and in case of hemorrhagic infarction, there are areas of inhomogeneous and hyperechoic echotexture (sonographic indication of intraparenchymal bleeding). Typically, the epididymis is enlarged and rendered hyperechoic by hemorrhage (Fig. 6.26) (29).

Duplex Doppler Ultrasonography

Although in general a critical view must be taken toward the value of **duplex Doppler ultrasonography** (DDUS) in diagnosing testicular torsion (30), DDUS may be a useful adjunct to clinical assessment if perfusion scintigraphy or color-coded duplex sonography is not available. This modality has been more helpful in adolescents and adults than in neonates or children, because of decreased flow in normal testis in pediatric patients. The diagnosis of torsion is based on comparison of the flow signal pattern of the testicle and spermatic cord on the affected side with that of the contralateral normal side. Acutely reduced or absent signals indicate torsion, whereas increased perfusion suggests an inflammatory condition (31). In addition, changes in blood flow occurring with compression of the spermatic cord can be evaluated by duplex pulsed Doppler, but this test is limited in restless patients with severe pain. One of the major pitfalls of duplex Doppler US is that the collateral blood supply to paratesticular tissue is reactively increased within a few hours of torsion and may be mistaken for the blood flow in the testicular artery. In

A

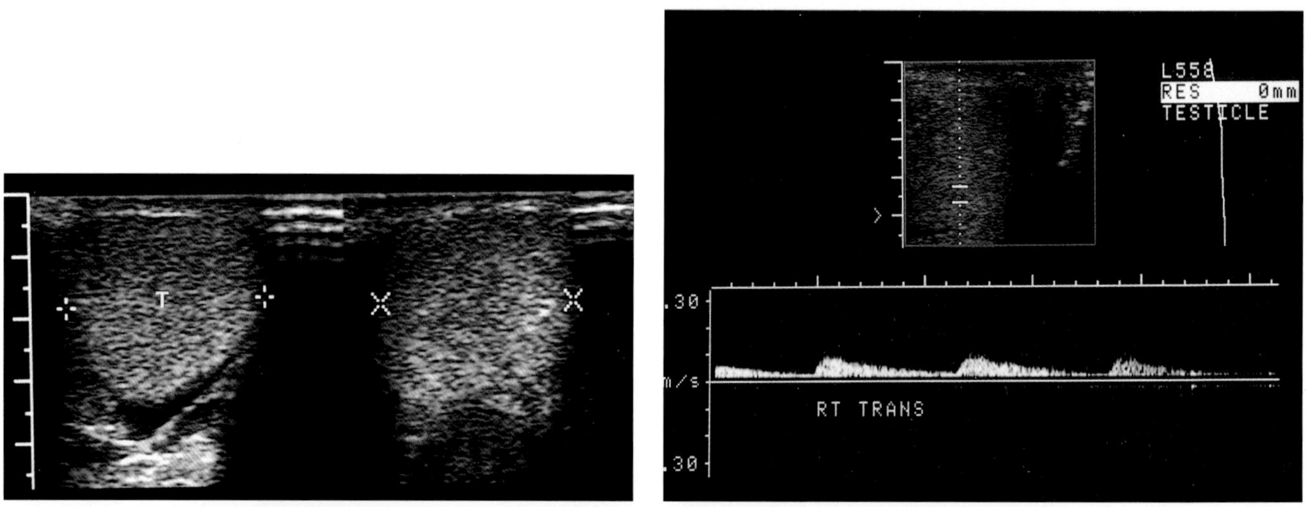

B

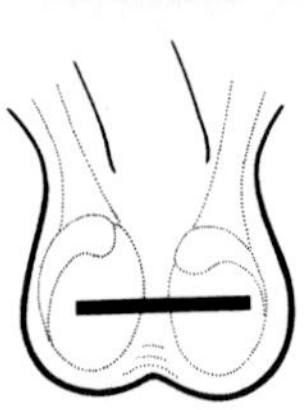

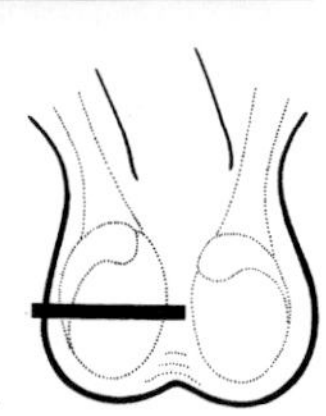

FIG. 6.25. Acute torsion of the right testis in a 16-year-old. **(A)** Transverse sonogram and **(B)** duplex Doppler demonstrate normal size, echogenicity, and flow of the right testis (T). The only abnormal finding is a small reactive hydrocele on the right. At surgery, there was 180° torsion.

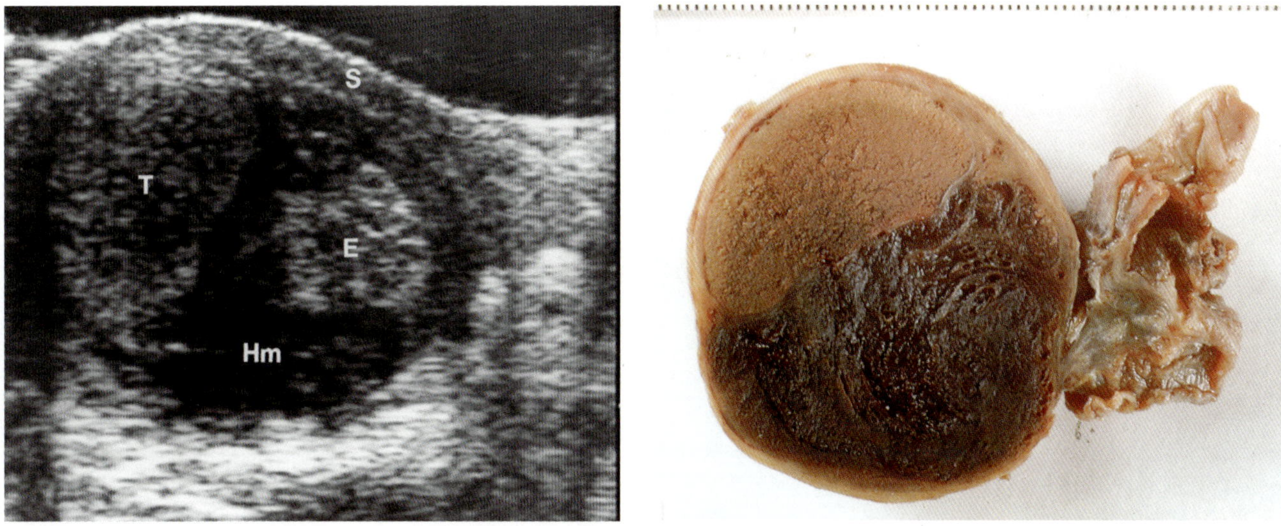

A B

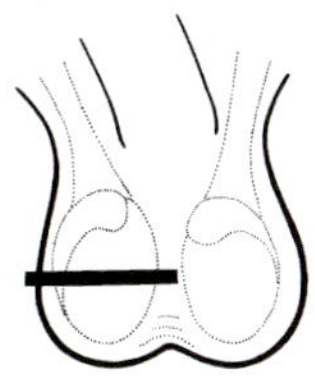

FIG. 6.26. Missed (8 days) testicular torsion in a 14-year-old patient. **(A)** Transverse sonogram demonstrates an echo-poor testicle (T), enlarged and hyperechoic epididymis (E), hematocele (Hm), and scrotal skin (S) edema. **(B)** Surgical specimen. Histologic examination confirmed a missed torsion with ischemic necrosis of the testis, hemorrhage into the epididymis, and hematocele.

addition, Doppler sonography may yield false-negative findings if the torsion is of less than 360° or if only venous congestion is present without impairment of arterial circulation during the early phase (Fig. 6.25). One other problem is that the vessels easiest and best integrated with duplex Doppler are those that can be directly visualized. The vessels in the testis are usually too small to resolve with gray-scale sonography. Another limitation of duplex Doppler US is that both late torsion with a reperfused testis and a detorsed testis demonstrate similar findings. Occlusion of the testicular artery at the level of the testis (mesorchial torsion) also may escape detection with this procedure.

Color-Coded Duplex Sonography

Color-coded duplex sonography (CCDS) is particularly useful in the diagnosis of torsion because it combines the strengths of gray-scale sonography (visualization of morphology) with those of scintigraphy (assessment of blood flow). As compared with duplex Doppler, color-coded technology of simultaneous display in a relatively large field of view is better for finding flow in small unseen vessels. Therefore, CCDS is now regarded by many as the modality of choice in the evaluation of patients with suspected testicular torsion (32–37). High-frequency (5.8 to 10.0 mHz) probe and patient cooperation are needed. Color is very sensitive to movement artifacts, and sedation is sometimes required. The normal testis and epididymis are characterized by the presence of isolated flow signals, and acute inflammation results in markedly increased blood flow (Fig. 6.27). In testicular torsion there is significantly diminished or absent organ perfusion (Fig. 6.28). The reactive hyperemia of the paratesticular structures and scrotal skin, however, can be seen (Fig. 6.29) (38,39). It is important to remember that the presence of blood flow in the testis does not exclude the possibility of torsion (Fig. 6.25) (40). The reduction of blood flow to the testis is generally not immediate or complete; rather, a gradual progression is seen as the edema increases. Therefore, not only is an absent blood flow an important diagnostic finding but so is a decreased one. Furthermore, incomplete or early torsion, for instance, may lead to false-negative results because of residual perfusion (37).

Color-coded duplex sonography is also useful in the identification of partial torsion and spontaneous detorsion. The former is characterized by reduced blood flow in the affected testicle relative to its normal counterpart, whereas the latter is characterized by increased reactive perfusion in the involved testis. Spontaneous detorsion can be differentiated from incipient epididymo-orchitis on the basis of the morphologic appearance and resolution of symptoms. Furthermore, in those cases, a "re-

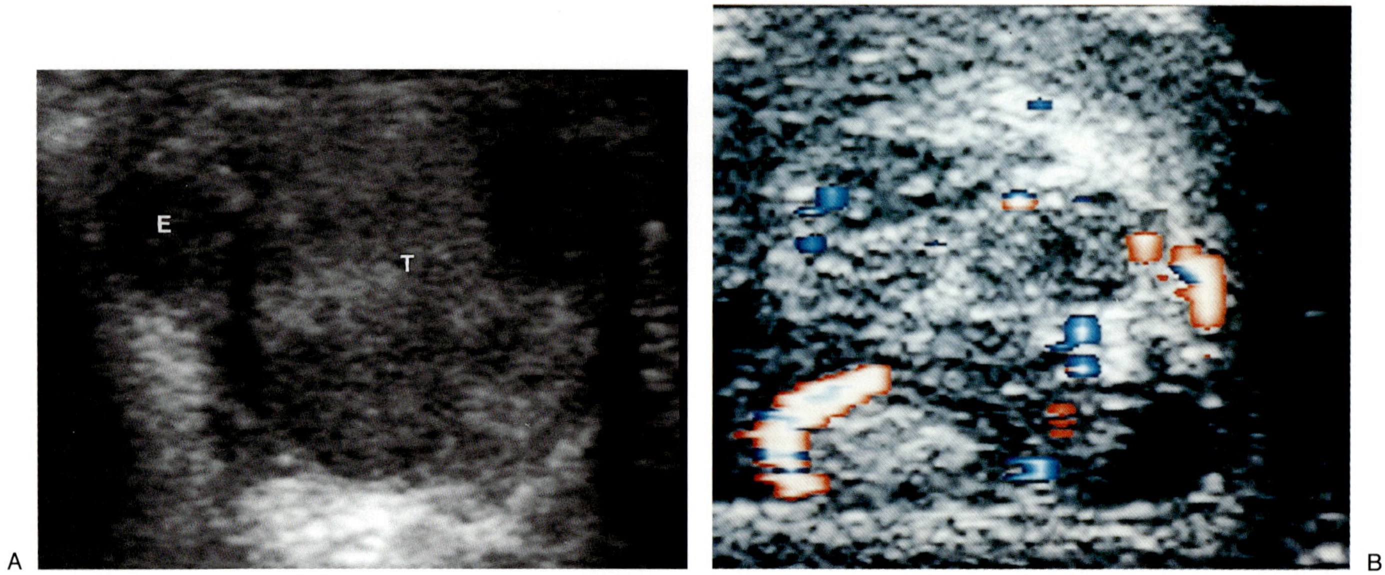

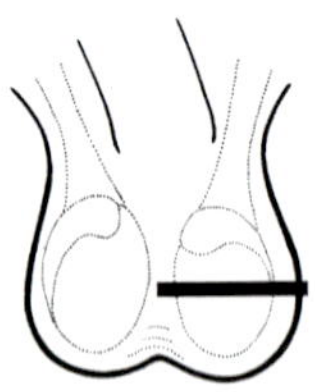

FIG. 6.27. Epididymo-orchitis. **(A)** Gray-scale and **(B)** color-coded Doppler scan show enlarged, heterogeneous echotexture of the left testis (T) and head of the epididymis (E) with marked increase in flow signals (red/blue).

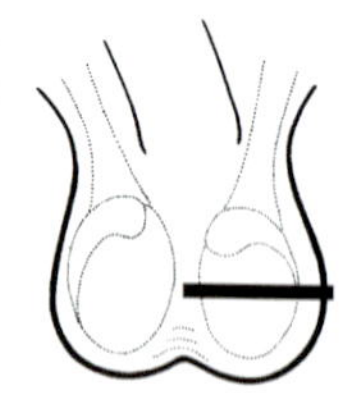

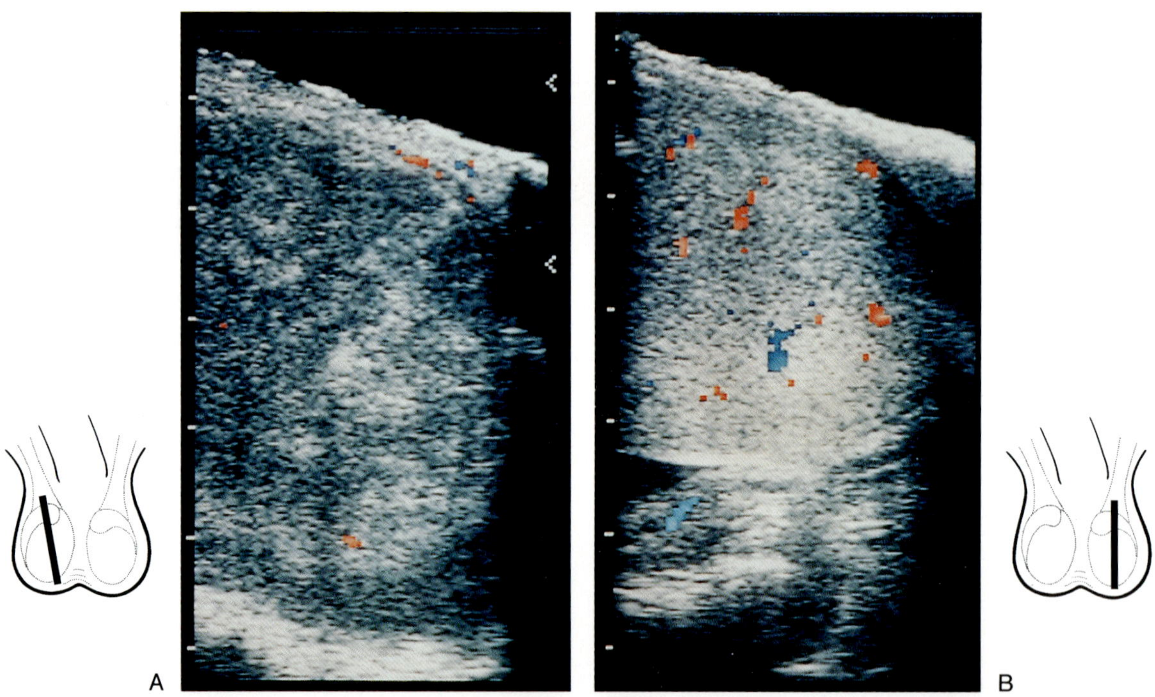

FIG. 6.28. Late testicular torsion (24 hours after the onset of symptoms) in a 42-year-old. Longitudinal color-coded duplex sonogram of the **(A)** right and **(B)** left testis. The torsed right testis is enlarged, is hypoechoic, and shows markedly diminished blood flow. Normal left testis.

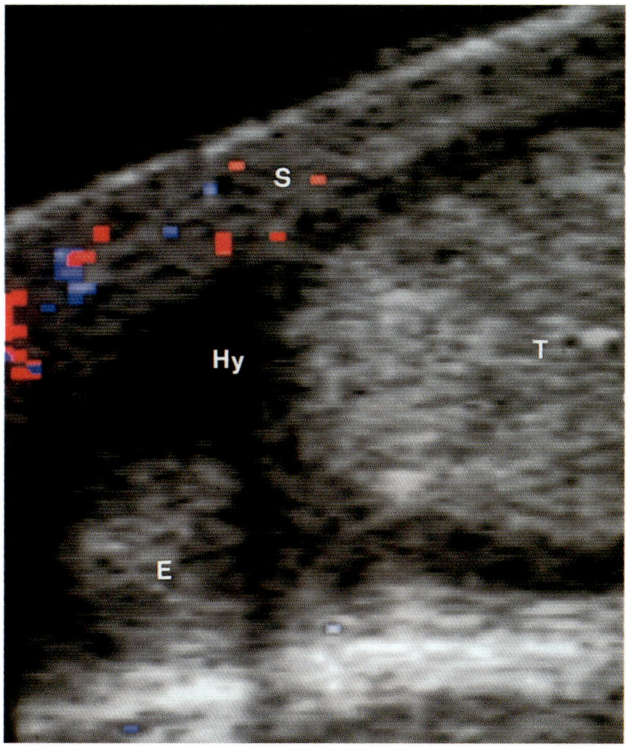

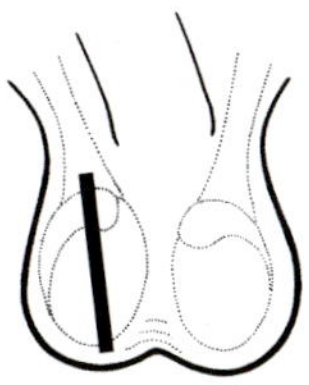

FIG. 6.29. Testicular torsion. Longitudinal CCDS showing enlargement of the epididymis (E) and testis (T) but no flow signals. Reactively increased perfusion of the scrotal skin (S) can be identified. (Hy, hydrocele)

bound effect" of arterial perfusion after detorsion may cause testicular hypervascularity (Fig. 6.30). Although useful, this distinction by CCDS is not always accurate. In addition, it is important to remember that CCDS yields only qualitative information on tissue perfusion. It is essential to compare the affected testicle with the unaffected side to identify the sometimes very subtle changes found in partial torsion (41). Detection of flow in the very small testis in normal infants or prepubertal children may also be difficult because of the small size and relatively little perfusion of the normal testis (42). Diagnosis of decreased perfusion associated with torsion is dependent on comparison with the normally perfused testicle. Therefore, in children whose testes are small and flow signals are normally difficult to detect, the diagnosis of torsion is more difficult. Overall, CCDS has a range of 82% to 90% sensitivity, but its specificity in diagnosing testicular torsion reaches 100% (37).

Magnetic Resonance Imaging in the Evaluation of Torsion

The reports on MRI findings in acute torsion in humans are sporadic and not well documented. The testis may be normal or enlarged and of heterogeneous signal intensity. In a study using an animal model, the acutely torsed testis was normal or enlarged and demonstrated either normal or diffuse heterogeneous low signal intensity on T2-weighted images (Fig. 6.31) (43). Much attention has been given to the appearance of the spermatic cord. With testicular torsion the spermatic cord may be enlarged, demonstrating a high signal intensity because of surrounding edema. However, it does not show hypervascularity, as it does in epididymitis. A twisted cord can be seen as multiple low-intensity curvilinear structures radiating in a "whirlpool" pattern, which is best seen in a plane perpendicular to its axis (44). The point of the twist may be seen as an area of signal void (**torsion knot**). In subacute and chronic torsion, the testis is usually small in size and has decreased cord vascularity (45). In patients with intermittent torsion, the testis is enlarged and demonstrates high signal intensity on both T1- and T2-weighted images. These findings correlate with the histologic findings of diffuse subacute hemorrhage. In chronic torsion, the testis shows a consistent low signal intensity on T2-weighted images, probably due to fibrosis and hemosiderin deposition following hemorrhagic infarction (43–45). The displaced epididymis is markedly thickened with edema and hemorrhage. The tunica albuginea is usually also thickened, especially in chronic disease, and there may be associated hematocele.

All these findings are helpful in differentiating torsion from epididymitis. Of them, vascularity of the spermatic cord is the most sensitive and specific (45,31). P MR spectroscopy has been reported to be helpful in the eval-

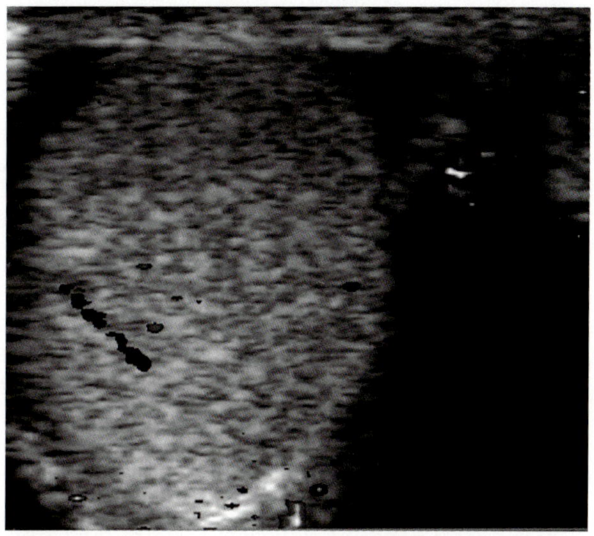

FIG. 6.30. "Rebound effect"—increased testicular hypervascularity immediately after manual detorsion. Doppler study of the right testis.

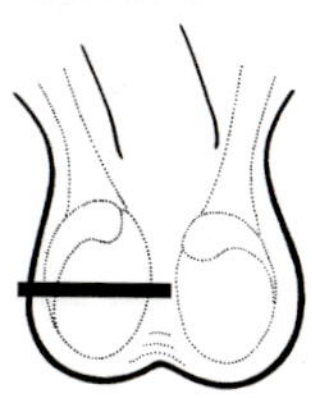

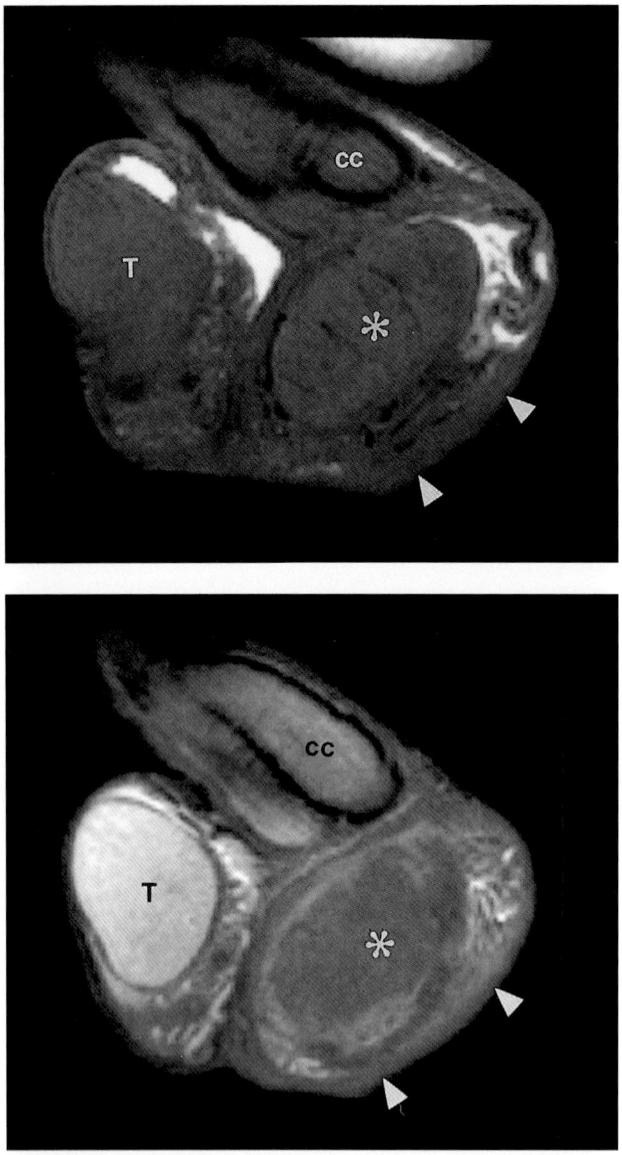

FIG. 6.31. Acute testicular torsion. Coronal **(A)** T1-weighted and **(B)** T2-weighted MR images. The left testis (*) is enlarged and of heterogeneous low signal intensity on T2 images. (*Arrowheads,* scrotal wall thickening and edema; T, normal right testis; cc, corpora cavernosa)

uation of acute torsion. In patients with spermatic cord torsion, levels of β-adenosine triphosphate (β-ATP) and phosphomonoester (PM) are markedly decreased, and inorganic phosphorus (P_i) is increased (46).

Nuclear Scintigraphy in the Evaluation of Torsion

In the early phase of testicular torsion, flow studies show normal or reduced vascularity in the spermatic cord, lack of visualization of vascularity in the pudendal vessels, and markedly decreased activity in the scrotum, both in the flow and in the static images. By the end of the early phase the spermatic cord flow may be normal, or a **"nubbin" sign** (pathognomonic for acute torsion) may be seen (47). The peripheral scrotal component of the flow study remains normal at this time, but the involved testis demonstrates absent activity in the static image. In the middle phase of acute torsion, cord activity is normal or again may show a nubbin sign. At this stage static images begin to show a "rim" of scrotal activity. After 24 hours—the late phase, or "missed torsion"—the **rim sign** is quite intense but gradually fades as the testicle undergoes necrosis and atrophy (48). At this very late stage scintigraphy may even become normal. The detorsed testicle, since it can appear perfectly normal on scan yet remains at high risk for torsion again in the future, is a particularly difficult problem (49). In the clinical setting a decrease in or disappearance of testicular pain may indicate spontaneous detorsion. Scintigraphy in such situations may show decreased, normal, or increased scrotal activity (10). A more detailed discussion of technique and nuclear scintigraphy findings can be found in Chapter 9.

Comparative Evaluation

Testicular torsion represents a surgical emergency. The decision to explore a patient with acute scrotal swelling is based mainly on physical examination and clinical history. A number of diagnostic tests have been advocated to reduce the number of unnecessary scrotal explorations. The main role of imaging is to exclude the diagnosis of torsion and to document normal testicular blood flow when conservative treatment is chosen. There is no one answer to the **best** imaging approach. The process of imaging depends on local expertise available. When imaging studies are needed for the diagnosis of torsion and for differentiation between torsion and epididymitis, color-coded duplex sonography and dynamic and static Tc-DTPA scintigraphy are the mainstays. Tc-DTPA is often preferred to CCDS in a pediatric patient because of poor flow signal of the normal prepubertal testis. A combination of these two modalities, however, is most accurate in the acute phases, where prompt diagnosis and surgery are necessary (43). Timing often prevents this luxury. Although Doppler ultrasound may be helpful in identifying detorsion (50,51), it is not always diagnostic (52). Magnetic resonance imaging plays a minor and questionable role but is advocated in the subacute phase (more than 24 hours) of torsion (44) In this time frame, MRI can be helpful in differentiating torsion from epididymitis. Despite high sensitivity and excellent tissue contrast, at present MR findings are not specific enough to diagnose acute torsion accurately.

APPENDICEAL TORSION

Four types of appendages represent vestigial embryologic structures: the appendix testis (sessile hydatid of Morgagni), the appendix epididymis (stalked or pedunculated hydatid of Morgagni), the paradidymis (organ of Giraldes), and the vas aberrans (organ of Haller). The appendix testis is commonly present (in 92% of normal subjects in one study), and the appendix epididymis, somewhat less common (34% in another study) (12). Acute scrotal symptoms may be produced by torsion of any of these intrascrotal appendages, but approximately 91% to 95% of appendiceal torsions affect the appendix testis (accounting for about 5% of patients with an acute scrotum), and most of the rest involve the appendix epididymis (12). Twisting of the vas aberrans or the paradidymis is less common (Fig. 6.32).

In children, appendiceal torsion is nearly as common as testicular torsion, accounting for 20% to 40% of cases of acute scrotum in the pediatric age group (14,53,54). The peak incidence is between 7 and 14 years of age.

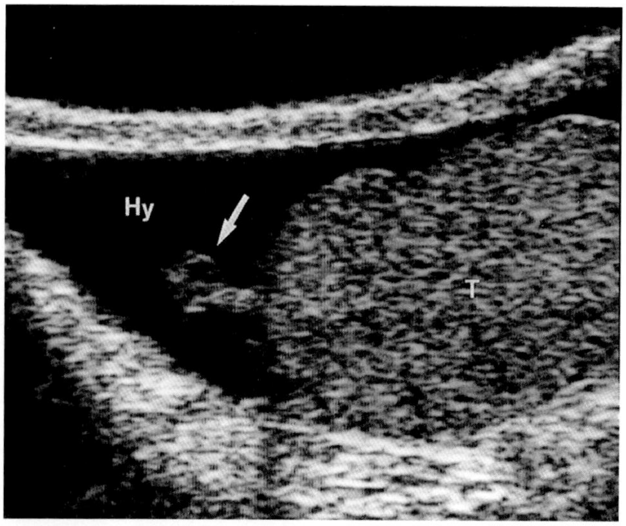

FIG. 6.33. Stalked hydatid in a 37-year-old patient. The appendage (*arrow*) is displayed against the surrounding hydrocele (Hy).

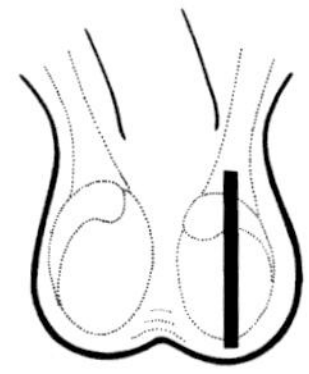

Clinical Presentation

Torsion of an appendage may be asymptomatic (missed torsion), with subsequent atrophy or spontaneous twisting off of the affected appendage. Parts thus separated may calcify, and some are discovered as an incidental finding on ultrasound or during an operation (hydrocele concretion, see p. 141).

More commonly, however, torsion of an appendage presents with the signs of an acute scrotum. The onset of symptoms is less sudden, and initially appendiceal torsion may not cause any discomfort or impair physical activity. Clinical examination may not reveal any scrotal abnormalities. The testis, epididymis, and spermatic cord are not painful; the cremasteric reflex is preserved; and fever and leukocytosis are absent. After several hours, or sometimes days, the initial presentation is obscured by more or less severe secondary alterations leading to the picture of acute scrotum. Formation of a reactive hydrocele leads to swelling of the affected side with erythema and scrotal edema, rendering the clinical examination extremely difficult. There is also pain, initially restricted to the upper aspect of the affected hemiscrotum, but it can radiate into the groin or into the upper abdomen. Nausea and vomiting are far less common than in testicular torsion, where there is direct peritoneal irritation.

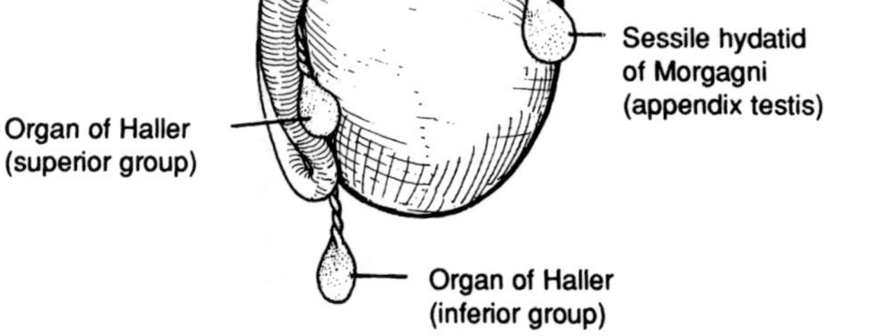

FIG. 6.32. Hydatids and other intrascrotal appendages.

Early in appendiceal torsion, the tender torsed appendix can be palpated near the upper pole of the testis, and a characteristic blue dot can be seen through the scrotal skin (15). This so-called **blue dot sign** is pathognomonic for torsion of an appendage. In later stages, the entire testis becomes swollen. Torsion of the epididymal appendix causes acute pain and hemiscrotal hydrocele.

Accurate diagnosis of torsion of the appendices depends on differentiation of testicular torsion from appendiceal torsion, since patients with torsion of the appendices may have symptoms sufficiently intense to suggest an acute testicular torsion.

Torsion of testicular or epididymal appendages is usually treated by simple excision with or without contralateral exploration.

Ultrasound in the Evaluation of Appendiceal Torsion

Under normal conditions the small intrascrotal appendages are seldom seen on ultrasound. On occasion they may be recognized as small, pedunculated structures floating in a hydrocele (Fig. 6.33). A torsed, swollen appendage is seen as a "third structure" in addition to the testis and epididymis. The latter two are of normal

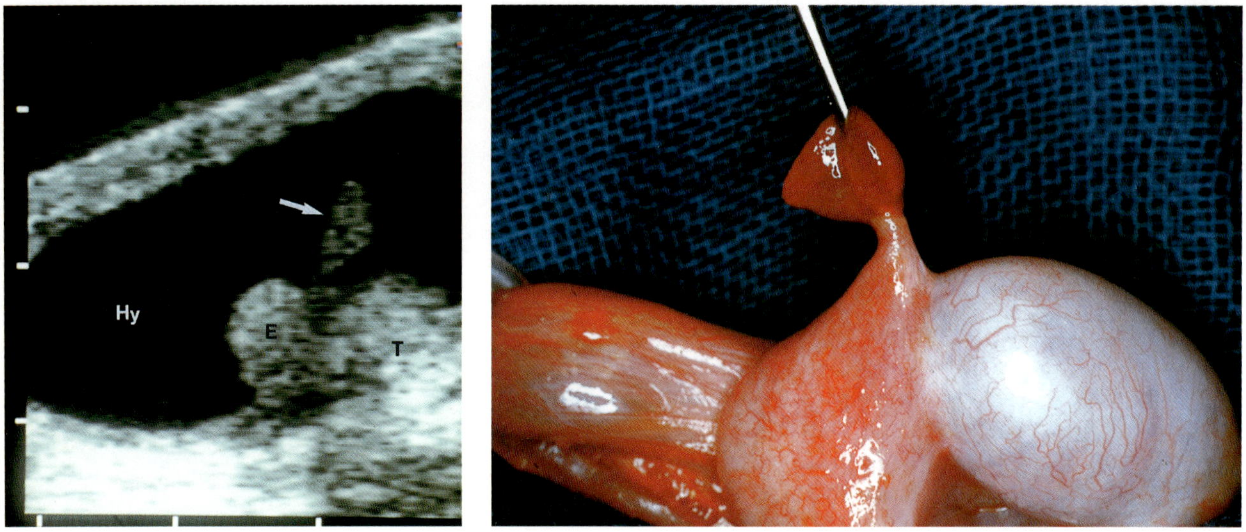

A B

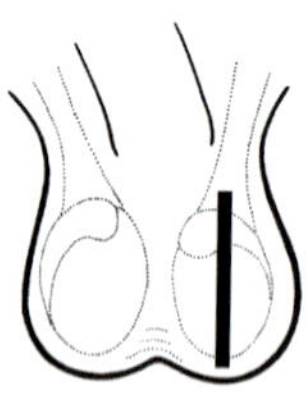

FIG. 6.34. Hydatid torsion in a 13-year-old patient presenting with acute scrotum. **(A)** Three structures—the testis (T), the enlarged epididymis (E), and a hydatid (*arrow*)—are seen against the background of a large hydrocele (Hy). **(B)** Intraoperative view.

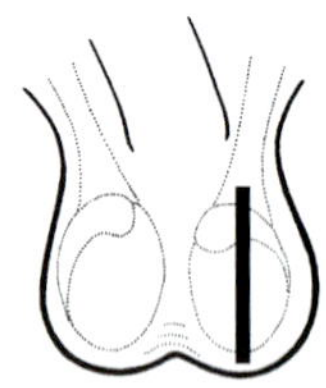

shape and echogenicity (Fig. 6.34). When present, reactive hydrocele and edema of the scrotal skin are also demonstrated on US. Occasionally, torsion of the appendix epididymis is associated with edematous enlargement of the adjacent head of the epididymis.

Doppler Ultrasonography

As intrascrotal blood flow is also preserved in other clinical entities (e.g., epididymitis), the duplex Doppler signals are not diagnostic or specific for appendiceal torsion. **Color-coded duplex sonography** (CCDS) is useful in the diagnosis of appendiceal torsion because preservation of normal testicular and epididymal blood flow differentiates it from testicular torsion. A moderate increase in epididymal blood flow is a sign of reactive hyperemia and can be confused with epididymitis.

Magnetic Resonance Imaging in the Evaluation of Appendiceal Torsion

Similar to ultrasound, normal intrascrotal appendages are rarely identified on MRI. When detected, testicular appendices are seen around the testicular margin and epididymal appendices are seen around the head of the epididymis. Torsion of the testicular or epididymal appendices can be identified on MR scans by their typical location and the signal characteristics of hemorrhage.

Nuclear Scintigraphy in the Evaluation of Appendiceal Torsion

Testicular scintigraphy may show augmented flow and a focal area of increased activity on the static images. However, the study is frequently normal.

Comparative Evaluation

When findings on physical examination need reinforcement, the imaging modality of choice for appendiceal torsion is ultrasound. Similar to the approach of testicular torsion, the main role of imaging is to exclude other causes of acute scrotum (e.g., epididymo-orchitis or testicular torsion). Scintigraphy plays a minor role in the evaluation of appendiceal torsion, and MRI is not used for the diagnosis of this entity.

REFERENCES

1. Chen DC, Holder LE, Melloul M. Radionuclide scrotal imaging: further experience with 210 new patients. Part 2: Results and discussion. *J Nucl Med* 1983;24:841–853.
2. Lutzker LG. Scrotal scintigraphy. In Tauxe WN, Dubovsky, EV, eds. *Nuclear medicine in clinical urology and nephrology*. Norwalk, CT: Appleton-Century-Crofts; 1985:321–346.
3. Chen DC, Holder LE, Melloul M. Radionuclide scrotal imaging: further experience with 210 patients. Part 1: Anatomy, pathophysiology, and methods. *J Nucl Med* 1983;24:735–742.
4. Sharer WC. Acute scrotal pathology. *Surg Clin North Am* 1982;62: 955–970.

5. Prater JM, Overdorf BS. Testicular torsion: a surgical emergency. *Am Fam Physician* 1991;44:834–840.
6. Barker K, Raper FP. Torsion of the testis. *Br J Urol* 1964;36:35–41.
7. Atallah MW, Ippolito JJ, Rubin BW. Intrauterine bilateral torsion of the spermatic cord. *J Urol* 1976;116:128–129.
8. Hricak H. The testis. In: Hricak H, Carrington BM. *MRI of the pelvis: a text atlas*. London: Martin Dunitz; 1991:343–381.
9. Scorer CG, Farrinton GH. Torsion of the testis. In: Scorer CG, Farrinton GH. *Congenital deformities of the testis and epididymis*. New York: Appleton-Century-Crofts; 1971:118–135.
10. Lutzker LG, Zuckier LS. Testicular scanning and other applications of radionuclide imaging of the genital tract. *Semin Nucl Med* 1990;20:159–188.
11. Bellinger MF. The blind-ending vas: the fate of the contralateral testis. *J Urol* 1985;133:644–645.
12. Williamson RC. Torsion of the testis and allied conditions. *Br J Surg* 1976;63:465–476.
13. Haynes BE, Bessen HA, Haynes VE. The diagnosis of testicular torsion. *JAMA* 1983;249:2522–2527.
14. Knight PJ, Vassy LE. The diagnosis and treatment of the acute scrotum in children and adolescents. *Ann Surg* 1984;200:664–673.
15. McAninch JW. Disorders of the testis, scrotum, and spermatic cord. In: Tanagho EA, McAninch JW. *Smith's general urology*, 13th ed. Norwalk, CT: Appleton & Lange, 1992:616–624.
16. Rajfer J. Congenital anomalies of the testis. In: Walsh PC, Retik AB, Stamey TA, Vaughan ED, eds. *Campbell's urology*, 6th ed, vol 2. Philadelphia: WB Saunders; 1992:1543–1562.
17. Harrison RH. Testicular torsion. In: Glenn JF, ed. *Urologic surgery*, 3rd ed. Philadelphia: JB Lippincott; 1983:1067–1076.
18. Laor E, Fisch H, Tennenbaum S, Sesterhenn I, Mostofi K, Reid RE. Unilateral testicular torsion: abnormal histological findings in the contralateral testis—cause or effect? *Br J Urol* 1990;65:520–523.
19. Mizrahi S. Shtamler B. Surgical approach and outcome in torsion of testis. *Urology* 1992;39:52–54.
20. Chen DC, Holder LE, Kaplan GN. Correlation of radionuclide imaging and diagnostic ultrasound in scrotal diseases. *J Nucl Med* 1986;27:1774–1781.
21. Finkelstein MS, Rosenberg HK, Snyder HM, Duckett JW. Ultrasound evaluation of scrotum in pediatrics. *Urology* 1986;27:1–9.
22. Hricak H, Jeffrey RB. Sonography of acute scrotal abnormalities. *Radiol Clin North Am* 1983;21:595–603.
23. Martin B, Conte J. Ultrasonography of the acute scrotum. *J Clin Ultrasound* 1987;15:37–44.
24. Stoller ML, Kogan BA, Hricak H. Spermatic cord torsion: diagnostic limitations. *Pediatrics* 1985;76:929–933.
25. Brown SM, Casillas VJ, Montalvo AM, Albores-Saavedra J. Intrauterine spermatic cord torsion in the newborn: sonographic and pathologic correlation. *Radiology* 1990;177:755–757.
26. Zerin JM, DiPietro MA, Grignon A, Shea D. Testicular infarction in the newborn: ultrasound findings. *Pediatr Radiol* 1990;20:329–330.
27. Bird K, Rosenfield AT, Taylor KJW. Ultrasonography in testicular torsion. *Radiology* 1983;147:527–534.
28. Hricak H, Lue T, Filly RA. Experimental study of the sonographic diagnosis of testicular torsion. *J Ultrasound Med* 1983;2:349–356.
29. Vick CW, Bird K, Rosenfield AT, et al. Extratesticular hemorrhage associated with torsion of the spermatic cord: sonographic demonstration. *Radiology* 1986;158:401–404.
30. Haynes BE. Doppler ultrasound failure in testicular torsion. *Ann Emerg Med* 1984;13:1103–1107.
31. Jequier S, Patriquin H, Filiatrault D, et al. Duplex Doppler sonographic examinations of the testis in prepubertal boys. *J Ultrasound Med* 1993;12:317–322.
32. London NJ, Smart JG, Kinder RB, Watkin EM, Rees Y, Haley P. Prospective study of routine scrotal ultrasonography in urological practice. *Br J Urol* 1989;63:416–419.
33. Fowler RC, Chennells PM, Ewing R. Scrotal ultrasonography: a clinical evaluation. *Br J Radiol* 1987;60:649–654.
34. Kass EJ, Stone KT, Cacciarelli AA, Mitchell B. Do all children with an acute scrotum require exploration? *J Urol* 1993;150:667–669.
35. Erden MI, Ozbek SS, Aytac SK, Adsan O, Suzer O, Safak SM. Color Doppler imaging in acute scrotal disorders. *Urol Int* 1993;50:39–42.
36. Fitzgerald SW, Erickson S, DeWire DM, et al. Color Doppler sonography in the evaluation of the adult acute scrotum. *J Ultrasound Med* 1992;11:543–548.
37. Wilbert DM, Schaerfe CW, Stern WD, Strohmaier WL, Bichler KH. Evaluation of the acute scrotum by color-coded Doppler ultrasonography. *J Urol* 1993;149:1475–1477.
38. Rifkin MD, Kurtz AB, Pasto ME, Goldberg BB. Diagnostic capabilities of high-resolution scrotal ultrasonography: prospective evaluation. *J Ultrasound Med* 1985;4:13–19.
39. Fobbe F, Heidt P, Hamm B, et al. Verbesserung der Diagnostik skrotaler Erkrankungen mit der farbkodierten Duplexsonographie. ROFO 1989;150:629–634.
40. Steinhardt GF, Boyarsky S, Mackey R. Testicular torsion: pitfalls of color Doppler sonography. *J Urol* 1993;150:461–462.
41. Cunningham JJ. Sonographic findings in clinically unsuspected acute and chronic scrotal hematoceles. *AJR* 1983;140:749–752.
42. Atkinson GO Jr, Patrick LE, Ball TI Jr, Stephenson CA, Broecker BH, Woodard JR. The normal and abnormal scrotum in children: evaluation with color Doppler sonography. *AJR* 1992;158:613–617.
43. Tzika AA, Vigneron DB, Hricak H, Moseley ME, James TL, Kogan BA. P-31 MR spectroscopy in assessing testicular torsion: rat model. *Radiology* 1989;172:753–757.
44. Mattrey R, Trambert M. MR imaging of the scrotum and testis. In: Edelman RR, Hesselink JR, eds. *Clinical magnetic resonance imaging*. Philadelphia: WB Saunders; 1990:952–979.
45. Trambert MA, Mattrey RF, Levine D, Berthoty DP. Subacute scrotal pain: evaluation of torsion versus epididymis with MR imaging. *Radiology* 1990;175:53–56.
46. Chew WM, Hricak H, McClure RD, Wendland MF. In vivo human testicular function assessed with P-31 MR spectroscopy. *Radiology* 1990;177:743–747.
47. Holder LE, Melloul M, Chen D. Current status of radionuclide scrotal imaging. *Semin Nucl Med* 1981;11:232–249.
48. Dunn EK, Chen PC, Lipschitz SS, Glassberg KI, Sarkar SD, Strashun AM. Testicular scintigraphic findings two to three months after torsion. Correlation with sonography and histopathology. *Clin Nucl Med* 1991;16:37–39.
49. Willgress ER, Camponova EJ, Kistler AM, Goyer PF, Silverman ED. Spontaneous reduction of testicular torsion during scrotal imaging. *Clin Nucl Med* 1989;14:540.
50. Middleton WD, Melson GL. Testicular ischemia: color Doppler sonographic findings in five patients. *AJR* 1989;152:1237–1239.
51. Middleton WD, Siegel BA, Melson GL, Yates CK, Andriole GL. Acute scrotal disorders: prospective comparison of color Doppler US and testicular scintigraphy. *Radiology*, 1990;177:177–181.
52. Feld R, Middleton WD. Recent advances in sonography of the testis and scrotum. *Radiol Clin North Am* 1992;30:1033–1051.
53. Anderson PA, Giacomantonio JM. The acutely painful scrotum in children: review of 113 consecutive cases. *Can Med Assoc J* 1985;132:1153–1155.
54. Tanaka T, Mishkin FS, Datta NS. Radionuclide imaging of the scrotal contents. In: Freeman LM, Weissmann HS, eds. *Nuclear medicine annual*. New York: Raven Press; 1981:195–219.

C. Scrotal Trauma

TRAUMA

Scrotal trauma usually results from either direct injury (e.g., a kick to the scrotum) or from straddle injuries (1). The diagnosis can be confidently established on the basis of anamnestic data and the generally impressive clinical presentation. Direct traumatic injury or forceful compression of the testis against the pubic ramus may result in infarction of the testis or epididymis, testicular torsion, or rupture of the tunica albuginea, with the testicular parenchyma bulging through the tear. Treatment of blunt scrotal trauma depends upon the extent of the injury. Because testicular rupture and massive intratesticular hematoma usually require surgical treatment, assessment of the integrity of the tunica albuginea and the extent of scrotal hematoma are important.

Clinical Presentation

Marked scrotal swelling, hematoma, or open injuries limit the physical examination. On transillumination the testicular shadow is nearly always concealed by an intrascrotal hematoma or a hematocele.

Ultrasound in the Evaluation of Scrotal Trauma

Patients with open and penetrating scrotal injuries undergo immediate surgery and are not candidates for sonography. In cases of blunt trauma, ultrasound is used to (1) confirm or exclude testicular rupture, (2) differentiate a soft tissue hematoma from a hematocele (6), and (3) follow up patients undergoing conservative therapy

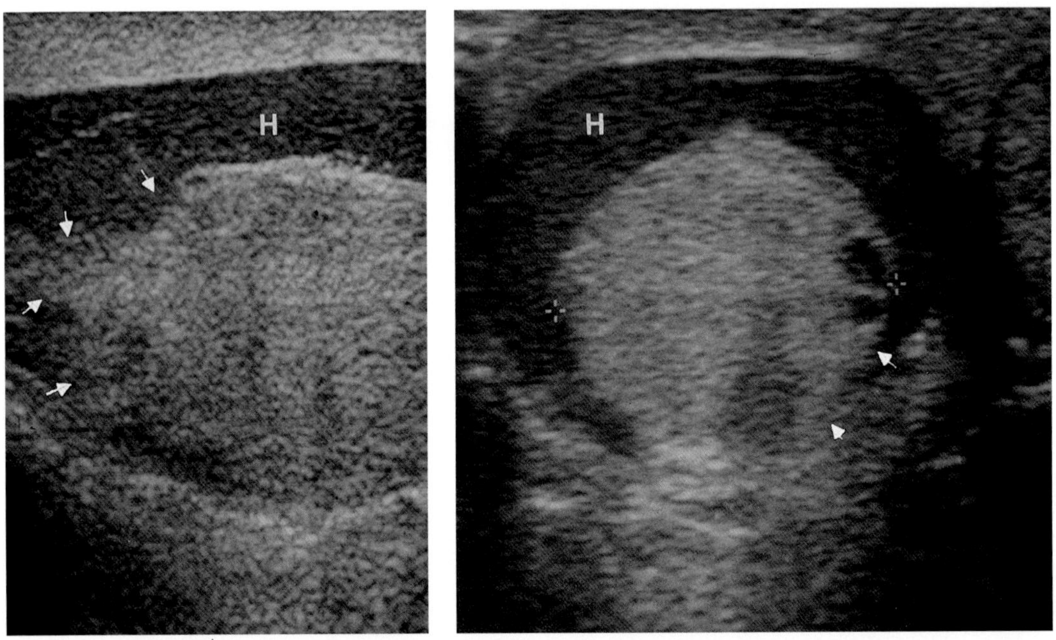

A B

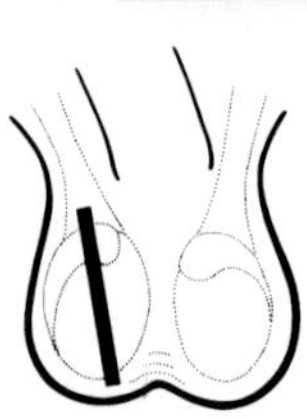

FIG. 6.35. Testicular rupture following direct injury to the scrotum. **(A)** Longitudinal and **(B)** transverse scan of the right hemiscrotum. Heterogeneous testicular echogenicity indicates testicular injury, and irregularities of testicular contour (*arrows*) indicate testicular rupture. Fluid with homogeneous internal echoes surrounds the testis, indicating hematocele (H).

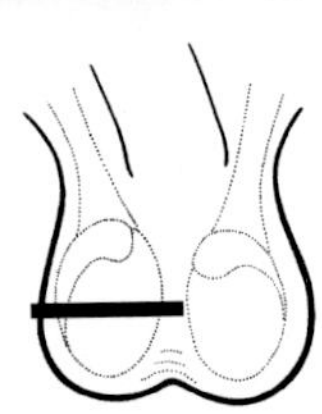

(1–8). The diagnosis of testicular rupture (a surgical emergency) and the identification of a large hematoma requiring intervention are of particular importance because sonographic findings have a decisive influence on clinical management (7–11). If testicular rupture is left untreated, serious complications, such as ischemic atrophy or infection, may supervene.

Testicular rupture from traumatic injury to the testis is generally easy to identify on ultrasonography. Irregularities of testicular contour and either hypo- or hyperechoic heterogeneous areas are characteristic of testicular injury (Fig. 6.35) (12). Histologically, these parenchymal lesions correspond to areas of hemorrhage or infarction. Direct visualization of fracture lines on ultrasonography is rare, but visualization of a mixed solid/liquid intrascrotal mass and absence of testislike structures are indicative of testicular fragmentation (Fig. 6.36). Delicate tears in the tunica albuginea without intratesticular hemorrhages and without extrusion of testicular tissue may escape sonographic detection (7,13). Hematoceles usually accompany testicular rupture, but their absence does not exclude this diagnosis (14). Even when testicular rupture is excluded by the demonstration of a normal testicular echotexture, sonographic follow-up is recommended in patients with blunt trauma to the scrotum as long as a hematocele is present. Intratesticular hemorrhage—hematoma—represents a diagnostic challenge. Intratesticular hematomas are usually sharply demarcated and have homogeneous decrease in echogenicity (Fig. 6.37). The main differential diagnosis is incidental testicular tumor, and careful clinical correlation (hematoma renders normal clinical examination while tumor most commonly has hard consistency) and short-term follow-up are mandatory.

The sonographic appearance of a **scrotal hematoma** between the layers of the scrotal coverings or in the scrotal septum depends on its size and duration. Acutely, the only change noted is thickening of soft tissue. Later, hypoechoic areas, indicating liquefaction, can be seen. The size of a hematoma and the status of underlying testis are accurately evaluated on sonograms (Fig. 6.38).

Injuries of the penis involving the corpus spongiosum result in **extravasation of urine**, which may seep into the scrotum. Perforation of the urethra can be demonstrated by urethrography. Sonography of the scrotum shows a characteristic "onion peel" distention of the scrotal coverings produced by the urine extravasated into the soft tissue structures.

The presence of numerous small internal echoes distinguishes a **hematocele** from a serous hydrocele (Fig. 6.35). In a chronic hematocele thick septa and wall thickening are demonstrated (Fig. 6.39) (15). Occasionally, calcified areas may be seen within a chronic hematocele. Testicular atrophy is commonly seen with a long-standing hematocele (Fig. 6.40). Since the sonographic appearance of a chronic hematocele may resemble that

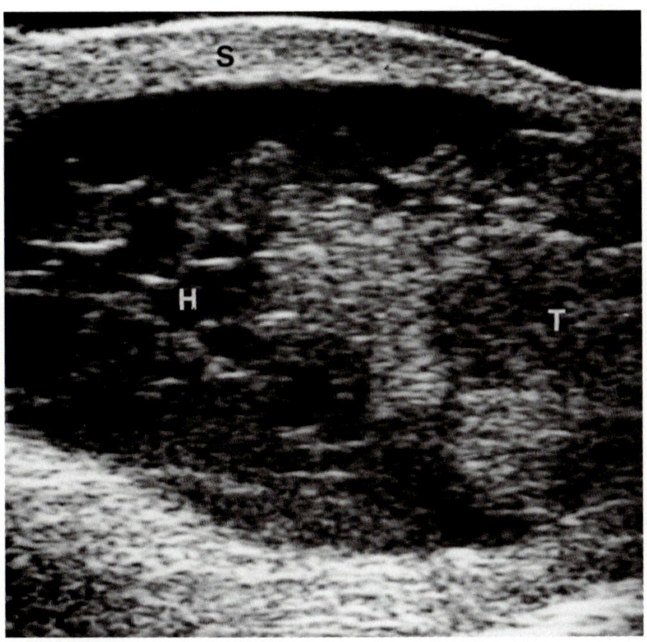

A

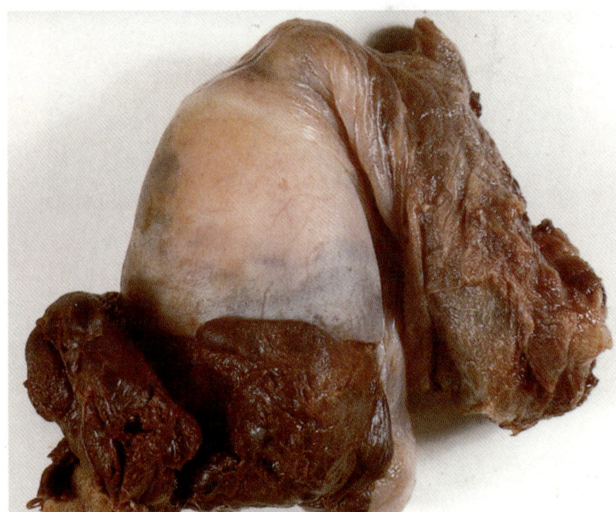

B

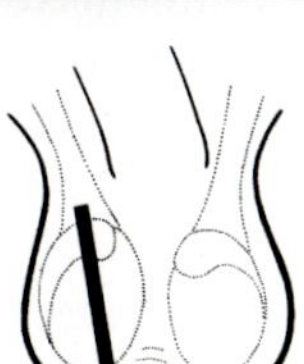

FIG. 6.36. Rupture of the testis in a 20-year-old patient after an automobile accident. **(A)** Sonography shows an irregular testicular contour with hypoechoic inhomogeneous intratesticular areas (T) and accompanying hematocele (H). (S, scrotal skin) **(B)** Surgical specimen.

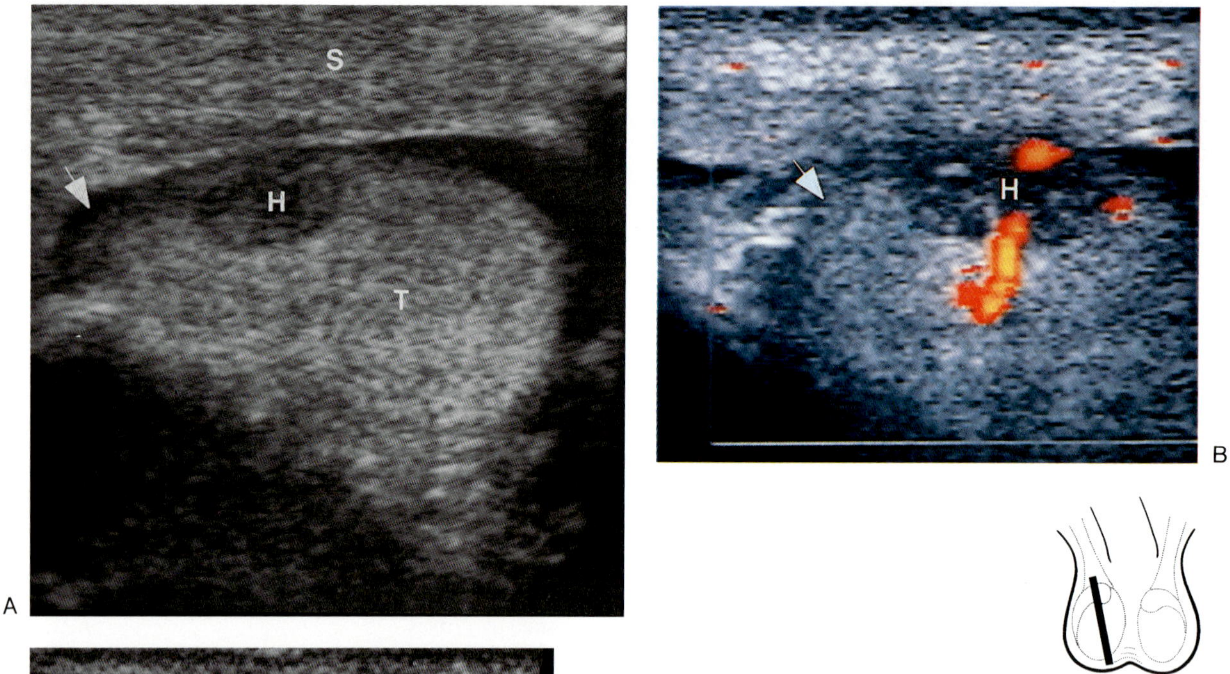

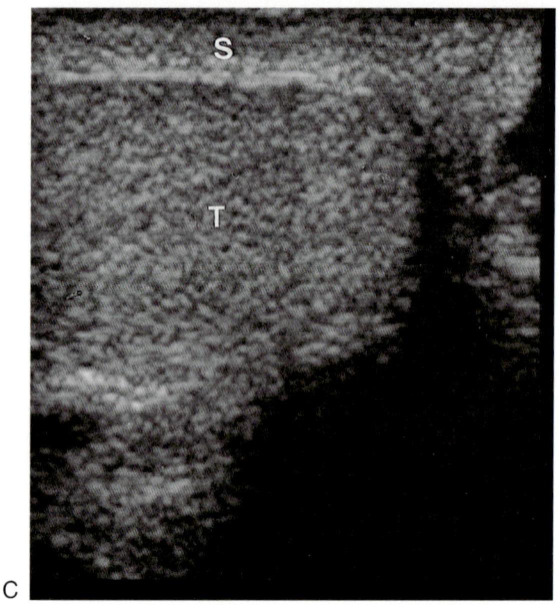

FIG. 6.37. Patient with direct injury to the scrotum seen 1 week after the incidence. **(A)** and **(B)** are gray-scale and color-coded duplex sonograms, respectively, at the time of initial examination; **(C)** is a gray-scale sonogram 6 weeks later. Sharply marginated hypoechoic mass (H) in the right testis (T) indicates an intratesticular tumor or hematoma. There is a second area of intratesticular hemorrhage (*arrow*). Follow-up sonogram shows normal right testis (T) and complete resolution of intratesticular hematoma. Scrotal skin (S) edema is also no longer seen. (T, testis)

of a chronic hydrocele or pyocele, differentiation between them requires clinical correlation (16). An infected hematocele after trauma must also be considered.

Color-Coded Duplex Sonography

In patients with severe scrotal trauma, rupture of the tunica albuginea and subsequent bleeding may cause a reduction or absence of testicular perfusion. Even in cases with extensive hematoma, CCDS can accurately demonstrate the vascular status of the scrotal contents and may be helpful in making decisions about surgical treatment.

Magnetic Resonance Imaging in the Evaluation of Scrotal Trauma

Magnetic resonance imaging can detect testicular injury and can help diagnose testicular rupture. The diagnosis of testicular rupture is facilitated by MR depiction of tunica albuginea. The integrity of the tunica albuginea is best judged on T2-weighted or contrast-enhanced T1-weighted images. Multiple planes of imaging are often needed for thorough evaluation. Testicular injury can be detected on T2-weighted images (the signal intensity of the injured testis is lower than normal) but is even better seen on postcontrast study. On contrast-enhanced T1-

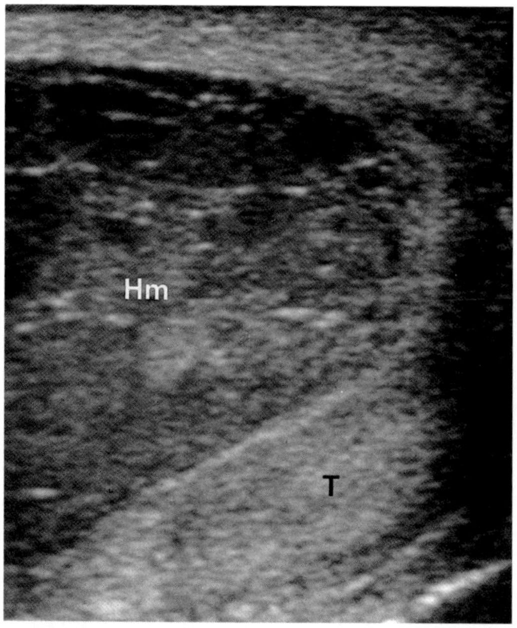

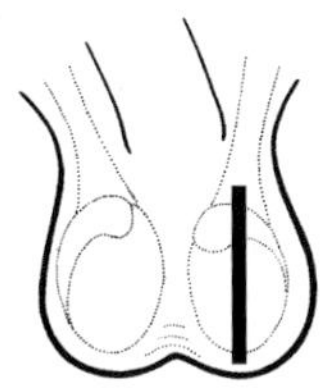

FIG. 6.38. A scrotal hematoma (Hm) demonstrates heterogeneous echotexture. Testis (T) is displaced. Longitudinal sonogram.

weighted images, the intratesticular injury demonstrates decreased enhancement (Fig. 6.41). Magnetic resonance imaging is also valuable in the detection of intratesticular hematoma. Signal intensity of the testicular hematoma depends on the time interval between bleeding and MR scan. In the acute phase low or medium signal intensity is seen on T1-weighted images, and high signal intensity is seen on T2-weighted images. In the chronic phase high signal intensity occurs on both T1- and T2-weighted images. Since hemorrhage may also be present in testicular tumor, differential diagnosis relies on the presence of an associated tumor mass, tumor necrosis, and petechial hemorrhages of varying age. Sometimes contrast-enhanced MR imaging is helpful for the differentiation, as tumors will enhance, whereas the area of hemorrhage will not.

Hematoceles may be difficult to diagnose on ultrasound examination, as sonographic findings of hematocele, pyocele, and chronic hydrocele may mimic each other. Hematocele, however, is readily identified on MR scans. As with intratesticular hemorrhage, the signal intensity varies with the age of the hemorrhagic fluid. At first, hematocele usually exhibits medium signal intensity on T1-weighted images and high signal intensity on T2-weighted images. Chronic hematocele usually demonstrates high signal intensity on both T1- and T2-weighted images.

Nuclear Scintigraphy in the Evaluation of Scrotal Trauma

A **hematocele** can be seen as a semilunar cold defect but cannot be differentiated from hydrocele or pyocele. **Hematomas** of the testis also produce a cold defect on static images, but the defect is somewhat irregular along its border. Flow is usually augmented through the cord. If the flow study is done while there is bleeding, there can be extravasation into the scrotum (1). Testicular ischemia may also result from trauma (17).

Comparative Evaluation

Early surgical intervention is important in testicular trauma. Today sonography is a mainstay imaging modality in the evaluation of scrotal injury. Gross rupture of the testis is accurately assessed sonographically, but a minor tear of the tunica albuginea can be missed. Other

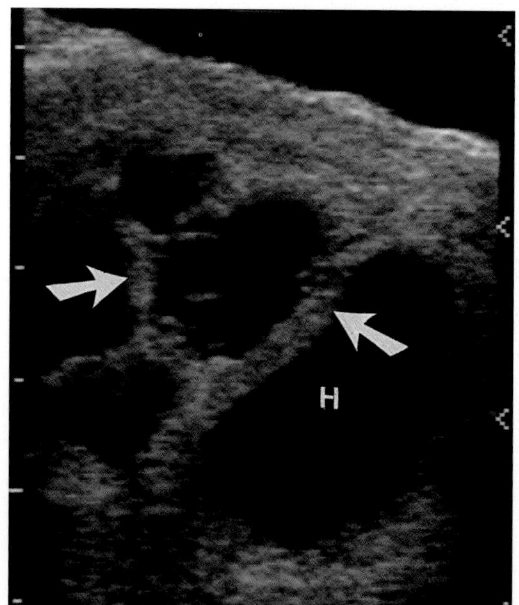

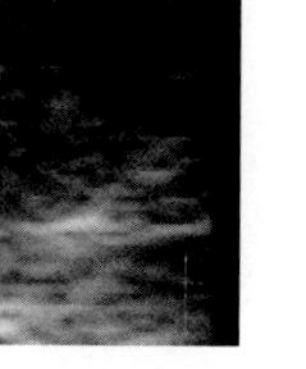

FIG. 6.39. Chronic hematocele (H) demonstrates thick septa (*arrows*). (T, testis)

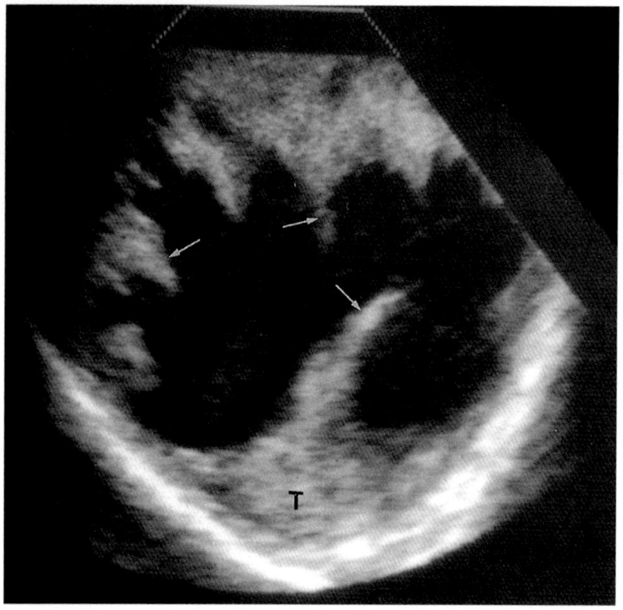

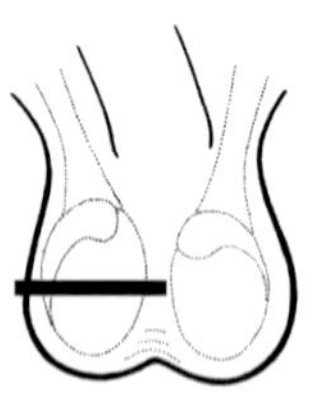

FIG. 6.40. Chronic hematocele (H) with numerous thick septa (*arrows*) and small atrophic testis (T).

sequels of trauma—hematocele and hematoma—are also well evaluated sonographically. Although ultrasound is usually an initial and often the only study requested in the work-up of scrotal trauma, several reports have recently been published questioning the accuracy of ultrasound in the diagnosis of **testicular rupture** (16). Scintigraphy also can play a role in evaluating this group of patients (17). There are, however, only a few anecdotal reports comparing color Doppler sonography and scintigraphy, and such studies are now essential. Scintigraphy has technical demands, but the studies are quite easy to perform, and the entire area can be evaluated on the flow and static images. Ultrasound, however, combines superb morphologic display and with the use of CCDS offers evaluation of testicular perfusion. Although sonography appears to be used more frequently than scintigraphy in this clinical setting, the definitive study comparing the merits of both modalities has not been performed. Magnetic resonance imaging also offers only anecdotal reports on its accuracy and superiority over ultrasound (Fig. 6.41). Although the large field of view, excellent contrast resolution, and (with the use of contrast media) assessment of vascularity are all advantages of MRI, MRI is expensive and rarely immediately available. This is a big disadvantage in this acute clinical setting.

A

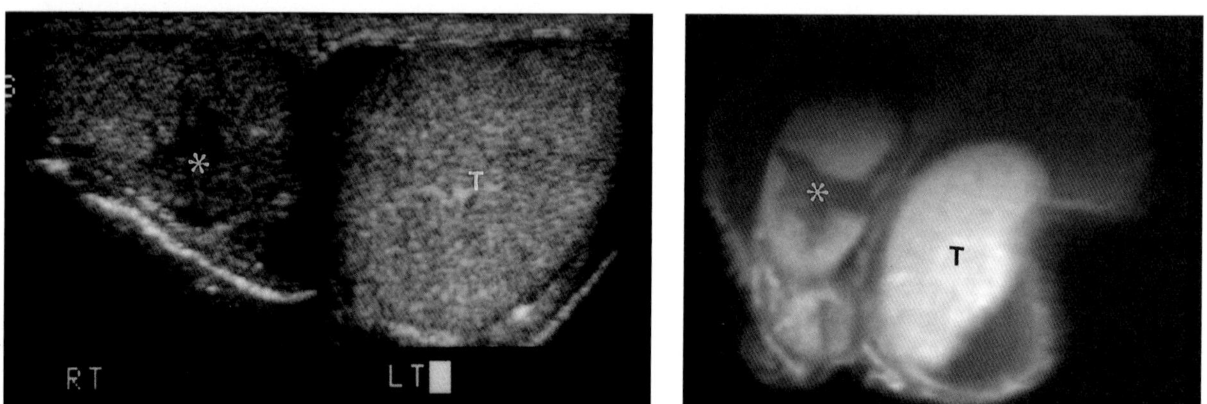

B

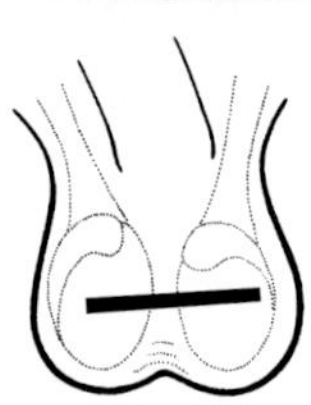

FIG. 6.41. Testicular fracture. **(A)** Sonogram and **(B)** coronal plane contrast-enhanced T1-weighted MR image. Irregular hypoechoic abnormality (*) seen on ultrasound indicates a tumor, infarct, or intratesticular hematoma. The diagnosis of testicular rupture (*) is better and more confidently diagnosed on MRI. (T, normal left testis).

REFERENCES

1. McConnell JD, Peters PC, Lewis SE. Testicular rupture in blunt scrotal trauma: review of 15 cases with recent application of testicular scanning. *J Urol* 1982; 128:309–311.
2. Elgazzar AH, Fernandez-Ulloa M, Black RR, Silberstein EB. Incidental detection of obstructive uropathy during scrotal imaging. *Clin Nucl Med* 1988; 13:823–825.
3. Charron M, Mandell JB, Kolodny GM. Detection of a rare complication of appendicitis by scrotal imaging. *Clin Nucl Med* 1988; 13:761–762.
4. Vieco PT, Stern J, Herschorn S. Patent processus vaginalis. *Clin Nucl Med* 1990; 15:263.
5. Edelsberg JS, Surh YS. The acute scrotum. *Emerg Med Clin North Am* 1988;6:521–546.
6. Schaffer RM. Ultrasonography of scrotal trauma. *Urol Radiol* 1985;7:245–249.
7. Anderson KA, McAninch JW, Jeffrey RB, Laing FC. Ultrasonography for the diagnosis and staging of blunt scrotal trauma. *J Urol* 1983; 130:933–935.
8. Fournier GR, Laing FC, McAninch JW. Scrotal ultrasonography and the management of testicular trauma. *Urol Clin North Am* 1989; 16:377–385.
9. Kratzik C, Hainz A, Kuber W, et al. Has ultrasound influenced the therapy concept of blunt scrotal trauma? *J Urol* 1989; 142:1243–1246.
10. MacDermott JP, Gray BK, Stewart PA. Traumatic rupture of the testis. *Br J Urol* 1988;62:179–181.
11. Hricak H, Jeffrey RB. Sonography of acute scrotal abnormalities. *Radiol Clin North Am* 1983;21:595–603.
12. Lupetin AT, King W, Rich PJ, Lederman RB. The traumatized scrotum. *Radiology* 1983; 148:203–207.
13. Jeffrey RB, Laing FC, Hricak H, McAninch JW. Sonography of testicular trauma. *AJR* 1983; 141:993–995.
14. Sanders LM, Premkumar A, Amis ES, Cohen M, Newhouse JH. Trauma-induced testicular torsion: ultrasonographic features and pathologic correlation. *J Clin Ultrasound* 1989; 17:538–541.
15. Cunningham JJ. Sonographic findings in clinically unsuspected acute and chronic scrotal hematoceles. *AJR* 1983; 140:749–752.
16. Ugarte R, Spaedy M, Cass AS. Accuracy of ultrasound in diagnosis of rupture after blunt testicular trauma. *Urology* 1990; 36:253–254.
17. Lutzker LG, Zuckier LS. Testicular scanning and other applications of radionuclide imaging of the genital tract. *Semin Nucl Med* 1990;20:159–188.

D. Miscellaneous Acute Conditions

There are other less common scrotal disorders presenting with acute scrotum. They represent a clinical challenge, as physical examination is limited not only by painful scrotum but also by history and laboratory data. Yet imaging can help greatly. In an infant, meconium periorchitis should be considered, along with extravaginal torsion, hernia, or tumor. In a child and young adolescent, testicular vasculitis secondary to Henoch-Schoenlein-Purpura (HSP) is a known cause of unnecessary surgical scrotal exploration. Similarly, vasculitis with testicular infarcts can cause an acute scrotum and should be considered in patients who have polyarteritis nodosa, rheumatoid arthritis, or HIV disease. Lastly, necrosis of the intrascrotal fatty tissue is a surgical emergency. Crepitations, when present, are specific clinical findings but sonographic findings may precede and help in this life-threatening condition.

MECONIUM PERIORCHITIS

Meconium periorchitis is the consequence of a meconium peritonitis. Meconium peritonitis can occur secondary to bowel perforation, obstruction (such as volvulus), atresia or tumor, or may be due to mesenteric vascular insufficiency (1,2). Spillage of the meconium into the peritoneum provokes a sterile inflammation with subsequent calcifications and fibrosis. Clinically, there are two forms of meconium peritonitis: a severe form that requires surgical intervention at birth (it presents with bowel obstruction, abdominal distention, and pneumoperitoneum), and a mild and self-limiting form (the only symptom is usually scrotal mass). The meconium migrates into the scrotal sac through a patent processus vaginalis. The peritonitis has usually healed by the time of birth, and in the immediate postpartum period, a newborn boy presents with enlarged scrotum that transilluminates and mimics a hydrocele. Rapid foreign body reaction and calcification occurring during the first month of life harden the contents of the scrotum into a tumorlike lesion that mimics testicular neoplasia. Meconium periorchitis undergoes spontaneous resolution, including the resorption of the calcifications (3).

Clinical Presentation

Meconium periorchitis is usually diagnosed in an infant (median age: 4 weeks). Neonatal torsion, tumor, and hernia are the main differential diagnosis. Clinical diagnosis can be suspected when a newborn with a reducible scrotal mass returns at 4 weeks of age with hard scrotal mass, and scrotal calcifications are noted on roentgenographic examination. If no preceding physical examination is available, the diagnosis may be difficult. The findings of calcifications are helpful but not diagnostic, as scrotal calcifications in an infant can also be seen in a testicular tumor, teratoma, or gonadoblastoma. Torsion followed by hemorrhagic infarction can also demonstrate calcification. Correct pretreatment diagnosis is essential, as meconium periorchitis does not require surgical intervention.

Ultrasound

Ultrasound is an ideal imaging modality to ascertain the differential diagnosis of enlarged scrotum in an infant. With a high degree of accuracy, sonography will differentiate between meconium periorchitis and tumor or torsion. In meconium periorchitis, the testis is normal and, as such, well visualized sonographically (1,4,5). The surrounding soft tissue mass often demonstrates acoustic shadowing, indicating calcifications (Fig. 6.42). The diagnosis will be reinforced by comparing the ultrasonographic study with plain film radiograph. Stipled calcifications will be seen in the scrotum and in the abdomen (Fig. 6.42). Sometimes it is difficult to differentiate between tumor and torsion. In a newborn the torsion is extravaginal, usually occurring in utero, and at the time of clinical discovery the testis is often infarcted. Intratesticular hemorrhage and necrosis cause the testis to appear heterogeneous on the sonogram. A hyperechoic rim is often seen in extravaginal torsion and has not been

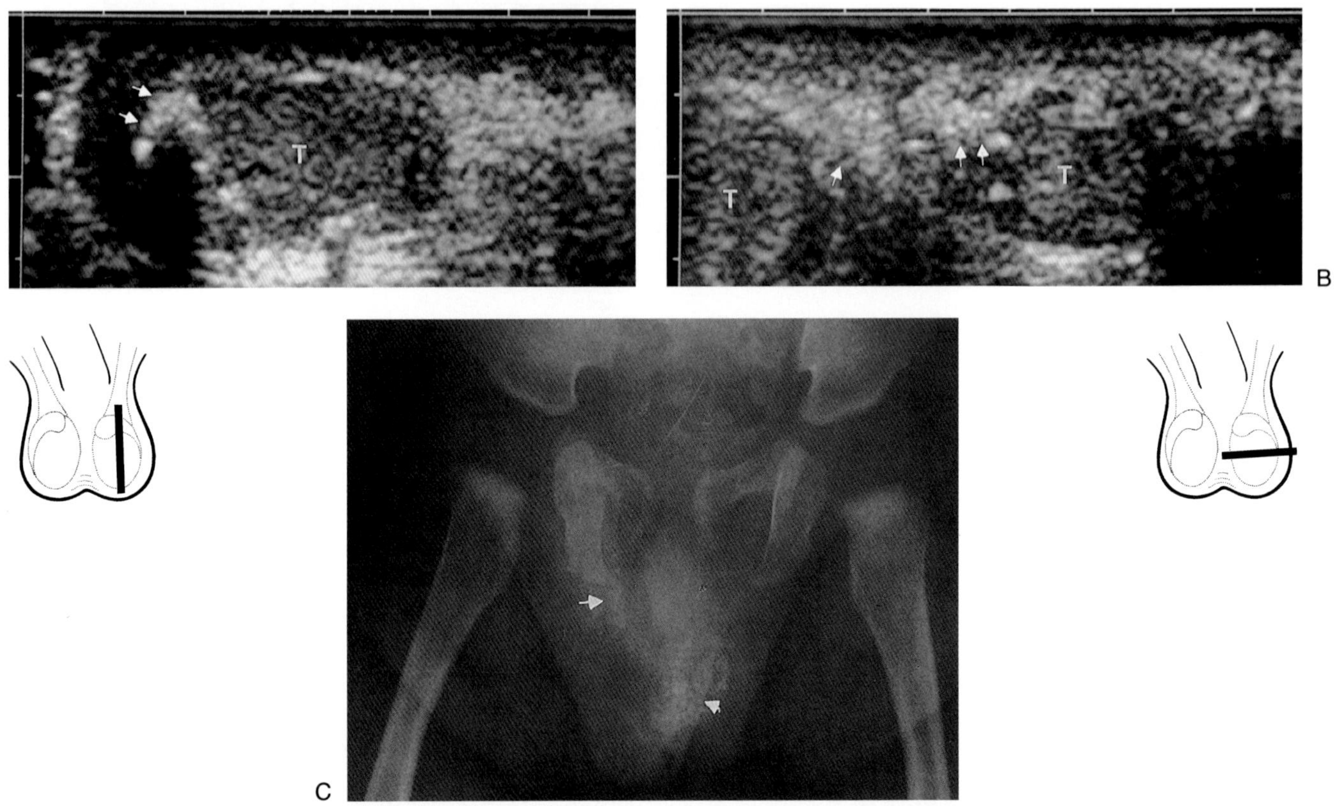

FIG. 6.42. Meconium periorchitis in a 4-week-old infant. **(A)** Longitudinal and **(B)** transverse sonograms, and **(C)** radiograph. Both right and left testis (T) are normal. There is peritesticular echogenic tissue (*arrows*) with acoustic shadowing. Stipled calcifications (*arrows*) in the scrotum are seen on the radiograph.

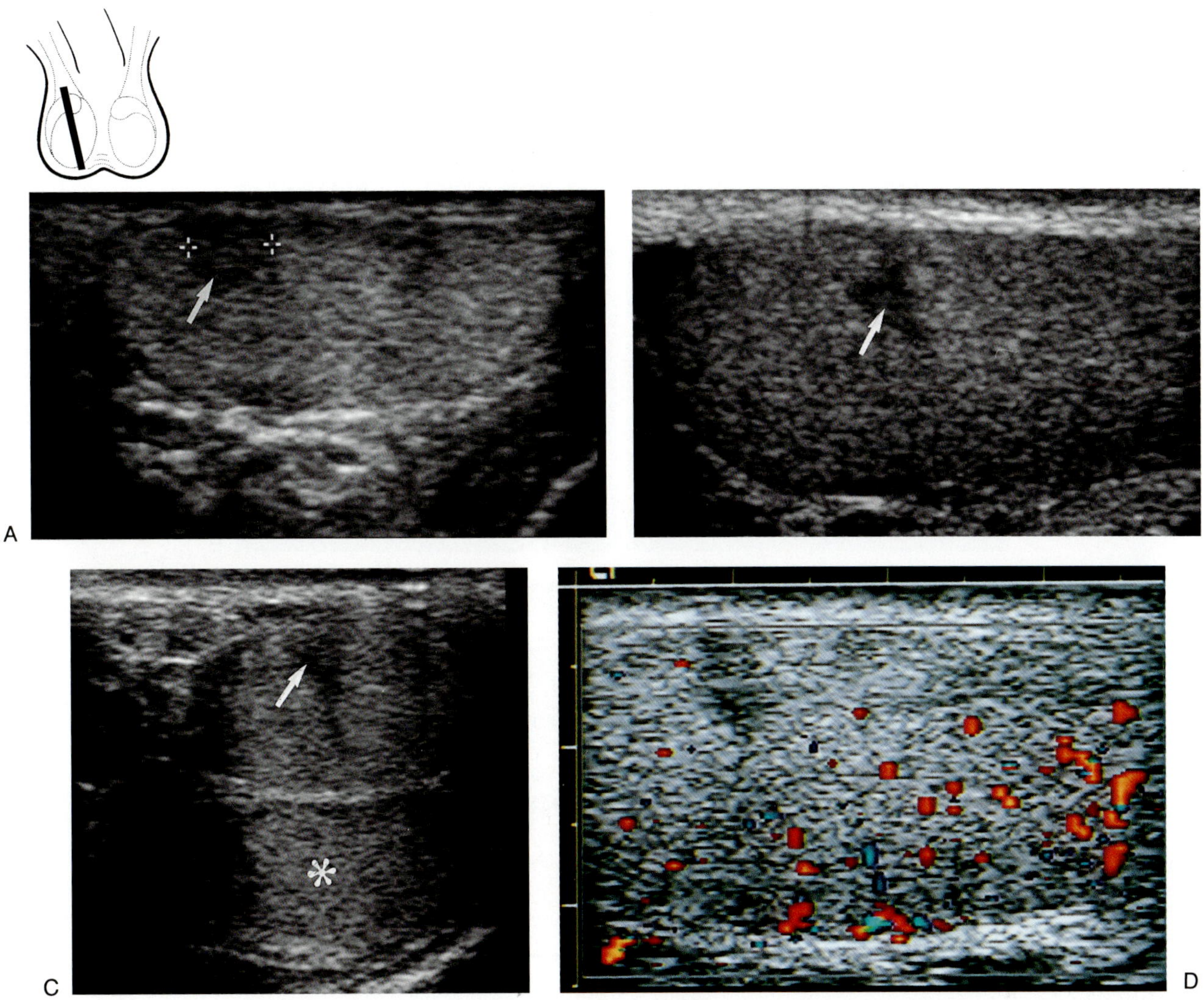

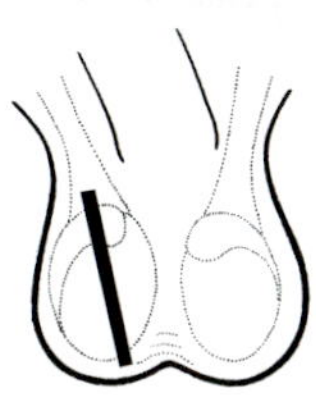

FIG. 6.43. Temporal changes of a testicular infarct in a 28-year-old patient with HIV disease. **(A)** Longitudinal sonogram at the time of clinical presentation of acute scrotum, and **(B)**, **(C)**, and **(D)** are longitudinal, coronal sonograms, and longitudinal color Doppler sonograms 6 weeks later. Round hypoechoic mass (*arrow*) indistinguishable from tumor was seen initially. Wedge-shaped peripheral hypoechoic lesion (*arrow*), much more suggestive of an infarct, is seen on follow-up study. No flow within an infarcted area is detected on color Doppler scan. Normal left testis (asterisk).

reported in cases of testicular tumor. Except for ultrasound, no other cross-sectional imaging modality plays a role in the evaluation of meconium periorchitis.

TESTICULAR VASCULITIS

Necrotizing vasculitis affecting the testis can be seen (in decreasing incidence) in patients with polyarteritis nodosa, Henoch-Schoenlein-Purpura, rheumatoid arthritis, HIV, and dermatomyositis (6–12). Patients present with an acute scrotum and, in rare instances, involvement of the testis is the only clinical manifestation of the disease (8,12). The potential for testicular involvement in polyarteritis nodosa is well established and was first reported in 1905 (6). It includes arteritis, infarctions of various duration, hematoma, hemorrhage, and aneurysm formation. Involvement of the testis can be seen in as many as 86% of patients with systemic polyarteritis nodosa (5). However, clinical manifestations of the disease are only seen in up to 18% of patients (7). Testicular involvement, therefore, although common, is rarely the presenting manifestation of the disease. Because of the high incidence of arteritis involving the testis at autopsy, random biopsies of the testis to establish the diagnosis have been proposed. Random biopsies, however, were diagnostic in only 22% of patients with polyarteritis nodosa (8); therefore, this diagnostic method has been abol-

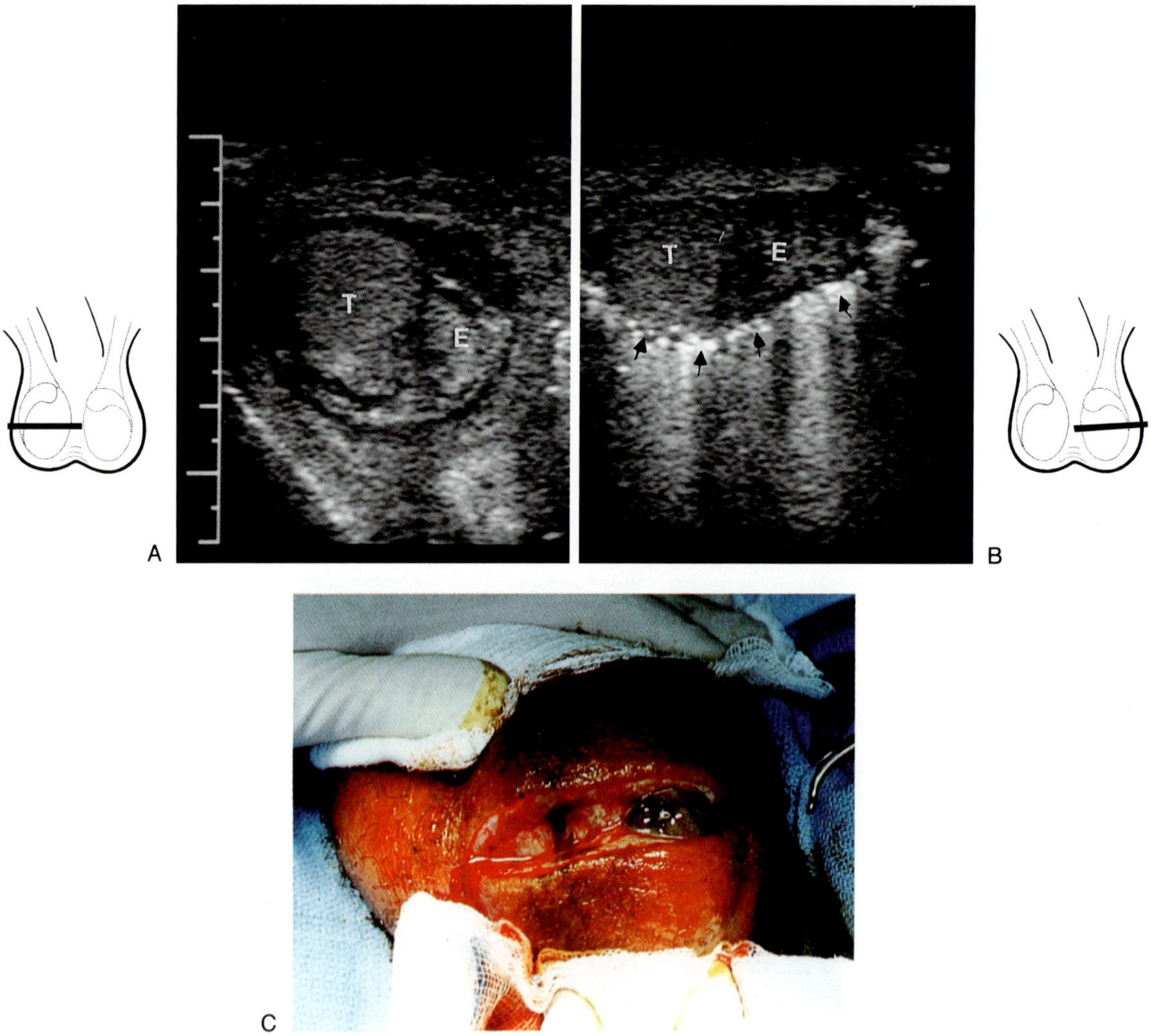

FIG. 6.44. Fournier-Gangrene in a 37-year-old patient with HIV disease. Transverse **(A)**, **(B)** sonograms, and **(C)** intraoperative view. There is bilateral epididymitis (both epididymis [E] are enlarged). Testes (T) are normal. Echogenic foci (*arrows*) with acoustic shadowing ("dirty shadowing") indicate air and, therefore, necrotizing fasciatis. Pus and necrosis seen during surgery. Bilateral orchiectomy and scrotal section were performed.

ished. In all patients with testicular vasculitis, the presenting clinical symptoms are usually diffusely enlarged, painful testis, and associated hematocele that transilluminates. Sometimes a localized intraparenchymal mass can be palpated (8). The missed diagnosis of vasculitis has caused many unnecessary surgical explorations. Imaging findings, clinical history, and the consideration of this disease can help in diagnosis. However, even a skilled examiner may be unable to exclude testicular torsion on physical examination in a child who presents with acute scrotal pain, and emergency exploration may be necessary (11). Diagnostic adjunct studies—mainly ultrasound—may be of assistance.

Ultrasound Evaluation

Sonographically, the only abnormality detected may be enlarged testis with unremarkable echotexture. Diffuse hypoechoic echotexture can also be seen. When infarcts occur they will often be seen as various-sized hypoechoic foci. They are usually sharply marginated, wedge shaped, peripheral in location, and septal in distribution; they do not cause a mass effect (Fig. 6.43). Round hypoechoic mass can, however, be seen early in the course of infarct (Fig. 6.43). However, sonographically, infarcts are difficult to differentiate from tumor, and close clinical correlation is essential.

Magnetic Resonance Imaging

Magnetic resonance imaging can be helpful in the diagnosis of vasculitis and testicular infarcts. The appearance of testicular infarct depends on its age. On the T1-weighted image, infarct may demonstrate medium or low signal intensity in its acute phase and high signal intensity with low-signal-intensity rim in its subacute phase. On the T2-weighted image, infarct is usually seen as a poorly marginated low-signal-intensity focus abutting the tunica albuginea. The peripheral location of intratesticular foci in combination with their configuration and signal intensity on T1- and T2-weighted images are suggestive of infarcts. MRI is also helped by the use of contrast media where lack of perfusion is identified. Close clinical correlation, however, is essential, and if suspicion of malignancy remains, open biopsy should be performed (9).

Comparative Evaluation

The diagnosis of vasculitis and testicular infarct is a difficult one, and high clinical suspicion is required. Ultrasound is usually employed as the initial imaging modality. Ultrasound will demonstrate hypoechoic, wedge-shaped, peripheral lesions, but sonographic findings are not specific enough to differentiate testicular infarcts from tumors. It has been reported that MRI is more sensitive than sonography for this application (9). Higher tissue contrast and use of contrast media are the advantages of MRI over US, but open biopsy may still be required.

FOURNIER-GANGRENE-NECROTIZING FASCIATIS

Necrotizing fasciatis of the scrotal wall with associated fat necrosis is a rare but potentially fatal disorder. The term *Fournier's gangrene* has been classically used to describe a particularly fulminant gangrene involving the scrotum. It usually occurs at middle age or later in life and has an explosive presentation that includes fever, chills, prostration, and painful erythematous edematous scrotum. Predisposing factors include diabetes melitus, chronic alcoholism, immunocompromise (patient with AIDS or underlying debilitating illnesses) (13,14). Necrotizing fasciatis and scrotal fat necrosis constitute a true urologic emergency mandating aggressive initial care, including early recognition, institution of broad-spectrum antibiotics, followed by debridements and often orchiectomy. On physical examination, the scrotum is enlarged, erythematous, and painful. Because of gas formation, crepitation of the scrotum is a specific clinical finding.

Ultrasound Findings

Ultrasound can be helpful in ascertaining the diagnosis. Underlying epididymo-orchitis is usually present and demonstrated sonographically. In addition, the scrotal skin is thickened and the characteristic echogenic foci with ill-defined shadowing indicating gas can be detected. Sonographic findings of gas formation can be present before clinical presentations of crepitations (Fig. 6.44).

Other than ultrasound, no other cross-sectional imaging modality has been used in the diagnosis of this rare but life-threatening condition.

REFERENCES

1. Pan EY, Chen LY, Yang JZ, Lee Z, Wang ZZ. Radiographic diagnosis of meconium peritonitis. A report of 200 cases including six fetal cases. *Pediatr Radiol* 1983; 13:199.
2. Tibboel D, Gaillard JL, Molenaar JC. The importance of mesenteric vascular insufficiency in meconium peritonitis. *Hum Pathol* 1986; 17:411–416.
3. Berdon WE, Baker DH, Becker J, De Sanctis P. Scrotal masses in healed meconium peritonitis. *N Engl J Med* 1967; 14:585–587.
4. Boccon-Gibod L, Roucayrol A. Meconium periorchitis. *Ped Pathol* 1992; 12:851–856.
5. Patalano VJ, Sommers SC. Biopsy diagnosis of periarteritis nodosa. *Arch Path* 1961; 72:1.
6. Monckeberg JG. Uber periarteritis nodosa. *Beitr Path Anal* 1905; 38:101.
7. Dahl EV, Baggenstoss AH, DeWeerd JH. Testicular lesions of periarteritis nodosa, with special reference to diagnosis. *Am J Med* 1960; 28:222.
8. Huisman T, Collins W, Voulgarakis G. Polyarteritis nodosa masquerading as a primary testicular neoplasm: A case report and review of the literature. *J Urol* 1990; 144:1236–1238.
9. Hayward I, Trambert MA, Mattrey RF, Saltzstein SL, Demby AM. MR imaging of vasculitis of the testis. *J Comput Assist Tomogr* 1991; 15(3):502–504.
10. Singer JI, Kissoon N, Gloor J. Acute Testicular Pain: Henoch—Schoenlein Purpura versus Testicular Torsion. *Ped Emerg Care* 1992; 8(1):51–53.
11. Balslev T. Schoenlein–Henoch syndrome with acute scrotal condition simulating torsion of the testis. *Ugeskr Laegaer* 1990; 152(10): 678.
12. Jalleh RP, Swift RI, Sundaresan M, Toma A. Necrotising testicular vasculitis associated with dermatomyositis. *Br J Urol* 1990; 66(6): 660.
13. Murphy M, Buckley M, Corr J, Vinayagamoorthy S, Grainger R, Mulcahy FM. Fournier's gangrene of scrotum in a patient with AIDS. *Genitourin Med* 1991; 67(4):339–341.
14. Paty R, Smith AD. Gangrene and Fournier's gangrene. *Urol Clin N Am* 1992; 19(1):149–162.

CHAPTER 7

The Epididymis, Spermatic Cord, and Paratesticular Tissue: Congenital Anomalies and Tumors

CONGENITAL ANOMALIES

Malformations of the epididymis are frequently associated with cryptorchidism and rarely occur without concomitant testicular anomalies. Conditions include dissociation of the testis and epididymis, complete or partial aplasia of the epididymis, epididymal cysts, bifid epididymis, fibrotic stenoses of the epididymal duct, and segmental obliteration or complete absence of the deferent duct. These disorders are generally asymptomatic and are nearly always discovered incidentally during surgery or in patients undergoing examination for fertility disorders.

As a rule, imaging rarely provides additional information in the evaluation of congenital anomalies of the epididymis or the ductus (vas) deferens. Agenesis of the epididymis is often associated with agenesis of the ipsilateral ductus deferens. The diagnosis is usually clinical but can be confirmed by CT or MRI. Both modalities will demonstrate an empty, often small spermatic cord. Associated agenesis of seminal vesicles is often present and can be detected on cross-sectional images—either CT or MRI.

TUMORS

Both benign and malignant tumors of the epididymis, spermatic cord, and paratesticular tissues are relatively rare and are primarily seen in older patients. Tumors of the epididymis and spermatic cord occur only about one-tenth as often as tumors of the testis (1). For this reason tumors of the ductus deferens, the rete testis, the epididymis, the spermatic cord, the tunica albuginea, the appendices, and the supporting structures are all covered under a single heading in the WHO classification. With the exception of cystadenoma, most tumors of the epididymis are of mesenchymal origin (2). Although benign tumors may arise from any mesenchymal tissues, their origin is most often the mesothelium of the tunica (2,3). It is sometimes difficult to determine whether a tumor originated from the epididymis, the spermatic cord, or the tunica vaginalis.

Other tumorlike lesions of the epididymis, such as spermatocele and epididymal cysts, are discussed in Chapter 8.

Benign Tumors

Adenomatoid tumors account for about 30% of the tumors arising from the paratesticular region and are the most common benign tumor. They originate from the mesothelium of the tunica vaginalis and are most often located in the epididymis (usually in the tail but sometimes at or near the head) and less frequently in the tunica albuginea (2,4). They most often occur in men over the age of 20 (the mean age is 40 to 45 years) (5,6), and they are usually asymptomatic. An adenomatoid tumor is palpated as a firm, painless epididymal mass. Malignant forms have been reported but are extremely rare (5).

The second most common benign tumor of the epididymis is **papillary cystadenoma**. It usually occurs in young adults, and it is bilateral in one third of cases, typically located in the head of the epididymis, and frequently seen in patients with von Hippel–Lindau disease (3,7). (Approximately 10% to 40% of patients with von Hippel–Lindau disease have epididymal involvement) (7). Patients may be asymptomatic or may have mild discomfort. The differential diagnosis based on clinical examination includes epididymal cysts, spermatocele, teratoma, adenomatoid tumor, and metastatic disease (7). Treatment is local excision because recurrence has not been observed.

Lipomas are the most frequent benign tumor of the spermatic cord. They present as a soft lesion and show considerable variation in size. Occasionally, it is difficult to distinguish a lipoma from a mesenteric hernia.

Malignant Tumors

Among the malignant tumors involving the epididymis and spermatic cord (30% of spermatic cord tumors are malignant), **paratesticular rhabdomyosarcomas** are the most common, representing 6% of all non–germ cell intrascrotal tumors. They arise from the paratesticular tissues, including the epididymis and the spermatic cord. Rhabdomyosarcomas occur predominantly in children and adolescents, with two peaks of increased incidence, one at the age of 4 and one at the age of 16 years (8–13). They are characterized by rapid and invasive growth, with early metastatic spread along lymphatic channels.

Other mesenchymal sarcomas arising in the paratesticular tissues—including **leiomyosarcoma**, **liposarcoma**, **fibrosarcoma**, **malignant fibrous histiocytoma**, and **malignant mesenchymoma**—most commonly occur in the spermatic cord (9). They are more common than their benign counterparts and most occur in patients more than 40 years of age. Local invasion of adjacent tissue and distant metastasis are often seen. Their occurrence in the epididymis follows rhabdomyosarcoma in frequency, but is so rare that most reports in the literature are anecdotal.

Mesothelioma, an uncommon tumor originating from the tunica vaginalis, is most often found in older patients, usually over 18 years of age (9,14). Approximately 15% of mesotheliomas have been reported to be malignant, presenting as metastases (15,16). **Metastases** from prostate, renal, or gastric carcinoma have also been reported, but their occurrence is rare.

Clinical Presentation

Most of these rare tumors present with similar clinical symptoms. In most cases, there is a slow-growing, solid, painless, intrascrotal mass. Palpation may offer a clue to the anatomic origin, and imaging generally permits distinction between intra- and extratesticular lesions. Surgical exploration (required in all patients with a suspected intrascrotal tumor) and histologic examination, however, are needed to make a definite diagnosis. Whereas most testicular tumors are malignant, the majority of extratesticular tumors are benign. Determination of benign or malignant status is important for management.

Rhabdomyosarcomas usually present with an acutely developing, painless swelling of the scrotum, and symptoms are primarily determined by the rapid growth of the tumor. They are usually painless (scrotal pain is present in only 7% of cases [10]) and are palpated as firm masses typically located above the testis. The treatment of choice for rhabdomyosarcoma is tumor excision and unilateral orchiectomy by inguinal incision (12,17). Although the value of retroperitoneal lymphadenectomy is controversial (17,18), adjuvant chemotherapy (because of the recent development of successful regimens) is now considered mandatory, even in low-stage tumors (8,10,12). Rhabdomyosarcomas generally carry a poor prognosis.

Mesotheliomas often present with long-standing hydrocele that gradually distends the scrotal sac. The overall prognosis of paratesticular mesothelioma is better than when the tumor is located in the pleura or peritoneum (15). Other mesenchymal tumors—leiomyosarcoma, liposarcoma, and fibrosarcoma—all have a similar nonspecific clinical presentation, and surgical excision—including radical orchiectomy with wide local incision and high ligation of the spermatic cord—is indicated in all. Although cross-sectional imaging can help in defining the extent of the tumor and in evaluating the underlying testis, it will seldom contribute to patient management and is therefore rarely performed.

Ultrasound in the Evaluation of Epididymal, Spermatic Cord, and Paratesticular Tumors

Ultrasound clearly differentiates the epididymis and other paratesticular structures from the testis and can therefore be used to confirm the paratesticular origin of a suspected epididymal tumor (19,20). Because these tumors are unusual, clinical findings rarely permit their precise assignment to a particular structure, and ultrasonography is performed to (1) delineate the lesion from the testis and epididymis, (2) confirm a suspected tumor by demonstration of a solid mass, and (3) exclude the presence of a cystic lesion such as spermatocele or funiculocele or a hernia. In addition, the solid consistency of most epididymal tumors produces internal echoes on ultrasound, a reliable criterion for distinguishing them from epididymal cysts or simple spermatocele (both of which present clinically as spherical, circumscribed masses). Cystadenomas, which usually have a cystic component, are the exception.

Sonographically, **adenomatoid tumors** are seen as round lesions, typically demarcated by smooth borders. They are usually hyperechoic and homogeneous (6) but may be hypoechoic or heterogeneous, compared to adjacent testicular tissue (Fig. 7.1). Occasionally, they may appear completely anechoic, mimicking epididymal cysts or spermatoceles (21). Hydrocele is associated in

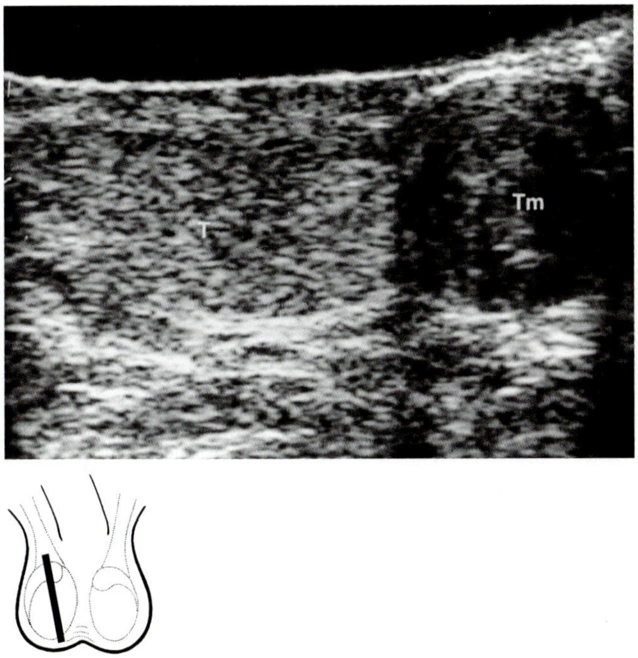

A

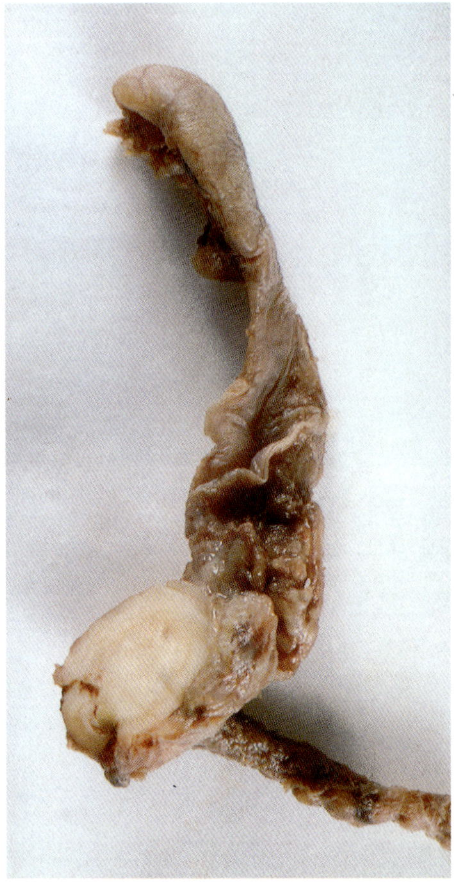

B

FIG. 7.1. Adenomatoid tumor in a 53-year-old patient. **(A)** Solid, hypoechoic mass (Tm) in the area of the tail of the epididymis. The tumorous lesion (Tm) can be clearly differentiated from the testis (T). **(B)** Surgical specimen (excised epididymis).

15% to 20% of cases (6). Adenomatoid tumors may be difficult to distinguish from an **epididymal granuloma** (sperm granuloma or granuloma secondary to vasectomy). The latter is palpated as a circumscribed mass and presents on ultrasound as a focal, typically hypoechoic or isoechoic, paratesticular lesion (an appearance that is also suspicious for tumor) (Fig. 7.2). A history of previous inflammation, trauma, or surgery (vasectomy) helps in establishing the diagnosis of epididymal granuloma.

Papillary cystadenomas are usually seen in the head of the epididymis. They may have a hypoechoic, nodular appearance. A multiseptated cystic appearance has also been described (7). When the mass is predominantly cystic, the differentiation between papillary cystadenoma or spermatocele may be in question.

The most frequent tumor of the spermatic cord, **lipoma**, presents on ultrasound as a circumscribed, homogeneous hypo- to hyperechoic structure that alters its shape when compressed with the transducer (Fig. 7.3). The echogenicity of lipomas varies according to the ratio of fat cells to interstitial tissue (22). Lipomas should be distinguished from **spermatic cord lipomatosis**, which chiefly occurs in obese patients. This condition can be best described as a pasty, compressible, and diffuse deposition of fat within the spermatic cord. Its echogenicity is of medium intensity. Cord lipoma or lipomatosis can readily be distinguished from a hernia by the demonstration of peristalsis in the intestinal loops. Omental fatty tissue in the inguinal canal communicates with the peritoneal cavity at the level of the internal inguinal ring. It is important to remember that a sonographically demonstrated circumscribed hypoechoic structure in the inguinal canal may also correspond to an undescended testicle, especially in patients with an empty scrotal compartment.

Invasive **malignant tumors** of the epididymis are characterized by poorly defined borders. In advanced tumor stages, the epididymis and testis can no longer be delineated confidently. Paratesticular and spermatic cord tumors have no uniform sonographic appearance.

Rhabdomyosarcomas are usually seen as circumscribed unilateral lesions without a capsule, 1 to 2 cm in size. Ultrasound demonstration of any solid mass (usually hypoechoic) is highly suspicious for tumor, and, especially in childhood, should alert the examiner to the possibility of a rhabdomyosarcoma. The majority of these lesions are separate from the testis, whereas delineation from the delicate structures of the epididymis may be difficult.

Sonographically, **mesotheliomas** are seen as multiple nodular homogeneous, either hyper- or isoechoic, paratesticular masses, usually associated with a hy-

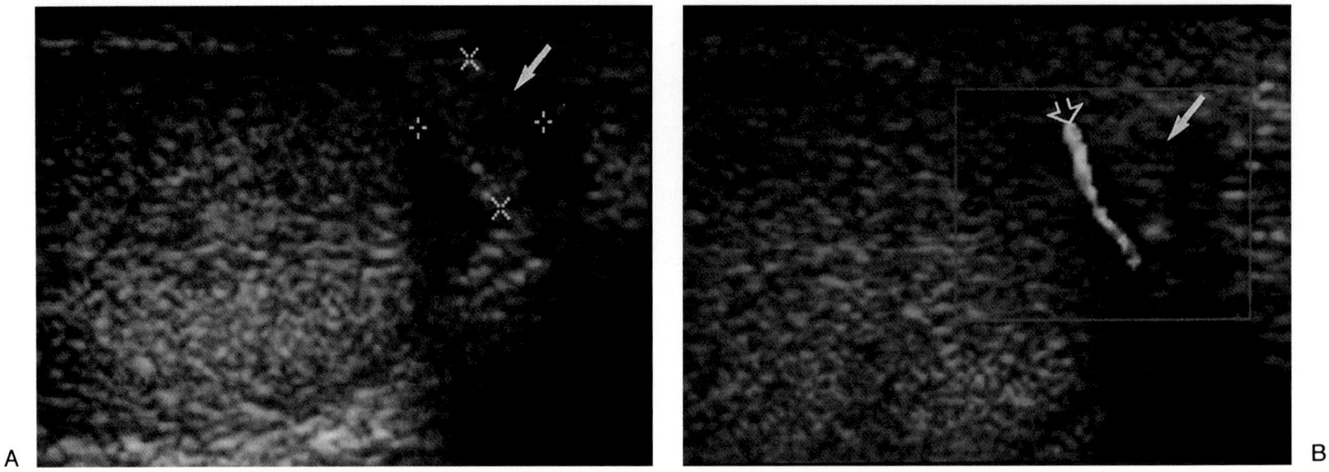

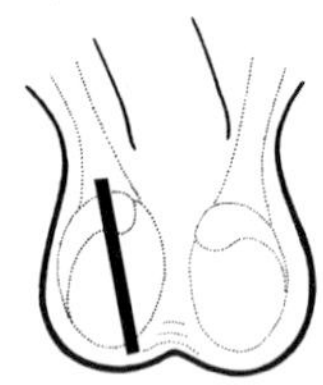

FIG. 7.2. Epididymal sperm granuloma in a 46-year-old patient. **(A)** Gray-scale and **(B)** color Doppler ultrasonogram showing solid paratesticular lesion (*arrow*), located in the tail of the epididymis. Demonstration of capsular artery (*open arrowhead*) helps in the demonstration of lesion paratesticular location.

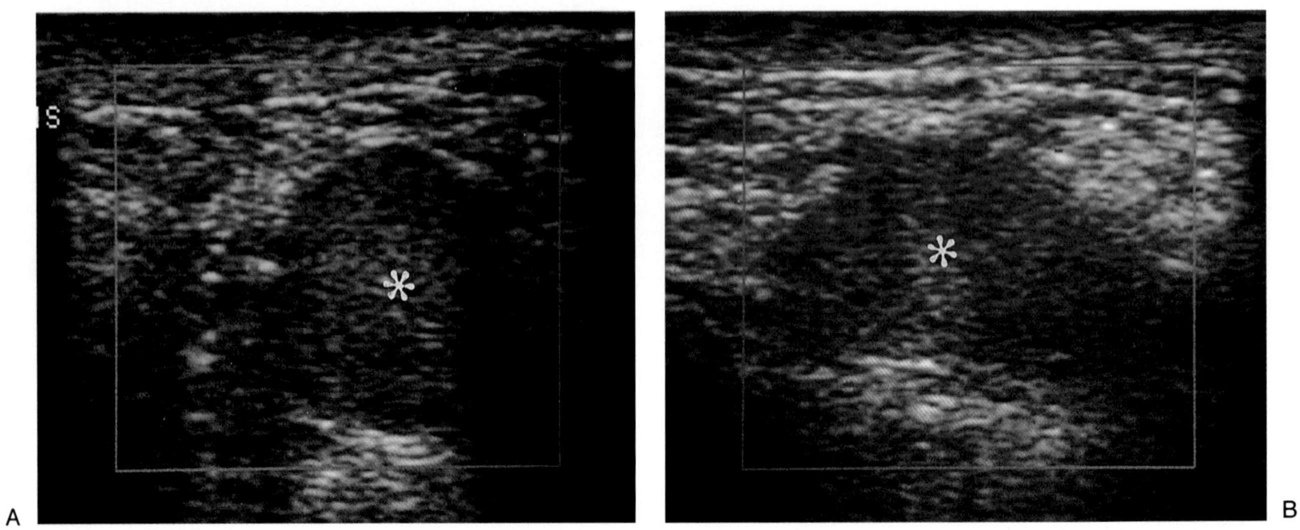

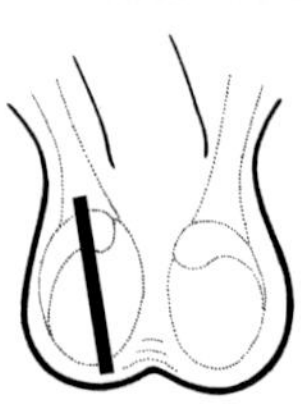

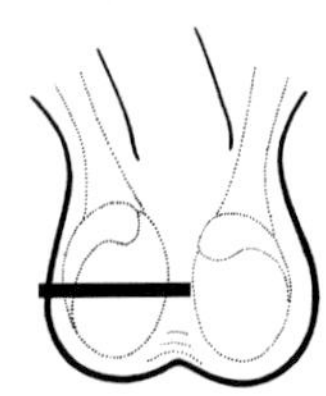

FIG. 7.3. Lipoma (*) of the spermatic cord in a 28-year-old man. **(A)** Longitudinal, and **(B)** transverse sonogram demonstrating a compressible lesion of medium echogenicity.

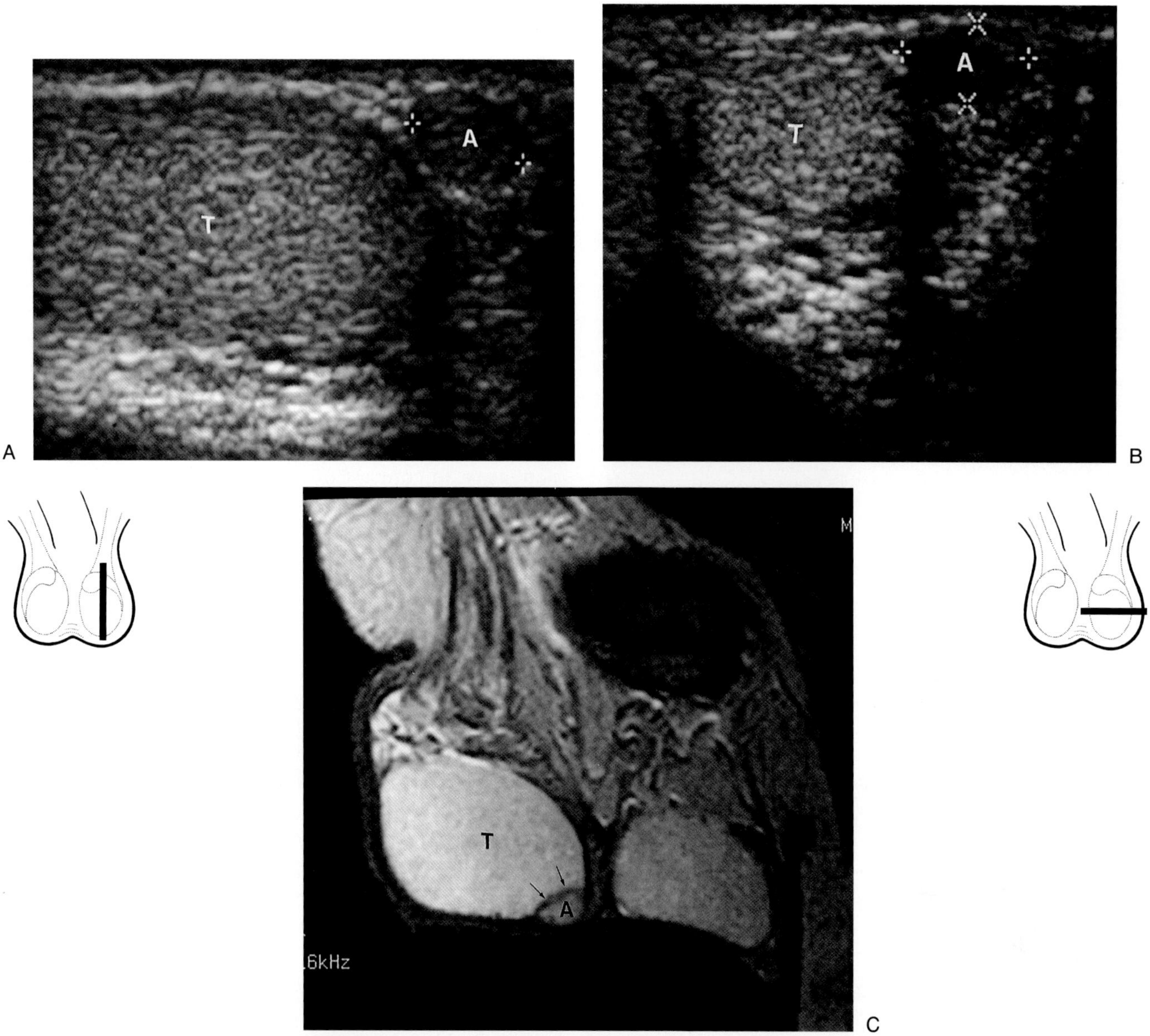

FIG. 7.4. Adenomatoid tumor in a 49-year-old patient. **(A)** Longitudinal, **(B)** transverse sonogram, and **(C)** coronal plane T1-weighted MR image. Adenomatoid tumor (A) is hypoechoic as compared with the testis (T). On the T2-weighted MR image, the tumor (A) paratesticular location is clearly seen by demonstration of interposed low-signal-intensity tunica albuginea (*small arrows*). Tumor (A) signal intensity is similar to the testis (T).

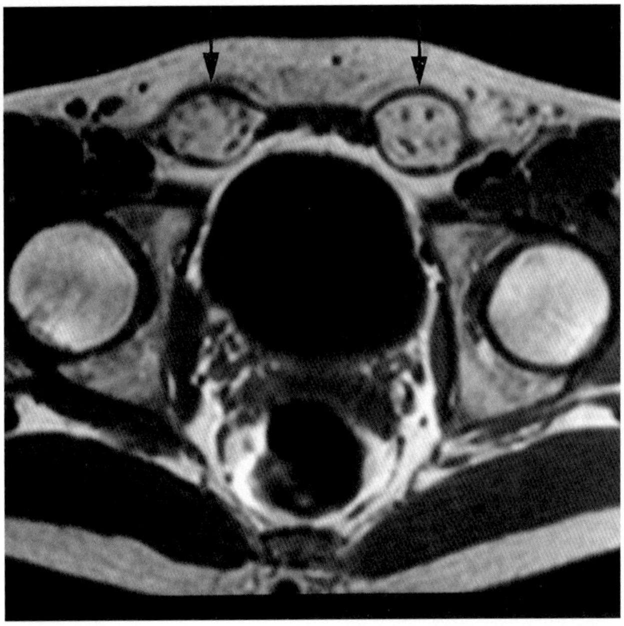

FIG. 7.5. Fatty herniation (*arrows*)—indirect mesenteric fat herniation in the spermatic cord. Transverse T1-weighted MR image.

drocele (23). Malignant mesotheliomas can be differentiated from benign tumors by the rapid reaccumulation of fluid and the presence of larger nodular or papillary lesions and complicated (bloody) hydrocele (16).

There are only anecdotal reports on the sonographic appearance of mesenchymal tumors—**leiomyosarcoma, liposarcoma,** or **fibrosarcoma** (24,25). In all, ultrasound will most commonly detect a predominantly solid, ill-defined, inhomogeneous, disorganized mass. Depending on tumor locoregional extent, the epididymis and testis can also be infiltrated (25).

Magnetic Resonance Imaging in the Evaluation of Epididymal, Spermatic Cord, and Paratesticular Tumors

Magnetic resonance imaging plays a minor role in the evaluation of epididymal, spermatic cord, and paratesticular tumors. An adenomatoid tumor is seen as a solid, sharply outlined mass, usually less than 4 to 5 cm in diameter and often detected in the tail of the epididymis. It demonstrates medium signal intensity (similar to the epididymis) on T1-weighted images. Its separation from the epididymis is facilitated on the T2-weighted image, where the normal epididymis demonstrates low signal intensity, in contrast to the adenomatoid tumor, which demonstrates high signal intensity. Differentiation of tumor from the testis is also best seen on T2-weighted images by depiction of low-signal-intensity tunica albuginea surrounding the testis (Fig. 7.4). MRI is also highly accurate in the detection and characterization of lipoma. Lipomas demonstrate high signal intensity (similar to the adjacent fat) on both T1- and T2-weighted images. On the T2-weighted image, their signal intensity sometimes can be higher than that of adjacent fat. If the diagnosis on conventional T1- and T2-weighted images is in question, a fat suppression sequence should be obtained. A lipoma can be differentiated from spermatic cord lipomatosis by identification of cord structures. In cord lipomatosis or in fatty herniation (Fig. 7.5), the cord is expanded by fatty tissue transversed by the ductus deferens, vessels, and lymphatics. In lipoma, the tumor

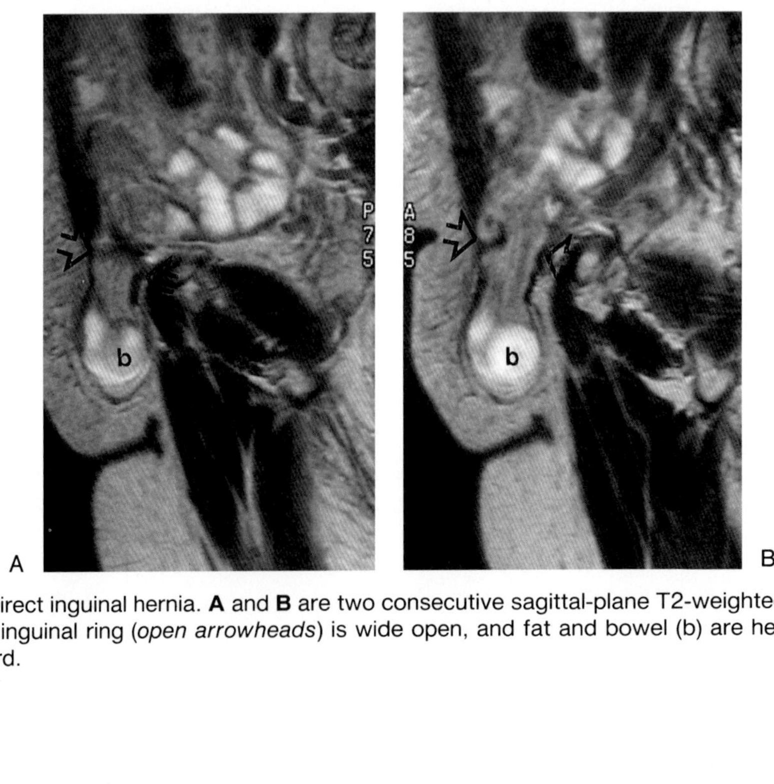

FIG. 7.6. Indirect inguinal hernia. **A** and **B** are two consecutive sagittal-plane T2-weighted MR images. The external inguinal ring (*open arrowheads*) is wide open, and fat and bowel (b) are herniated to the spermatic cord.

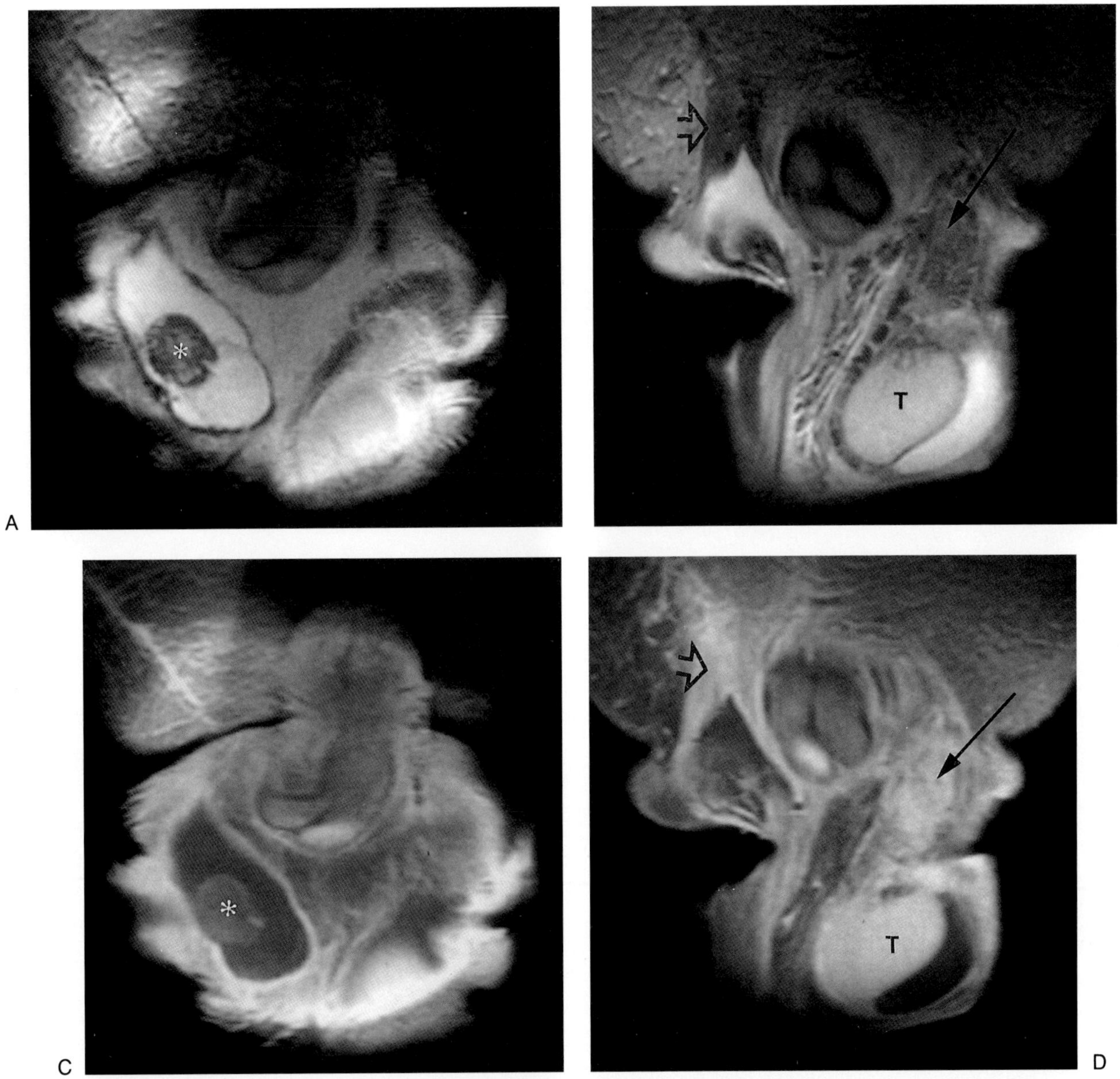

FIG. 7.7. Recurrent mesothelioma, coronal plane of section. **A** and **B** are T2-weighted MR images, and **(C)** and **(D)** are contrast-enhanced T1-weighted MR images. Patient had right-side orchiectomy for scrotal mesothelioma 4 months prior to MR study. There is a recurrent tumor (*) in the right hemiscrotum. The left spermatic cord (*arrow*) is thickened and shows enhancement. Left testis (T) is normal. There is also thickening and enhancement of the right spermatic cord (*open arrow*). At surgery, there was recurrent mesothelioma in the right scrotum and both spermatic cords.

capsule can sometimes be detected, and, in addition, the ductus deferens, vessels, nerves, and lymphatics are displaced asymmetrically. Differentiation between cord lipomatosis and mesenteric fat hernia can be accomplished by identifying changes at the level of the internal inguinal ring, which should be widely open in the case of hernia and of normal size in cord lipomatosis (Fig. 7.6).

There is very little experience in MR imaging of malignant paratesticular tumors. In most, the main contribution of MRI is not in the diagnosis but in the evaluation of the locoregional extent of the tumor, especially to the testis or scrotal skin (Fig. 7.7).

Computed Tomography in the Evaluation of Epididymal, Spermatic Cord, and Paratesticular Tumors

Similar to MRI, CT is seldom indicated as a primary imaging modality for epididymal, spermatic cord, or paratesticular tumors. Benign tumors of the epididymis

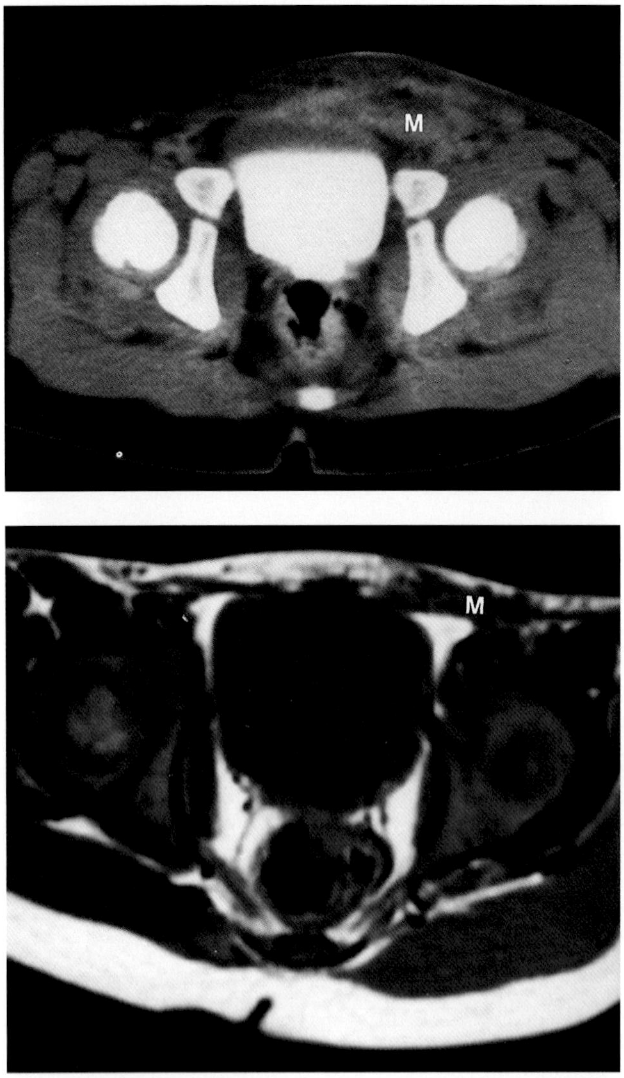

FIG. 7.8. Rhabdomyosarcoma of the left spermatic cord in a 9-year-old boy. Axial plane of section. **(A)** Contrast-enhanced CT and **(B)** T1-weighted MR image. There is a soft tissue mass (M) enlarging the spermatic cord and infiltrating the surrounding tissue. Considering the patient's age, the invasive appearance of the lesion, and the lack of clinical symptoms of inflammation, malignant tumor is the leading diagnosis.

or spermatic cord are usually an incidental finding. They are seen as sharply defined masses with an attenuation value reflecting their histologic composition. Lipomas have a specific negative attenuation value. Malignant tumors are usually poorly marginated, solid tumors with heterogeneous attenuation value (Fig. 7.8). Fat in the liposarcoma can be identified, but absence of fatty tissue does not exclude the diagnosis (26). The primary role of CT is not in diagnosing but rather in staging the neoplasm and design of surgical extent (Fig. 7.9). Lymphatic spread in the tumors of the spermatic cord follows the course of drainage of spermatic cord structures: The ductus deferens lymphatics drain into the external iliac system; the other spermatic cord structures drain via the testicular lymphatics along the course of the testicular vein.

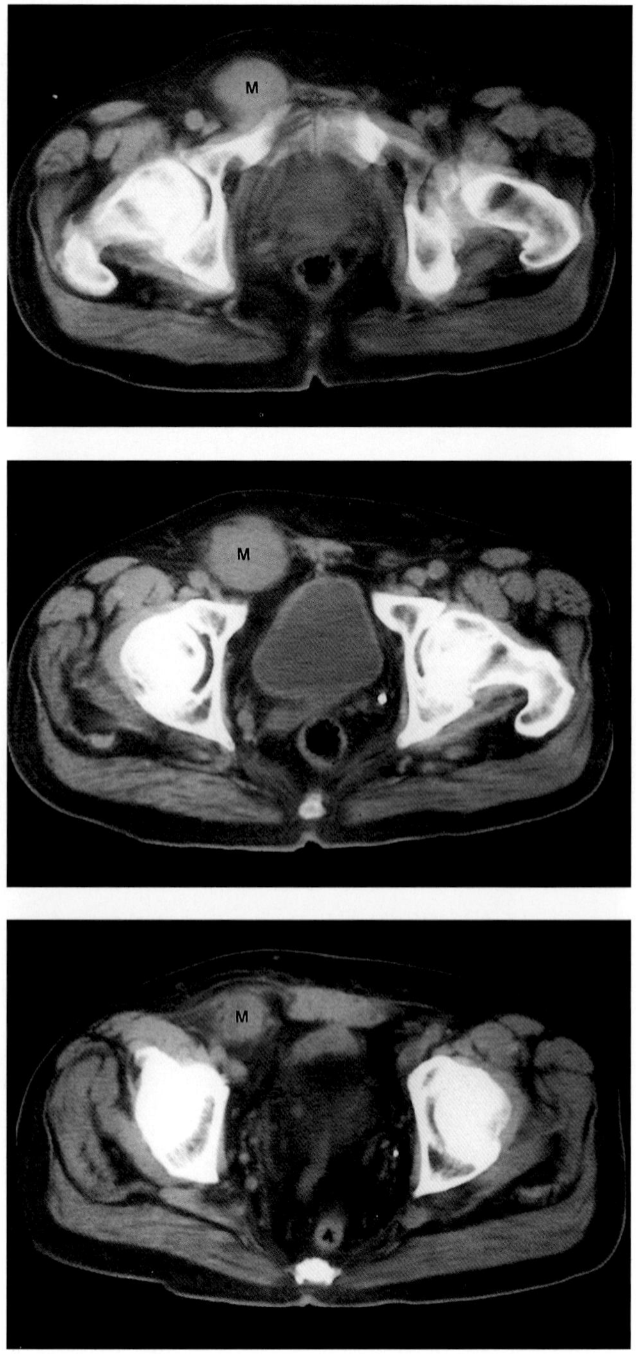

FIG. 7.9. Poorly differentiated myxoid liposarcoma of the right spermatic cord. A noncontrast CT scan at the level of the **(A)** superficial inguinal pouch (*high scrotal location*), **(B)** external ring of the inguinal canal, and **(C)** internal ring of the inguinal canal. Left spermatic cord is normal. A homogeneous soft tissue attenuation mass (M) is seen within the right spermatic cord extending into the inguinal canal. Because of the irregular margins of the tumor and the likelihood of its malignant nature (being primary spermatic cord tumor), the most likely CT diagnosis is spermatic cord sarcoma. Fat cannot be identified within the mass; thus, the specific diagnosis of liposarcoma on CT could not be made. (Courtesy Dr. J. P. Heiken.)

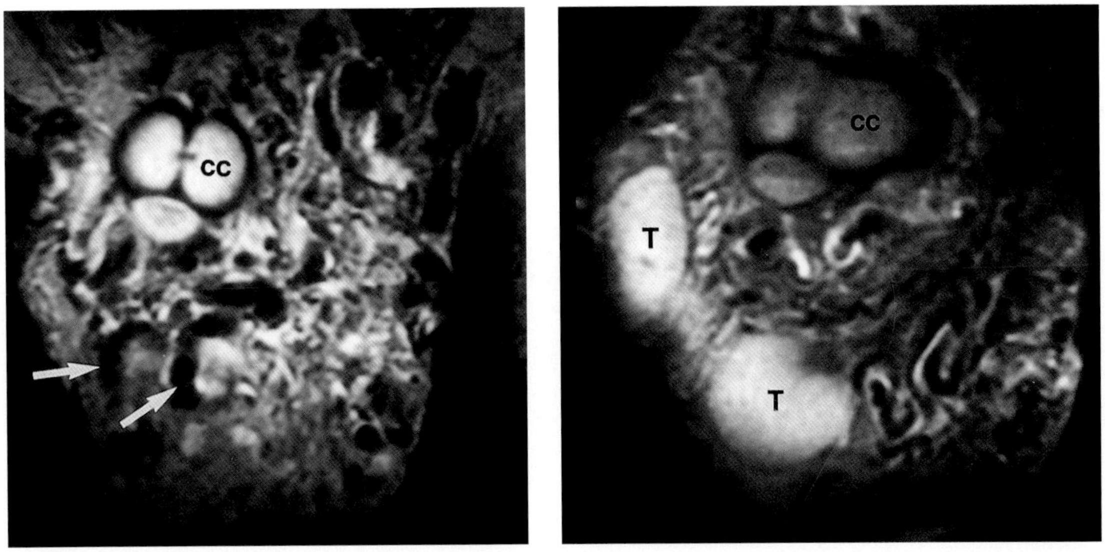

A B

FIG. 7.10. Arteriovenous malformation of the left hemiscrotum. **A** and **B** are coronal plane T2-weighted MR images. Numerous serpiginous, enlarged vessels (*arrows*) are seen. Testis (T) and penis (cc, corpora cavernosa) are not involved.

Therefore, for staging purposes, CT of the abdomen and pelvis is required.

Comparative Evaluation

Ultrasound is the primary imaging modality when an intrascrotal mass is identified and, based on clinical findings, the intra- or paratesticular origin of the mass is difficult to assess. Solid tumors of the epididymis are visualized on ultrasound, and their separation from the testis can be demonstrated with a high level of confidence, especially when gray-scale examination is coupled with CCDS. The latter will help in identifying the capsular artery, which is located between the testis (including the tunica albuginea) and the epididymis. The differentiation, however, between various types of benign tumors—adenomatoid tumor, epididymal granuloma, papillary cystadenoma—is often difficult to impossible. Furthermore, it may sometimes be difficult to differentiate between a benign and a malignant tumor type. When a tumor demonstrates infiltrative borders, irregular margins, and marked heterogeneity, its malignant nature is more obvious. Magnetic resonance imaging is rarely requested in the evaluation of the epididymal tumor, but if taken, differentiation between intra- and paratesticular lesions can be done with a high level of confidence. In a malignant tumor of the epididymis or spermatic cord, the role of MRI and CT surpasses that of ultrasound, as tumor locoregional extent and presence of metastatic disease can be evaluated.

Vascular Lesions of the Scrotum

Vascular lesions of the scrotum include varicocele, hemangioma, lymphangioma, and arteriovenous malformation. Varicoceles are the most common of the group. They are easily diagnosed and distinguished from the others because they are confined to the spermatic cord. For further discussion of clinical and imaging features of varicocele, see Chapters 8 and 10. Scrotal hemangiomas and lymphangiomas are rare, with fewer than 50 cases of each reported (27). Although both neoplasms have been reported in newborns, the peak age incidence is the third to fifth decades (27). Both lymphangioma and hemangioma are believed to be congenital, but the latter may also result from trauma. Complete surgical excision (laser surgery is preferred today) is the treatment of choice for both. Scrotal arteriovenous malformations are the rarest vascular neoplasms of the scrotum. Only four cases have been reported in the literature (28). In each case the lesion was solitary. There was a bruit heard on auscultation, and there was no known association with the cutaneous angiomatous syndrome. Angioembolization followed by surgical incision is the recommended treatment. Pretreatment imaging for diagnostic purposes is rarely indicated, its main use being the evaluation of the underlying testis or penis. Ultrasound can be applied, but MRI—because of its large field of view, better tissue contrast, and high sensitivity to flow—has an even more important role (Fig. 7.10).

REFERENCES

1. Schroder R, Hedinger C: Paratestikulre Tumoren. *Schweiz Med Wschr* 1970;100:1281–1287.
2. Elsser E. Epididymal tumors. *Recent Results Cancer Res* 1977;60:163–175.
3. Gowing NFC. Paratesticular tumours of connective tissue and muscle. In: Pugh RCB eds. *Pathology of the testis*. Oxford: Blackwell; 1976:317–333.

4. Restrepo C. Surgical pathology of the male adnexa and diseases of the soft tissue. In: Javadpur N, Basky S, eds. *Surgical pathology of urologic disease*. Baltimore: Williams Wilkins; 1987:247–260.
5. Mäkäräinen HP, Tammela TL, Karttunen TJ, Mattila SI, Hellstrom PA, Kontturi MJ. Intrascrotal adenomatoid tumors and their ultrasound findings. *J Clin Ultrasound* 1993;21:33–37.
6. Leonhardt WC, Gooding GA. Sonography of intrascrotal adenomatoid tumor. *Urology* 1992;39:90–92.
7. Alexander JA, Lichtman JB, Varma VA. Ultrasound demonstration of a papillary cystadenoma of the epididymis. *J Clin Ultrasound* 1991;19:442–445.
8. Hays DM. Rhabdomyosarcoma and other soft tissue sarcoma. In: Hays DM, ed. *Pediatric surgical oncology*. New York: Grune & Stratton; 1986:87–122.
9. Richie JP. Neoplasms of the testis. In: Walsh PC, Retik AB, Stamey TA, Vaughan ED, eds. *Campbell's urology*, 6th ed, vol 2. W B Saunders; 1992:1222–1263.
10. Stewart LH, Lioe TF, Johnson SR. Thirty-year review of intrascrotal rhabdomyosarcoma. *Br J Urol* 1991;68:418–420.
11. Mostofi FK, Sesterhenn IA, Davis CJ. Pathology of testicular tumors. In: Javadpur N, ed. *Principles and management of testicular cancer*. New York: Thieme; 1986:33–72.
12. Hamilton CR, Pinkerton R, Horwich A. The management of paratesticular rhabdomyosarcoma. *Clin Radiol* 1989;40:314–317.
13. Nativ O, Graif M, Goldwasser B. Rhabdomyosarcoma of the cord: ultrasonic evaluation. *Urol Radiol* 1983;5:131–132.
14. Pfister M, Sáez D, Celeste F. Sonographic appearance of malignant mesothelioma of the tunica vaginalis testis in a child. *J Clin Ultrasound* 1992;20:129–131.
15. Tyagi G, Munn CS, Kiser LC, Wetzner SM, Tarabulcy E. Malignant mesothelioma of tunica vaginalis testis. *Urology* 1989;34:102–104.
16. Fields JM, Russell SA, Andrew SM. Case report: ultrasound appearance of a malignant mesothelioma of the tunica vaginalis testis. *Clin Radiol* 1992;46:128–130.
17. Blyth B, Mandell J, Bauer SB, et al. Paratesticular rhabdomyosarcoma: results of therapy in 18 cases. *J Urol* 1990;144:1450–1453.
18. Catton CN, Cummings BJ, Fornasier V, O'Sullivan B, Quirt I, Warr D. Adult paratesticular sarcomas: a review of 21 cases. *J Urol* 1991;146:342–345.
19. Hricak H, Filly RA. Sonography of the scrotum. *Invest Radiol* 1983;18:112–121.
20. Krone KD, Carroll BA. Scrotal ultrasound. *Radiol Clin North Am* 1985;23:121–139.
21. Vick CW, Klein FA, Schneider V. Adenomatoid tumor of epididymis simulating benign cyst on scrotal ultrasound. *Urology* 1991;38:369–371.
22. Gooding GAW. Sonography of the spermatic cord. *AJR* 1988;151:721–724.
23. Aquino NM, Vazquez R, Matari H. Ultrasound demonstration of a benign mesothelioma of tunica vaginalis testis. *J Clin Ultrasound* 1986;14:310–311.
24. Hellstrom PA, Makarainen H, Tammela TL, Laurila A. Spermatic cord liposarcoma: Ultrasound for diagnosis and follow-up. Case report. *Scand J Urol Nephrol* 1991;25(4):321–324.
25. Sonksen J, Hansen EF, Colstrup H. Liposarcoma of the spermatic cord. Case report. *Scand J Urol Nephrol* 1991;25(3):239–240.
26. Fox LA, Forman HP, Heiken JP, Levitt RG, Andriole GL. Inguinal mass in a 66-year-old man. *Urol Radiol* 1992;14:62–64.
27. Petersen RO. Scrotum. In: *Urologic pathology*, Philadelphia: JB Lippincott: 1986:713–714.
28. Sule JD, Lemmers MJ, Barry JM. Scrotal arteriovenous malformation: case report and literature review. *J Urol* 1993;150(6):1917–1919.

CHAPTER 8

Extratesticular Fluid Collections

Extratesticular fluid collections include abnormal fluid accumulation between two layers of tunica vaginalis, such as hydrocele (serous fluid), hematocele (hemorrhagic fluid), or pyocele (infected fluid); cystic structures of the epididymis (spermatocele and epididymal cyst), dilatation of the pampiniform plexus (varicocele), and inguinal hernias. The main clinical task is to differentiate extra- from intratesticular pathology and to assure that the underlying testis is normal. When clinical examination is difficult or inconclusive, imaging modalities, specifically ultrasound, are required and represent an important diagnostic tool.

HYDROCELE

An abnormal accumulation of serous fluid between the two layers of the tunica vaginalis testis is known as *hydrocele.* Normally, the processus vaginalis closes by the end of the first year of life, the fluid exchange is interrupted, and the retained fluid is absorbed. A *congenital* hydrocele is due to failure of the processus vaginalis to close, which allows serous fluid to communicate between the abdominal cavity and the scrotum. Congenital hydrocele is therefore a *communicating hydrocele.* It commonly occurs in infancy, and about 6% of full-term boys have a congenital hydrocele (1). A *reactive* or *acquired hydrocele* is a *noncommunicating hydrocele* that results from impaired fluid reabsorption. It may occur in conjunction with an inflammatory process (epididymitis or orchitis), as a sequel to trauma or torsion, or in the presence of a testicular tumor (in about 10% of cases), or its etiology may be idiopathic. Fluid retention in one or more unobliterated segments of the processus vaginalis gives rise to a funicular hydrocele (*funiculocele*).

Clinical Presentation

Young boys with communicating hydrocele present with a typical history of a cystic scrotal mass limited to one hemiscrotum that is larger and tenser at night than in the morning (2). Hydroceles are usually painless, although palpation of the underlying testis is frequently inhibited. In communicating hydrocele resulting from a patent processus vaginalis, fluid can be moved during clinical examination. A communicating hydrocele usually decreases with pressure on the scrotum and increases with elevation of intra-abdominal pressure (1). It is important not to overlook potential herniation of bowel segments in evaluating communicating hydrocele.

A **noncommunicating hydrocele** is not affected by palpation or position change (1). An acute hydrocele transilluminates, and therefore can be easily diagnosed clinically. **Chronic hydrocele** represents a clinical challenge. It usually has a thick wall and therefore does not transilluminate. Imaging is essential for making a diagnosis in this situation.

In **funiculocele** palpation findings include demonstration of a normal testis and epididymis and a spherical, tense-elastic lesion situated near the inguinal ring. A funiculocele can be distinguished from a communicating hydrocele by the fact that the latter empties in the recumbent position.

Because hydrocele causes enlarged scrotum, it is essential to differentiate it from an intrascrotal tumor. Associated torsion or an inguinal hernia must also be considered. Careful physical examination and absence of scrotal pain and swelling may help in the differentiation. The diagnosis of a scrotal hernia is made by the demonstration of bowel loops in the scrotal area. Unlike a hydrocele, an inguinal hernia cannot be delineated from the spermatic cord, extends into the inguinal canal, and does not transilluminate. Another condition to be considered in the differential diagnosis of a hydrocele is a spermatocele, which is usually palpated as a painless, spherical lesion in the area of the epididymal head, and the testis is displaced inferiorly.

Ultrasound in the Evaluation of Hydrocele

In cases of suspected hydrocele, a sonographic examination is indicated to (1) confirm the presence of a fluid collection in patients with unclear clinical findings, (2)

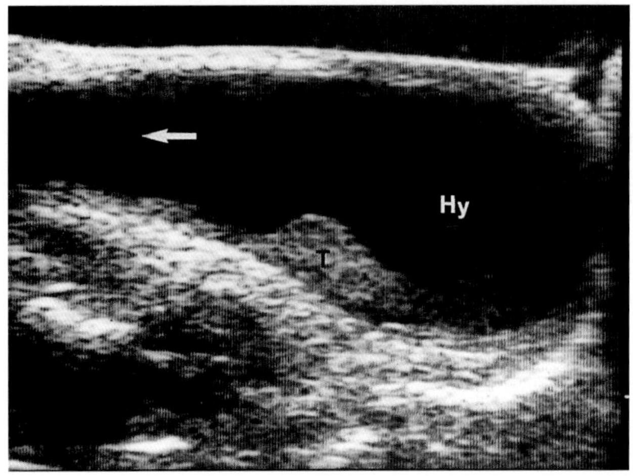

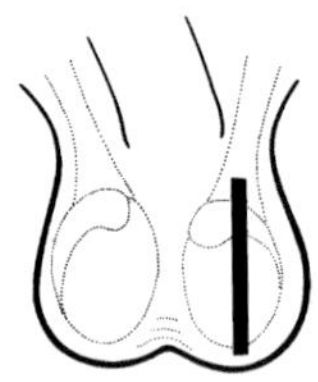

FIG. 8.2. A large abdominoscrotal hydrocele (Hy) in a newborn. The hydrocele extends up into the spermatic cord (*arrow*). The testis (T) is normal.

differentiate a hydrocele from a testicular tumor reliably, (3) evaluate the testis and epididymis if palpation is limited, (4) exclude a testicular tumor (an advantage over transillumination), and (5) differentiate better a suspected funiculocele from a tumor of the spermatic cord.

The characteristic appearance of hydrocele, an anechoic fluid collection within the scrotal sac, makes the sonographic diagnosis straightforward (Fig. 8.1). Using the hydrocele as an acoustic window, there is good visualization of both the testis and the epididymis, and focal testicular lesions can be reliably excluded (3). In hydrocele the testis and epididymis are laterally displaced by the adjacent, crescentlike fluid collection.

In abdominoscrotal (communicating) hydroceles (Fig. 8.2), scanning should be performed both in the standing position (filling of the involved hemiscrotum) and in the supine position (emptying of the hydrocele). Fluid can also be detected along the spermatic cord in the presence of a communicating hydrocele, especially in infants with ascites.

A chronic inflammatory hydrocele is also filled with fluid and most commonly has anechoic appearance. Fine echoes through the hydrocele, however, can be present, and it is believed that these are due to crystals within a chronic hydrocele (Fig. 8.3). Chronic hydrocele is often septated, may show thickening of the wall, and may contain small calcifications (Fig. 8.4). In addition, a chronic hydrocele may lead to considerable compression of the testis, with resultant deformity (Fig. 8.4) and atrophy. Although palpation of chronic inflammatory hydroceles rarely permits delineation of the testis and epididymis, the sonographic examination nearly always ensures sufficient evaluation of these structures.

A funiculocele is displayed as an elongated or nodular anechoic structure around the spermatic cord (Fig. 8.5). Unlike communicating hydroceles, funiculoceles do not empty into the peritoneum in response to compression.

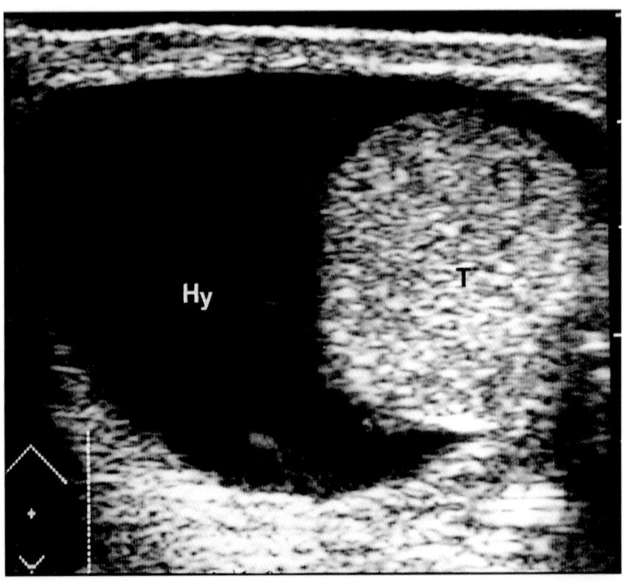

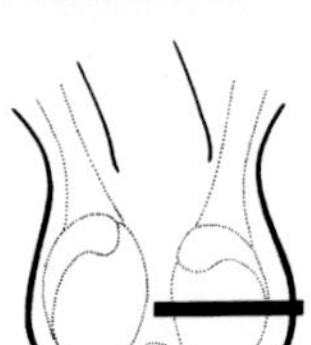

FIG. 8.1. Hydrocele in a 54-year-old patient. Anechoic fluid (Hy) surrounds the normal appearing testis (T) like a crescent.

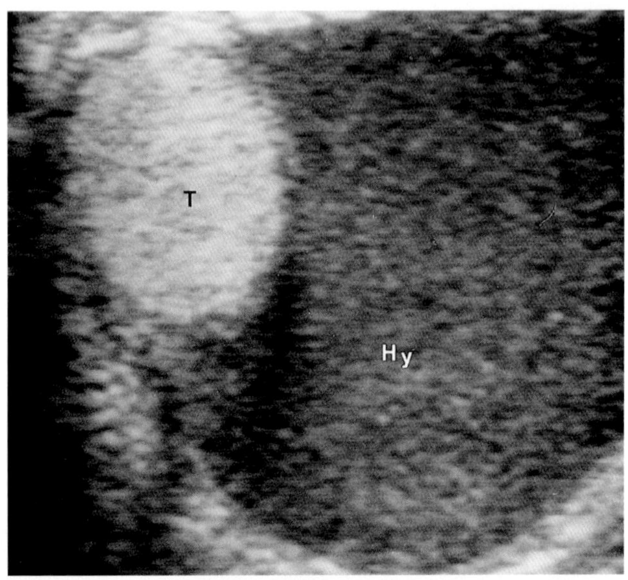

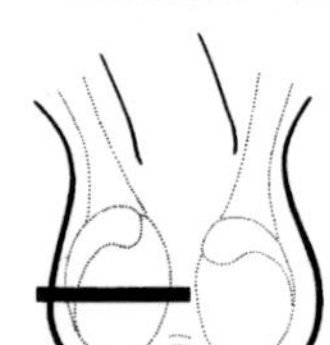

FIG. 8.3. Hydrocele in a 55-year-old patient with a clinical history of slowly enlarging hemiscrotum. The testis (T) is normal. Dispersed fine echoes are seen throughout the hydrocele (Hy).

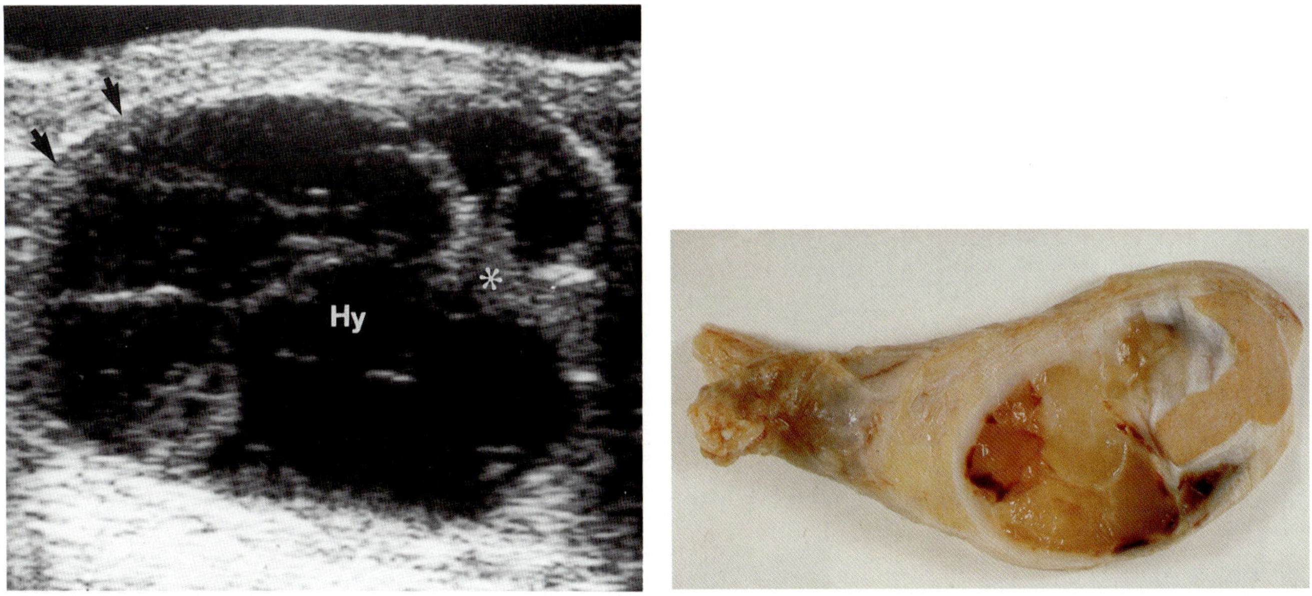

A B

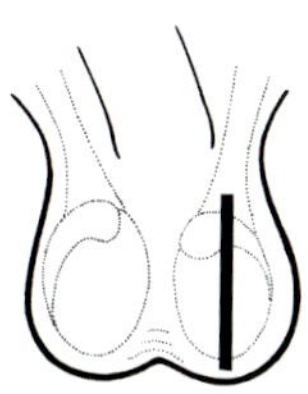

FIG. 8.4. Chronic inflammatory hydrocele secondary to recurrent epididymitis in a 40-year-old patient. **(A)** A thick-walled (*arrows*) septated hydrocele (Hy). The testicle (*) is small and deformed. Histologic examination showed chronic inflammatory epididymitis and a septated hydrocele. **(B)** Surgical specimen.

Occasionally, a so-called **hydrocele concretion**, which is a small, mobile concretion in the serous cavity of the scrotum, is discovered on ultrasound examination. It is characterized by high echogenicity and posterior acoustic shadowing, and it can be moved during scanning (Fig. 8.6). A hydrocele concretion may also be seen without a fluid collection. Such concretions may be due to a calcified missed appendiceal torsion; they have no pathologic significance, and their etiology is often uncertain. They often escape detection by palpation, since they are easily displaced, and their demonstration by ultrasound is incidental (4).

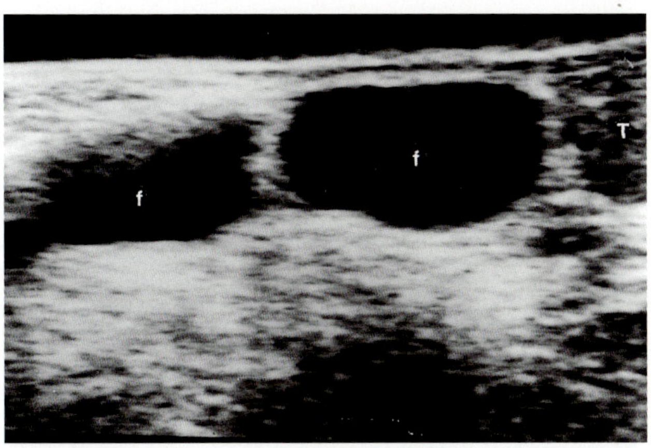

FIG. 8.5. Funiculocele. Two loculated fluid collections (f) are seen within a spermatic cord. (T, testis)

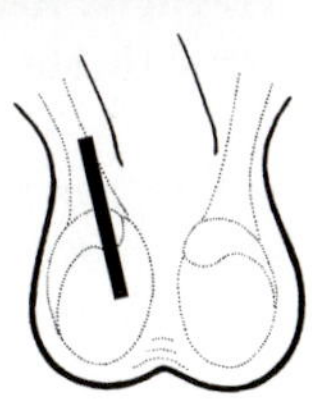

Ultrasound is particularly useful in differentiating hydrocele from other conditions that may cause similar clinical findings. Hernia, which is one of the most important conditions to be considered in the differential diagnosis, can be excluded with sonography and the diagnosis of hydrocele confirmed. Hematoceles and pyoceles (see pp. 142 and 145), which are also fluid collections in the cavum serosum, may demonstrate internal echoes and septations and may be difficult to differentiate from chronic hydrocele based on sonographic features. Clinical correlation is often needed to distinguish these two entities from hydrocele. An intrascrotal lymphocele, which has the same sonographic appearance as a hydrocele, is rare and is usually encountered 2 weeks to 6 months after ipsilateral renal transplantation (5). Spermatocele is differentiated from hydrocele by its anatomic location and consequent eccentric and inferior displacement of the testis.

Magnetic Resonance Imaging in the Evaluation of Hydrocele

Magnetic resonance imaging is almost never indicated for the diagnosis of hydrocele. On MRI the finding of a hydrocele is incidental.

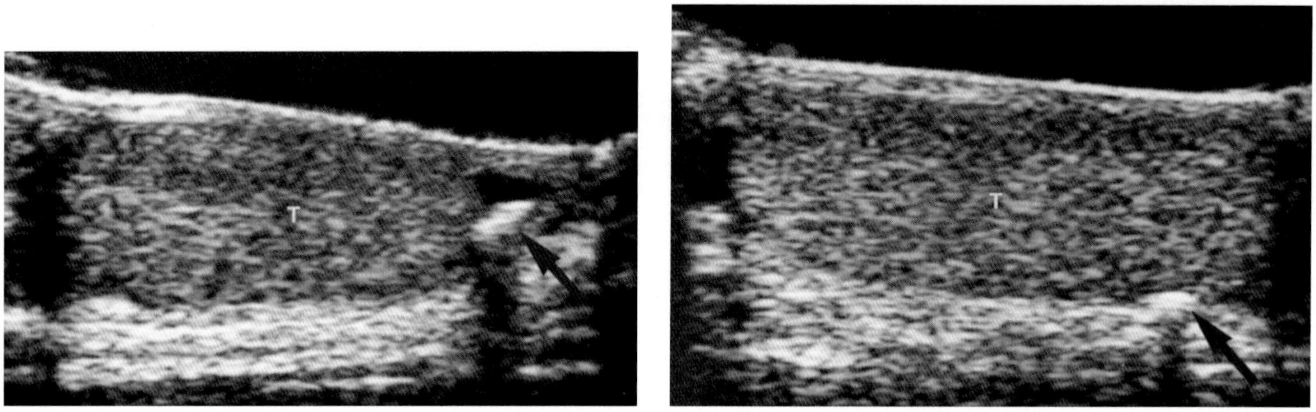

A B

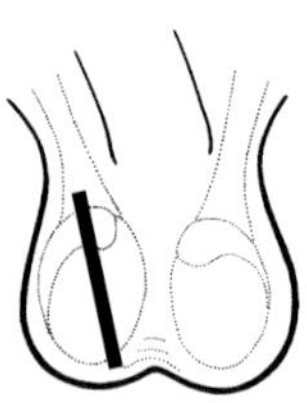

FIG. 8.6. A hydrocele concretion in the cavum serosum in a 27-year-old patient. **(A)** The sonogram shows an incidentally detected concretion (*arrow*) with dorsal acoustic shadowing. **(B)** The concretion is displaced by palpation. (T, testis)

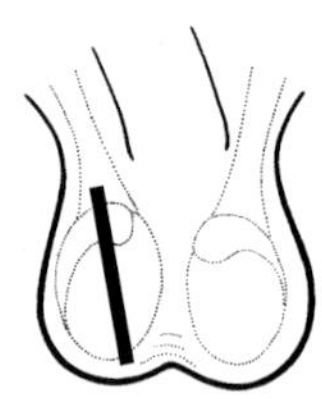

The signal characteristics of hydroceles are typical for fluid: low signal intensity on T1-weighted images and high signal intensity on T2-weighted images (Fig. 8.7) (6). The fluid collection is usually unilocular, but multilocular, septated hydroceles may also be seen. The fibrous septa within a hydrocele are best visualized on T2-weighted images. The T2-weighted image also allows optimal differentiation between the testis, hydrocele, and wall of the scrotum (6–8). The scrotal skin demonstrates low signal intensity on T2-weighted images (Fig. 8.7), and thickening of the scrotal wall, if present, is depicted against a high-signal-intensity hydrocele.

Computed Tomography in the Evaluation of Hydrocele

Computed tomography, similar to magnetic resonance imaging, is not used for the diagnosis of hydrocele. Hydroceles (Fig. 8.8) and spermatoceles can be seen as water density within the scrotal sac. However, it is often impossible to differentiate them from one another by computed tomography.

Comparative Evaluation of Hydrocele

Ultrasound is an extension of the physical examination and is an initial imaging study when clinical diagnosis of a hydrocele needs reinforcement. The sonographic diagnosis of hydrocele is straightforward. The differentiation between a hematocele, pyocele, and hydrocele often requires clinical correlation. The differentiation between hydrocele and spermatocele is based on the anatomic features of fluid location and testis displacement. Hydrocele surrounds the testis except in its "bare" position, whereas spermatocele "caps" the testis, displacing it inferiorly. The use of MRI for the diagnosis of hydrocele is rare except in patients in whom ultrasound is unable to differentiate between chronic hydrocele and hematocele and clinical history is not helpful. Better tissue–fluid characterization by MRI allows such differentiation more accurately. CT is not used for the diagnosis of hydrocele.

HEMATOCELE

Presence of hemorrhagic fluid between the parietal and visceral layer of the tunica vaginalis is called a **hematocele**. Hematocele can be seen in association with trauma (often present with testicular rupture or hematoma), torsion, testicular infarcts, and tumors. Similar to chronic hydrocele or pyocele, hematoceles most commonly do not transilluminate.

Ultrasound in the Evaluation of Hematocele

Hematocele sonographically may have an anechoic appearance similar to that of hydrocele, but more commonly, fine, dispersed echoes are seen throughout. In a chronic hematocele, numerous irregular thick septa can be identified (Fig. 8.9), and the underlying testis is often atrophic. Occasionally, calcified areas may be seen within a chronic hematocele. Sonographically, hematocele, pyocele, and chronic hydrocele often resemble each other, and clinical correlation is essential.

Magnetic Resonance Imaging in the Evaluation of Hematocele

The signal intensity of a hematocele depends on the time interval between the onset of bleeding and MR scan. In the acute phase, the signal intensity is often nonspecific and similar to hydrocele (low to medium signal

A

B

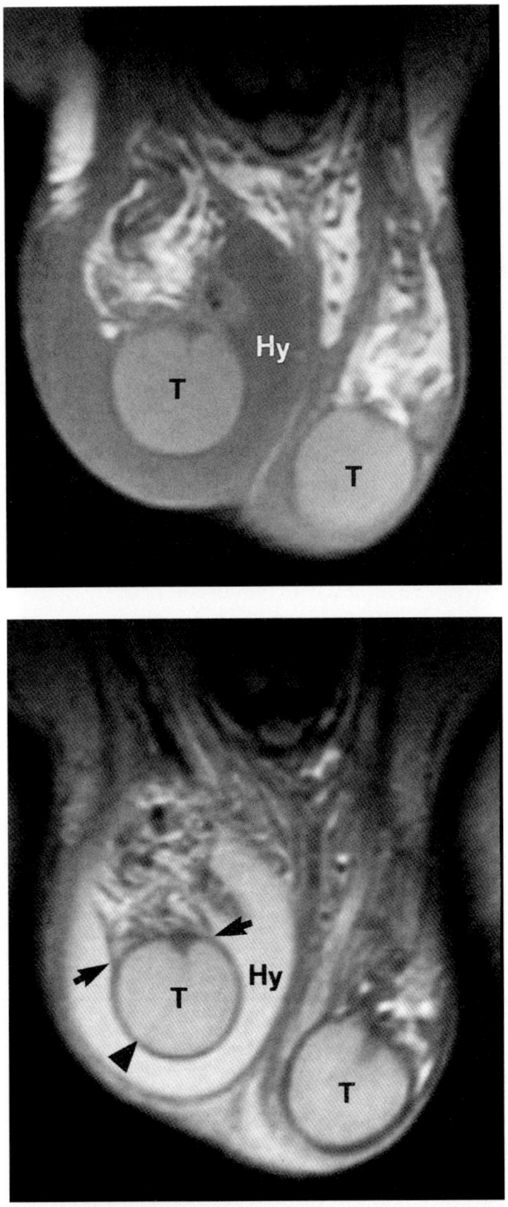

FIG. 8.7. Right hydrocele (Hy). **(A)** Coronal proton density, and **(B)** T2-weighted images. On the T2-weighted image, the tunica albuginea (*arrowhead*) is clearly visualized in contrast to the high-signal-intensity fluid (hydrocele). (*Arrows*, bare area of the testis; T, testis)

intensity on T1-weighted images and high signal intensity on T2-weighted images). In the subacute and chronic phase, the MR appearance of hematocele is specific, demonstrating high signal intensity on the T1- and T2-weighted images (Fig. 8.10). Septa and nodular vegetations can be seen within a chronic hematocele.

Computed Tomography in the Evaluation of Hematocele

Computed tomography is not used for the diagnosis of hematocele. When scanning for other reasons is performed (e.g., multiple trauma), acute hematocele is demonstrated as scrotal fluid with characteristic high attenuation value.

Comparative Evaluation of Hematocele

Although ultrasound is used as a primary imaging approach for the diagnosis of scrotum and hematocele, the role of ultrasound in this specific diagnosis is limited, requiring clinical correlation. Ultrasound, however, is very useful in evaluating underlying testis in either trauma, torsion, infarcts, or tumors. In the diagnosis of chronic hematocele when clinical history is ambiguous, MR findings may offer a specific diagnosis. MRI is indicated in selective cases where the exact diagnosis of hematocele will influence patient treatment.

PYOCELE

A pyocele is an accumulation of pus or infected fluid between the two layers of the tunica vaginalis. It may occur in conjunction with intrascrotal abscess formation or with suppurative inflammatory conditions of the intrascrotal organs, or it may result from iatrogenic contamination (e.g., during hydrocele aspiration). Clinically, a pyocele presents as a fluctuant or tense–elastic intrascrotal swelling accompanied by signs of inflammation such as swelling, reddening, pain, fever, and leukocytosis.

Ultrasound in the Evaluation of Pyocele

Like a hydrocele, a pyocele is seen as a fluid collection in the cavum serosum. Most pyoceles, however, have

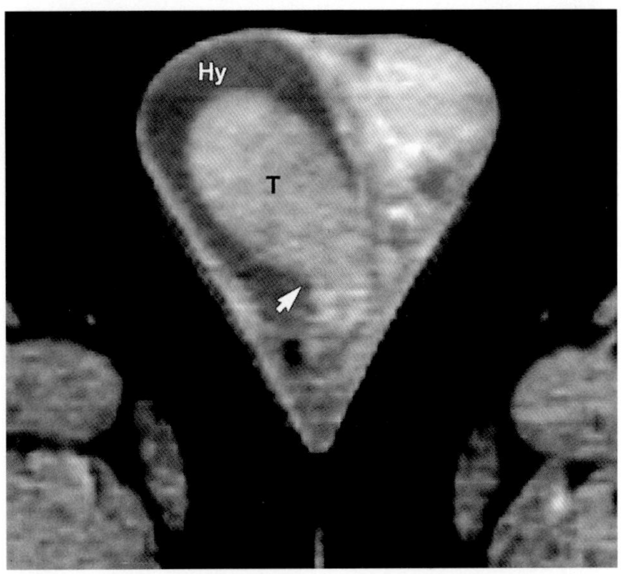

FIG. 8.8. Hydrocele (Hy) on CT scan is seen as a fluid collection around the right testis (T). Note the "bare area" (*arrow*) in the posterior aspect of the testis where the tunica vaginalis fails to cover the testis and the testis is intimately attached to the epididymis.

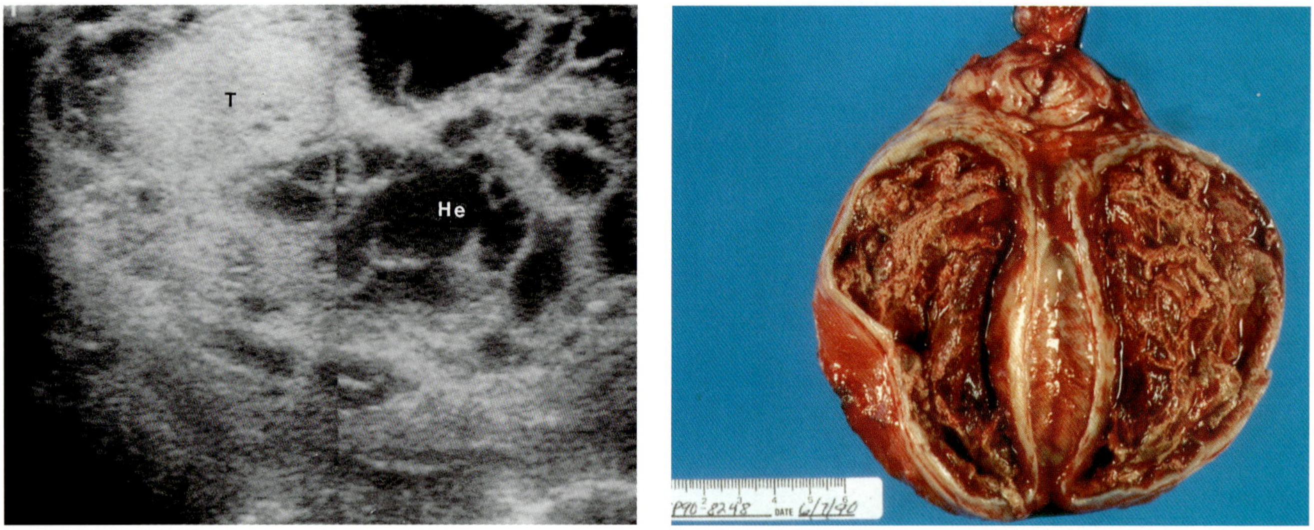

A B

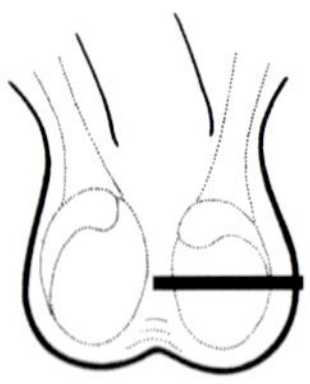

FIG. 8.9. Hematocele. **(A)** Ultrasound and **(B)** gross specimen. Testis (T) is normal. Surrounding the testis is a thick-walled fluid collection, a hematocele (He), traversed with numerous thick septa.

netlike septations formed of cellular debris and fibrin (Fig. 8.11), not of connective tissue. With good spatial resolution, small suspended particles can be seen in the fluid, a phenomenon that can be accentuated by slight lateral tapping. These particles could be blood, pus, or crystals. Tiny, bright, echogenic foci in the fluid may also correspond to minute bubbles produced by bacterial metabolism. These particles produce more internal echoes in a pyocele than are seen in the serous fluid of a hydrocele. Nevertheless, clinical and ultrasound findings should be considered together to distinguish reliably a pyocele from a chronic inflammatory reactive hydrocele.

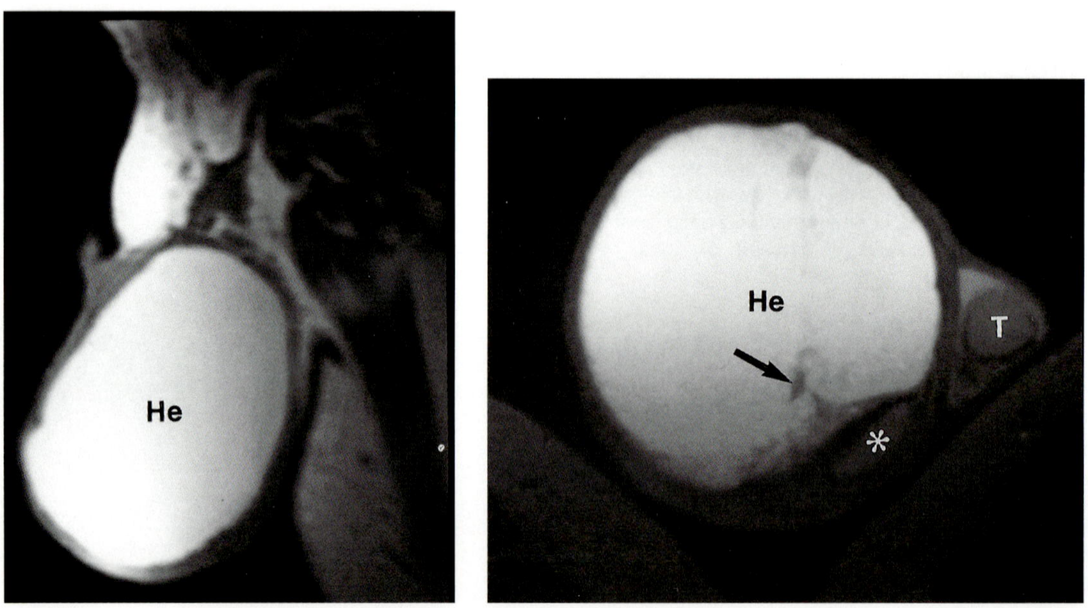

A B

FIG. 8.10. **(A)** Sagittal T1-weighted and **(B)** transaxial T2-weighted MR images. A fluid collection in the right hemiscrotum, hematocele (He), shows high signal intensity on both T1- and T2-weighted images. Intervening septa (*arrow*) within the hematocele are seen. The right testis (*) is displaced and compressed by the lesion. (T, left testis)

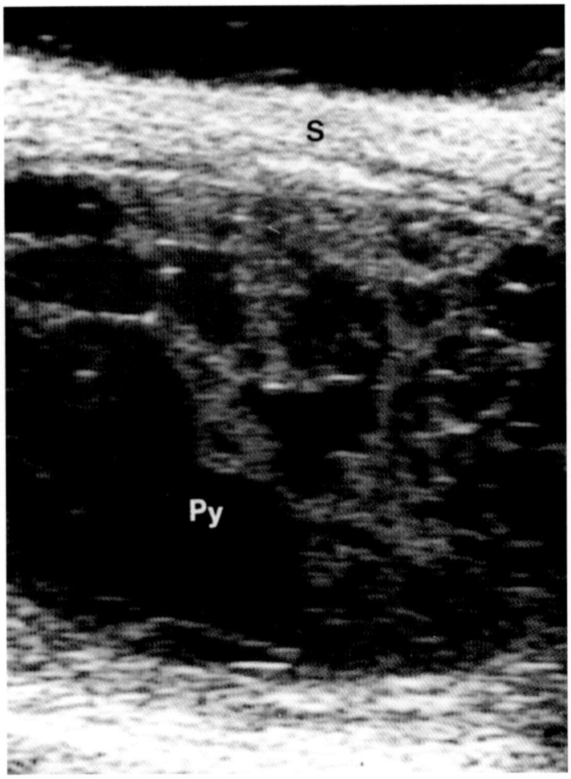

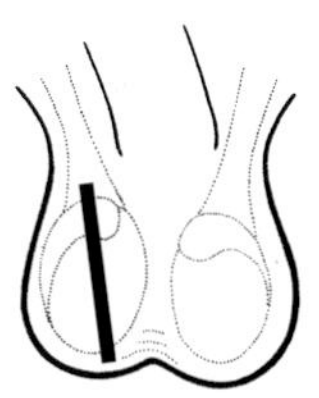

FIG. 8.11. A large pyocele (Py) demonstrating a thick wall and numerous septa in a 64-year-old patient. The testis is not shown. (S, scrotal skin)

In most cases a pyocele is associated with secondary inflammatory changes, such as thickening of the scrotal skin or swelling of the spermatic cord.

Magnetic Resonance Imaging in the Evaluation of Pyocele

The fluid collection in pyocele is usually multilocular and has multiple internal septations and infected debris. The fluid in the pyocele demonstrates medium (higher than hydrocele) signal intensity on T1-weighted image and high signal intensity on T2-weighted image. The septa and debris are often better seen on T2-weighted MR images. Based on imaging findings, chronic hydrocele and pyocele have similar features, and the differentiation is based on clinical findings of epididymo-orchitis.

Computed Tomography in the Evaluation of Pyocele

Computed tomography is not used in the diagnosis of pyocele. Sometimes the pyocele can be seen when scanning for extensive inflammatory disease or abscess. The attenuation value of infected fluid is higher than water density. Debris and septa are easily displayed as an associated finding of epididymal infection, and scrotal wall thickening can also be seen.

Comparative Evaluation of Pyocele

Although the diagnosis of pyocele can be made on either MRI or CT, ultrasound is the initial and often the only imaging modality needed in the diagnosis of pyocele and associated inflammatory changes, including a search for abscess.

SPERMATOCELE

Spermatoceles, retention cysts of small tubules that connect the rete testis to the head of the epididymis, are asymptomatic and are often discovered incidentally. They are relatively common, usually occurring in middle-aged men. The incidence increases with age. They may occur following vasectomy, inguinal herniorrhaphy, or epididymitis, which can cause obstruction of the sperm pathway (7). Spermatoceles are lined by epithelium and filled with fluid that contains sediment composed of cellular debris, immobile spermatozoa, and lipids. **Seminiferous tubular ectasia** of the rete testis and **testicular cysts** are often associated with spermatoceles (see Chapter 5).

Clinical Presentation

Most spermatoceles are discovered by patients themselves or during a routine physical examination. Patients commonly present with a painless cystic mass located just above and posterior to the testis. On occasion, patients describe a mild dragging sensation in the inguinal region radiating into the scrotum. On physical examination, spermatoceles are palpated as tense-elastic nodules in the area of the globus major (the head of the epididymis). The cystic mass is freely movable and usually transilluminates. The fluid in spermatoceles is grossly yellow but clear, and usually contains dead sperm. Spermatoceles show considerable variation in size. Most are 1 to 4 cm in diameter (2), but very large (giant) spermatoceles can be encountered as well.

Clinically, the differential diagnosis includes tumors arising around the spermatic cord, such as mesothelioma, fibroma, epididymal cyst, and loculated hydrocele. It is generally easy to differentiate a spermatocele from the testis. Only larger spermatoceles will transilluminate. Torsion of a spermatocele, which occurs very rarely, may present as an acute scrotum (9,10). Therapeutic management is required only in patients with large or painful spermatoceles.

The diagnosis of **epididymal cyst** is clinically indistinguishable from a spermatocele. Epididymal cyst is thought to be a congenital lesion, occurring in approximately 5% of normal males. It is often seen at 15–20 years of age. In utero exposure to diethylstilbestrol has been reported to be associated with an increased incidence (up to 21%) of epididymal cysts (11). Like spermatoceles, epididymal cysts are found most commonly in the head of the epididymis. They contain clear fluid, with a composition similar to that of spermatoceles, but they do not contain spermatozoa (12). They are usually smaller than 3 cm in diameter.

Ultrasound in the Evaluation of Spermatocele

In general, ultrasound is seldom needed to confirm the clinical diagnosis of a spermatocele. It is, however, a useful and simple procedure for demonstrating a spermatocele in patients with inconclusive clinical findings. In such cases, sonography can reliably differentiate the spermatocele from the solid mass suspected of being a tumor. Spermatoceles and/or epididymal cysts have been reported in as many as 70% of men who undergo high-resolution US examination (13). Spermatoceles are recognized on sonograms as anechoic and smoothly demarcated cystic structures (Fig. 8.12). Because of their cystic character, spermatoceles as small as 2 mm are easily displayed (Fig. 8.13). The differentiation between a spermatocele (Fig. 8.13) and an epididymal cyst (Fig. 8.14) can be difficult except when internal echoes or debris within a fluid collection are detected. These are assumed to represent dead sperm and thus allow a specific diagnosis of a spermatocele (Fig. 8.13). Furthermore, when the fluid collection is larger than 4 cm in diameter, it is probably a spermatocele.

Occasionally, a large spermatocele may be difficult to distinguish from a hydrocele, which is also anechoic (Fig. 8.15). Differentiation is facilitated by slight manual displacement of the testis in a cranial direction that causes a concomitant shift of the fluid retained in a hydrocele,

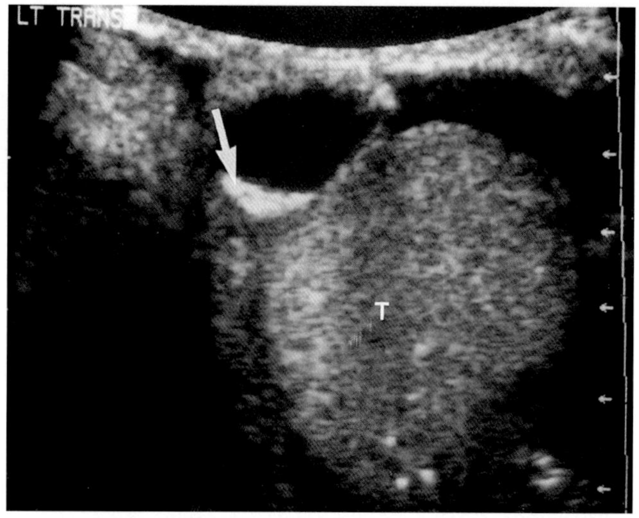

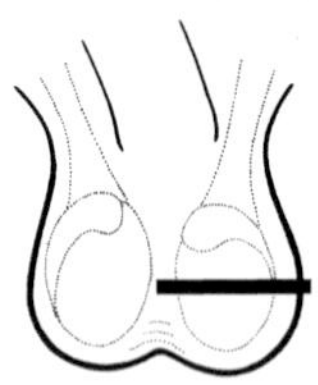

FIG. 8.13. Spermatocele in a 35-year-old patient. Debris (*arrow*) within a cystic lesion in the head of the epididymis is a differentiating feature between a spermatocele and epididymal cyst. (T, testis)

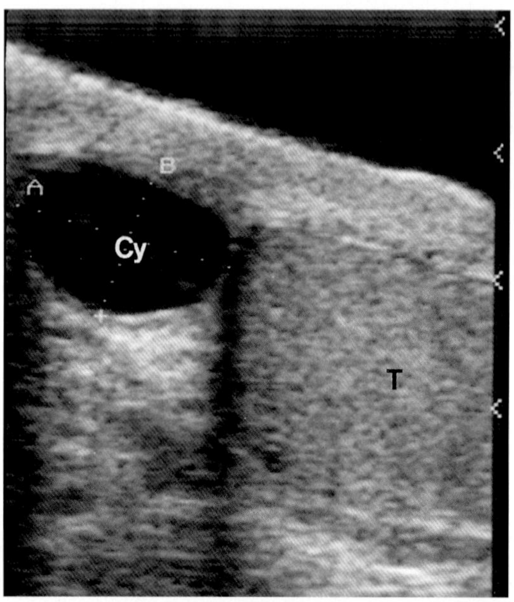

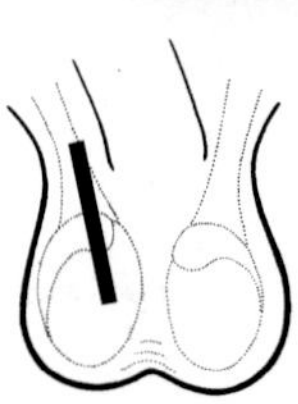

FIG. 8.12. Spermatocele or epididymal cyst in a 17-year-old patient. Longitudinal sonogram demonstrates an ovoid anechoic cystic lesion (Cy) in the epididymal head. (T, Normal testis)

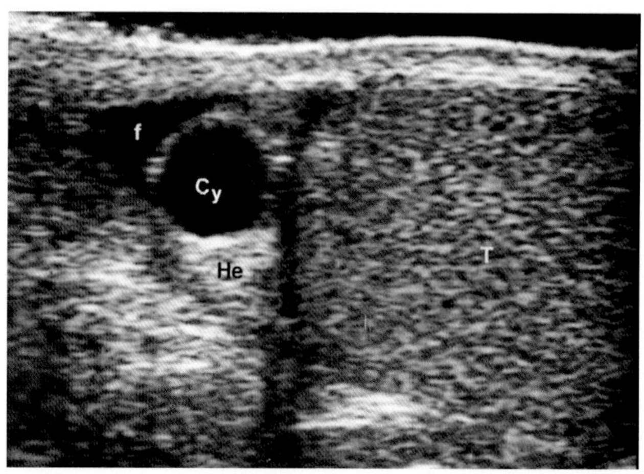

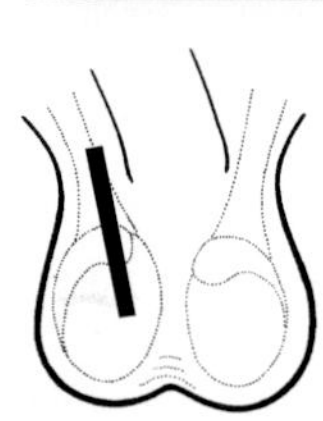

FIG. 8.14. Epididymal cyst (Cy) of the globus major in a 36-year-old patient. The small size and lack of internal echoes indicate an epididymal cyst. A slight, physiologic collection of fluid (f) in the serous cavity cranial to the epididymal head (He) can be identified. (T, testis)

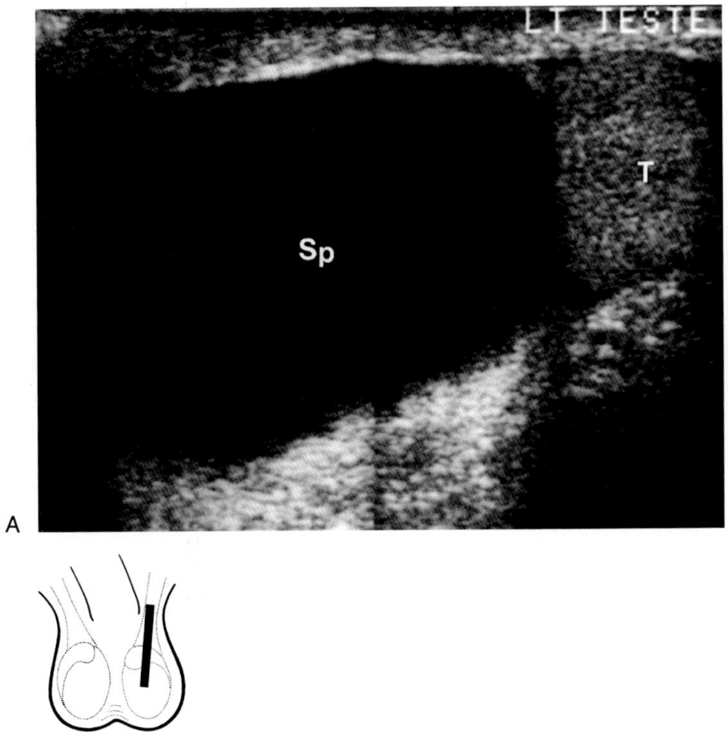

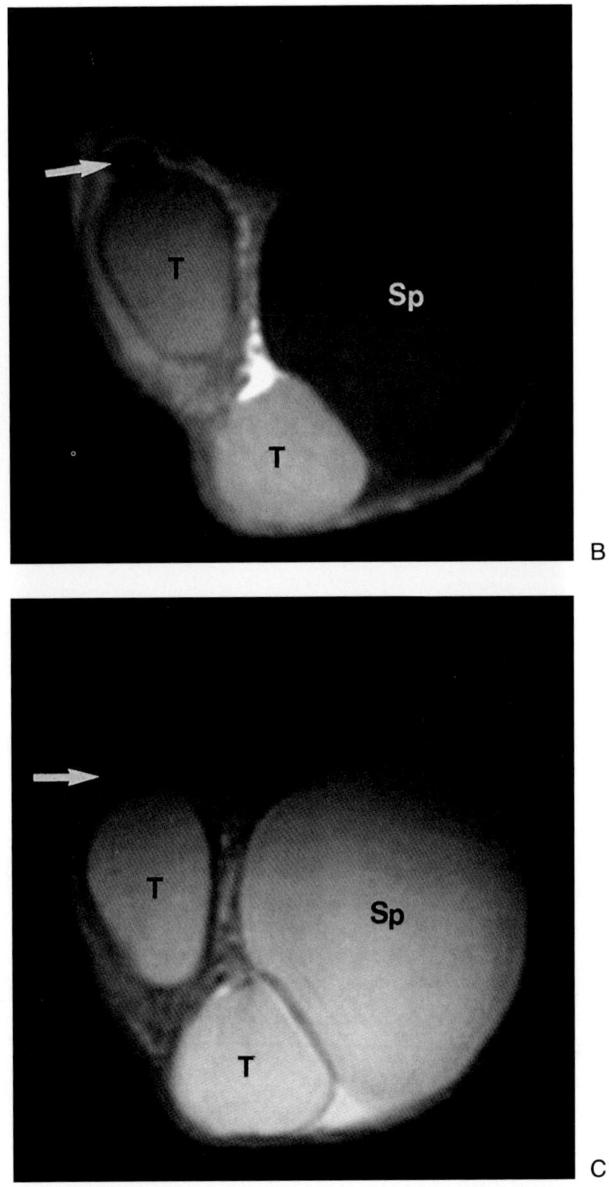

FIG. 8.15. Left spermatocele (Sp). **(A)** Ultrasonogram. **(B)** Contrast-enhanced T1-weighted and **(C)** T2-weighted MR images. The spermatocele (Sp) is seen as a discrete cystic mass in the region of the epididymal head, displacing the left testis downward and medially. The signal intensity of the spermatocele on MR resembles that of a hydrocele. (*Arrow*, right epididymis; T, testis)

but not in a spermatocele. In addition, hydroceles have a relatively flaccid consistency on palpation, whereas spermatoceles are palpated as circumscribed, tense-elastic lesions. Anatomic features such as fluid location and testicular displacement are other findings helpful in their differentiation. Differentiation of a spermatocele from the testis and from normal epididymal tissue is easily accomplished with ultrasonography.

Magnetic Resonance Imaging in the Evaluation of Spermatocele

On MR scans the diagnosis of spermatocele can be made by the typical location (usually in the head of the epididymis) of the fluid collection, inferior testicular displacement (Fig. 8.16), and signal intensity characteristics. Spermatoceles are round and well circumscribed, and the signal intensity is usually similar to water (Fig. 8.15). Depending upon the fluid contents (e.g., presence of blood or protein), however, spermatoceles may demonstrate various signal intensity on both T1- and T2-weighted images.

Computed Tomography in the Evaluation of Spermatocele

Spermatoceles can be seen as water density within the scrotal sac. However, it is often impossible to differentiate them from epididymal cyst or hydrocele by CT.

Scintigraphy in the Evaluation of Spermatocele

Spermatoceles are located along the superior aspect of the testicle (14,15), and a static scan shows a cold defect in this area (14,16,17).

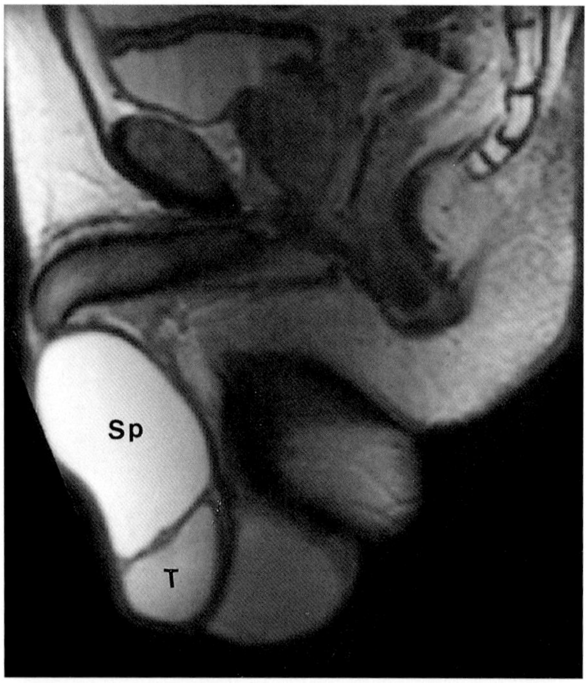

FIG. 8.16. Spermatocele. T2-weighted MR image, sagittal plane of section. A typical location of a spermatocele (Sp) in the region of the head of the epididymis and inferior displacement of the testis (T) are well displayed.

Comparative Evaluation of Spermatocele/Epididymal Cyst

Ultrasound is the initial imaging examination that will make a confident diagnosis of spermatocele in most patients. When US findings are inconclusive, differentiation between spermatocele and hydrocele is not feasible and an MRI study can be performed. Neither CT nor scintigraphy is indicated for the diagnosis of spermatocele.

VARICOCELE

Varicocele, a dilatation of the veins of the pampiniform plexus, is the most frequent cause of male infertility, occurring in approximately 10% to 15% of the general male population (18). This condition is more common on the left side and is thought to be caused by incompetence of the valves of the internal spermatic vein and the effect of gravity. Sometimes varicoceles are associated with renal cell carcinoma or a large retroperitoneal mass, which may compress or extend into the renal vein. Varicocele, demonstrated in 10% to 40% of all infertile men, is usually associated with decreased sperm count, motility, and abnormal sperm morphology. However, the severity of seminal abnormalities does not correlate with the size of the varicocele (18,19). As treatment improves sperm quality in as many as 53% of cases, the correct diagnosis of this disorder is of utmost clinical importance. Up to 24% of patients presenting with fertility disorders are reported to have nonpalpable, so-called subclinical varicoceles (18,20,21).

The most commonly used procedures for radiologic diagnostic evaluation of patients with a suspected varicocele is **sonography**. **Venography** and **thermography** can be used as well. The indications and the findings on venography and thermography are discussed in Chapter 10. Ultrasound, in particular color-coded duplex sonography (CCDS), has now become the procedure of choice and is discussed later. MR imaging findings have been described, but MRI is not recommended for the evaluation of varicocele. With CT, demonstration of varicocele is often impossible, unless the vessels are large or thrombosed and marked with phleboliths (22).

Clinical Presentation

The patient should first be examined standing up. With varicocele a mass of tortuous veins, which is sometimes tender, can be palpated in the posterior and superior aspects of the testis, up to the external inguinal ring. The filled and dilated veins in the area of the pampiniform plexus feel like a "bag of worms." On inspection a large varicocele has a bluish appearance through the skin. Normally, a varicocele empties and the dilatation decreases in a recumbent position and is aggravated with the Valsalva maneuver. If it does not, or if the patient reports spontaneous occurrence of the varicocele, the possibility of a **reactive (symptomatic) varicocele** secondary to a retroperitoneal mass lesion (such as a renal tumor, lymphoma, or other retroperitoneal mass) should be considered. The presence of a reactive varicocele can be confirmed or excluded by sonography by examining the scrotum and the retroperitoneum.

Early detection and treatment of varicoceles are important, since testicular tissue damage and resultant atrophy and infertility do not correlate with the size of the varicocele (23). To avoid infertility, surgical ligation or percutaneous embolization of the testicular vein is performed in selected patients. Clinical evaluation of the treatment is difficult, however, since the cordlike indurations of the pampiniform plexus (occurring in particular after sclerotherapy) do not allow exclusion of persistence of a varicocele based on palpation. Therefore, noninvasive diagnostic procedures play an important role in the follow-up of patients who have undergone treatment for a varicocele (21,23).

Ultrasound in the Evaluation of Varicocele

Real-Time Ultrasound

With real-time ultrasound it is possible to evaluate both the varicocele and the scrotal contents in a single

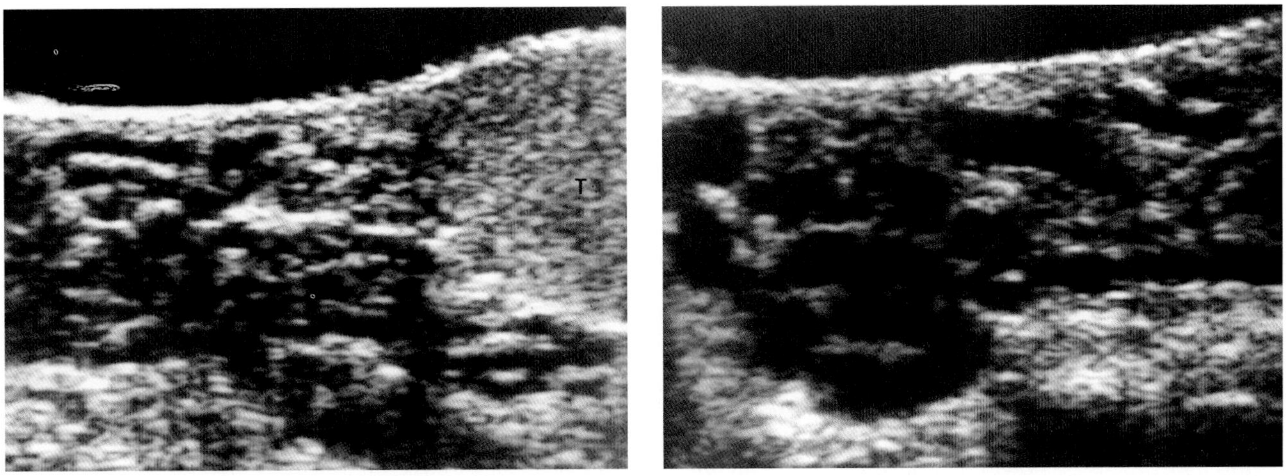

A

B

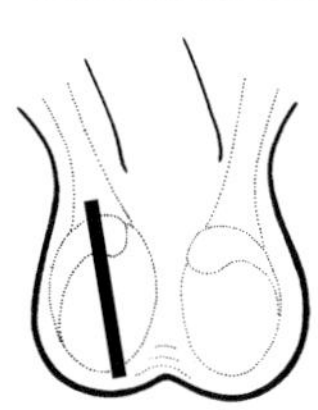

FIG. 8.17. Large varicocele in a 19-year-old patient. **(A)** Multiple distended veins are seen in the recumbent position. **(B)** There is considerable additional vascular dilatation when the patient stands. (T, testis)

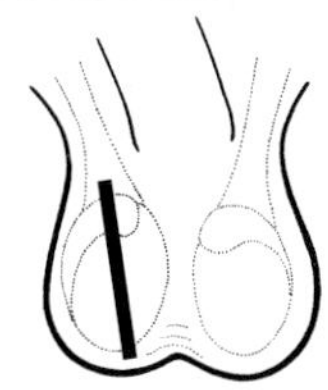

session. A sonographic diagnosis of varicocele can be made if the vessels of the pampiniform plexus are enlarged (greater than 2–3 mm in diameter) and if they further dilate when the patient, in standing position, performs the Valsalva maneuver (Fig. 8.17) (24,25). Based on this simple criterion, ultrasound has a sensitivity of 92% in diagnosing varicocele (24). Ultrasound is less useful in identifying subclinical varicoceles and in evaluating patients who have undergone sclerotherapy (23). Very small varicose veins (subclinical varicoceles) are usually 2–3 mm in diameter, their number is greater than 3, and they show no or only moderate enlargement during pressing or standing (Fig. 8.18) (26). They may escape detection by real-time sonography (26). Following treatment, sclerosed vessels present as hypoechoic structures for several months, making it impossible, without the use of color-coded duplex sonography, to determine the patency of individual veins (23).

Doppler, Duplex, and Color-Coded Duplex Sonography

Doppler ultrasound can be used to assess blood flow in the vessels of the pampiniform plexus. Under normal conditions there is only slow venous flow in a cranial direction. Varicoceles, however, are characterized by ret-

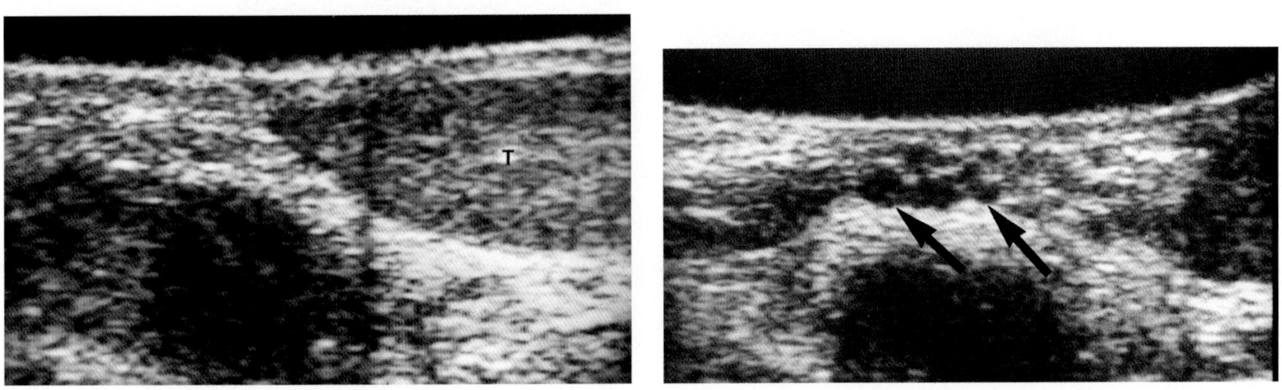

A

B

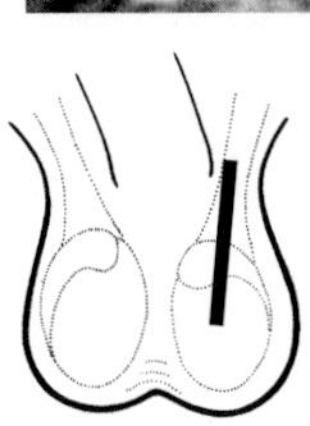

FIG. 8.18. Subclinical varicocele in a 32-year-old patient. **(A)** Normal sonographic appearance in the recumbent position. (T, normal testis) **(B)** Individual small veins become dilated (*arrows*) when the patient stands.

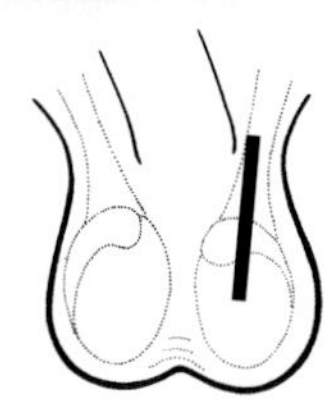

rograde filling of the testicular vein during the Valsalva maneuver (Fig. 8.19). This venous reflux can sometimes be detected in subclinical forms of varicocele (27,28). Continuous-wave Doppler is limited by the fact that only flow itself can be evaluated, not vessels. It is not possible, therefore, to rule out a varicocele with this modality, since evaluation of all veins of the pampiniform plexus is necessary. Even though an extensive varicocele is easily depicted by Doppler US, it is difficult to depict small, subclinical varicoceles.

Duplex ultrasound represents a theoretical improvement over continuous-wave Doppler, since it provides simultaneous assessment of soft tissue structures and blood flow. The frequency shift can only be derived from one point of the scan, however, and movement of the transducer and/or the patient limits measurement ability, especially from vessels with a small lumen. Sensitivity in the detection of subclinical varices is only 64% (29).

Color-coded duplex sonography represents a significant technological improvement. This technique simultaneously displays soft tissue morphology and blood flow characteristics over the entire B-scan area and registers venous flow in very small or partly thrombosed vessels. The direction-dependent assignment of red and blue colors to flowing blood simplifies and speeds up the diagnostic evaluation of varicoceles, with resultant sensitivity and specificity approaching 100% (30).

CCDS examination for varicocele is performed with the patient lying down. The pampiniform plexus is focused in the longitudinal or transverse plane, and the patient is asked to perform the Valsalva maneuver. If a varicocele is present, there is retrograde flow in the vessels of the pampiniform plexus, which is immediately identified by the increase in color flow (Fig. 8.19). Even small, subclinical (not palpable) varicoceles can be easily detected. This retrograde flow does not occur at rest or in healthy subjects.

With CCDS it is also possible to differentiate reactive or symptomatic varicoceles secondary to renal or retroperitoneal tumors from other varicoceles. In tumor-related conditions, compromised venous return via the renal vein, caused by tumor compression, causes flow in the vessels of the pampiniform plexus to be constantly high regardless of the breathing status (Fig. 8.20).

In contrast to its superiority in preoperative detection of clinically nonpalpable varicoceles, CCDS is not completely accurate in evaluating the effects of surgery in patients with varicocele (31).

Magnetic Resonance Imaging in the Evaluation of Varicocele

On MR images a varicocele is seen as a mass of serpiginous and tubular dilated vessels accompanied by an enlarged spermatic cord (Fig. 8.21). Signal intensity varies with the flow velocity. Because of slow flow, a varicocele commonly demonstrates medium signal intensity on

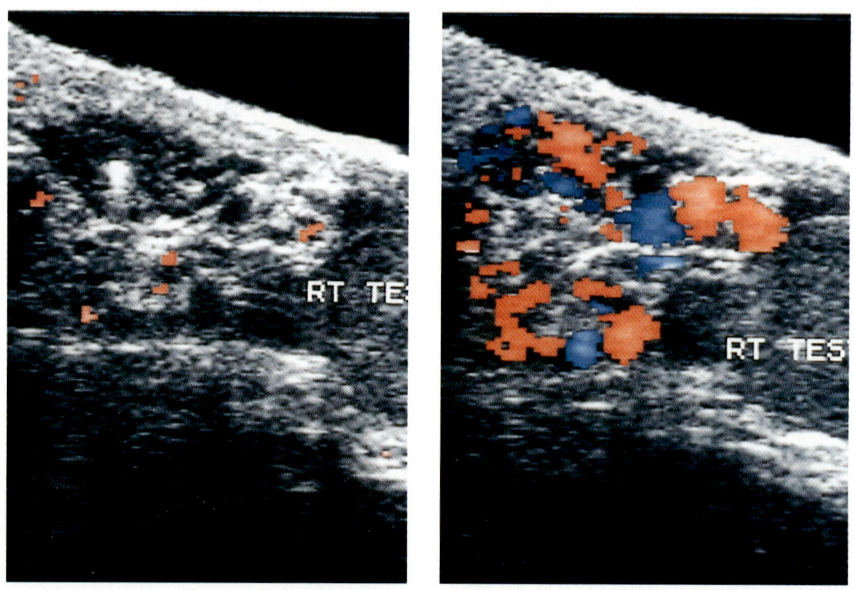

A B

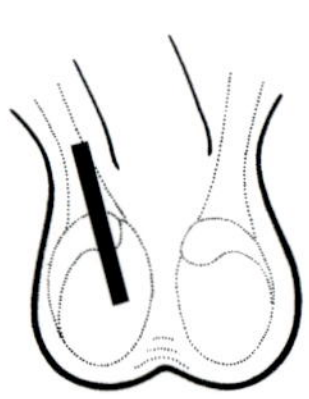

FIG. 8.19. Varicocele. **(A)** A longitudinal image of the pampiniform plexus at the upper pole of the testis during quiet respiration shows enlarged veins but minimized flow signals. **(B)** During the Valsalva maneuver, there is increased flow in the dilated veins. This retrograde flow can be visualized even in very small, impalpable varicoceles.

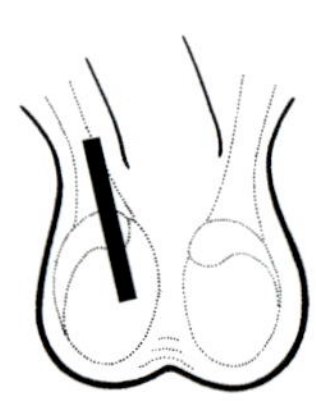

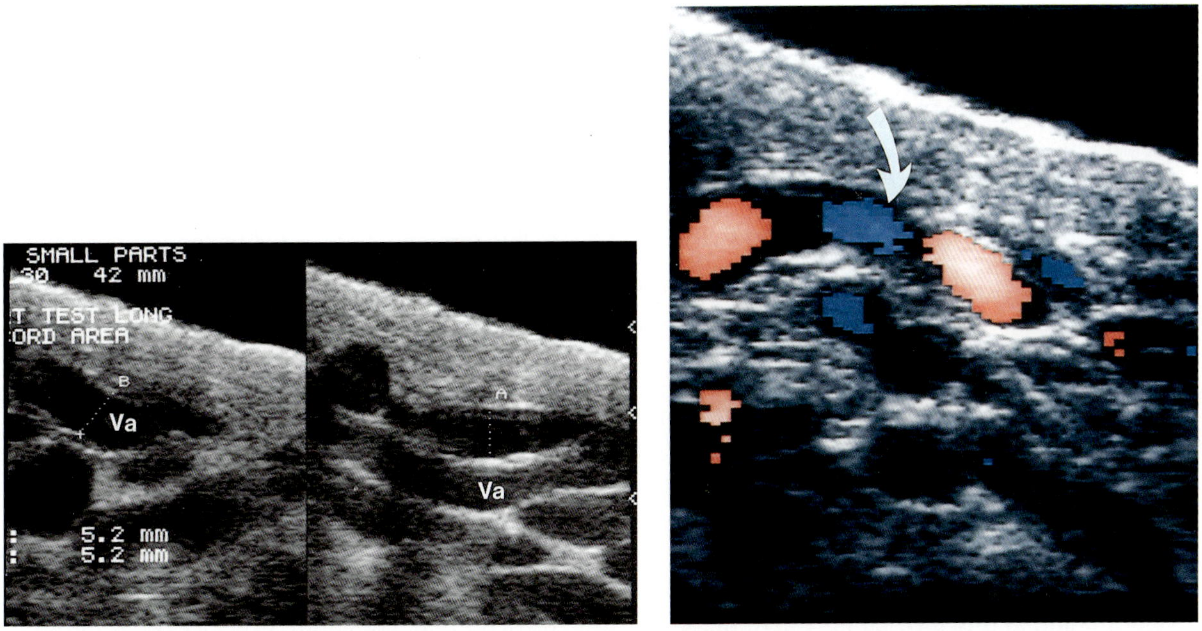

A B

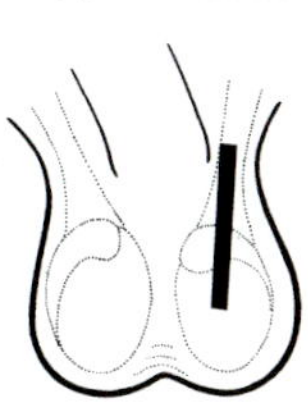

FIG. 8.20. Left varicocele in a patient with left-side renal cell carcinoma. **(A)** Longitudinal sonogram in left shows markedly dilated, tortuous vascular structures (Va) measures 5.2 mm in largest diameter. **(B)** Color-coded duplex sonogram demonstrates high flow (*arrow*) within the dilated veins of the pampiniform plexus regardless of the breathing status.

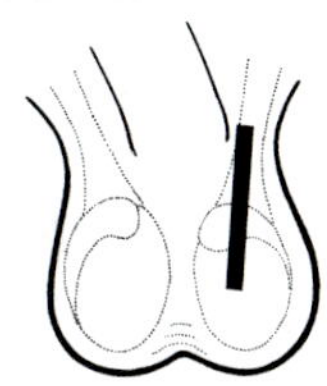

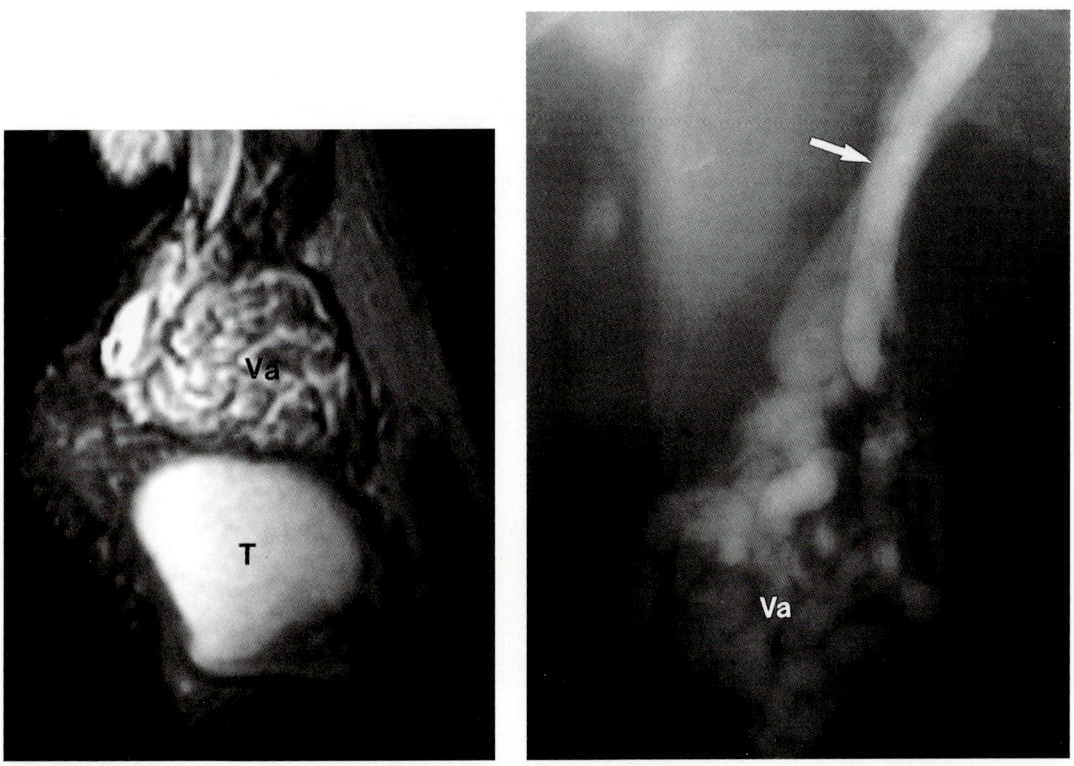

A B

FIG. 8.21. Left varicocele (Va). **(A)** Sagittal T2-weighted MR image and **(B)** testicular venogram. On the MR image, the varicocele is seen as a mass of serpiginous, dilated vessels above the testis (T). Venography confirms multiple tortuous, dilated vessels in the scrotum with dilatation of the testicular vein (*arrow*).

T1-weighted images and high signal intensity on T2-weighted images. For detection of subclinical varicoceles, veins can be distended by application of abdominal compression during a MR study (32). Gradient echo (GRE) technique can be helpful to confirm the presence of vascular structures. While a demonstration of a varicocele is possible with MRI, MRI is not used for its detection or evaluation of treatment.

Computed Tomography in the Evaluation of Varicocele

Varicocele, especially with new CT scanners and bolus injection, can be seen on CT. The added risk of radiation and contrast injection, however, limits the use of CT in this application.

Scintigraphy in the Evaluation of Varicocele

In 1979 Freund and Bautovich (33) were the first to describe the use of radionuclide scintigraphy for the evaluation of varicoceles. The presence of a varicocele can be seen during the flow study, in particular during the venous phase. Technetium-99m-labeled (Tc-99m) red blood cells are used in most studies, although Tc-99m human serum albumin may also be used. During the later part of the flow study, most patients with varicoceles will show reflux into the spermatic vein. On static images varicoceles appear as an area of linear and fusiform activity. (See Chapter 10 for details on the technique for use of nuclear medicine in the evaluation of varicocele.)

Comparative Evaluation of Varicocele

Ultrasound, especially when coupled with CCDS, is today considered an initial examination in the evaluation of varicoceles. Geatti and colleagues (19) studied 263 patients using a combination of thermography, ultrasound, venography, and scintigraphy; they found an excellent correlation. In a group of 96 patients, with phlebography used as the gold standard, sensitivity was 98% for scintigraphy, 100% for thermography, and 98% for ultrasound. Most of the varicoceles seen on venography were also seen by scintigraphy (23,34–38); in addition, scintigraphy had the advantage of demonstrating reflux of the spermatic vein. Despite this high sensitivity, scintigraphy is not widely utilized. The primary approach to the evaluation of varicocele is ultrasound followed by venography, if there is discrepancy between US examination and clinical findings or if percutaneous embolization of the testicular vein is planned. (The technique and success of percutaneous embolization are described in Chapter 10.) Venography is often considered as a standard of reference.

Ultrasound, however, is preferred to venography because it is noninvasive, does not utilize radiation, is widely available, is relatively inexpensive, and does not require the same special expertise as does venography.

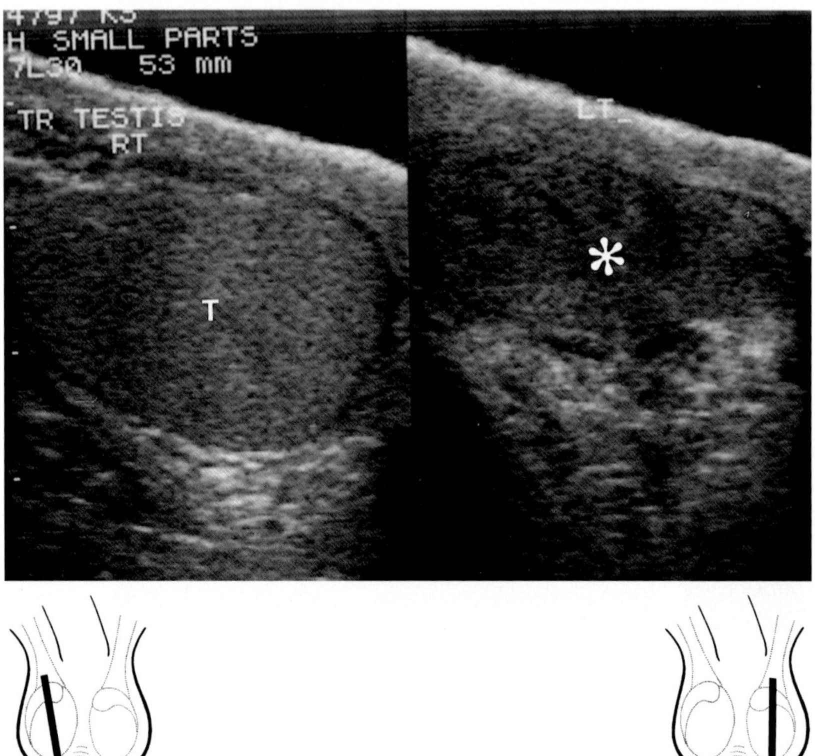

FIG. 8.22. Left testicular atrophy in a 41-year-old patient with left subclinical varicocele. Longitudinal scans of both testes show small left testis (*) with diffusely decreased echogenicity and small subclinical varicocele. The right testis (T) is normal.

Furthermore, ultrasound allows the evaluation not only of subclinical or clinical varicoceles but of echotexture of the underlying testis (Fig. 8.22). The use of MRI or CT is limited, unless technical breakthrough in the future bring new possibilities and change our approach.

INGUINAL HERNIA

Inguinal hernias are among the most common congenital disorders encountered in infants and children, with a reported incidence of 1% to 4.4% (39). The incidence is even higher in premature infants, and boys are 8 to 10 times more likely to be affected than girls (40). Inguinal hernias may be associated with cystic fibrosis; connective tissue disorders, such as Ehlers-Danlos syndrome; and mucopolysaccharidoses (40). They are caused by failure of the peritoneal pouches to obliterate, resulting in persistent communication between the peritoneal sac and the tunica vaginalis. Since testicular descent is closely related to obliteration of the processus vaginalis, more than 90% of patients with undescended testes have hernia sacs (1).

The actual incidence of bilateral inguinal hernia and the usefulness of routine bilateral exploration in cases of apparent unilateral hernia remain controversial issues (39,41). In one study a contralateral patent processus vaginalis was found in 50% to 90% of patients undergoing surgery for unilateral inguinal hernia. In another study subsequent development of a contralateral hernia was reported in approximately 20% of patients (40,42,43). Because testicular atrophy occurs in approximately 0.5% of

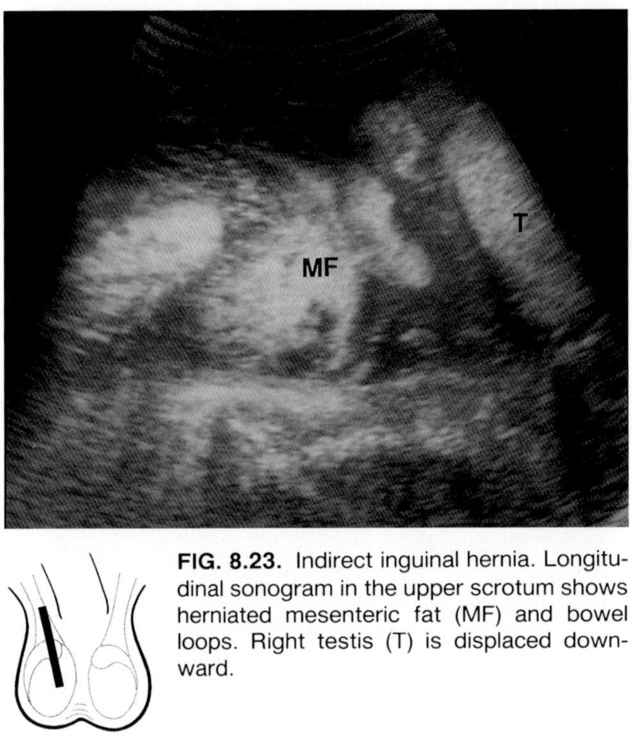

FIG. 8.23. Indirect inguinal hernia. Longitudinal sonogram in the upper scrotum shows herniated mesenteric fat (MF) and bowel loops. Right testis (T) is displaced downward.

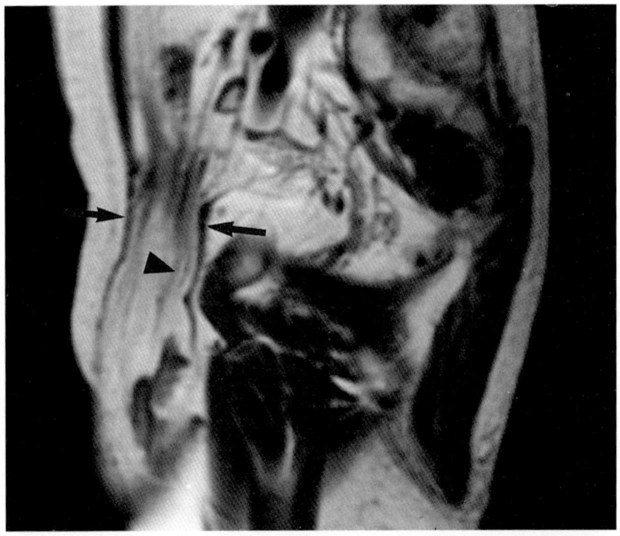

A

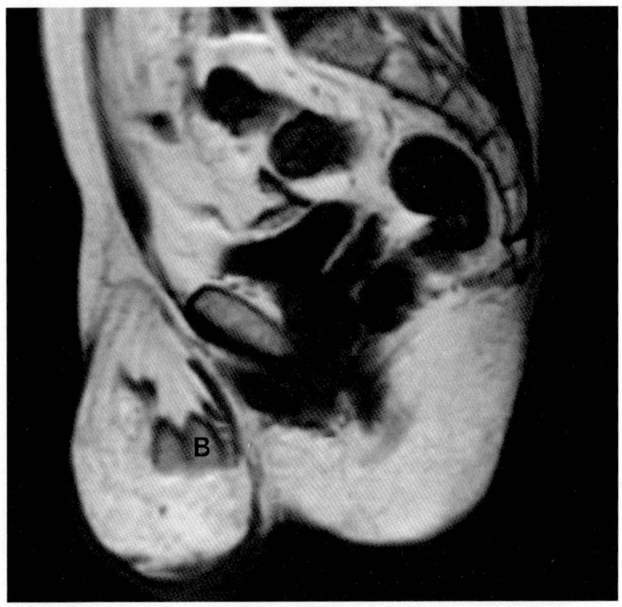

B

FIG. 8.24. Indirect inguinal hernia of small bowel. Sagittal T1-weighted images through **(A)** the hernial neck (*arrow*) and **(B)** the scrotal sac. Herniated small bowel (B), mesenteric vessels (*arrowhead*), and fat are easily identified.

patients following herniorrhaphy, the decision to perform bilateral exploration should be based on the patient's age, sex, and associated disorders.

Accurate diagnosis and timely corrective surgery for congenital inguinal hernia are important because the possible complications of incarceration and strangulation may result in loss of gonads, in segmental bowel loops, or even in death. In subjects with a wide and elastic inguinal ring, parts of the peritoneum, intestine, or omentum may bulge through the inguinal canal in response to increased intra-abdominal pressure and become incarcerated. In chronic scrotal hernias, there may be additional confinement of bowel contents. In either case, compromised venous return leads to edema and inflammation. If the hernia is not surgically repositioned, hemorrhagic infarction, gangrene, and perforation follow. Additional sequelae of a strangulated inguinal hernia include peritonitis and ileus.

Clinical Presentation

Most inguinal hernias present within the first year, and the diagnosis is usually made clinically. Infantile inguinal hernias present with a bulge in the groin that appears suddenly after crying, coughing, or straining (39). With the patient standing, palpation demonstrates invagination of the scrotum up to the external inguinal ring on the cough impulse. A thickened spermatic cord can be palpated against the pubic tubercle (**silk-glove sign**). The clinical diagnosis is usually straightforward, and imaging evaluation is not indicated. Occasionally, however, inguinal hernias may mimic other scrotal disorders, necessitating further examination. When sudden scrotal pain accompanies marked scrotal enlargement, however, it prevents thorough physical examination and necessitates imaging.

Both incarcerated inguinal hernia and chronic scrotal hernia may present with the symptoms of acute scrotum. The most common clinical symptom is sudden pain in the groin and scrotum. In children, vomiting and concomitant obstipation occur in 80% of cases. Palpation reveals a unilateral, painful, pasty swelling that cannot be repositioned by manipulation. The lesion does not transilluminate.

Ultrasound in the Evaluation of Inguinal Hernia

Sonographically, an inguinal hernia presents as a structure of varying shape and echotexture, which moves

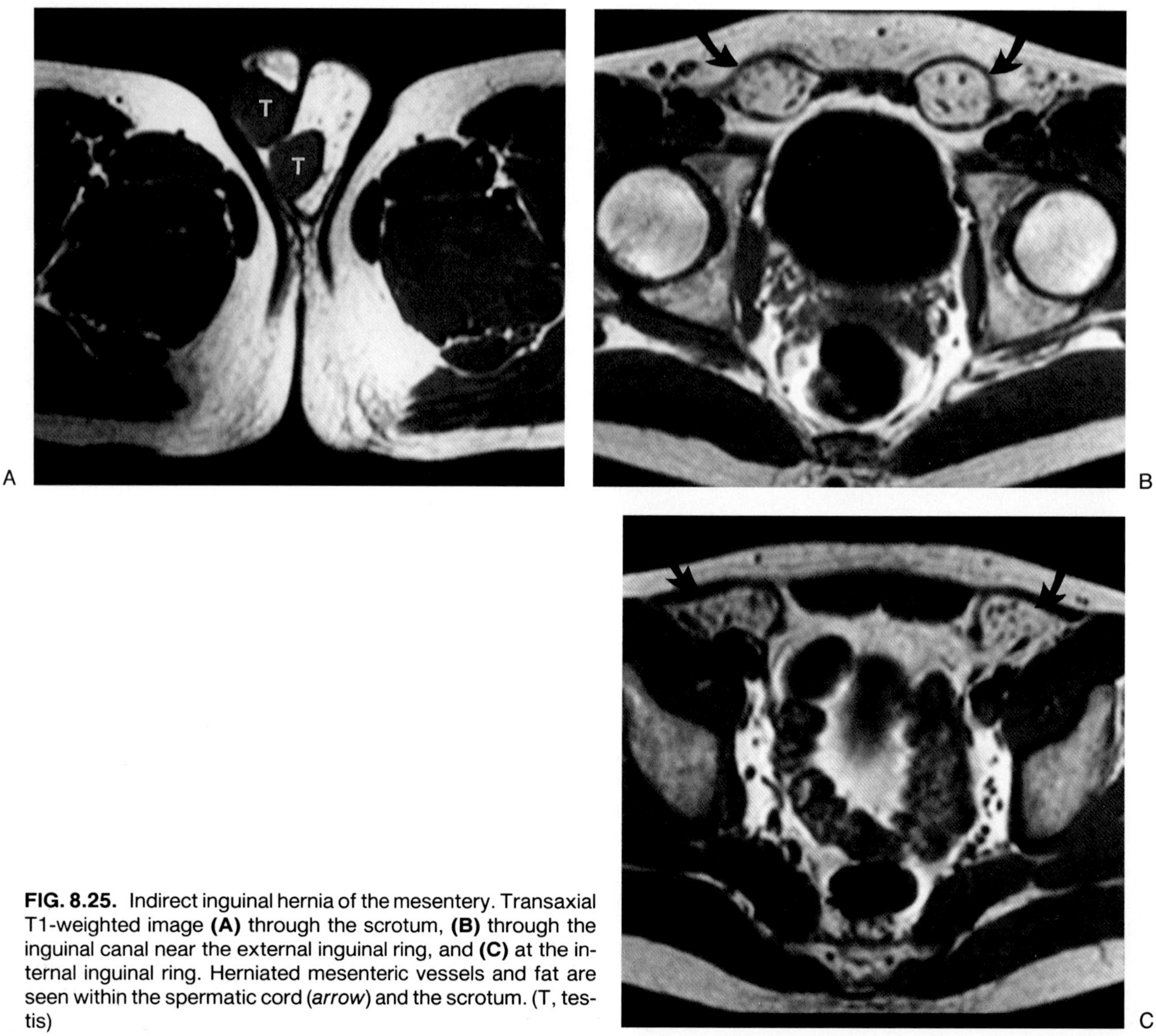

FIG. 8.25. Indirect inguinal hernia of the mesentery. Transaxial T1-weighted image **(A)** through the scrotum, **(B)** through the inguinal canal near the external inguinal ring, and **(C)** at the internal inguinal ring. Herniated mesenteric vessels and fat are seen within the spermatic cord (*arrow*) and the scrotum. (T, testis)

in the inguinal canal with breathing. In some cases the bowel loops have a garlandlike appearance (Fig. 8.23). The testis and epididymis should be delineated and retain their normal echotexture. Whereas uncomplicated inguinal or scrotal hernias usually do not represent a problem to sonographic diagnosis, an incarcerated hernia may present a challenge. Peristaltic activity in the bowel loops is diagnostic of a hernia, but in incarcerated hernia, peristalsis is only occasionally demonstrated, and that is only in early stages of incarceration. In more advanced cases of incarceration, multicystic alterations can be seen in the bowel loops resulting from edematous thickening of the walls, increasing accumulation of fluid in the lumen, and absence of peristalsis. The correct diagnosis is facilitated by the continuous visualization of the lesion in a cranial direction up into the inguinal canal.

Magnetic Resonance Imaging in the Evaluation of Inguinal Hernia

On MR scans, widening of the inguinal canal and spermatic cord (seen on sagittal, transaxial, or coronal plane images) and the contents of the hernial sac can be demonstrated. Depending on its contents, a complex mass lesion may be seen adjacent to the normal testis. Air or fluid in entrapped bowel loops (Fig. 8.24) and/or mesenteric fat (Fig. 8.25) may be recognized by typical MR signal intensity. Incarcerated hernia can be diagnosed on MRI with a high level of confidence.

Computed Tomography in the Evaluation of Inguinal Hernia

On CT examination, herniated omental fat (Fig. 8.26), bowel loops filled with air or contrast material (Fig. 8.27), or, on occasion, ascites may be seen along the course of the inguinal canal. Indirect inguinal hernias can be differentiated (on either CT or MRI) from direct inguinal and femoral hernias by their respective anatomic locations. In indirect inguinal hernias the sac is located lateral to the inferior epigastric vessels at the level of the internal inguinal ring and passes down the course of the inguinal canal anterior to the spermatic cord (or down the course of the round ligament to the labia in females) (Fig. 8.26) (44). In direct inguinal hernias, the neck is located medial to the inferior epigastric vessels at the level of the internal inguinal ring. In femoral hernias (which are more common in women) the hernia is located below and lateral to the pubic tubercle. Indirect

A B C

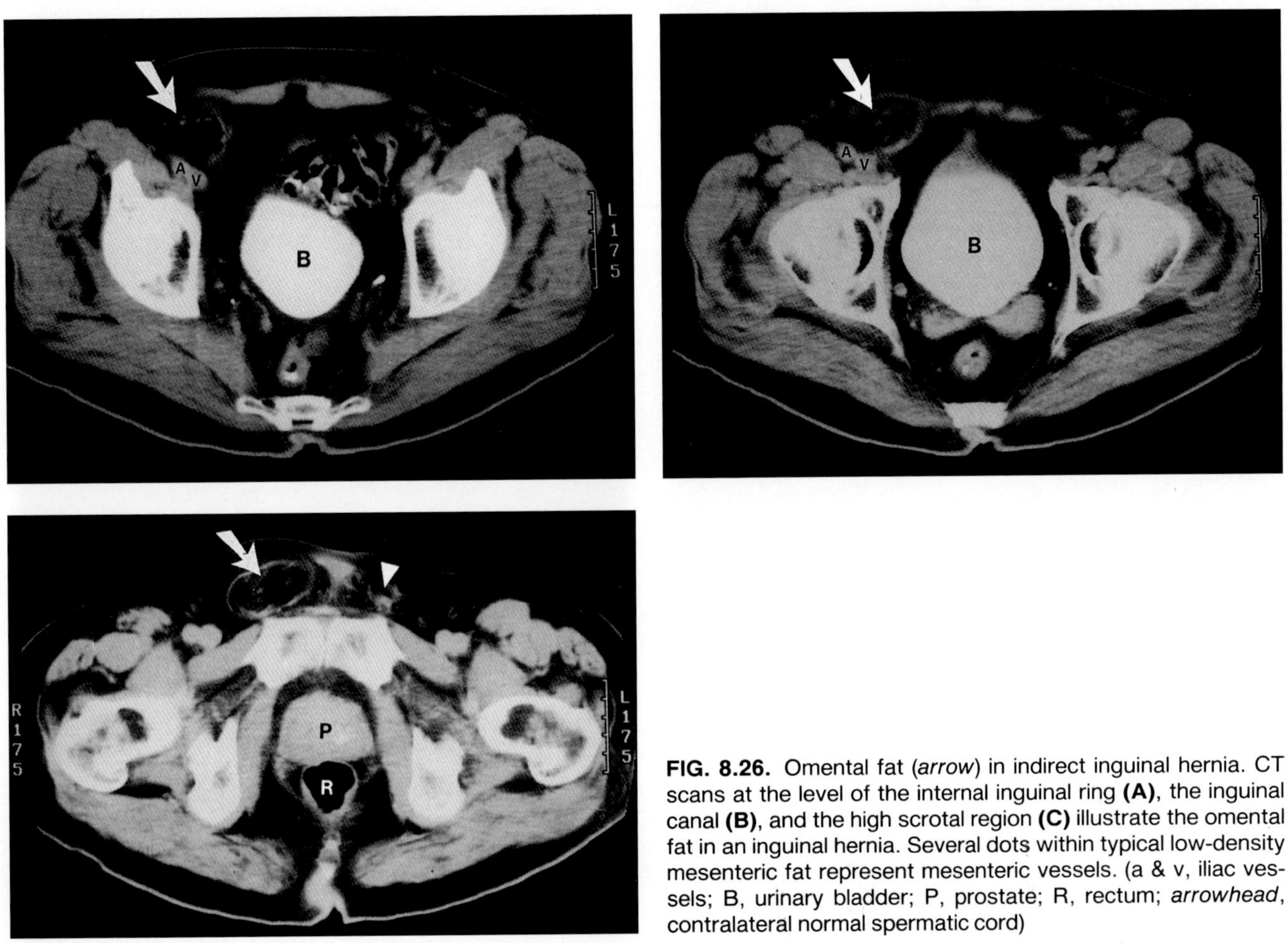

FIG. 8.26. Omental fat (*arrow*) in indirect inguinal hernia. CT scans at the level of the internal inguinal ring **(A)**, the inguinal canal **(B)**, and the high scrotal region **(C)** illustrate the omental fat in an inguinal hernia. Several dots within typical low-density mesenteric fat represent mesenteric vessels. (a & v, iliac vessels; B, urinary bladder; P, prostate; R, rectum; *arrowhead*, contralateral normal spermatic cord)

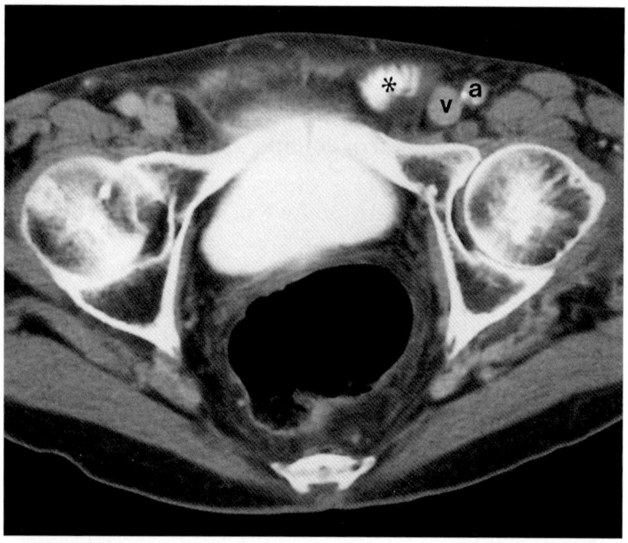

A

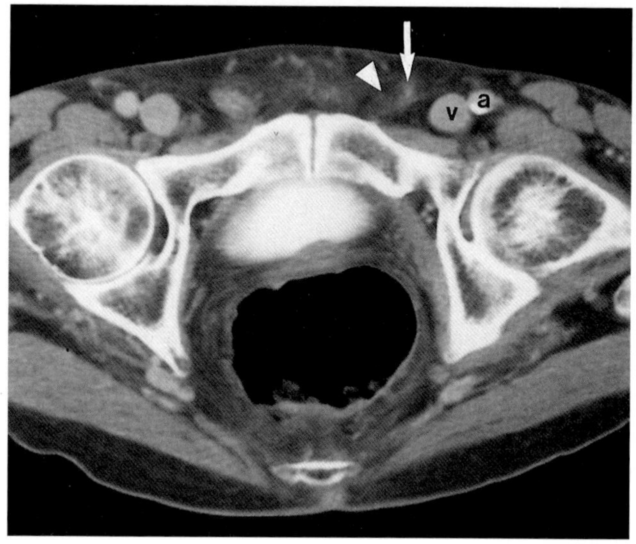

B

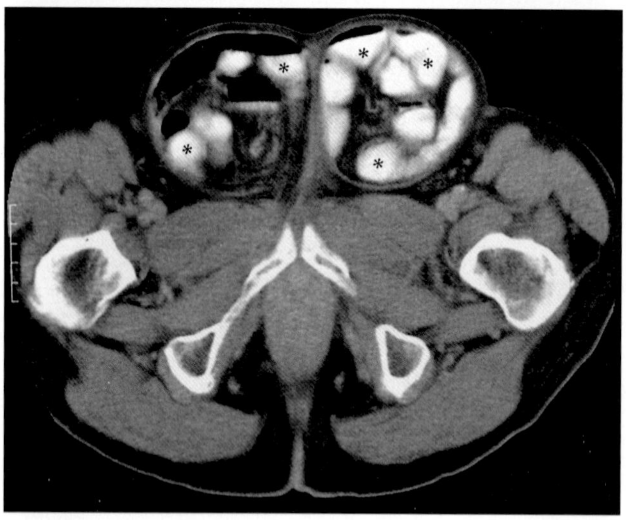

C

FIG. 8.27. **(A)** and **(B)** inguinal hernia, and **(C)** bilateral scrotal hernia. **A** and **B** are two consecutive sections below the external inguinal ring; contrast-filled bowel loop (*). The left spermatic cord (*arrow*) is displaced by herniating mesenteric fat (*arrowhead*). (a & v femoral vessels). **(C)** Bilateral scrotal hernias with multiple contrast-filled bowel loops (*).

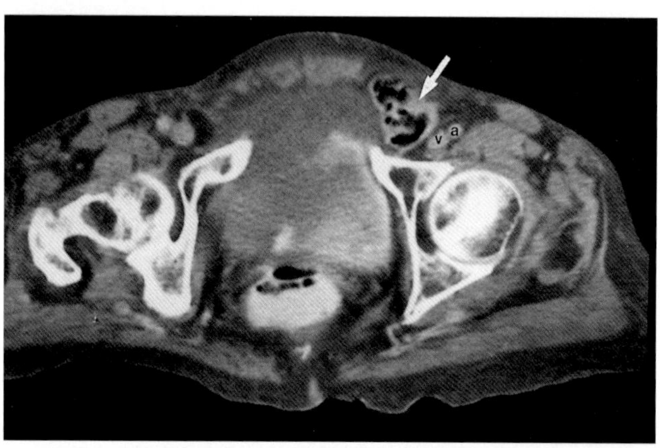

A

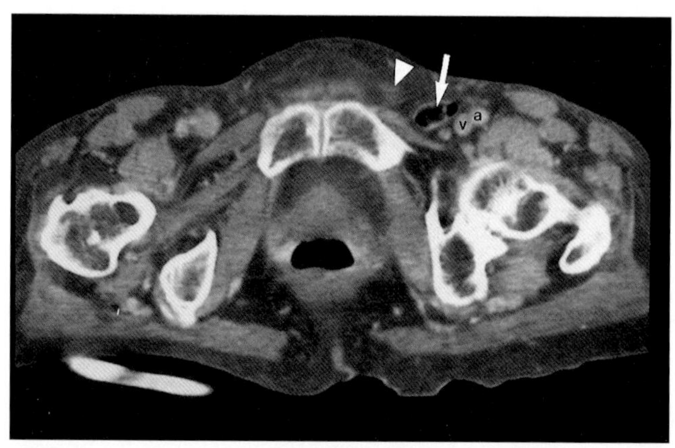

B

FIG. 8.28. Femoral hernia with gas-filled bowel loops (*arrow*) in a female patient. Two consecutive sections below the external inguinal ring **(A)** and **(B)**. Compared with the indirect inguinal hernia (see Fig. 8.27), the hernial sac is located lateral to the left round ligament of the uterus (*arrowhead*)—a female counterpart of the spermatic cord—close to the femoral vessels (a & v).

inguinal hernias lie above and medial to the tubercle (Fig. 8.28) (44). Because of excellent tissue contrast, when CT findings are combined with clinical symptoms, the diagnosis of incarcerated hernia can be achieved with high accuracy.

Comparative Evaluation of Inguinal Hernia

When physical examination is inconclusive or limited by scrotal swelling or pain, an ultrasound study should be ordered. In a large number of patients, ultrasound is the only imaging needed. In incarcerated hernia if the sonogram is limited or inconclusive, CT or MRI examination can be used. Large field of view, multiplanar imaging, and excellent soft tissue contrast rendered a higher confidence of diagnosis of hernia and its type on CT and MRI. However, MRI is still considered only a problem-solving modality. The former is often preferred because of its use of oral contrast, wide availability, and physician familiarity. Although the diagnosis of hernia often requires the use of cross-sectional imaging, the value of plain radiography should not be forgotten. The identification of air, fat, or calcification is valuable in hernia diagnosis. For example, in **meconium hernia**, which can be depicted by stippled calcifications on a radiograph (Fig. 8.29), it is sometimes difficult to make the diagnosis on US or MR examination. Therefore, the familiarity with

A 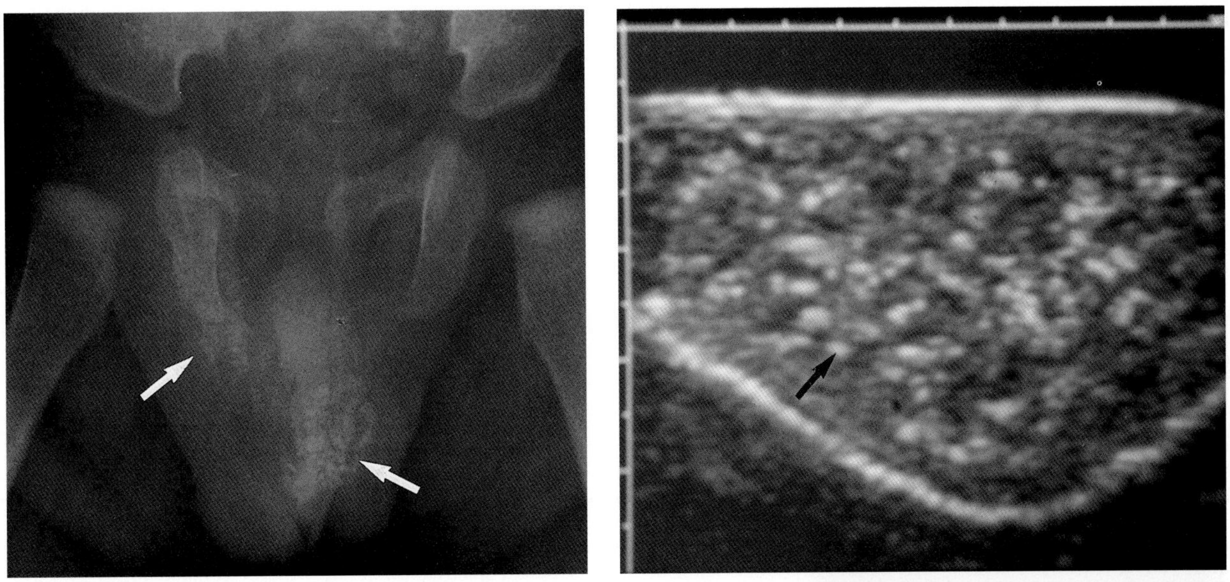 B

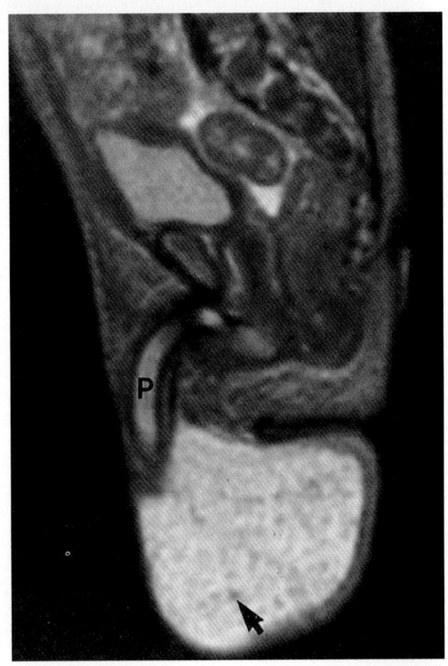

C

FIG. 8.29. Meconium hernia. **(A)** Plain radiograph, **(B)** ultrasonogram, and **(C)** sagittal T2-weighted image. Stippled calcifications (*arrows*), which are clearly seen on the radiograph, are seen as disseminated bright echos within the scrotum (*arrow*) on US and as low-intensity dots (*arrow*) on the MR image. (P, penis) imaging algorithms and the advantages and limitations of each modality with respect to clinical problems addressed is critical for successful approach.

REFERENCES

1. Scorer CG, Farrinton GH. Inguinal hernia and hydrocele in childhood. In: Scorer CG, Farrinton GH. *Congenital deformities of the testis and epididymis.* Norwalk, CT: Appleton-Century-Crofts; 1971:157–174.
2. McAninch JW. Disorders of the testis, scrotum, and spermatic cord. In: Tanagho EA, McAninch JW. *Smith's general urology,* 13th ed. Norwalk, CT: Appleton & Lange; 1992:616–624.
3. Hricak H, Filly RA. Sonography of the scrotum. *Invest Radiol* 1983;18:112–121.
4. Linkowski GD, Avellone A, Gooding GA. Scrotal calculi: sonographic detection. *Radiology* 1985;156:484.
5. Dierks PR, Moore PT. Scrotal lymphocele: a complication of renal transplant surgery. *J Ultrasound Med* 1985;4:91–92.
6. Thurnher S, Hricak H, Carroll PR, Pobiel RS, Filly RA. Imaging the testis: comparison between MR imaging and US. *Radiology* 1988;167: 631–636.
7. Baker LL, Hajek PC, Burkhard TK, et al. MR imaging of the scrotum: normal anatomy. *Radiology* 1987;163: 89–92.
8. Rholl KS, Lee JKT, Ling D, Heiken JP, Glazer HS. MR imaging of the scrotum with a high-resolution surface coil. *Radiology* 1987;163:99–103.
9. Jassie MP, Mahmood P. Torsion of spermatocele: a newly described entity with two case reports. *J Urol* 1985;133:683–684.
10. Kaye RI; Cromie WJ. Torsion of a spermatocele: a case report and review of the literature. *J Urol* 1990;143:786.
11. Kogan SJ. Acute and chronic scrotal swelling. In: Gillenwater JY, Grayhack JT, Howards SS, Duckett JW, eds. *Adult and pediatric urology.* St Louis: Mosby–Year Book; 1991:2189–2215.
12. Cooper TG, Raczek S, Yeung CH, Schwab E, Schulze H, Hertle L. Composition of fluids obtained from human epididymal cysts. *Urol Res* 1992;20:275–280.
13. Goldstein M. Surgery of male infertility and other scrotal disorders. In: Walsh PC, Retik AB, Stamey TA, Vaughan ED, eds. *Campbell's urology,* 6th ed, vol 3. Philadelphia: WB Saunders; 1992:3114–3147.
14. Eshghi M, Silver L, Smith AD. Technetium 99m scan in acute scrotal lesions. *Urology* 1987;30:586–593.
15. Burks DD, Barkey BJ, Burkhard TK, Balsara ZN, Haluszka MM, Canning DA. Suspected testicular torsion and ischemia: evaluation with color Doppler sonography. *Radiology* 1990;175:815–821.
16. Chen DC, Holder LE, Melloul M. Radionuclide scrotal imaging: further experience with 210 new patients. Part 2: Results and discussion. *J Nucl Med* 1983;24:841–853.
17. Fenner MN, Roszhart DA, Texter JH. Testicular scanning: evaluating the acute scrotum in the clinical setting. *Urology* 1991;38: 237–241.
18. Yarborough MA, Burns JR, Keller FS. Incidence and clinical significance of subclinical scrotal varicoceles. *J Urol* 1989;141:1372–1374.
19. Geatti O, Gasparini D, Shapiro B. A comparison of scintigraphy, thermography, and phlebography in grading of clinical varicocele. *J Nucl Med* 1991;32:2092–2097.
20. Basile-Fasolo C, Izzo PL, Canale D, Menchini Fabris GF. Doppler sonography, contact scrotal thermography and venography: a comparative study in evaluation of subclinical varicocele. *Int J Fertil* 1986;30:62–64.
21. Fobbe F, Hamm B, Sörensen R, Felsenberg D. Percutaneous transluminal treatment of varicoceles: where to occlude the internal spermatic vein. *AJR* 1987;149:983–987.
22. Gottlieb RH, Poster R, Subudhi MK. Computed tomographic, ultrasound, and plain film appearance of phleboliths in varicoceles. *J Ultrasound Med* 1989;8:329–331.
23. Hamm B, Fobbe F, Sörensen R, Felsenberg D. Varicoceles: combined sonography and thermography in diagnosis and posttherapeutic evaluation. *Radiology* 1986;160:419–424.
24. Gonda RL, Karo JJ, Forte RA, O'Donnell KT. Diagnosis of subclinical varicocele in infertility. *AJR* 1987;148:71–75.
25. Wolverson MK, Houttuin E, Heiberg E, Sundaram M, Gregory J. High-resolution real-time sonography of scrotal varicocele. *AJR* 1983;141:775–779.
26. McClure RD, Hricak H. Scrotal ultrasound in the infertile man: detection of subclinical unilateral and bilateral varicoceles. *J Urol* 1986;135:711–715.
27. Dhabuwala CB, Kumar AB, Kerkar PD, Bhutawala A, Pierce J. Patterns of Doppler recordings and its relationship to varicocele in infertile men. *Int J Androl* 1989;12:430–438.
28. Annoni F, Colpi GM, Marincola FM, Negri L. Doppler examination in varicocele: a standard method of evaluation. *J Androl* 1988;9:248–252.
29. Haller J, Gritzmann N, Czembirek H, et al. Fehleranalyse bildgebender Varikozelendiagnostik. *Radiologe* 1987;27:576–580.
30. Fobbe F, Heidt P , Hamm B, et al. Verbesserung der Diagnostik skrotaler Erkrankungen mit der farbkodierten Duplexsonographie. *ROFO* 1989;150:629–634.
31. Cvitanic OA, Cronan JJ, Sigman M, Landau ST. Varicoceles: postoperative prevalence—a prospective study with color Doppler US. *Radiology* 1993;187:711–714.
32. Ziffer JA, Nelson RC, Chesmar JL, et al. Subclinical varicoceles: detection with MRI. Presented at SMRI, 1989, Los Angeles, *Magn Res Imaging* 1989;7(suppl):78.
33. Freund J, Bautovich GJ: Varicocele detection by blood pool imaging. *Aust N Z J Med* 1979;9:628.
34. Freund J, Handelsman DJ, Bautovich GJ, Conway AJ, Morris JG. Detection of varicocele by radionuclide blood pool scanning. *Radiology* 1980;137:227–230.
35. Harris JD, McConnell BJ, Lipshultz LI, McConnell RW, Conoley PH. Radioisotope angiography in diagnosis of varicocele. *Urology* 1980;16:69–72.
36. Marmar JL, Zeiger LS, DeBenedictis TJ, Praiss DE. Comprehensive scrotal flow and scan technique for detection of varicoceles. *Urology* 1985;25:505–510.
37. Ramanna L, Waxman AD, Yoon J, Hyun M, Rothman C. Evaluation of scrotal varicocele with blood pool scintigraphy: correlation with contrast gonadal venography. *Clin Nucl Med* 1990;15:768.
38. Wheatley JK, Fajman WA, Witten FR. Clinical experience with the radioisotope varicocele scan as a screening method for the detection of subclinical varicoceles. *J Urol* 1982;128:57–59.
39. Rajfer J. Congenital anomalies of the testis. In: Walsh PC, Retik AB, Stamey TA, Vaughan ED, eds. *Campbell's urology,* 6th ed, vol 2. Philadelphia: WB Saunders; 1992:1543–1562.
40. Weber TR, Tracy TF. Groin hernia and hydroceles. In: Ashcraft KW, Holder TM, eds. *Pediatric surgery,* 2nd ed. Philadelphia: WB Saunders; 1993:562–570.
41. Sparkman RS. Bilateral exploration in inguinal hernia in juvenile patients. *Surgery* 1962;51:393–406.
42. Rathauser F. Historical overview of the bilateral approach to pediatric inguinal hernias. *Am J Surg* 1985;150:527–532.
43. Rowe MI, Copelson LW, Clatworthy HW. The patent processus vaginalis and the inguinal hernia. *J Pediatr Surg* 1969;4:102–107.
44. Wechsler RJ, Kurtz AB, Needleman L, et al. Cross-sectional imaging of abdominal wall hernias. *AJR* 1989;153:517–521.

CHAPTER 9

Nuclear Medicine

Eugene T. Morita, David C. Price, and Mailine H. Chew

Testicular scanning with radionuclides was first described by Nadel and colleagues (1), and these and other early studies were done with rectilinear scanners as the primary imaging device (2–4). With the advent of the Anger scintillation camera it became possible to perform an initial arterial bolus flow study (thus providing additional clinical information) and to obtain subsequent static images with greatly improved spatial resolution. Scrotal scintigraphy is still performed most effectively with Tc-99m pertechnetate and a state-of-the-art scintillation camera. The procedure can be done quickly, safely, and accurately, with low radiation exposure to the patient and with a high degree of confidence in the results.

Primary indications for radionuclide scintigraphy of the testicles include:

1. The acute scrotum (2,5–26), which may be caused by testicular torsion; epididymitis with or without orchitis; trauma; torsion of the appendices of the testis, the epididymis, the paradidymis, or the vas aberrans (20); referred groin pain (to rule out scrotal/testicular disease (5,27–31)), which may result from hernia (5), renal colic (32), appendicitis with secondary infection of the scrotum (27,31), or hip pain (29); and torsion of the undescended testis (33–35).
2. Varicoceles (2,36–45).
3. Assessment of testicular viability following surgery (46–49).

Additional miscellaneous reasons for testicular nuclear medicine studies include:

1. Reflux of urine into the vas deferens (10) (M. McBiles personal communication).
2. Tumors—either painless or painful (tumor necrosis and torsion).
3. Lymphoscintigraphy (see section on testicular tumors).
4. Monoclonal antibodies (see section on testicular tumors).

TECHNIQUES OF EXAMINATION

Radiopharmaceuticals

Technetium-99m (Tc-99m) pertechnetate is usually used for testicular scintigraphy. The injected dose is 20 millicuries (mCi) or 740 MBq for adults and is scaled down by weight in children (0.29 mCi/kg or 10.6 MBq/kg, with a minimum injected dose of 2 mCi [74 MBq]). Although adjusting the dose using body surface area provides a more accurate exposed radiation dose in small children, scaling by weight is mathematically much simpler.

Technetium-99m diethylenetriamine penta-acetic acid (Tc-99m DTPA) is preferred by some because the rapid renal clearance of this compound results in the patient experiencing lower radiation exposure (32). In vivo or in vitro Tc-99m-labeled autologous red blood cells may also be used, since the study is primarily one of tissue blood flow and vascularity. Because Tc-99m pertechnetate is trapped by the thyroid, patients are sometimes pretreated with 400 mg of perchlorate to reduce the thyroid radiation dose. However, the thyroid radiation dose from Tc-99m pertechnetate is quite low (51) (Table 9.1), and perchlorate pretreatment is generally not considered necessary. Use of Tc-99M-labeled autologous red blood cells is preferred for evaluation of varicoceles; the dosage is 20 mCi (740 MBq). A commercial kit for the preparation of red blood cells is now available, and in vivo tagging of red cells using preinjection of stannous pyrophosphate is no longer considered preferable. Gallium-67 citrate is very effective for the study of testicular malignancies; the dosage is 4 to 8 mCi (148 to 296 MBq), and images are obtained 24 or 48 hours after injection. Both

TABLE 9.1. ^{99m}Tc radiation dosimetry

Age of patient	1 year (rads/mCi)	1 year (mGy/MBq)	5 years (rads/mCi)	5 years (mGy/MBq)	10 years (rads/mCi)	10 years (mGy/MBq)	15 years (rads/mCi)	15 years (mGy/MBq)	Adult (rads/mCi)	Adult (mGy/MBq)
Upper large intestine	1.443	(0.39)	0.777	(0.21)	0.481	(0.13)	0.285	(0.077)	0.229	(0.062)
Thyroid	0.851	(0.23)	0.444	(0.12)	0.207	(0.056)	0.137	(0.037)	0.085	(0.023)
Testes	0.063	(0.017)	0.034	(0.0093)	0.022	(0.0059)	0.014	(0.0037)	0.010	(0.0027)
Red marrow	0.074	(0.020)	0.048	(0.013)	0.036	(0.0098)	0.026	(0.0071)	0.023	(0.0061)
Whole body	0.063	(0.017)	0.034	(0.0093)	0.022	(0.0060)	0.015	(0.0040)	0.013	(0.0034)

Data derived from Ref. 51.

indium-111 (In-111)– and Tc-99m-hexamethylpropyleneamineoxime (Tc-99m-HMPAO)–labeled white blood cells are used for evaluating acute inflammatory processes. In-111–labeled autologous white blood cells have been used to study patients with epididymitis (52); the usual dose is 500 μCi (18.5 MBq) (9). With Tc-99m-HMPAO–labeled white blood cells (dose 5–10 mCi [185 to 370 MBq]), flow as well as static images can be obtained (53). Another advantage of using technetium is the ability to study patients within 2 to 3 hours after injection. Two minicolloids, Tc-99m hydrogen sulfide sulfur colloid and Tc-99m antimony sulfide colloid, have been used to evaluate lymphatic drainage and regional lymph nodes following interstitial injection of 1 mCi (37 MBq) per injection site.

Equipment

For optimum spatial resolution and sensitivity, testicular scintigraphy should be performed with a state-of-the-art Anger scintillation camera. A computer interface is advantageous in case repeat photography or reformatting of the flow images at different time intervals is necessary for accurate interpretation (most likely to be needed when proper intensities have not been set on the photorecording device; discussed later). The study can be performed using either a low-energy all-purpose (LEAP) collimator, frequently optimized by electronic magnification of the image (mag., 1.2 to 1.5), or a converging collimator, which has the advantages of image magnification as well as greater sensitivity. When using the converging collimator it is essential that the camera head be centered exactly over the scrotum since geometric distortion can occur at the periphery of the collimator field. In very young patients, a pinhole collimator may be used after the flow study, to further magnify the image of the small testicles in this age group (54).

Patient Procedure

Acute Scrotum

The patient with acute scrotal pain is usually studied in the supine position with the legs abducted. The penis is taped suprapubically, or may be held cephalad in the midline by the patient if he is cooperative and able to keep his hand away from the area of interest. The scrotum is supported with a sling constructed to bring the contents forward as close as possible to the camera. An alternative is to support the scrotum with folded towels. The median raphe of the scrotum is positioned perpendicular to the gamma camera so both testes can be visualized without distortion in the anterior projection. Because the scrotum may be distorted by inflammation, paper tape may be used for positioning. The position should be checked to assure that all the areas of interest are in the camera's field of view (50).

Because the flow sequence is critical in analyzing the study, it is important to recheck all technical settings before injecting the tracer bolus. An incorrect setting may result in nondiagnostic images. A thin lead strip absorber placed over the median raphe prior to the start of the study can be helpful for marking the midline in the images.

Older scintillation cameras (analogue systems) take images and place them directly onto film. With these cameras, all the technical parameters—the isotope and energy settings, the image orientation and film intensities, and the patient position—must be correct before the study begins. Most systems are now interfaced with computers, which permit data to be stored for later analysis. Computers also provide an opportunity to improve the quality of the flow images by adding frames in the dynamic portion of the study (e.g., by acquiring 1 second frames and then adding groups to display the flow in 3- or 5-second intervals).

The flow study takes about 1 minute and the static study from 10 to 20 minutes to complete. The usual framing rate for the flow study is 3 to 5 seconds a frame following acquisition in 1-second frames, as mentioned earlier. Computer image storage enables reformatting and variable playback for optimum visual analysis. Flow curves can also be generated and analyzed (55). Static images should be acquired for 500,000 to 1,000,000 total counts. Placing a lead shield under the scrotum reduces background thigh activity and may thereby provide improved contrast. However, the lead shield can also produce distortion, making interpretation more complex (8,14,50).

The nuclear medicine physician should be present while the study is being performed. Appropriate physical assessment of the patient is necessary to place scrotal markers accurately, ensuring anatomic delineation of the areas of interest on the images.

Varicocele

In patients with varicoceles the technique described previously is somewhat modified (39,40,42). These patients are usually studied in the standing position facing the camera with their legs spread apart (some clinicians have found the supine position to be acceptable) (43). The radiopharmaceutical used in this case is Tc-99m-labeled autologous red blood cells. One technique is to perform the flow and initial static images in the supine position, followed by a static image in the standing position. Sometimes a further image during a Valsalva maneuver is beneficial (42).

In summary, careful positioning of the patient, appropriate camera and computer settings, sufficient counting statistics, and accurate determination of external landmarks are all important in obtaining high-quality diagnostic images.

RADIATION DOSIMETRY

The International Commission on Radiological Protection (ICRP) statistics on the dosimetry of Tc-99m pertechnetate to various organs and to the whole body (thyroid unblocked) are summarized in Table 9.1 (51). For example, the radiation exposure to a 15-year-old boy weighing 50 kg who received 11 mCi (407 MBq) Tc-99m pertechnetate is 3.1 rads (31 mGy) to the upper large intestinal wall, 1.5 rads (15 mGy) to the unblocked thyroid, 286 millirads (mrads) (2.9 mGy) to the red bone marrow, and 154 mrads (1.5 mGy) to the testes.

NORMAL ANATOMY

Because of the extremely low data density in 2-second scintigraphic flow images, no vascular flow pattern is normally seen in the spermatic cords (Fig. 9.1). Occa-

A

B

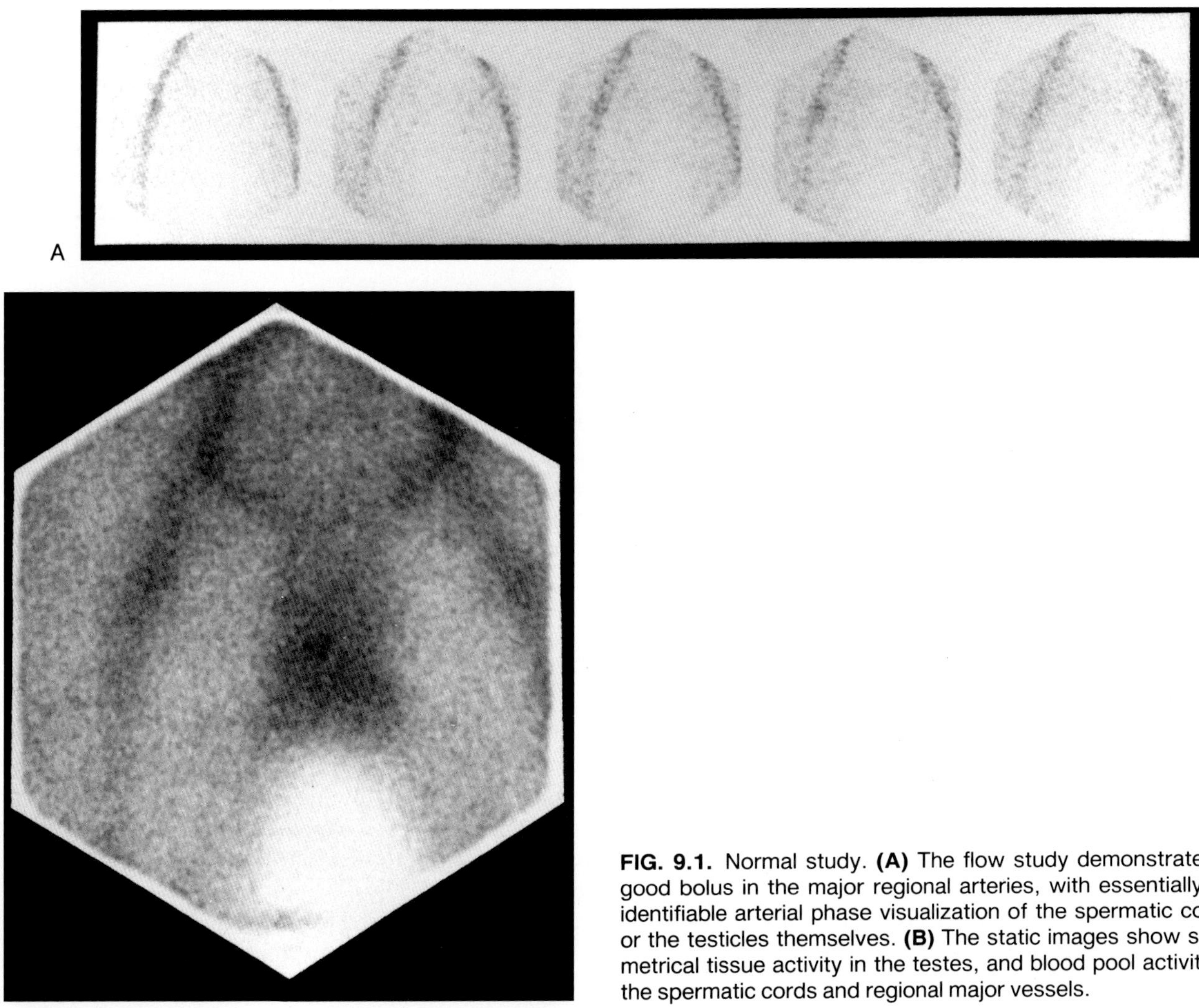

FIG. 9.1. Normal study. **(A)** The flow study demonstrates a good bolus in the major regional arteries, with essentially no identifiable arterial phase visualization of the spermatic cords or the testicles themselves. **(B)** The static images show symmetrical tissue activity in the testes, and blood pool activity in the spermatic cords and regional major vessels.

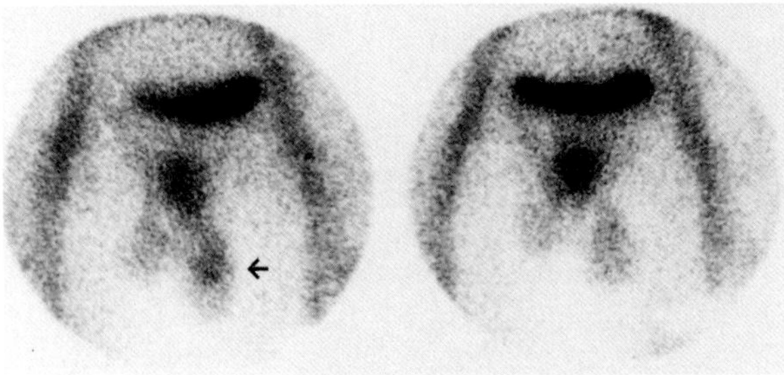

FIG. 9.2. Artifact. The static image on the left shows increased activity in the region of the left testicle (*arrow*). The image on the right shows normal testicular activity after the penis has been moved from its position overlying the left testicle and placed superiorly in the midline.

sionally, however, minimally visualized symmetrical perfusion may be seen. Summation of the flow study into a single arterial image may help define spermatic cord vascularity.

Static images often show a "hot" area around the base of the penis, which can mistakenly be interpreted as a focus of hypervascularity. An area of lucency around the "hot" spot may also be seen (13). Later images show bladder activity from renal clearance of the Tc-99m pertechnetate. Normal diffuse testicular activity is greater than thigh activity and increases with time. Testicular activity should be symmetrical, although asymmetric activity may be seen if one testis is smaller than the other.

Artifacts

The penis must be positioned away from (above) the testicles since it will confuse interpretation of the results (Fig. 9.2). In addition, coins, keys, and so on, can also result in a "cold" artifact. We routinely have the patient remove all clothes from the waist down. Checking for motion artifacts should be a routine part of the quality control of images.

THE ACUTE SCROTUM

Testicular Torsion

Anatomic Considerations

The testicle is supplied by three separate arterial vessels, the testicular, deferential, and cremasteric arteries. These vessels all merge in the spermatic cord. The scrotum is supplied by the internal and external pudendal arteries, which travel outside the cord. There is no significant collateral circulation between these two separate blood supplies (8,13,50).

Types of Torsion

There are two types of torsion of the testis (18,21). The first type, which is very uncommon, is outside the tunica vaginalis and occurs almost exclusively in newborns, before the testicle has had a chance to mature and become a more compact structure (7). It is thought that this type of torsion occurs in utero and often is present as a mass in the groin (56). The testicle is almost always necrotic. Because it is not associated with a congenital anomaly, orchiopexy is usually not necessary (19). The second and more common type of torsion is within the tunica vaginalis. As described in Chapter 1, the tunica vaginalis is an extension of the peritoneal cavity that embryologically invaginates into the scrotum to create the scrotal sac. Normally it separates from the peritoneal cavity, and both the testis and the gubernaculum descend into the scrotal sac. The testis and the epididymis adhere closely to one another and are connected to the posterolateral aspect of the scrotum by the broad and short mesorchium, so that the testis cannot rotate. Two additional structures fix the testis to the scrotum—the gubernaculum, which fixes the testis to the floor of the scrotum, and the parietal peritoneum of the tunica vaginalis, which covers the epididymis (14). Sometimes enlargement and extension of the tunica vaginalis envelop the testis and epididymis, creating a **"bell clapper" anomaly**, predisposing the testis and epididymis to torsion. A second type of congenital anomaly occurs when the testis and the epididymis are separated by an elongated mesorchium. In this situation torsion occurs because the testis can rotate around the mesorchium.

Diagnosis and Clinical Presentation

The diagnosis of testicular torsion is one of the most important made in the clinical setting of the acute scrotum because testicular viability is at risk. If the torsed testicle is detorsed within 2 hours, function will almost always be preserved. Significant salvage still occurs when diagnosis and repair occur between 2 and 4 hours. By 12 to 24 hours after the onset of symptoms, however, only 20% salvage is possible. After 24 hours, although testicular salvage can still occur, loss of function is generally the rule (7,57). The degree of torsion of the testicle is a modifying factor in the viability of the testis. Three twists of the cord result in loss of function in a few hours, whereas partial torsion may give longer viability (58). It is interesting to note that Leydig cells (involved in testosterone secretion) are more resistant to ischemia than the seminiferous tubules (involved in sperm production) (57).

Diagnosis of torsion of the testicle on clinical grounds is difficult and is made only about 50% of the time. Torsion appears to be related to adolescence, deep sleep, physical exertion, sexual activity, and, occasionally, trauma (58). In the series by Chen and colleagues (8,50), torsion was found to occur most frequently in boys and young men 11 to 20 years of age, followed by men 21 to 30 years of age. More commonly, the two groups with increased frequency of torsion are neonates and prepubertal and pubertal boys (6,7). An increase in testicular size probably accounts for the increased likelihood of torsion during adolescence (59).

A history of acute onset of testicular pain, or a history of such pain, and the physical findings of loss of the ipsilateral cremasteric reflex, palpable twist of the cord, abnormal elevation, and alteration of the axis of the involved as well as the contralateral testicle may be sufficient cause to perform surgery (10,60). Another important finding is referred pain to the abdomen from torsion of the testis (60). The physical finding of a negative **Prehn's sign** (pain relieved on raising a torsed testicle) is not considered reliable in the clinical diagnosis of torsion (10). Fenner and colleagues (61) considered clinical assessment to be the most important diagnostic factor and imaging an adjunctive procedure to be used when the clinical findings are equivocal. Cass and colleagues (58) advocate immediate operation on young males with testicular pain. Although they achieve significant salvage with this protocol, a significant number of patients in their study proved to have epididymitis and did not require surgery. Because of its high predictive value, nuclear scintigraphy plays an important role in the diagnosis of the acutely torsed testicle and in identifying patients who do not, in fact, require operations (24). Nuclear scintigraphy should be available 24 hours a day and be performed within 1 hour of the request.

Scintigraphic Findings (Table 9.2)

In the first 7 hours, the early phase of testicular torsion, flow studies show normal or reduced vascularity in the spermatic cord, failure to visualize vascularity in the pudendal vessels, and markedly decreased activity in the scrotum, both in the flow and the static images (Fig. 9.3). From 4 to 7 hours, the end of the early phase, the spermatic cord flow may be normal or a **"nubbin" sign** (pathognomonic for acute torsion) may be seen (11). The peripheral scrotal component of the flow study remains normal at this time, but the involved testis demonstrates absent activity in the static image. From 7 to 24 hours, the middle phase of acute torsion, cord activity is normal or again may show a nubbin sign. At this stage there is increased activity in the scrotum and pudendal vascular activity increases. Static images begin to show a "rim" of scrotal activity. After 24 hours, the late phase or "missed torsion," the rim sign is quite intense (Fig. 9.4), but gradually fades as the testicle undergoes necrosis and atrophy (62). At this very late stage scintigraphy may even become normal. The **rim sign** is the hyperemic response of the dartos of the scrotum to the ischemia of torsion. If the rim shows greater activity than the femoral vessels, the testicle is considered unsalvageable. A rim equal in intensity to the femoral vessels also indicates a low likelihood of ultimate testicular survival (8). A complicating necrotic abscess may also occur at this time. Other conditions may mimic the rim sign, an appearance usually produced by central areas of decreased activity but without a true hyperemic rim. Such false-positive rim signs may be caused by tumors with central necrosis, abscesses, hydroceles with epididymitis, and hernias (28,44,63–66).

Other pitfalls in evaluating the acute scrotum for torsion include bilateral symmetrical torsion, bilateral epididymo-orchitis, epididymo-orchitis with abscess, and unilateral testicular atrophy (67). A particularly vexing problem is the detorsed testicle, since it can appear perfectly normal on scan yet remain at high risk for torsion again in the future (68). Because of this risk, such normal scans are considered false negatives when evaluating the sensitivity and specificity of testicular scintigraphy for torsion (Table 9.3). In the clinical setting, a decrease in or disappearance of testicular pain may indicate spontaneous detorsion. Scintigraphy in such situations may show decreased, normal, or increased scrotal activity (14). Although Doppler ultrasound may be helpful in this situation (69,70), it is not always diagnostic for detorsion (71). In the presence of a large hydrocele, nuclear scans show a large central negative defect, further complicating the interpretation. The use of a lead shield as

TABLE 9.2. *Testicular scintigraphic findings in torsion*[a]

Scan	0–7 hours	7–24 hours	Late	Torsion followed by detorsion
Flow: spermatic cord	N, or nubbin	N, or nubbin	N, or nubbin	Decrease, N, or increase
Flow: pudendal vessels	N	Min increase	Min to mod increase	N
Flow: scrotum	Decrease	Min rim	Marked rim	Decrease, N, or increase
Static: scrotum	Decrease	Decrease in center, early increased rim	Marked rim, cold center	Decrease, N, or increase

[a] N, normal pattern. Flow is symmetric, usually nonvisualized; static is symmetric, equal to other soft tissues.

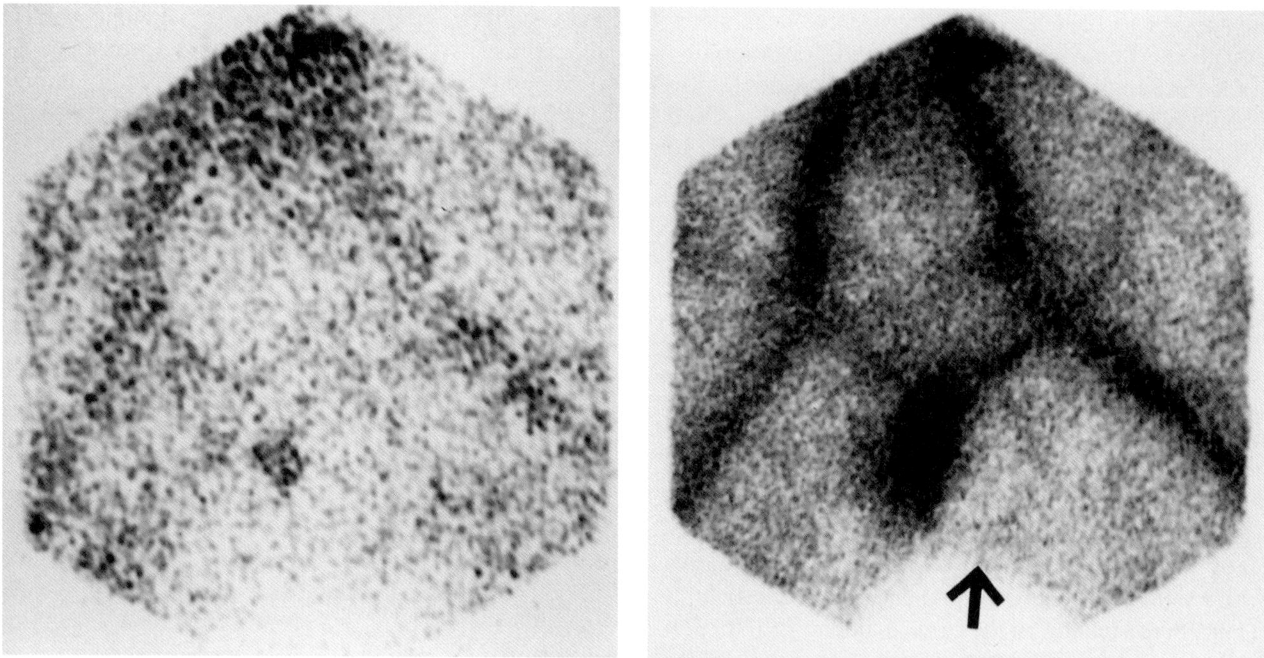

A B

FIG. 9.3. Early torsion of the testis. **(A)** The flow study shows slightly decreased perfusion to the involved left side, particularly notable in the left spermatic cord. The localized midline focus of vascular activity is increased at the base of the penis, a common normal finding that should not be misinterpreted as increased scrotal vascularity. **(B)** The static image shows markedly decreased activity in the left scrotum (*arrow*). At surgery, an acute torsion of the left testicle was found.

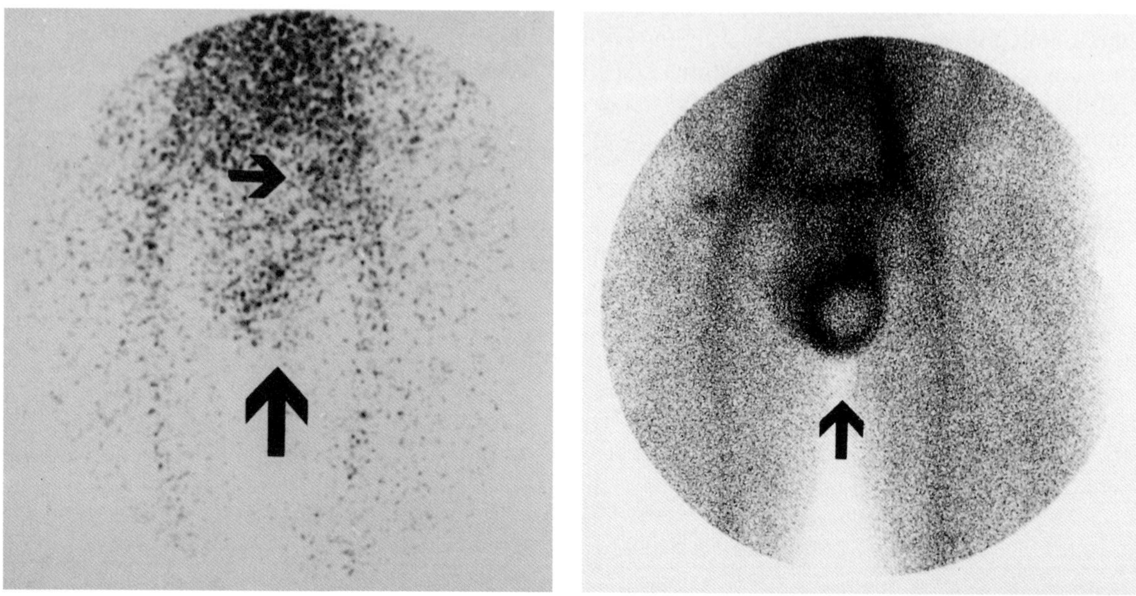

A B

FIG. 9.4. Missed torsion. **(A)** The flow study demonstrates a "nubbin" sign (*arrow*). Moderately increased perfusion is noted around the hyperemic dartos of the left testicle (*small closed arrow*). The larger closed arrow marks the right side of the patient. **(B)** The static images show markedly increased uptake around the left testicle (*arrow*).

TABLE 9.3. *Sensitivity of testicular scintigraphy for torsion*

Reference	Year	Number of patients	Sensitivity: Acute torsion	Sensitivity: Missed torsion	False positives	Comments
Hahn (2)	1975	28	3/3		1	Rectilinear; 1 hydrocele (FP)
Mukerjee (3)	1975	28	1/1			Rectilinear
Riley (4)	1976	98	24/25		2	Rectilinear
Hitch (78)	1976	21	7/8			1 Spontaneous detorsion (FN)
Holder (79)	1977	74	9/9	3/3		
Boedecker (80)	1979	32	6/6			
Abu-Sleiman (5)	1979	43	11/13		4	3 Hydroceles and 1 hernia (FP); 2 described as torsion (FN)
Orovan (73)	1979	34	5/8			
Falkowski (81)	1980	18	4/4			
Wasnick (82)	1980	34	5/5	6/6		
Tanaka (23)	1981	410	48/50		6	Specificity for torsion: 98% (354/360)
Bailey (83)	1981	16	6/6		2	1 Abscess (FP)
Stage (84)	1981	72	13/14		1	1 Hernia (FP)
Dunn (85)	1981	9		9/9		
Valvo (86)	1982	46	6/6	12/12		
Chen (50)	1983	246	19/19	16/16	1	1 Hydrocele (FP)
Blacklock (87)	1983	33	3/3			
Thomas (55)	1983	80	7/7	9/9	3	3 Testicular tumors (FP)
Wise (88)	1983	42	10/10	0/1	1	1 Hematocele (FP); 1 described as acute epididymitis (FN)
Nakielny (89)	1984	106	4/7			1 Normal, 2 spontaneous detorsion (FN)
Golimbu (90)	1985	62	11/11			
Mendel (91)	1985	75	3/5	12/13		2 Incomplete torsion (FN); 1 4-day-old infant (FN) (missed)
Dunn (67)	1986	57	12/13	15/15	2	1 Bilateral epididymitis plus unilateral hydrocele (FP); 1 abscess (FP)
Chen (92)	1986	52	1/1	4/4		
Eshghi (47)	1987	155	11/11			
Mueller (93)	1988	43	5/7		3	2 Spontaneous detorsion (FN); 3 hydroceles (FP)
Burks (94)	1990	17	1/1	2/2		
Middleton (70)	1990	28	4/5	2/2	1	1 Partial torsion (FN)
van Ahlen (95)	1991	108	23/23	14/14		
Fenner (61)	1991	44	11/11			
Atkinson (96)	1992	23	2/2	4/4		
Totals		2134	275/294 (93.5%)	108/110 (98.1%)	27	

FN, false negative; FP, false positive.

well as longer image times for higher total count acquisition may show a vaguely defined viable testicle medially in the central cold area (14).

Repeat imaging with the same dose can be helpful in evaluating postmanipulative viability following manual detorsion of the testis (72). Successful manual detorsion confirmed by scan is useful because it provides relief of the acute problem and permits corrective surgery on a less urgent basis.

Epididymitis

Patients with acute epididymitis are likely to wait longer before seeking help than those with acute torsion. In these patients testicular pain is frequently accompanied by dysuria, pyuria, and fever. Epididymitis can be classified into three types: nonspecific, specific, and traumatic. Nonspecific cases are the most common, and frequently the causative organism is not found or not looked for. Causes include gonorrhea, syphilis, tuberculosis, *H. influenzae*, or fungi. Epididymitis can occur following instrumentation of the genitourinary tract or may occur as a result of minimal trauma that reactivates a dormant infection (23). For the most part, patients are postpubertal. In this age group, 80% of patients with an acute scrotum have epididymitis and only 15% have torsion (58). Epididymitis is distinctly uncommon in young boys and may occur with orchitis. Acute torsion may mimic the findings of epididymitis, and the separation of these two entities is important because torsion is an operative emergency, whereas epididymitis is almost invariably managed medically. In epididymitis the flow study shows augmented flow through the cord and hyperemia to the area of the epididymis (Fig. 9.5). The activity may extend inferiorly and can involve the testis.

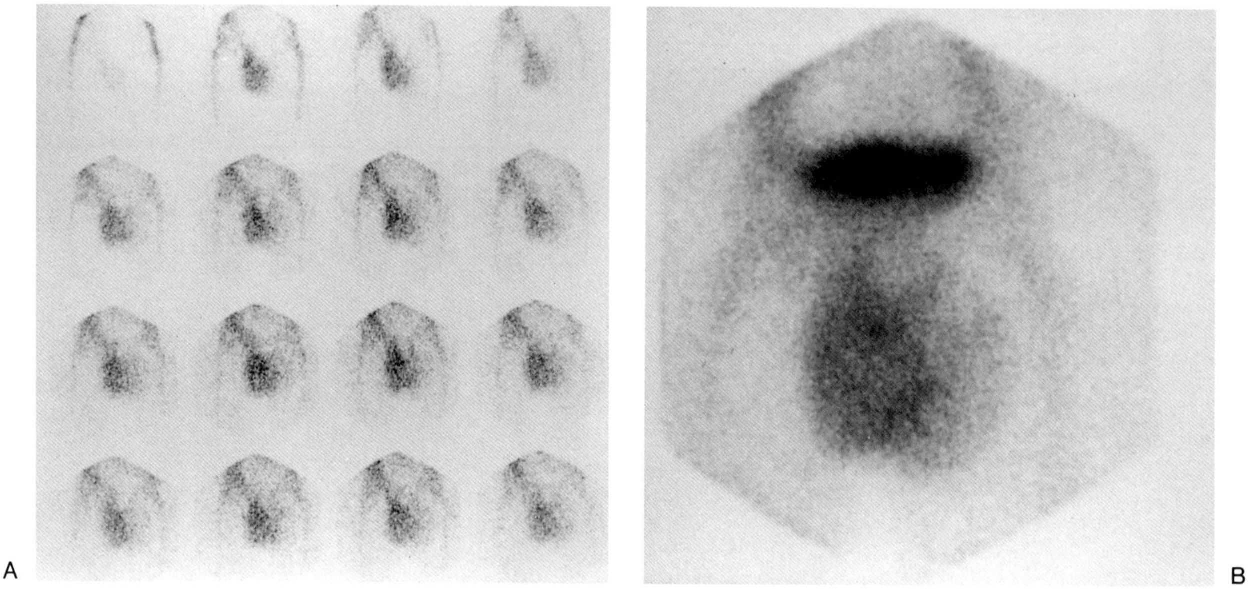

FIG. 9.5. Epididymo-orchitis. **(A)** The flow study shows marked increase in perfusion of the right spermatic cord, epididymis, and testicle. **(B)** The postflow static image demonstrates diffusely increased activity throughout the right epididymis and testis.

With epididymitis there may be an associated reactive hydrocele with a semilunar shape that is generally diagnostic (5,50,74). When large enough, the hydrocele may appear as a torsed testicle (50,67). In addition to orchitis, abscess formation may develop, in which case the scan pattern shows a "cold" defect. Testicular infarction, related to compression of the cord by inflammation, may also complicate epididymitis (73–76). Abscess formation and/or torsion should be considered when the patient shows no improvement on antibiotics. The sudden onset of increased pain, a history of epididymitis, and thickening of the cord may be indicators of progression to abscess formation and/or infarction of the testis (74). In one scintigraphy series, Vordermark and colleagues (24) found five patients who demonstrated hydroceles, with the smallest being 1 cm in diameter. Testicular scintigraphy can be quite helpful in the diagnosis of epididymitis and its complications.

Torsion of Appendices

As mentioned earlier, the acute scrotum may also be caused by torsion of the appendices of the testicle, the epididymis, the paradidymis, or the vas aberrans. Torsion of the testicular appendices occurs in about 5% of patients with an acute scrotum. In the pediatric age group, however, the incidence is 20% to 40% in the setting of an acute scrotum (6,23,60). Accurate diagnosis of torsion of the appendices depends on differentiation of testicular torsion from appendiceal torsion, since patients with torsion of the appendices may have symptoms sufficiently intense to suggest an acute testicular torsion. Of the four appendices, the most frequently torsed is the appendix of the testis, followed by the appendix of the epididymis. Torsion of the appendices of the paradidymis or the vas aberrans occurs rarely (10). Testicular scintigraphy may show augmented flow and a focal area of increased activity on the static images. However, the study is frequently normal.

Scrotal Trauma

Trauma to the scrotum may result in infarction of the testis or epididymis, or in testicular torsion. Trauma usually results from direct testicular trauma (e.g., a kick to the scrotum) or from straddle injuries (77). A hematocele can be seen as a semilunar cold defect. Hematomas of the testis also produce a cold defect on static images, but the defect is somewhat irregular along its border. Flow is usually augmented through the cord. If the flow study is done while there is bleeding, extravasation into the scrotum can occur (77). Testicular ischemia may result from trauma (14). Most studies indicate that early surgical intervention is important in trauma, and testicular scintigraphy can play an important role in evaluating this group of patients (77).

Referred Groin Pain

Acute and subacute pain in the scrotum may be related to pathology outside the scrotum. Acute renal colic may cause referred testicular pain, and there is one report of hydronephrosis diagnosed on a testicular study (32). In a patient presenting with hip pain, acute epididymitis was found on the flow study of a three-phase bone scan of the hips (29). Hernias through the inguinal canal may also mimic late torsion. Abscesses associated with acute appendicitis have been reported to enter the scrotum via a patent tunica vaginalis (27,30). Testicular pain on urination can be related to reflux of urine into the vas deferens, considered a predisposing factor for epididymitis (normally, reflux is prevented by the oblique angle at which the vas deferens enters the prostate (10). M. McBiles has studied a patient in whom reflux of urine into the vas deferens on voiding was documented by scintigraphy (personal communication).

Torsion of the Undescended Testis

Torsion of the undescended testis can be extremely difficult to diagnose. Clinical assessment is critical in determining the cause of inguinal pain in these patients. The finding of an absent testicle in the scrotum on physical examination is very helpful. If the undescended testicle is in the retroperitoneum, diagnosis by scintigraphy is impossible. The incidence of an undescended testicle is higher in premature than in full-term infants. The incidence of testicular torsion in the undescended testicle ranges from 7% to 13% (33,35). Of three case reports of the diagnosis of torsion of an undescended testicle by scintigraphy, two cases were accurately diagnosed and one was missed (33–35). The use of pinhole and converging collimators can be helpful in visualizing torsion. A torsed redux testicle (one that retracts into the canal) has also been found by scintigraphy (34). The possibility of a torsed undescended testicle should be suspected when no testicle is found in the scrotum and a painful mass is present in the groin.

Review of the Literature on Acute Scrotum

A review of 32 papers that contain patient data referable to testicular torsion (Table 9.3) (2–5,20,23,47, 50,55,61,67,73,78–96) and epididymitis (Table 9.4) (2–5,23,24,47,50,55,61,67,70,73,78–84,86–97) summarizes data from more than 2,000 patient studies. In acute torsion, the sensitivity of radionuclide scintigraphy was 93.5% (294 patients), and in delayed torsion it was 98.1% (110 patients) (Table 9.3). False negatives were usually the result of spontaneous detorsion (70,78,91,97), very small testicles (in neonates or young boys), or—occasionally—epididymitis (5,88). As mentioned earlier, detorsions are classified as false negatives (in Table 9.3) because of the high likelihood of recurrence and frequent association with the developmental "bell clapper" abnormality in the contralateral testicle. False negatives for torsion may also be due to epididymitis, but these result in an operative procedure that excludes acute torsion, resulting in relatively little harm. False-positive studies for torsion were due to large hydroceles, hernias, abscesses, hematoceles, bilateral epididymitis with a hydrocele, and tumors (5,50,55,67,83,84,88). Although a true figure for specificity is not easy to extract from many of the published series, Tanaka and colleagues (23), in one of the largest series, found a specificity of 98.3% (354 of 360 cases).

The sensitivity of radionuclide scintigraphy for epididymitis was 96.3% (948 patients) (Table 9.4). Among patients with surgical confirmation of epididymitis, usually operated on for suspected torsion or abscess, there were few false negatives. Most of the false negatives were the result of mild epididymitis without scintigraphic abnormality (78,97). Other causes of false negatives include torsed appendix, testicular torsion diagnosed on scintigraphy as epididymitis with hydrocele, and testicular abscess (73,80,83). False positives were usually a result of misinterpretation of testicular torsion, epididymitis, varicocele, inflammatory tumor, or postoperative changes (5,67,88).

Radionuclide Scintigraphy in Relation to Other Modalities

Early studies using B-mode ultrasound and Doppler showed poor clinical correlation, and ultrasound was not initially recommended as a diagnostic tool in the acute scrotum (86,87). Recently, however, the introduction of color and duplex Doppler ultrasound has significantly improved diagnostic imaging in the acute scrotum. In fact, in one study in dogs, color Doppler was able to detect partial torsion in subjects in whom scintigraphy did not clearly define the process (98). In addition, detorsion of the testis has been noted on Doppler by observation of intratesticular and peritesticular arterial vessels and an increase in the diastolic component on spectral analysis (94,99). The question of how confident one can be in the diagnosis of detorsion by color Doppler remains (70).

Unfortunately, there are only a few studies comparing color Doppler and scintigraphy, and such studies are now essential. Ultrasound clearly has an advantage in the diagnosis of hydroceles and hematoceles. One disadvantage of ultrasound is the necessity to place the probe on a painful testicle. Scintigraphy has technical demands, but the studies are quite easy to perform. An additional advantage of scintigraphy is the ability to see the entire area being imaged on the flow and static images. As with all new technical developments, further comparisons between ultrasound and scintigraphy and correlation with surgical outcomes is essential.

TABLE 9.4. *Sensitivity of testicular scintigraphy for epididymitis*

Reference	Year	Number of patients	Sensitivity	False positives	Comments
Hahn (2)	1975	28	20/20		Rectilinear
Muskerjee (3)	1975	28	2/3		Rectilinear; 1 called torsion (FN)
Riley (4)	1976	98	40/40		
Hitch (78)	1976	21	4/5		1 Normal scan (FN)
Holder (79)	1977	74	22/22		
Kogan (97)	1979	22	5/6		1 Normal scan (FN)
Boedecker (80)	1979	32	25/25		
Abu-Sleiman (5)	1979	43	12/13	2	2 Torsions (FP); 1 epididymitis plus hydrocele (FN)
Orovan (73)	1979	34	13/15		2 Normal scans (FN)
Falkowski (81)	1980	18	1/1		
Wasnick (82)	1980	34	18/18		
Tanaka (23)	1981	410	214/218		
Bailey (83)	1981	16	8/10		2 Called torsion (FN)
Stage (84)	1981	72	48/48		
Vordermark (24)	1981	79	65/69		4 Normal scans (FN)
Valvo (88)	1982	46	28/28		
Chen (50)	1983	246	69/69		
Blacklock (87)	1983	33	14/14		
Thomas (55)	1983	80	30/30		
Wise (88)	1983	42	15/15	3	2 Varicoceles and 1 torsion (FP)
Nakielny (89)	1984	106	42/42		
Golimbu (90)	1985	62	18/18	1	1 Inflammatory tumor (FP)
Mendel (91)	1985	75	29/35		6 Normal to near normal scans (FN)
Dunn (67)	1986	57	17/20	3	3 Normal (FN); 1 torsion, 2 indeterminate (FP)
Chen (92)	1986	52	16/16		
Eshghi (47)	1987	155	48/49		1 Called abscess (FN)
Mueller (93)	1988	43	16/16		
Burks (94)	1990	17	7/7		
Middleton (70)	1990	28	13/15		2 Normal scans (FN)
van Ahlen (95)	1991	108	42/49		4 Normal; 3 epididymal abscess with ischemia (FN)
Fenner (61)	1991	44	8/8		
Atkinson (96)	1992	23	4/4		
Totals		2,226	913/948 (96.3%)	9	

POSTOPERATIVE EVALUATION OF TESTICULAR PERFUSION

Testicular scintigraphy may be helpful in evaluating testicular perfusion following operations such as herniorrhaphy, varicocelectomy, postoperative repair of torsion of the testis, and orchipexy of an undescended testis (8,46–49). The incidence of loss of testicular vascular supply after a herniorrhaphy is 2.5% (48). Surgical correction of an undescended testicle involves ligation of the testicular artery and mobilization of the vas deferens and the testicle into the scrotum. The collateral circulation from the vas deferens can maintain the viability of the testis. Nuclear scintigraphy plays a small but important role in the assessment of these postoperative patients. If collaterals are adequate, scintigraphy should show normal blood flow and testicular activity.

VARICOCELE

In 1979, Freund and Bautovich (36) were the first to describe the use of radionuclide scintigraphy for the evaluation of varicoceles. Diagnosis of varicocele is important in the evaluation of the infertile or subfertile male, although varicoceles do not invariably cause infertility (40). Loss of testicular mass as well as abnormalities in sperm morphology and sperm count have been shown in patients with varicoceles. A sperm count that is not corrected following varicocelectomy is occasionally the result of unsuspected bilateral varicoceles (39). The left spermatic vein drains into the left renal vein at a right angle, whereas the right spermatic vein drains directly into the inferior vena cava at an acute angle. The difference in flow dynamics results in a higher incidence of varicoceles on the left side (41). The association of varicoceles with a reduced sperm count is presumed to be related to temperature and stasis effects on spermatogenesis. Varicoceles develop during sexual maturation; the finding of a varicocele before puberty is unusual. Lyon and colleagues (41) considered the duration of the varicocele, rather than its size, to be more predictive of the deleterious effect on sperm production.

The scintigraphic technique for evaluation of varicoceles is different from that used to evaluate the acute scrotum. The presence of a varicocele can be seen during the flow study, in particular during the venous phase (Fig. 9.6). Technetium-99m–labeled red blood cells are used in most studies, although Tc-99m human serum albumin may also be used. As previously described, the patient is studied in the standing position for the flow study and in both the standing and supine positions for the static images. During the later part of the flow study, most patients with varicoceles will show reflux into the spermatic vein. Usually, reflux is due to incompetence of the valves of the spermatic vein, although obstruction to venous drainage at the level of the hypogastric or iliac veins may also be a causative factor (38). On static images varicoceles appear as an area of linear and fusiform activity.

Correlation of scintigraphy results with other modalities is impressive, most of the varicoceles seen on venography are also seen by scintigraphy (37–39,42,43,45, 100). In one study 13 of 15 patients with suspected or poorly palpable lesions were found to have varicocele on contrast venogram. Of this group, 11 were found by scintigraphy (42). Geatti and colleagues (38) studied 263 patients using a combination of thermography, ultrasound, venography, and scintigraphy, and found excellent correlation. In a group of 96 patients, with phlebography as the standard, sensitivity was 98% for scintigraphy, 100% for thermography, and 98% for ultrasound. Scintigraphy had the added advantage of demonstrating reflux of the spermatic vein. In another study of 83 patients with infertility, 29 had palpable varicocele, and of this group 22 had positive scans (90% sensitivity) (37). These sensitivity statistics are impressive, and scintigraphy deserves closer examination in the assessment of patients with infertility.

TESTICULAR TUMORS

Testicular scintigraphy with Tc-99m pertechnetate is of little or no value in patients with testicular neoplasms. Most frequently these patients present with painless swelling, and the issue of testicular scanning never arises. If performed, technetium scanning may show normal perfusion and blood pool patterns, although reduced vascularity may be present, particularly if the tumor is large and necrotic (Fig. 9.7). Increased blood flow and blood pool can be seen if the tumor is highly vascular. In the case of a vascular tumor with a necrotic center or a hypovascular tumor with an inflammatory reaction surrounding it, scanning may show increased vascularity with a cold center, mimicking torsion.

Occasionally, a patient with acute testicular symptoms and a nondiagnostic testicular scan may be misdiagnosed as having epididymitis and may respond to conservative management, only to have a painless underlying neoplasm become evident some time later (101).

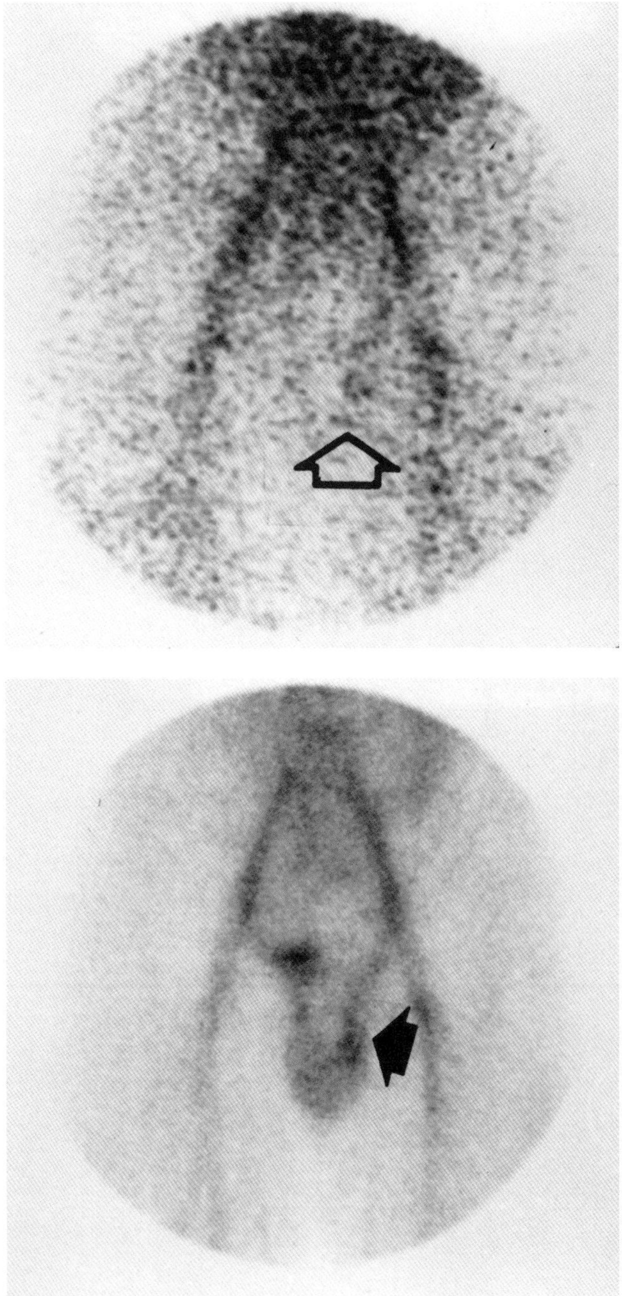

A

B

FIG. 9.6. Varicocele. **(A)** The late venous phase image in the flow sequence shows increased venous pooling on the left side (*open arrow*). **(B)** The static image shows increased vascular activity consistent with a varix (*closed arrow*). Note also the previously mentioned focus of normal vascular activity above the right testicle, which is at the base of the penis.

However, tumor-involved testes can and do present with torsion, as described by Cos and colleagues (102). This occurs most frequently with an undescended testicle or in association with other developmental testicular anomalies. Pain can also be the presenting complaint in a testicular neoplasm with acute necrosis, increasing the

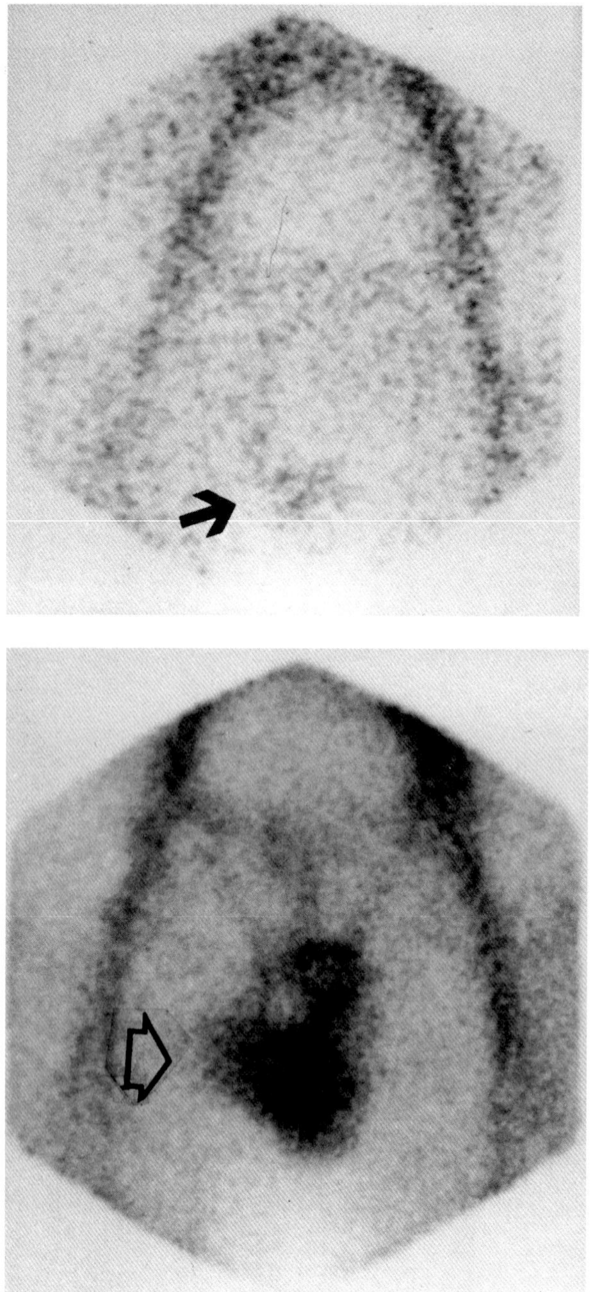

A

B

FIG. 9.7. Testicular neoplasm. **(A)** The scintigraphic flow study is characterized by a moderate focal increase in flow to the right testicular seminoma (*arrow*). **(B)** The postflow static image shows the mass as a region of tracer-containing activity. The tumor has anatomically distorted the right testicle (*open arrow*).

likelihood in this unusual circumstance of a misdiagnosis of acute torsion due to the central cold focus.

Gallium-67 scanning has been found to be very useful in patients with seminoma testis, demonstrating a sensitivity of 83% and a specificity of 95% (103). With other testicular neoplasms, however, sensitivity was only 26% and specificity only 50%. In a study by Sauerbrunn and colleagues (104), none of six primary testicular tumors was found to be positive with Ga-67. However, 53% (30 out of 56) of metastatic sites were correctly identified. The highest sensitivity, 75%, was for embryonal carcinoma (18 of 24 patients) and the lowest sensitivity, 21%, was for teratoma (4 of 19 patients). When positive, gallium scanning can be extremely useful in identifying the presence and extent of regional tumor spread (105). It has no place in the evaluation of the primary site, however, because of its low sensitivity and the potential for false positives with inflammatory lesions. In another study, Haddy and colleagues (106) found positive gallium uptake in patients with testicular lymphomas, two of which were first identified as bilateral on the gallium scan.

As the incidence of skeletal and hepatic metastases is so low, there is no place in the work-up of testicular tumors for the routine use of bone scans (107) or liver scans (108). Shulkin and colleagues (109) have described a very interesting, but most unusual, patient who developed bilateral testicular infiltration with neuroblastoma and a strikingly positive I-123 metaiodobenzylguanidine (MIBG) scan of the testicles.

Tc-99m sulfur colloid or antimony sulfide colloid lymphoscintigraphy has been used to characterize the extent of regional lymph node involvement with testicular metastases (110,111). This approach to lymph node visualization is worthy of consideration because the only other lymphatic procedure, lymphangiography, is technically much more difficult, is associated with higher morbidity, and can have sensitivities as low as 77% for the presence of metastatic disease. In lymphoscintigraphy the radiopharmaceutical is administered in two deep perianal injections into the right and left ischiorectal fossae, with iliopelvic scintigraphy performed 3 hours later. In a study of lymph node metastases in 15 patients with nonseminomatous germ cell tumors, Kaplan and colleagues (111) demonstrated a sensitivity of 89% and a specificity of 83%. Despite these findings, lymphoscintigraphy has not gained widespread acceptance. Although direct injection of microcolloid into the testicles can provide information on testicular lymphatic drainage itself (112), this cannot be considered a clinically useful procedure.

Scanning for tumors with radiolabeled antitumor antibodies has become of particular interest in the last decade, and this scintigraphic approach to testicular neoplasms has been explored by several investigators. Epenetos and colleagues (113) labeled an antibody to testicular placental-like alkaline phosphatase (PLAP) with radioiodine and studied 12 patients with germ cell tumors of the testes. Their findings were positive in 6 of 10 patients, a sensitivity of 60%. Khazaeli and colleagues (114) produced an antibody to a testicular embryonal cell carcinoma with choriocarcinoma components, and they found that the radiolabeled antibody was effective in scanning nude mice transplanted with human embryonal carcinoma cell lines. Wahl and colleagues

(25) demonstrated that in animals this radioiodinated antibody (5F9.3) was even more effective when injected subcutaneously rather than intravenously. Hitchins and colleagues (115) evaluated an I-131 labeled antibody to the oncofetal antigen alpha-fetoprotein (AFP). They studied 22 patients with testicular tumors and identified an overall sensitivity of 57% for metastatic sites. Finally, Kalofonos and colleagues (116) have further pursued the use of the anti-PLAP antibody H17E2 labeled with In-111 and I-123 in 33 patients, and have demonstrated excellent sensitivity for the presence of testicular tumors. At present there is no commercially available radiolabeled antitumor antibody for scanning testicular neoplasms, nor is one likely to be approved by the FDA for a number of years, but this approach to tumor localization remains very interesting and worthy of much further exploration.

MISCELLANEOUS DISORDERS

Spermatoceles are located along the superior aspect of the testicle (47,94), and a static scan shows a cold defect in this area (8,47). Fenner and colleagues (61) have described identification of a hemorrhagic spermatocele in one patient. Scintigraphy in a patient with allergic scrotitis has been described and showed a normal pattern (78). The diagnosis is usually made clinically in a young boy with an inflamed scrotum and a history of allergies but no scrotal pain.

CONCLUSION

Testicular scintigraphy is highly sensitive and specific in the evaluation of acute scrotal pain and can be very helpful in the postoperative assessment of the patient who has recently undergone testicular surgery. Unfortunately, it tends to be seriously underutilized considering its effectiveness. Testicular blood pool scintigraphy provides characteristic findings in varicocele, and gallium-67 scanning and iliopelvic lymphoscintigraphy play an important role in testicular neoplasms. The role of radiolabeled antitumor antibodies in such malignancies, however, remains to be established.

REFERENCES

1. Nadel NS, Gitter MH, Hahn LC, Vernon AR. Preoperative diagnosis of testicular torsion. *Urology* 1973;1:478–479.
2. Hahn LC, Nadel NS, Gitter MH, Vernon A. Testicular scanning: a new modality for the preoperative diagnosis of testicular torsion. *J Urol* 1975;113:60–62.
3. Mukerjee MG, Vollero RA, Mittemeyer BT, Borski AA. Diagnostic value of 99mTc in scrotal scan. *Urology* 1975;6:453–455.
4. Riley TW, Mosbaugh PG, Coles JL, Newman DM, Van Hove ED, Heck LL. Use of radioisotope scan in evaluation of intrascrotal lesions. *J Urol* 1976;116:472–475.
5. Abu-Sleiman R, Ho JE, Gregory JG. Scrotal scanning: present value and limits of interpretation. *Urology* 1979;13:326–330.
6. Anderson PA, Giacomantonio JM. The acutely painful scrotum in children: review of 113 consecutive cases. *Can Med Assoc J* 1985;132:1153–1155.
7. Barker K, Raper FP. Torsion of the testis. *Br J Urol* 1964;36:35–41.
8. Chen DC, Holder LE, Melloul M. Radionuclide scrotal imaging: further experience with 210 new patients. Part 2: Results and discussion. *J Nucl Med* 1983;24:841–853.
9. Datta NS, Mishkin FS. Radionuclide imaging in intrascrotal lesions. *JAMA* 1975;231:1060–1062.
10. Edelsberg JS, Surh YS. The acute scrotum. *Emerg Med Clin North Am* 1988;6:521–546.
11. Holder LE, Melloul M, Chen D. Current status of radionuclide scrotal imaging. *Semin Nucl Med* 1981;11:232–249.
12. Holder LE, Martire JR, Schirmer HK. Clinical applications of testicular radionuclide angiography and scrotal scanning. *JAMA* 1981;245:2526–2429.
13. Lutzker LG. Scrotal scintigraphy. In: Tauxe,WN, Dubovsky EV, eds. *Nuclear medicine in clinical urology and nephrology*. Norwalk, CT: Appleton-Century-Crofts; 1985:321–346.
14. Lutzker LG, Zuckier LS. Testicular scanning and other applications of radionuclide imaging of the genital tract. *Semin Nucl Med* 1990;20:159–188.
15. May DC, Lesh P, Lewis S, Anderson RJ. Evaluation of acute scrotum pain with testicular scanning. *Ann Emerg Med* 1985;14:696–699.
16. Mishkin FS. Differential diagnostic features of the radionuclide scrotal image. *AJR* 1977;128:127–129.
17. Mishkin FS. Increased scrotal activity. *Semin Nucl Med* 1981;11:315.
18. Noronha PA, Demir RH. Differentiating the acute scrotum. *Hosp Pract* 1984;19:216–217,223–242.
19. O'Brien WM, Lynch JH. The acute scrotum. *Am Fam Physician* 1988;37,239–247.
20. Palestro CJ, Manor EP, Kim CK, Goldsmith SJ. Torsion of a testicular appendage in an adult male. *Clin Nucl Med* 1990;15:515–516.
21. Sharer WC. Acute scrotal pathology. *Surg Clin North Am* 1982;62:955–970.
22. Smith SP, King LR. Torsion of the testis: techniques of assessment. *Urol Clin North Am* 1979;6:429–443.
23. Tanaka T, Mishkin FS, Datta NS. Radionuclide imaging of the scrotal contents. In: Freeman LM, Weissmann HS, eds. *Nuclear Medicine Annual*. New York: Raven Press; 1981:195–219.
24. Vordermark JS, Buck AS, Brown SR, Tuttle WK. The testicular scan. Use in diagnosis and management of acute epididymitis. *JAMA* 1981;45:2512–2514.
25. Wahl RL, Laino L, Fisher S, Schteingart M, Beierwaltes WH. Improved radioimmunolocalization of human tumor xenografts following subcutaneous delivery of monoclonal antibodies. *Eur J Nucl Med* 1988;13:530–536.
26. Williamson RC. The continuing conundrum of testicular torsion [editorial]. *Br J Surg* 1985;72:509–510.
27. Charron M, Mandell JB, Kolodny GM. Detection of a rare complication of appendicitis by scrotal imaging. *Clin Nucl Med* 1988;13:761–762.
28. Melton JW, Chung CJ, Gordon L. Pseudobullseye sign of the testicle. A window to the peritoneum. *Clin Nucl Med* 1991;16:604–605.
29. Schauwecker DS. Three-phase bone scan reveals epididymo-orchitis. *Clin Nucl Med* 1989;14:468–469.
30. Vieco PT, Stern J, Herschorn S. Patent processus vaginalis. *Clin Nucl Med* 1990;15:263.
31. Wilkins SA, Holder LE, Raiker RV, Wilson TH. Acute appendicitis presenting as acute left scrotal pain: diagnostic considerations. *Urology* 1985;25:634–636.
32. Elgazzar AH, Fernandez-Ulloa M, Black RR, Silberstein EB. Incidental detection of obstructive uropathy during scrotal imaging. *Clin Nucl Med* 1988;13:823–825.
33. Dravid VS, Heyman S. Torsion of an undescended testis not detected on testicular imaging. *Clin Nucl Med* 1991;16:275–277.
34. Fink-Bennett D, Uppal TK, Conway GF. Redux testis: potential pitfall in testicular imaging. *J Urol* 1979;121:821–822.
35. Ueno K, Hayashi H, Oohama K, Asano S. Missed torsion of an

undescended testis detected with testicular imaging [letter]. *J Nucl Med* 1987; 28:1061.

36. Freund J, Bautovich GJ: Varicocele detection by blood pool imaging. *Aust NZ J Med* 1979;9:628.
37. Freund J, Handelsman DJ, Bautovich GJ, Conway AJ, Morris JG. Detection of varicocele by radionuclide blood pool scanning. *Radiology* 1980; 137:227–230.
38. Geatti O, Gasparini D, Shapiro B. A comparison of scintigraphy, thermography, ultrasound and phlebography in grading of clinical varicocele. *J Nucl Med* 1991;32:2092–2097.
39. Harris JD, McConnell BJ, Lipshultz LI, McConnell RW, Conoley PH. Radioisotope angiography in diagnosis of varicocele [editorial comment]. *Urology* 1980; 16:69–72.
40. Hirokawa M, Iwamoto T, Iwasaki A, Yamazaki A, Tosaka A, Asakura S, Matsushita K. Clinical observations of fertile males with varicocele. *Eur Urol* 1989; 16:23–27.
41. Lyon RP, Marshall S, Scott MP. Varicocele in youth. *West J Med* 1983; 138:832–834.
42. Marmar JL, Zeiger LS, DeBenedictis TJ, Praiss DE. Comprehensive scrotal flow and scan technique for detection of varicoceles. *Urology* 1985;25:505–510.
43. Ramanna L, Waxman AD, Yoon J, Hyun M, Rothman C. Evaluation of scrotal varicocele with blood pool scintigraphy: correlation with contrast gonadal venography. *Clin Nucl Med* 1990; 15: 768.
44. Turetsky DB, Wilf LH. Epididymal cyst simulating missed torsion by scrotal scintigraphy. *Clin Nucl Med* 1990; 15:846–847.
45. Wheatley JK, Fajman WA, Witten FR. Clinical experience with the radioisotope varicocele scan as a screening method for the detection of subclinical varicoceles. *J Urol* 1982; 128:57–59.
46. Datta NS, Tanaka T, Zinner NR, Mishkin FS. Division of spermatic vessels in orchiopexy: radionuclide evidence of preservation of testicular circulation. *J Urol* 1977; 118:447–449.
47. Eshghi M, Silver L, Smith AD. Technetium 99m scan in acute scrotal lesions. *Urology* 1987;30:586–593.
48. Nagle C, Clark K, Browning HR, Murphy J. Testicular ischemia and infarction following herniorrhaphy or varicocelectomy: evaluation by radionuclide imaging. *Clin Nucl Med* 1989; 14:243–248.
49. Thurston A, Whitaker R. Torsion of testis after previous testicular surgery. *Br J Surg* 1983;70:217.
50. Chen DC, Holder LE, Melloul M. Radionuclide scrotal imaging: further experience with 210 patients. Part 1: Anatomy, pathophysiology, and methods. *J Nucl Med* 1983;24:735–742.
51. International Commission on Radiological Protection. Radiation dose to patients from radiopharmaceuticals. ICRP Publication 53. *Ann ICRP* 1987; 18:197–199.
52. Debatin JF, Beytas EM. Indium-111 white blood cell imaging of epididymitis. *Eur J Nucl Med* 1990; 17:286–289.
53. Lantto EH, Lantto TJ, Vorne M. Fast diagnosis of abdominal infections and inflammations with technetium-99m-HMPAO labeled leukocytes. *J Nucl Med* 1991;32:2029–2034.
54. Gelfand MJ, Williams PJ, Rosenkrantz JG. Pinhole imaging: utility in testicular imaging in children. *Clin Nucl Med* 1980;5:237–240.
55. Thomas WEG, Williamson RCN. Diagnosis and outcome of testicular torsion. *Br J Surg* 1983;70:213–216.
56. Atallah MW, Ippolito JJ, Rubin BW. Intrauterine bilateral torsion of the spermatic cord. *J Urol* 1976; 116:128–129.
57. Smith GI. Cellular changes from graded testicular ischemia. *J Urol* 1955;73:355–362.
58. Cass AS, Cass BP, Veeraraghavan K. Immediate exploration of unilateral acute scrotum in young male subjects. *J Urol* 1980; 124: 829–832.
59. Stoller ML, Kogan BA, Hricak H. Spermatic cord torsion: diagnostic limitations. *Pediatrics* 1985;76:929–933.
60. Knight PJ, Vassy LE. The diagnosis and treatment of the acute scrotum in children and adolescents. *Ann Surg* 1984;200:664–673.
61. Fenner MN, Roszhart DA, Texter JH. Testicular scanning: evaluating the acute scrotum in the clinical setting. *Urology* 1991;38: 237–241.
62. Dunn EK, Chen PC, Lipschitz SS, Glassberg KI, Sarkar SD, Strashun AM. Testicular scintigraphic findings two to three months after torsion. Correlation with sonography and histopathology. *Clin Nucl Med* 1991; 16:37–39.
63. Boedecker RA, Glicklich M, Sty JR. Rim sign in entodermal sinus tumor. *Clin Nucl Med* 1979;4:130–131.
64. Gips S, Mecz Y, Hardoff R. Scintigraphic 'rim sign' in a patient with epididymitis associated with fluid collection. *Clin Nucl Med* 1991; 16:952.
65. Mishkin FS. Bullseye sign in scrotal imaging. *Semin Nucl Med* 1981; 11:316.
66. Vieras F, Kuhn CR. Nonspecificity of the "rim sign" in the scintigraphic diagnosis of missed testicular torsion. *Radiology* 1983; 146:519–522.
67. Dunn EK, Macchia RJ, Chauhan PS, Laungani GB, Solomon NA. Scintiscan for acute intrascrotal conditions. *Clin Nucl Med* 1986; 11:381–388.
68. Willgress ER, Camponova EJ, Kistler AM, Goyer PF, Silverman ED. Spontaneous reduction of testicular torsion during scrotal imaging. *Clin Nucl Med* 1989; 14:540.
69. Middleton WD, Melson GL. Testicular ischemia: color doppler sonographic findings in five patients. *AJR* 1989; 152:1237–1239.
70. Middleton WD, Siegel BA, Melson GL, Yates CK, Andriole GL. Acute scrotal disorders: prospective comparison of color doppler US and testicular scintigraphy. *Radiology*, 1990; 177:177–181.
71. Feld R, Middleton WD. Recent advances in sonography of the testis and scrotum. *Radiol Clin North Am* 1992;30:1033–1051.
72. Diaz-Ball FL, Moreno AJ, Toney MA, Rodriguez A, Turnbull GL. One-dose technetium-99m pertechnetate imaging in acute testicular torsion followed by manual detorsion. *Clin Nucl Med* 1990; 15:76–79.
73. Orovan WL, McLorie GA. Testicular scanning: its efficacy in diagnosing intrascrotal lesions. *Can J Surg* 1979;22:477–480.
74. Vordermark JS, Favila MQ. Testicular necrosis: a preventable complication of epididymitis. *J Urol* 1982; 128:1322–1324.
75. Eisner DJ, Goldman SM, Petronis J, Millmond SH. Bilateral testicular infarction caused by epididymitis. *AJR* 1991;157:517–519.
76. Vieras F. Evolution of acute epididymitis to testicular infarction. Scintigraphic demonstration. *Clin Nucl Med* 1986; 11:158–160.
77. McConnell JD, Peters PC, Lewis SE. Testicular rupture in blunt scrotal trauma: review of 15 cases with recent application of testicular scanning. *J Urol* 1982; 128:309–311.
78. Hitch DC, Gilday DL, Shandling B, Savage JP. A new approach to the diagnosis of testicular torsion. *J Pediatr Surg* 1976; 11:537–541.
79. Holder LE, Martire JR, Holmes ER, Wagner HN. Testicular radionuclide angiography and static imaging: anatomy, scintigraphic interpretation and clinical indications. *Radiology* 1977; 125:739–752.
80. Boedecker RA, Sty JR, Jona JZ. Testicular scanning as a diagnostic aid in evaluating scrotal pain. *J Pediatr* 1979;94:760–762.
81. Falkowski WS, Firlit CF. Testicular torsion: the role of radioisotopic scanning. *J Urol* 1980; 124:886–888.
82. Wasnick RJ, Pohutsky KR, Macchia RJ. Testicular torsion and usefulness of radionuclide scanning. *Urology* 1980; 15:318–320.
83. Bailey GA, Lane JW. Testicular scanning at Memorial Division Charleston Area Medical Center. *W Va Med J* 1981;77:133–136.
84. Stage KH, Schoenvogel R, Lewis S. Testicular scanning: clinical experience with 72 patients. *J Urol* 1981; 125:334–337.
85. Dunn EK, Macchia RJ, Solomon NA. Scintigraphic pattern in missed testicular torsion. *Radiology* 1981; 139:175–180.
86. Valvo JR, Caldamone AA, O'Mara R, Rabinowitz R. Nuclear imaging in the pediatric acute scrotum. *Am J Dis Child* 1982; 136: 831–835.
87. Blacklock ARE, Kwok HKY, Mason GR, Mills JA, Taylor DN. Radionuclide imaging in scrotal swellings. *Br J Urol* 1983;55: 749–753.
88. Wise PA, Mann H, Sagar VV, Meckelnburg RL. Scrotal scintigraphy: a review of 42 cases. *Del Med J* 1983;55:421–424.
89. Nakielny RA, Thomas WEG, Jackson P, Jones M, Davies ER. Radionuclide evaluation of acute scrotal disease. *Clin Radiol* 1984;35:126–129.
90. Golimbu M, Fiorio FE, Al-Askari S, Morales PA, Passalaqua A.

Value of scrotal scanning. Report of 62 cases. *Urology* 1985;25: 89–92.
91. Mendel JB, Taylor GA, Treves S, Cheng TH, Retik A, Bauer S. Testicular torsion in children: scintigraphic assessment. *Pediatr Radiol* 1985;15:110–115.
92. Chen DCP, Holder LE, Kaplan GN. Correlation of radionuclide imaging and diagnostic ultrasound in scrotal diseases. *J Nucl Med* 1986;27:1774–1781.
93. Mueller DL, Amundson GM, Rubin SZ, Wesenberg RL. Acute scrotal abnormalities in children: diagnosis by combined sonography and scintigraphy. *AJR* 1988;150:643–646.
94. Burks DD, Barkey BJ, Burkhard TK, Balsara ZN, Haluszka MM, Canning DA. Suspected testicular torsion and ischemia: evaluation with color doppler sonography. *Radiology* 1990;175:815–821.
95. van Ahlen H, Bockisch A, van Stauffenberg A, Bruhl P. Static and dynamic radionuclide imaging in the diagnosis of the acute scrotum. *Urol Int* 1991;47:20–24.
96. Atkinson GO Jr, Patrick LE, Ball TI Jr, Stephenson CA, Broecker BH, Woodard JR. The normal and abnormal scrotum in children: evaluation with color Doppler sonography. *AJR* 1992;158: 613–617.
97. Kogan SJ, Lutzker LG, Perez LA, Novich I, Schneider KM, Hanna MK, Levitt SB. The value of the negative radionuclide scrotal scan in the management of the acutely inflamed scrotum in children. *J Urol* 1979;122:223–225.
98. Mevorach RA, Lerner RM, Greenspan BS, Russ GA, Heckler BL, Orosz JF, Rabinowitz R. Color Doppler ultrasound compared to a radionuclide scanning of spermatic cord torsion in a canine model. *J Urol* 1991;145:428–433.
99. Lerner RM, Mevorach RA, Hulbert WC, Rabinowitz R. Color doppler US in the evaluation of acute scrotal disease. *Radiology* 1990;176:355–358.
100. Hamm B, Fobbe F, Sorensen R, Feisenberg D. Varicoceles: combined sonography and thermography in diagnosis and posttherapeutic evaluation. *Radiology* 1989;160:419–424.
101. Donoghue GD, Prezio JA, Ricci PE. Early diagnosis of testicular tumor using Tc-99m pertechnetate scrotal imaging. *Clin Nucl Med* 1983;8: 630–631.
102. Cos LR, Peartree RJ, Descalzi M, Rabinowitz R. Torsion of intrascrotal malignant testis tumors. *J Urol* 1983;130:145–147.
103. Willan BD, Penney H, Castor WR, McGowan DG. The usefulness of gallium-67 citrate scanning in testicular seminoma. *Clin Nucl Med* 1987;12:813–815.
104. Sauerbrunn JL, Andrews GA, Hubner KF. Ga-67 citrate imaging in tumors of the genito-urinary tract: report of cooperative study. *J Nucl Med* 1978;19:470–475.
105. Bekerman C, Hoffer PB, Bitran JD. The role of gallium-67 in the clinical evaluation of cancer. *Semin Nucl Med* 1984;14:296–323.
106. Haddy TB, Sandlund JT, Magrath IT. Testicular involvement in young patients with non-Hodgkin's lymphoma. *Am J Pediatr Hematol/Oncol* 1988:10:224–229.
107. Merrick MV. Bone scintigraphy in testicular tumors. *Br J Urol* 1987;60:167–169.
108. Harbert JC. Efficacy of liver scanning in malignant diseases. *Semin Nucl Med* 1984;14:287–295.
109. Shulkin BL, Geatti O, Hattner RS, Ablin AR, Hutchinson RJ, Shapiro B. Bilateral testicular neuroblastoma. Scintigraphic depiction and therapy with I-131 MIBG. *Clin Nucl Med* 1992;17: 638–642.
110. Kaplan WD. Iliopelvic lymphoscintigraphy. *Semin Nucl Med* 1983;13:42–53.
111. Kaplan WD, Garnick MB, Richie JP. Iliopelvic radionuclide lymphoscintigraphy in patients with testicular cancer. *Radiology* 1983;147:231–235.
112. Yeh SDJ, Morse MJ, Grando R, Kleinert EL, Whitmore WF. Lymphoscintigraphic studies of lymphatic drainage from the testes. *Clin Nucl Med* 1986;11:823–827.
113. Epenetos AA, Carr D, Johnson PM, Bodmer WF, Lavender JP. Antibody-guided radiolocalisation of tumours in patients with testicular or ovarian cancer using two radioiodinated monoclonal antibodies to placental alkaline phosphatase. *Br J Radiol* 1986;59:117–125.
114. Khazaeli MB, Beierwaltes WH, Pitt GS, Kabza GA, Rogers KJ, LoBuglio AF. Development and characterization of a monoclonal antibody to human embryonal carcinoma. *J Urol* 1987: 137:1295–1299.
115. Hitchins RN, Begent RHJ, Green AJ, Searle F, van Heyningen V, Bagshawe KD. Clinical value of imaging using antibody to alpha fetoprotein in germ cell tumors. *Nuklear Medizin* 1989;28:29–33.
116. Kalofonos HP, Kosmas C, Pawlikowska TR, et al. Immunolocalisation of testicular tumors using radiolabelled monoclonal antibody to placental alkaline phosphatase. *J Nucl Med Allied Sci* 1990;34:294–298.

CHAPTER 10

Angiography

With the advent and general acceptance of other less invasive methods of evaluation of the scrotum and its contents, only two indications remain for angiography (testicular venography):

1. Diagnosis and treatment of varicoceles
2. Impalpable testis

TECHNIQUES OF EXAMINATION

Angiography requires puncture of the femoral vein at the inguinal ligament and selective probing of the testicular vein through the inferior vena cava and renal vein. In healthy subjects, the valves prevent retrograde filling of the vessel with contrast material. In the presence of a varicocele, however, there will be retrograde filling in a caudal direction up to the inguinal canal. Visualization of the pampiniform plexus itself is not required. (The testes have to be protected from radiation exposure by lead pads.) The left testicular vein opens into the medial segment of the left renal vein, and is relatively easily probed with catheter with a Hopkins curve. The right testicular vein normally opens into the inferior vena cava at an acute angle, directly caudal to the right renal vein. It occasionally joins the vena cava more caudally or opens directly into the renal vein (in 10% of cases). A so-called cobra or sidewinder catheter is used to selectively probe the testicular vein on the right, but the acute angle and variable joining sites make this procedure more difficult and time-consuming than on the left (1,2).

RISKS AND BIOEFFECTS

For the experienced angiographer, 2 or 3 minutes of fluoroscopy is usually sufficient for visualization of the left testicular vein. Probing of the right vein may require 5 to 10 minutes. Total radiation exposure can be kept to a minimum by reducing the fluoroscopic field to a minimum. The testis should be protected from radiation exposure by lead pads. Serious side effects are rare if the patient is adequately informed and low-osmolar contrast agents are used (3).

NORMAL ANATOMY

The testicular artery arises from the aorta just below the renal artery and descends in the retroperitoneum to meet the spermatic cord at the internal inguinal ring. Within the spermatic cord, the testicular artery runs downward and anastomoses with the cremasteric and deferential arteries. Below the inguinal canal, it divides into two branches, the internal testicular artery and the inferior testicular artery. However, this division may occur in the spermatic cord (6% to 8% of cases) or in the retroperitoneum (4). Another branch of the testicular artery, the epididymal artery, arises variably above the epididymis and supplies the head and body of the epididymis.

The veins from the testis and epididymis form a venous network (pampiniform plexus). The testicular vein is formed by the joining of the pampiniform plexus veins. Usually, a single vessel or two vessels remain on passage through the inguinal canal. Cranial to the internal inguinal canal, the testicular vein commonly has a variety of branches with connections to other retroperitoneal veins (the paralumbar, renal capsular, and iliac veins) (5,6).

Whereas the testis and the anterior part of the epididymis drain into the pampiniform plexus, the blood from the posterior part of the epididymis, the vas deferens, and the paratesticular tissues drains into the cremasteric, deferential, and funicular veins. The cremasteric vein drains into the internal saphenous or the inferior epigastric vein, and the deferential vein, which courses along the vas deferens, drains into the venous plexus of the spermatic cord or the prostatic and vesical plexus (4). The funicular vein drains the posterior part of the epididymis into the inferior epigastric vein.

VARICOCELE

Clinical Presentation

Varicoceles are characterized by dilatation, elongation, and increased tortuosity of the veins of the pampiniform plexus. It is one of the few treatable causes of male infertility, and it is estimated that up to 10% of men in the United States suffer from this condition (7). The majority of varicoceles occur on the left side, and right-sided varicoceles are very rare. The true incidence of bilateral varicoceles is controversial and has been reported to range from 5% to 44% (8–10). The higher reported incidence is probably due to the detection of more subclinical varicoceles with high-resolution ultrasonography. Most varicoceles are asymptomatic, although some patients report a sensation of pressure in the affected hemiscrotum or a dragging pain that occurs predominantly when standing.

Several factors are implicated as causes of varicoceles: absence or incompetence of valves in the testicular vein; compression of the caudal segment of the left testicular vein by feces in the descending colon; opening of the left testicular vein into the left renal vein at the hemodynamically unfavorable angle of 90°; and compression of the left renal vein between the superior mesenteric artery and the aorta. The three latter factors are assumed to impede venous return. The predilection of varicoceles for the left side is attributed to both the obtuse-angled opening into the renal vein on the left (as opposed to the acute-angled infrarenal opening of the right testicular vein) and compression of the left renal vein where it crosses the aorta (11). In some instances, a varicocele may be caused by occlusion of the testicular draining veins by a malignant tumor (so-called symptomatic vs. idiopathic varicocele). Wilms' tumor in children or renal cell carcinoma with invasion of the renal vein in adults are the most common tumors.

Venous stasis in the scrotum leads to hyperthermia of the testes, which is assumed to impair spermiogenesis by changing sperm morphology and motility. Extensive varicoceles in children and adolescents have been associated with testicular atrophy. However, not all patients with a varicocele are infertile, and it is still unclear why the testes react differently to higher temperatures. Surgical treatment or embolization is reported to improve the spermiogram in the majority of patients (12–14).

In large varicoceles, inspection of the scrotum with the patient standing reveals tortuous vessels in the area of the pampiniform plexus. The vessels are palpated as cord-like, elastic, and nontender structures. The veins empty with the patient supine and breathing smoothly and refill during a Valsalva maneuver. Extensive varicoceles may surround the entire testis, but even nonpalpable, so-called subclinical (i.e., functional) varicoceles can cause infertility (8). The extent of a varicocele is usually described by three grades, with no generally accepted definition (15). All definitions are based on the subjective evaluation of morphology and accompanying clinical symptoms. However, because the indication for treatment is typically established on the basis of clinical symptoms (sterility or pain), these grading systems are of little practical relevance.

Diagnostic Evaluation

Most large varicoceles are easily palpated and require no diagnostic evaluation other than physical examination (unless a varicocele secondary to a renal or retroperitoneal tumor is suspected). Small varicoceles almost always require diagnostic procedures in addition to physical examination. Additional studies are especially important in patients with a pathologic spermiogram (suspicion of a subclinical varicocele) and in cases where palpation is limited (e.g., lipomatosis of the spermatic cord). The procedures available for diagnostic evaluation of patients with a suspected varicocele are **venography**, **thermography**, and **ultrasound**. Color-coded duplex sonography (CCDS) has now become the procedure of choice (discussed in Chapter 8).

Venography

In about 85% of patients with varicoceles, there is typically one large main vessel that joins the left renal vein at the usual site (Figs. 10.1 and 10.2). In the remaining patients, there are only multiple small and more tortuous vessels that join the renal vein separately or the testicular vein cannot be visualized at all (despite sonographically proven varicocele) (Fig. 10.3). In such cases, the testicular vein probably opens into a lateral vein from the renal capsule (which does not fill with contrast material when a conventional venographic technique is used) or into an iliac vein. Similar problems are encountered in cases of persistent or recurrent varicoceles: Following occlusion of the testicular vein in the cranial third, the collaterals maintaining the varicocele may be connected with renal capsular veins or other retroperitoneal veins, which cannot be visualized by venography. Although testicular venography provides a good survey of the anatomic situation, it is an invasive procedure and cannot be performed in patients with certain vessel variants and in some patients after unsuccessful surgical ligation. Color-coded duplex sonography (CCDS), however, is noninvasive and can be used regardless of the anatomy of the testicular vein. Because of the advantages of CCDS, ven-

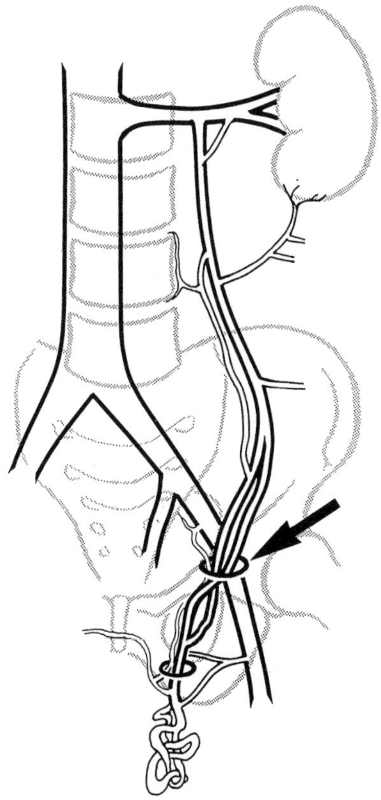

FIG. 10.1. Schematic drawing of the anatomy of the left testicular vein (5) (*Straight arrow*, internal inguinal ring).

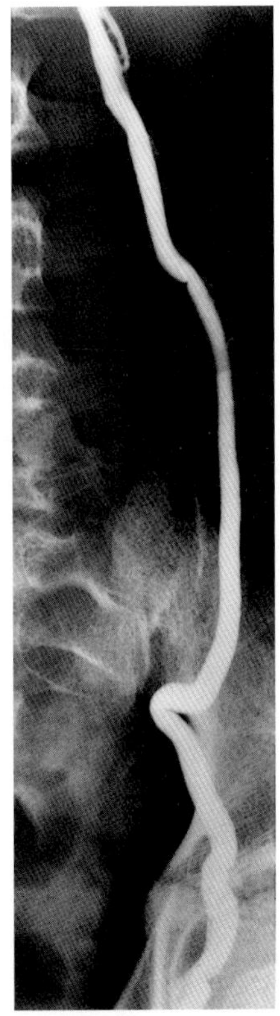

FIG 10.2. Phlebogram of the left testicular vein.

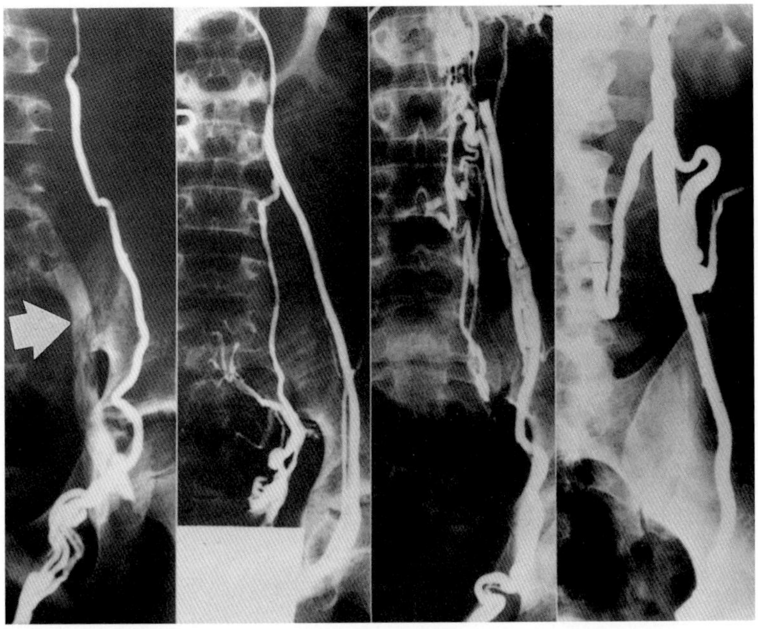

FIG. 10.3. Phlebography of the testicular vein: Anatomic variants with different collaterals to retroperitoneal and pelvic veins. (*Arrow*, common iliac vein).

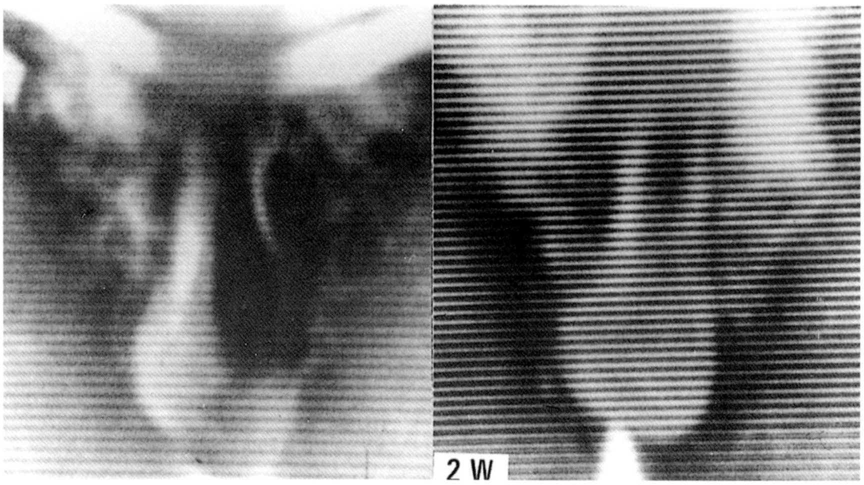

FIG. 10.4. Thermography. The illustration on the left illustrates hyperthermia on the left side of the scrotum in a patient with varicocele (*black area*). The illustration on the right was obtained two weeks after successful sclerotherapy. Note the equal heat radiation on both sides of the hemiscrotum.

ography is now indicated only in those patients who are scheduled to undergo embolization and sclerotherapy.

Thermography

Thermography is based on the assumption that venous stasis in the vessels of the pampiniform plexus leads to hyperthermia of the affected hemiscrotum relative to the contralateral side. Two procedures, contact thermography and telethermography, are available for measuring heat reflection. Because of the anatomic location of the scrotum, contact thermography is rather limited in registering its heat radiation. Telethermography has a high sensitivity for varicoceles (Fig. 10.4), but has a low specificity, since regional hyperthermia can also be caused by other pathologic conditions such as inflammation or tumor. Thus, patients with temperature differences between the left and right hemiscrotum must always undergo additional gray-scale ultrasonography to exclude other disorders. Another disadvantage of this technique is the rather long examination time. (The scrotum needs to be cooled for at least 10 minutes prior to measurement [8].)

Comparison of Imaging Techniques for Varicocele

The evaluation of a varicocele should not be limited to the vessels of the pampiniform plexus. Bilateral examination of the testis, epididymis, and kidneys is necessary to exclude associated disorders.

Of the examination techniques just described, CCDS is the method of choice. Although the underlying (retroperitoneal) cause of an idiopathic varicocele cannot be assessed, the procedure reliably demonstrates the morphologic and functional changes in the scrotum (10,16).

Percutaneous Interventional Treatment of Varicocele

Percutaneous interventional procedures for treating varicoceles have the same aim as surgery, that is, occlusion of the testicular vein at the level of the internal inguinal ring. Because of highly developed collaterals and connections to the renal capsular and paralumbar veins, the occlusion site should be located as far caudally as possible. In addition, as the different branches coalesce after exiting from the inguinal canal, occlusion at this level interrupts connections to other retroperitoneal veins (5). Interventional procedures are performed directly after diagnostic venography. The intervention requires only mild sedation in addition to local anesthesia of the puncture site. The testicular vein can be occluded by **embolization** or **sclerotherapy**.

Embolization

The material used for embolization may be a coil, a detachable balloon, or glue (e.g., bucrylate). Therapeutic success depends on proper positioning in the caudal segment of the testicular vein right above the internal inguinal ring. With modern coaxial catheter systems and maneuverable guide wires, it is usually not difficult to probe the testicular vein selectively up to this position. Both the glue and the coil can be deposited via a coaxial catheter. The balloons that are presently available are attached to the catheter tip and must be positioned without a guide wire. In the presence of a curved vessel, therefore, it is not always possible to advance the balloon far enough caudally.

There are a number of **disadvantages** to embolization of the testicular vein. A primary problem is that only the vessel in which the embolic material was delivered is occluded. Embolization of larger collaterals, which in some cases is also possible, prolongs the intervention and the duration of fluoroscopy. After the first embolization, collaterals typically have rather small calibers and may not be visualized at all. Furthermore, they continue to develop over the course of time (5). In such cases treatment can only be performed in a second session several weeks later (Fig. 10.5). Another risk is that the material used for embolization cannot be as firmly fixed in the soft wall of the testicular vein as it is in arteries, and it may become dislocated and cause pulmonary embolism (2). In addition, embolization material is more expensive than sclerosing agents. Implantation of a noninert foreign body, such as a metal coil, may be problematic especially in younger patients because of possible unknown long-term effects.

Sclerotherapy

Agents used for sclerotherapy are ethanol solutions (e.g., Ethoxysclerol) that have been used in the treatment of superficial varices of the legs for many years. These agents induce local thrombosis and inflammation of the vessel wall with subsequent occlusion of the lumen. The sclerosing agent is applied by means of a coaxial catheter.

Typically, a number 7 French guide catheter (with a Hopkins curve) with an inflatable balloon at the tip is anchored in the orifice of the testicular vein. To avoid vascular spasm, the catheter tip is advanced only a few centimeters into the vessel lumen. Through this guiding catheter a second smaller catheter (e.g., SOS wire) is then advanced coaxially down to the internal inguinal ring, where approximately 3 ml of the sclerosing agent is deposited. Cranial advancement of the sclerosing agent is prevented by prior inflation of the balloon at the tip of the guiding catheter (17). Most patients report a dragging pain after application of the sclerosing agent, which subsides after 5 to 10 minutes. The total fluoroscopy time (including diagnostic venography) for sclerotherapy of a left-sided varicocele is 5 to 10 minutes.

Sclerotherapy has a number of **advantages** over embolization. For one, with sclerosing agents it is possible to occlude collateral veins as well as the main vessel. For this to take place, however, the sclerosing agent must be applied at the level of the internal inguinal ring, where the individual veins are interconnected. Only rarely is additional probing and sclerosing of a collateral vein necessary. In addition, sclerotherapy is not associated with the risk of embolization, and sclerosing agents are relatively inexpensive.

A possible **disadvantage** of sclerotherapy is local in-

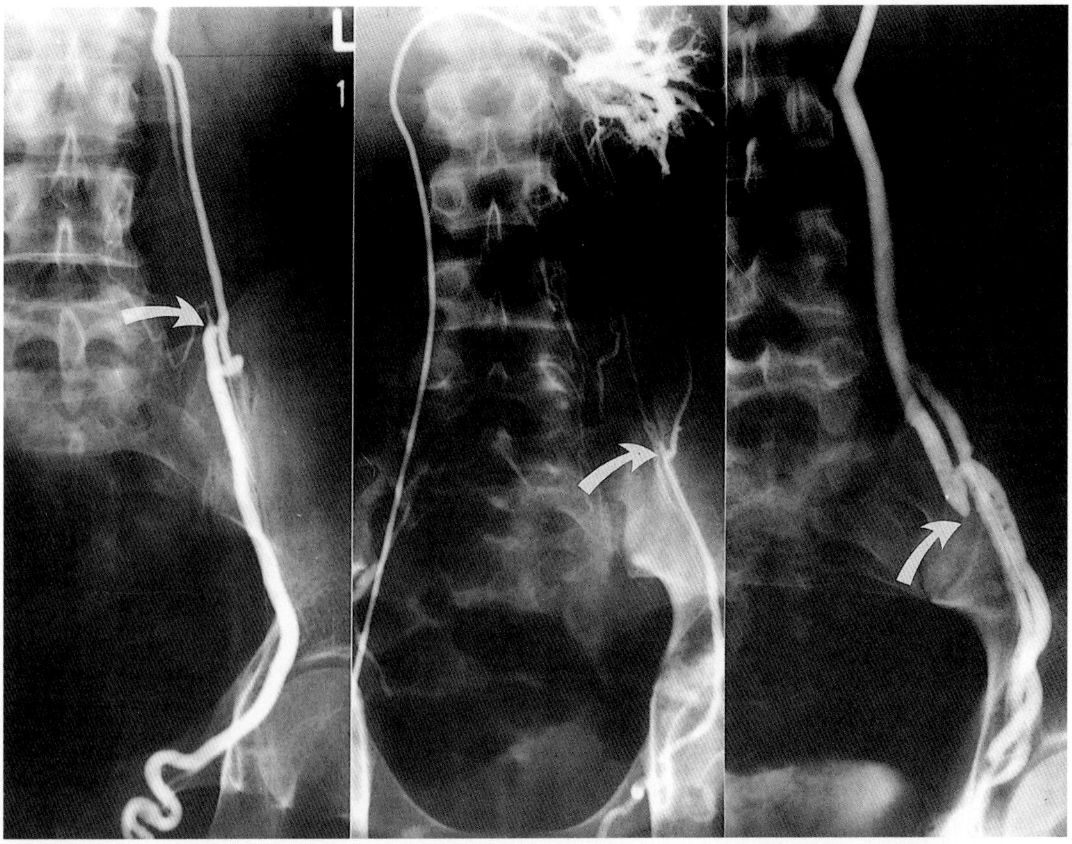

FIG. 10.5. Phlebogram after unsuccessful treatment of varicocele. The occlusion is bridged via collaterals. (*Arrows*, site of former occlusion).

flammation induced by the ethanol solution. If the sclerosing agent is applied too far caudally, it advances into the pampiniform plexus, where it may induce pronounced swelling. This swelling subsides after 2 to 3 days and has not been found to cause damage to the testicle (8).

As with surgical treatment, there is considerable variation in the data on persistence of varicoceles after transfemoral treatment. Although there are several studies in which patients were followed up for persistence of varicocele (2,5), in some only palpation or sonography were used and neither of these examination techniques can definitely exclude persistence of a varicocele. A persistence rate of about 10% is expected after distal sclerotherapy. In most cases, at least some improvement in the findings is seen even with persistence of a varicocele. However, it is not known to what extent varicocele reduction improves semen profiles. In unclear cases sclerotherapy can be repeated.

Sclerotherapy appears to be the method of choice for the treatment of varicoceles. Only patients in whom sclerotherapy is not possible (e.g., unfavorable vessel course) should undergo surgery.

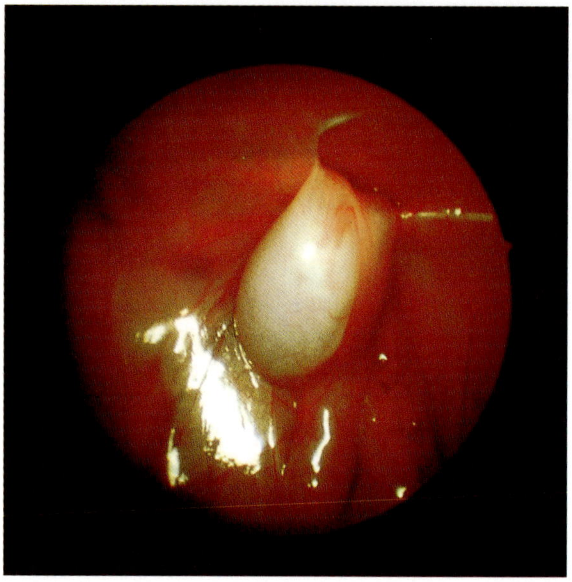

FIG. 10.7. Laparoscopic demonstration of an intra-abdominal testis in a boy with right-sided cryptorchidism. (Courtesy of D. Fahlenkamp, Charité, Humboldt-Universität zu Berlin.)

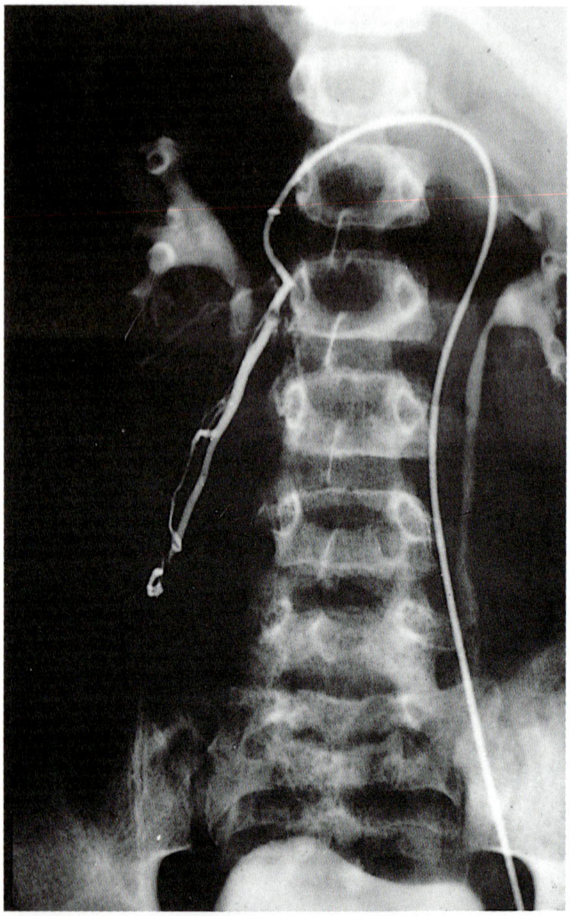

FIG. 10.6. Testicular venography in a boy with an impalpable right testis. The testicular vein is demonstrated, but the finding does not permit a reliable decision about whether a testicle is present or not. (Photo courtesy of D. Fahlenkamp, Charité, Humboldt-Universität zu Berlin.)

IMPALPABLE TESTES

Approximately 20% of undescended testes are impalpable (18). Some are located in the inguinal canal and are not palpable because of their small size or the surrounding tissue. Others are situated in the abdominal cavity or may be absent.

For many years the most widely used diagnostic procedure was testicular venography (17,19–21). When successfully performed, testicular venography significantly reduces the need for surgical exploration. Three distinct radiographic findings have been reported in the literature.

1. Demonstration of a pampiniform plexus (Fig. 10.6)
2. Demonstration of the testicular parenchyma
3. Demonstration of a blind-ending testicular vein

These findings, however, do not allow one to determine whether or not a testicle is present. If a pampiniform plexus is demonstrated, it is most likely that a testicle is present (22). If there is a blind-ending testicular vein, it is most unlikely that a testicle is present.

There are a number of **disadvantages** to testicular venography. It requires a highly skilled angiographer, especially in children, and even so, in 30% to 40% of cases the origin of the testicular vein cannot be found or the flow of the contrast material is obstructed by the presence of valves (22). Radiation exposure is five to ten times higher than that received when computerized tomography is used to search for an impalpable testis. In addition, venography is an invasive procedure, which may require sedation or anesthesia when performed in young children. Other major drawbacks of testicular venography are a high rate of unsuccessful procedures and the inability to distinguish cryptorchidism from testicular agenesis (since the testis is not visualized directly). As a result, testicular venography is rarely used nowadays and laparoscopy has become the procedure of choice for evaluating patients with impalpable testes (23). Laparoscopy is highly reliable in demonstrating intra-abdominal testes (Fig. 10.7) and at the same time allows mobilization of the undescended testis and orchiectomy of an atrophic or hypoplastic testis. An experienced examiner can perform a diagnostic laparoscopy in about 15 minutes and needs a total of about 30 minutes when additional endoscopic orchiectomy is performed.

REFERENCES

1. Kadir S. *Diagnostic angiography.* Philadelphia: WB Saunders; 1986:486–488.
2. Zeitler E. Testicular vein occlusion for the treatment of infertility. In: Kadir S, ed. *Current practice of interventional radiology.* Philadelphia: Decker; 1991:709–715.
3. Katayama H, Yamaguchi K, Kozuka T, Takashima T, Seez P, Matsuura K. Adverse reactions to ionic and nonionic contrast media. *Radiology* 1990;175:621–628.
4. Hinman F. *Atlas of urosurgical anatomy.* Philadelphia: WB Saunders; 1993:471–503.
5. Fobbe F, Hamm B, Sörensen R, Felsenberg D. Percutaneous transluminal treatment of varicoceles: where to occlude the internal spermatic vein. *AJR* 1987;149:983–987.
6. Riedl P. Radiologic anatomy of the left testicular vein in varicoceles. In: Jecht EW, Zeitler E, eds. *Varicocele and male infertility: recent advances in diagnosis and therapy.* Berlin: Springer-Verlag; 1982:49–58.
7. Gillenwater JY, Grayhack JT, Howards SS, Ducket JW, eds. *Adult and pediatric urology,* 2nd ed. St Louis: Mosby–Year Book; 1991: 1453–1477.
8. Hamm B, Fobbe F, Sörensen R, Felsenberg D. Varicoceles: combined sonography and thermography in diagnosis and posttherapeutic evaluation. *Radiology* 1986;160:419–424.
9. Gonda RL, Karo JJ, Forte RA, O'Donnell KT. Diagnosis of subclinical varicocele in infertility. *AJR* 1987;148:71–75.
10. Macek DH, Levran Z, Jafri SZ, Madrazo BL, Goldman KA. Value of color Doppler in detection of varicoceles in infertile men. RSNA '93 Scientific Program. *Radiology* 1993;189 (suppl):376.
11. Verstoppen GR, Steeno OP. Varicocele and the pathogenesis of the associated subfertility. A review of the various theories. I: Varicocelogenesis. *Andrologia* 1977;9:133–140.
12. McClure RD, Khoo D, Jarvi K, Hricak H. Subclinical varicocele: the effectiveness of varicocelectomy. *J Urol* 1991;145:789–791.
13. Verstoppen GR, Steeno OP. Varicocele and the pathogenesis of the associated subfertility. A review of the various theories. II: Results of surgery. *Andrologia* 1977;9:293–305.
14. Pollack HM, ed. *Clinical urography: an atlas and textbook of urological imaging.* Philadelphia: WB Saunders; 1990:2994–2996.
15. Geatti O, Gasparini D, Shapiro B. A comparison of scintigraphy, thermography, ultrasound and phlebography in grading of clinical varicocele. *J Nucl Med* 1991;32:2092–2097.
16. Petros JA, Andriole GL, Middleton WD, Picus DA. Correlation of testicular color Doppler ultrasonography, physical examination and venography in the detection of left varicoceles in men with infertility. *J Urol* 1991;145:785–788.
17. Amin M, Wheeler CS. Selective testicular venography in abdominal cryptorchidism. *J Urol* 1976;115:760–761.
18. Levitt SB, Kogan SJ, Engel RM, Weiss RM, Martin DC, Ehrlich RM. The impalpable testis: a rational approach to management. *J Urol* 1978;120:515–520.
19. Diamond AB, Meng CH, Kodroff M, Goldman SM. Testicular venography in the nonpalpable testis. *AJR* 1977;129:129–135.
20. Greenberg SH, Ring EJ, Oleaga J, Wein AJ. Gonadal venography for preoperative localization of nonpalpable testis in adults. *Urology* 1979;13:453–455.
21. Weiss RM, Glickman MG. Localization and management of nonpalpable undescended testes. *Surg Clin North Am* 1980;60:1253–1263.
22. Khan O, Krausz T, Williams G. Testicular venography in impalpable testis. *Eur Urol* 1993;9:341–342.
23. Fahlenkamp D, Raatz D, Schönberger B. Laparoscopic diagnosis and therapy of cryptorchidism. *Urologe* 1992;31:328–332.

Self-Examination Atlas

TIPS FOR USING THE ATLAS

The purpose of this self-examination atlas is to test and improve skills in the analysis of scrotal images. The following cases cover a wide range of pathologic alterations of the scrotum.

The atlas will be most helpful if it is used to simulate clinical practice as closely as possible. We recommend, therefore, that you first cover the text portion and try to interpret the images on the basis of the case history and clinical findings alone. Then, step by step, compare your own interpretation and analysis with the description given in the text. For each case, the diagnosis (conclusion) from the imaging findings and the final diagnosis (based on histologic examination or the clinical course) are given. There is an occasional addition of notes highlighting areas of interest. Case presentations are grouped by modalities.

To minimize bias in each subgroup, cases are presented in a random order, just as in daily clinical routine, rather than according to anatomic aspects or clinical pictures. Frequent disorders and entities that may pose problems in differential diagnosis are presented most often and very rare disorders are not included. Cases in each subsection are presented in order of difficulty. For better orientation, each sonogram is provided with a small drawing indicating the position of the transducer. The left margin of the figure is oriented toward the patient's head for longitudinal scans through the scrotum and toward the patient's right side for transverse scans. The presented images, the data from the patient's history, and the physical findings as well as a description of the imaging findings are restricted to the relevant features of each case.

Case 1

A 28-year-old patient presents with vague bilateral scrotal pain. He has had no prior episodes of infection.

Physical Examination. The scrotal contents are normal to palpation and there is increased tenderness of both testes.

Ultrasound. Longitudinal view (Fig. 1A) and transverse view (Fig. 1B) of the left testis. The homogeneous echotexture is interrupted only by a hyperechoic band.

Conclusion. The hyperechoic intratesticular band is the mediastinum testis.

Notes. This eccentrically located, hyperechoic band that increases in thickness caudally to cranially is the typical sonographic appearance of the mediastinum testis. In the majority of cases, it is not displayed as clearly as in this patient.

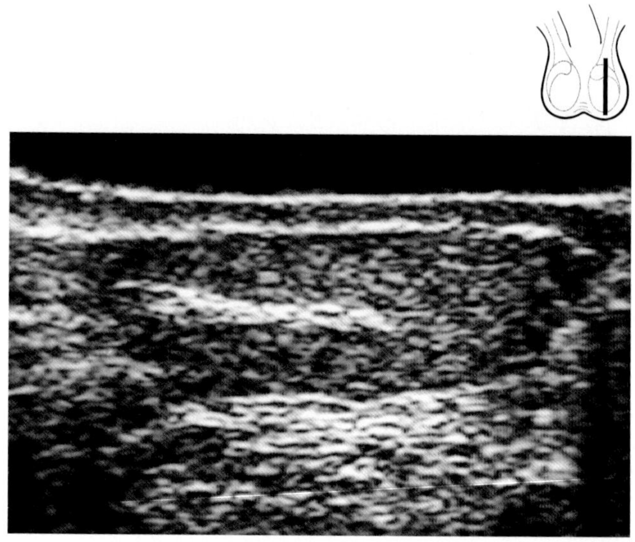

A

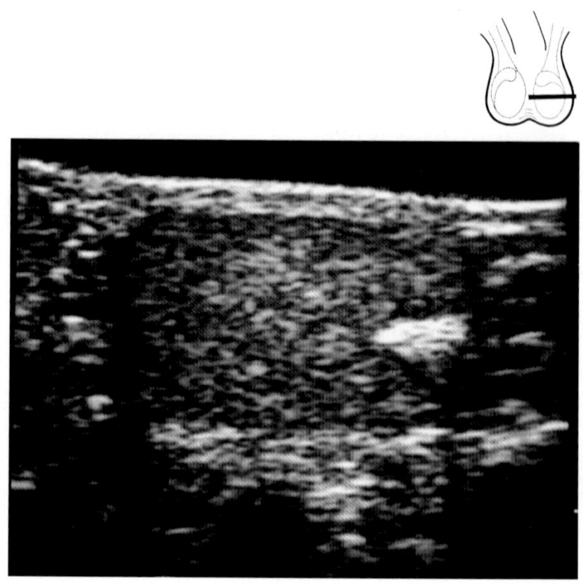

B

Case 2

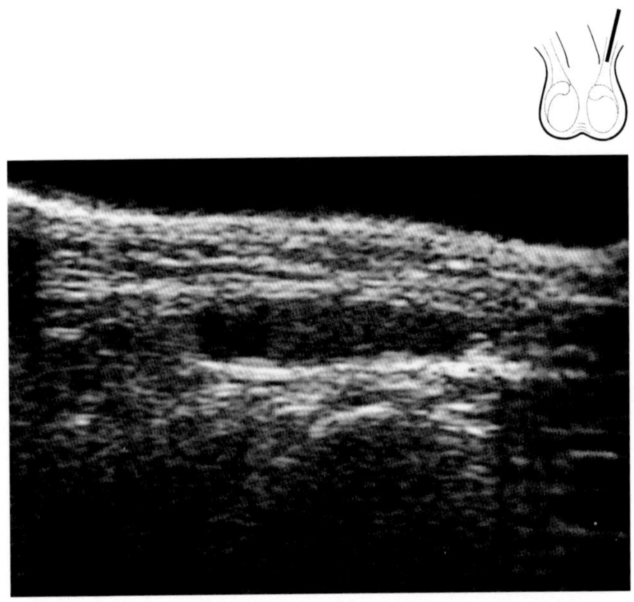

A 31-year-old patient presents with left-sided cryptorchidism.

Physical Examination. The left testis is palpable in the inguinal canal. Evaluation of testicular consistency is limited.

Ultrasound. Longitudinal view of the left testis in the inguinal canal (Fig. 2). A small, elongated testis of uniformly decreased echogenicity can be identified. The hypoechoic epididymal head is displayed at the upper pole of the testis. The undescended testis is mobile on coughing.

Conclusion. Cryptorchid, hypoplastic testis on the left without suspicion of tumor.

Notes. Homogeneously decreased echogenicity is typical of the immature undescended testis and testicular atrophy.

Case 3

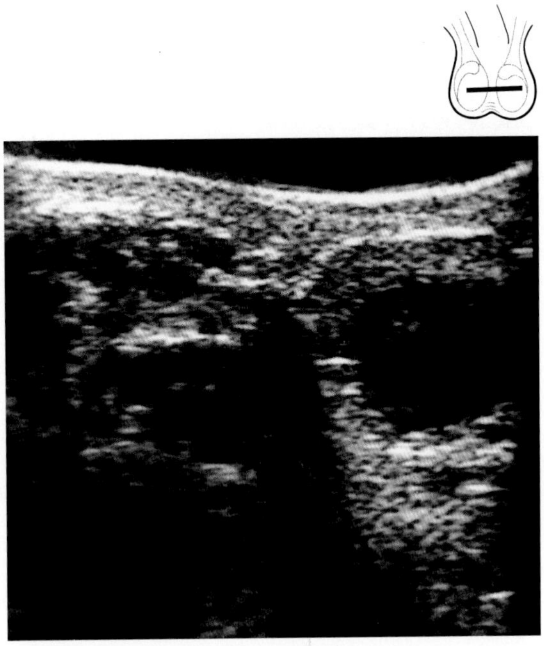

A 32-year-old patient with a 2-year history of recurrent right testicular swelling now presents with an additional inflammatory component.

Physical Examination. There is a large, moderately tender indurated right hemiscrotum. The right testis cannot be palpated separately and there is slight erythema and edema of the scrotal skin. There is no transillumination. The left testis is of normal shape and size, but it is of slightly increased consistency.

Ultrasound. Transverse view of both testes (Fig. 3). The right testis contains a large, inhomogeneous mass with multiple cystic spaces. The thickness of the scrotal skin on the right is slightly increased. In addition, a nodular and well-defined lesion of markedly decreased echogenicity is seen in the normal-sized left testis.

Analysis. The extensive, irregular destruction of the right testis leaves no doubt about the diagnosis of a tumor, particularly since there are no inflammatory changes such as epididymal enlargement or homogeneously decreased echogenicity of the testicular tissue. The abnormality of the left testis, which was barely noted during the physical examination (the testis was indurated and only slightly painful), suggests an additional tumor on the left.

Conclusion. Bilateral testicular tumor.

Histology. Mature teratoma and embryonal cell carcinoma of the right testis and seminoma of the left testis.

Case 4

A 33-year-old patient presents with painless swelling of the left testis following antibiotic treatment for left epididymo-orchitis.

Physical Examination. Firm, painful mass in the normal-sized left testis. The left epididymis is of normal shape and size and can be separated from the testis.

Ultrasound. Longitudinal scan of the left testis (Fig. 4A) and transverse scan of both testes (Fig. 4B). The left testis is of normal size and shape and contains an intratesticular, hypoechoic lesion with well-defined borders. Only a thin rim of normal testicular parenchyma is identified. The epididymal head is unremarkable (see Figure 4A). There is a minimally increased amount of fluid in the serous cavity consistent with a hydrocele.

Analysis. Despite the reported inflammation 3 weeks previously, clinical findings indicate a tumor and are confirmed by the sonographic demonstration of a focal intratesticular lesion.

Conclusion. Testicular tumor.

Histology. Seminoma (Fig. 4C).

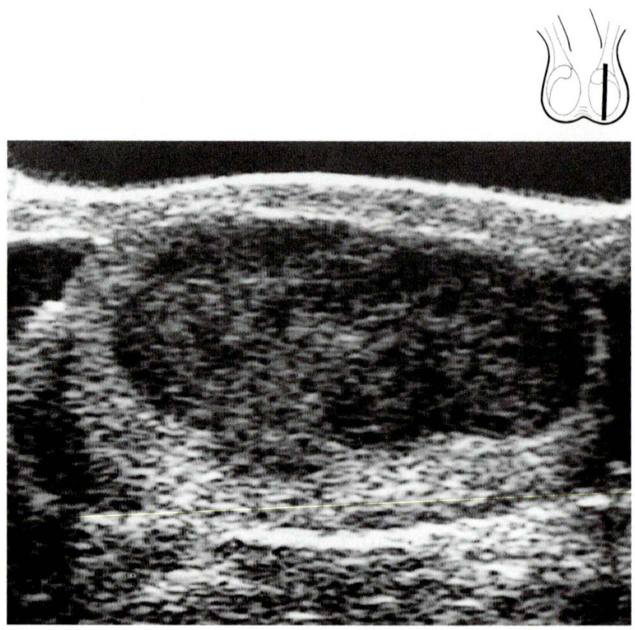

A

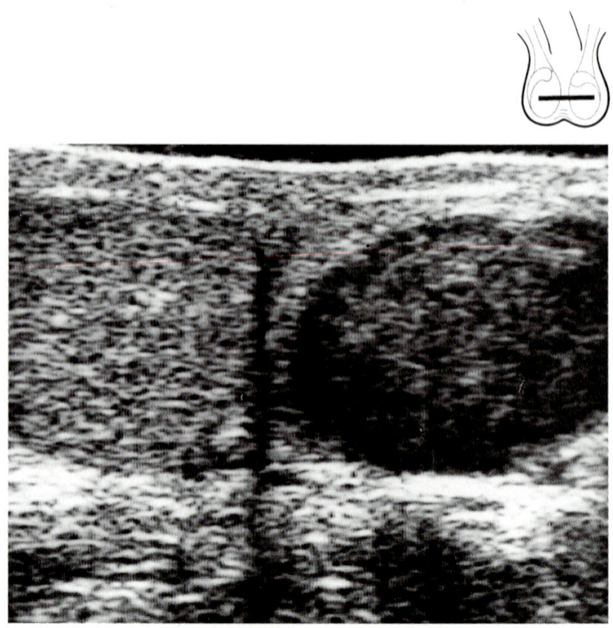

B

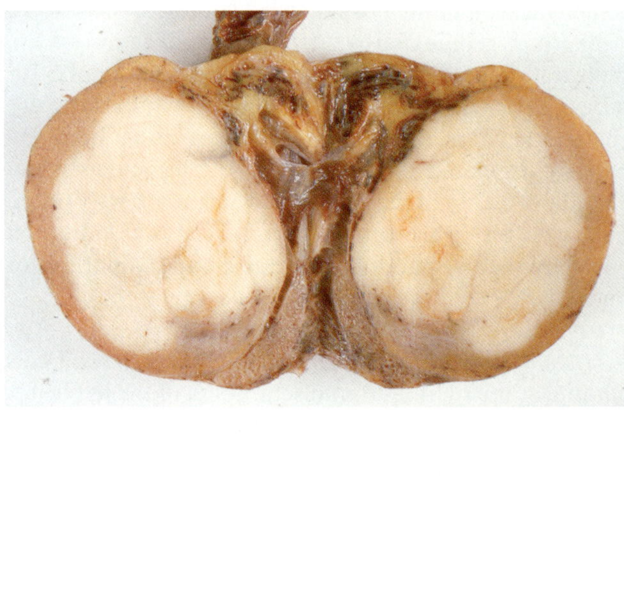

C

Case 5

A 42-year-old patient reports unchanged swelling of the left testis following scrotal trauma 6 weeks earlier.

Physical Examination. There is nontender enlargement and induration of the left testis. The hemiscrotum does not transilluminate.

Ultrasound. Longitudinal scan of the left testis (Fig. 5A) and transverse scan of both testes (Fig. 5B). The left testis is enlarged and demonstrates predominantly hypoechoic echotexture.

Analysis. Palpation and sonographic demonstration of an intratesticular, solid lesion are highly suggestive of tumor. The patient's history might suggest an intrascrotal hematoma or hematocele.

Conclusion. Left testicular tumor.

Histology. Seminoma.

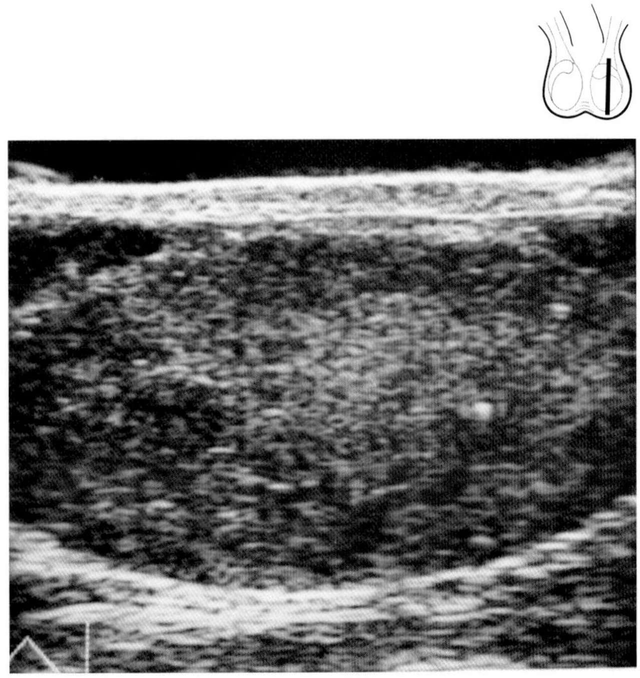

A

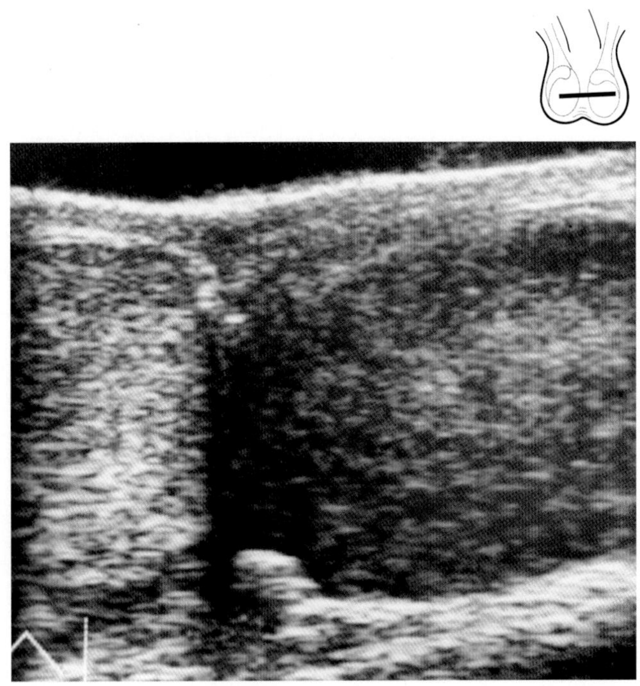

B

Case 6

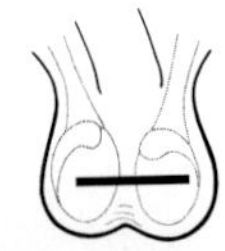

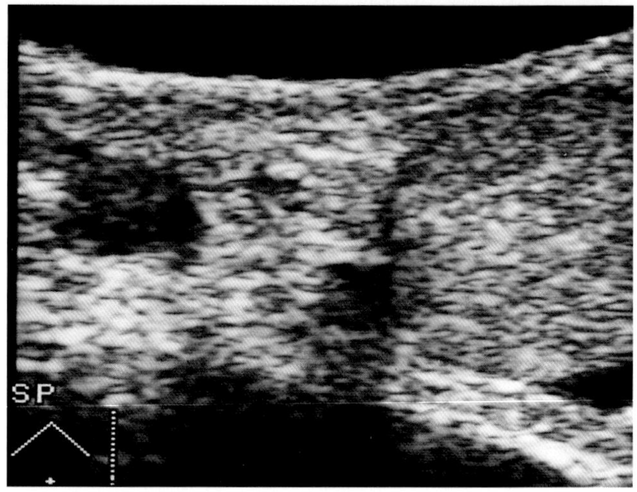

A 63-year-old patient presents with a history of right herniotomy (several years previously) and subsequent atrophy of the ipsilateral testis. He is now referred for a suspected testicular tumor on the left.

Physical Examination. Moderately tender testis on the left, no mass. Left epididymis can be delineated. Very small, soft testis on the right.

Ultrasound. Transverse scan of both testes (Fig. 6). The left testis is normal in size and echogenicity. The right testis is very small and hypoechoic.

Conclusion. Right testicular atrophy following herniotomy. Normal left testis.

Case 7

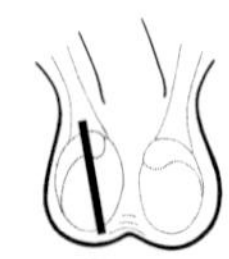

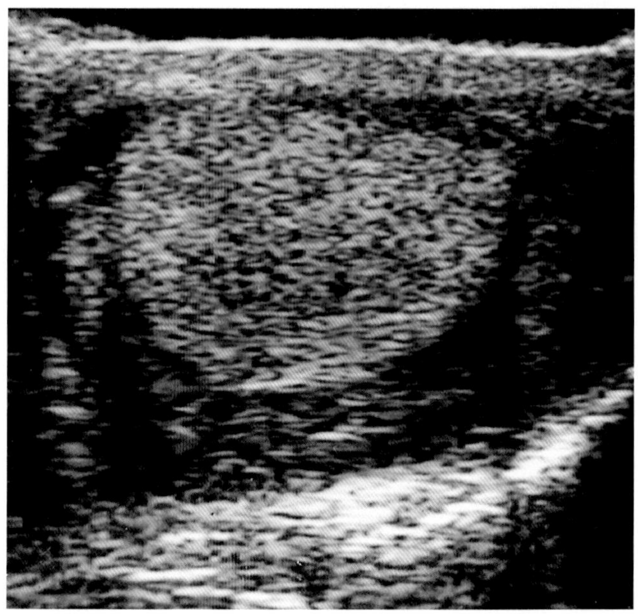

A 31-year-old diabetic patient presents with painful swelling of the right hemiscrotum, fever, and leukocytosis.

Physical Examination. The right epididymis, especially the tail, is enlarged and extremely painful. There is edema and erythema of the scrotal skin. The hemiscrotum does not transilluminate.

Ultrasound. Longitudinal scan of the right testis (Fig. 7). The tail and body of the epididymis are markedly enlarged and hypoechoic with nearly normal size and echogenicity of the epididymal head. The testis appears normal, but there is scrotal skin edema.

Conclusion. Acute epididymitis on the right.

Clinical Course. The further course was uneventful with antibiotic treatment.

Notes. Despite the clinically convincing picture of epididymitis, an underlying testicular tumor should be excluded. This can be reliably achieved by ultrasound scanning.

Case 8

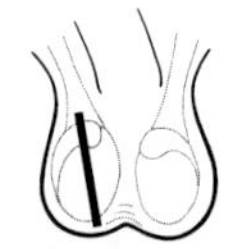

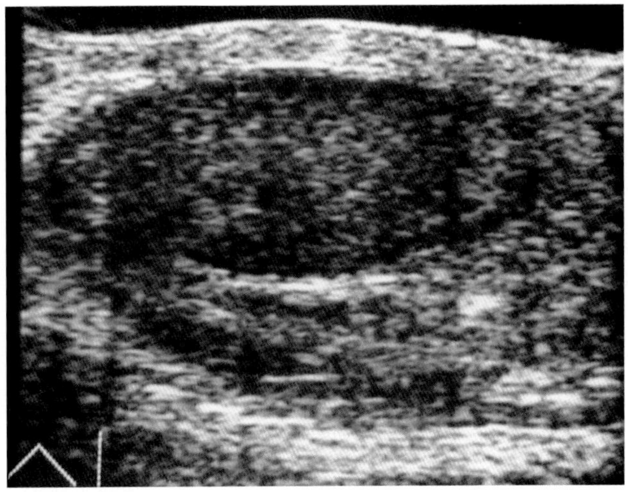

A 53-year-old patient presents with a painful swelling of the right testis of 6 days' duration. There is leukocytosis and fever.

Physical Examination. There is swelling of the right scrotum. The testis and epididymis are not separately discernible.

Ultrasound. Longitudinal scan of the right testis (Fig. 8). The epididymis is enlarged (predominantly the tail and body). The testis is uniformly hypoechoic and there is scrotal skin edema.

Conclusion. Epididymo-orchitis.

Clinical Course. Resolution of symptoms with antibiotic treatment.

Case 9

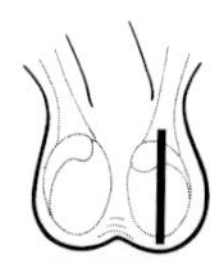

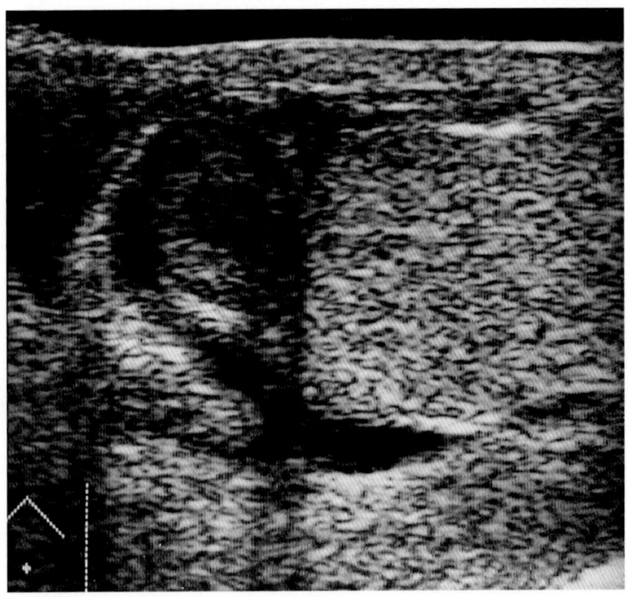

A 33-year-old patient presents with a 2-week history of painful testicular swelling.

Physical Examination. There is a markedly indurated and very tender swelling in the area of the left upper pole of the testis (most likely related to the epididymal head). Pain is relieved by elevation and cooling.

Ultrasound. Longitudinal scan of the left testis (Fig. 9). The left epididymal head is enlarged and hypoechoic and is clearly delineated from the adjacent testicular parenchyma. The testis is normal. There is a small hydrocele.

Conclusion. Acute epididymitis on the left, mainly affecting the head.

Clinical Course. Resolution of symptoms with antibiotic treatment.

Notes. In this case the ultrasound examination reliably excludes a possible tumor in the area of the upper pole of the testis.

Case 10

A 42-year-old patient presents with a painful, acute swelling of the right testis.

Physical Examination. The right scrotum is tender and swollen. Severe pain prevents palpation, but there is erythema and swelling of the scrotal skin and fever. The hemiscrotum does not transilluminate.

Ultrasound. Longitudinal scan of the right testis (Fig. 10A). There is massive enlargement of the testis and epididymis with markedly reduced echogenicity and mild irregularity of the testicular echotexture. Pronounced scrotal skin edema can also be seen.

Analysis. There is clear clinical evidence of epididymo-orchitis. The slightly inhomogeneous echotexture of the testicular tissue can be explained by the severity of the inflammatory process.

Conclusion. Severe epididymo-orchitis.

Clinical Course. Even with antibiotic treatment, there is only slow resolution of symptoms. Ultrasound follow-up after 2 weeks (Fig. 10B) demonstrates reduction of testicular swelling but persistence of hypoechoic testicular tissue and scrotal skin edema. Sonographic follow-up after 8 months (Fig. 10C) displays postinflammatory testicular atrophy.

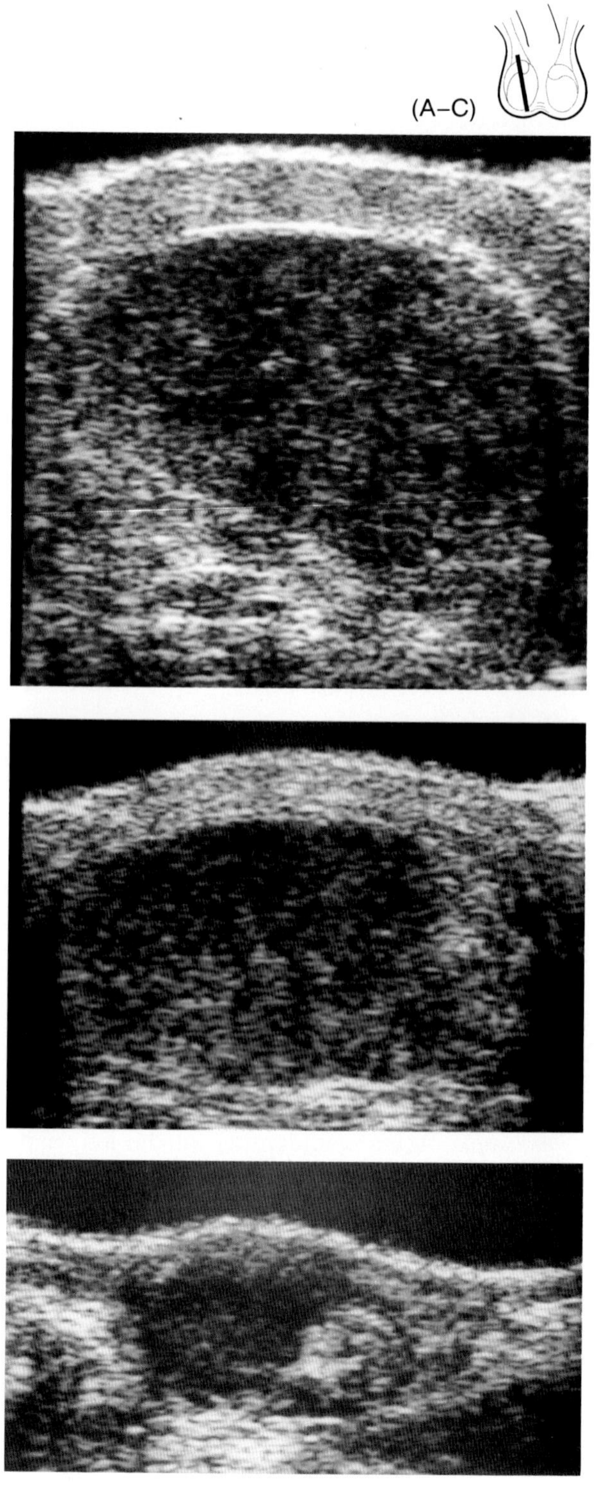

(A–C)

A

B

C

Case 11

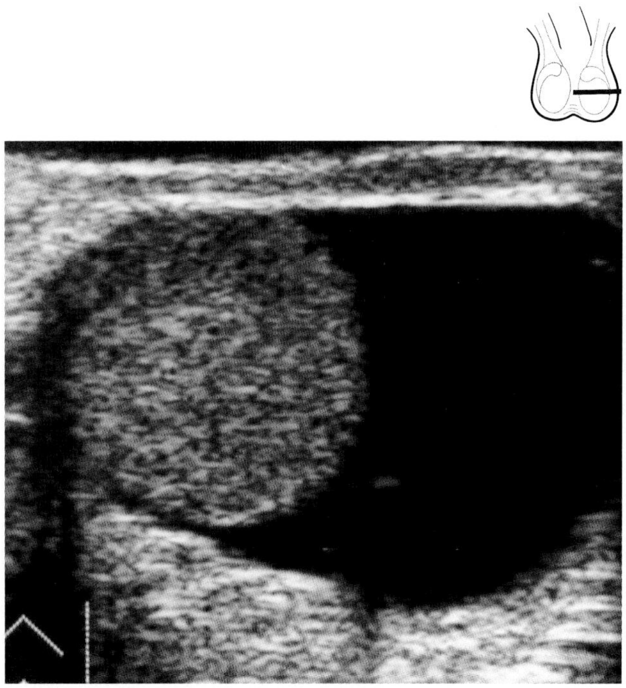

A 21-year-old patient with slow, painless swelling of the left hemiscrotum, first noticed 4 months before presentation.

Physical Examination. The left scrotum is tense but not tender. The testis cannot be differentiated from the epididymis. The left hemiscrotum transilluminates, and there are no signs of inflammation.

Ultrasound. Transverse scan of the left hemiscrotum (Fig. 11). There is a large collection of fluid—hydrocele. The testis and epididymis (not shown) are normal.

Conclusion. Hydrocele. Exclusion of testicular tumor.

Case 12

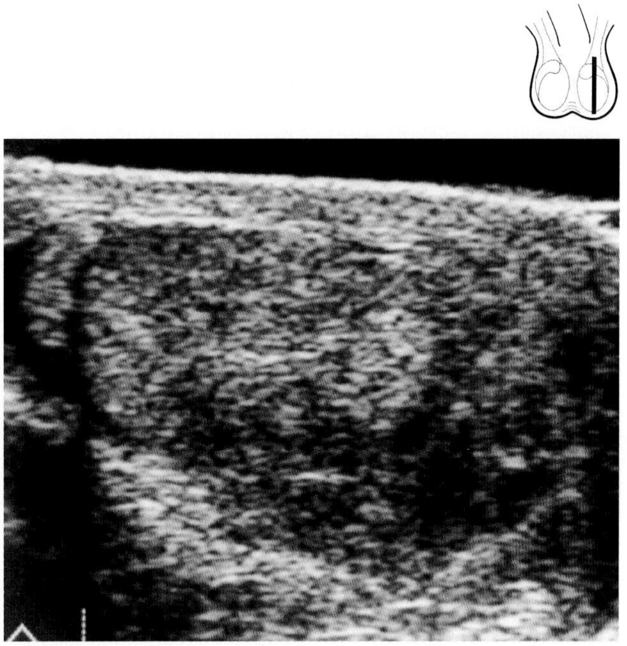

A 31-year-old patient presents with swelling and pain following blunt scrotal trauma 2 days previously.

Physical Examination. There is very tender swelling of the left hemiscrotum. The testis and epididymis cannot be palpated separately, and there is no transillumination, fever, or leukocytosis.

Ultrasound. Longitudinal scan of the left testis (Fig. 12). There is an inhomogeneous, partly hypoechoic, enlarged epididymal tail. Delineation from the adjacent lower pole of the testis is unclear. The epididymal head appears normal.

Analysis. In light of the patient's history and clinical findings, the swelling of the epididymis is most likely caused by a traumatic hemorrhage. There may also be small hemorrhages into the adjacent testicular tissue. Since there is no increased fluid (hematocele), testicular rupture seems to be unlikely.

Conclusion. Hemorrhages in the body and tail of the epididymis and suspected small intratesticular hemorrhages secondary to trauma.

Intraoperative Findings and Histology. Extensive hemorrhages and partial necroses of the epididymis. No rupture of the testis.

Case 13

A 73-year-old patient presents with asymptomatic enlargement of the right hemiscrotum.

Physical Examination. There is painless swelling of the right hemiscrotum, consistent with a hydrocele, and a firm, spherical mass in the area of the head of the right epididymis. The testis is normal to palpation and clearly separate from the epididymis. There are no signs of inflammation.

Ultrasound. Longitudinal view of the upper pole of the right testis (Fig. 13). A roundish, smoothly demarcated and nearly anechoic lesion can be seen in the head of the right epididymis. Some echoes, however, are seen in its dependent portion. There is hydrocele anterior to the epididymal head. The testis appears normal.

Conclusion. Spermatocele of the epididymal head. Presence of internal echoes favors the diagnosis of a spermatocele over an epididymal cyst. Also seen is a hydrocele.

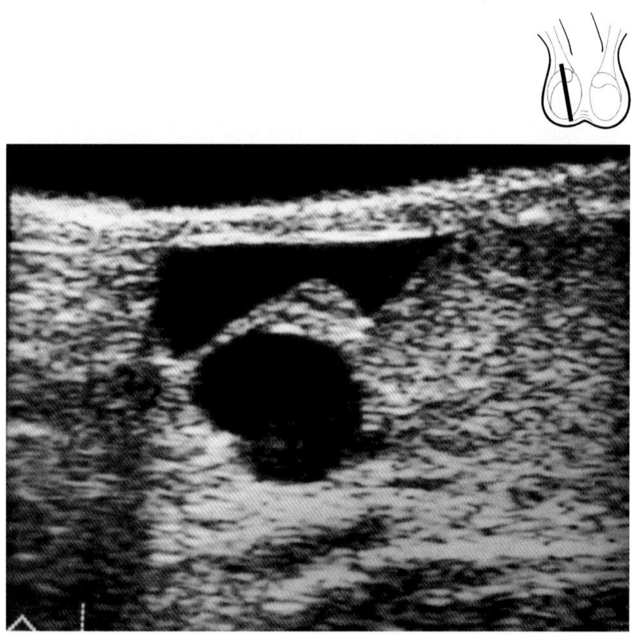

Case 14

A 28-year-old patient reports a slight feeling of heaviness in the area of the left testis.

Physical Examination. The testis and epididymis appear normal on both sides. There is an engorgement of the spermatic cord with the patient standing.

Ultrasound. Longitudinal scan showing the upper pole of the testis and the spermatic cord on the left (Fig. 14). Tortuous, dilated veins of the pampiniform plexus can be seen with a Valsalva maneuver or when the patient stands. Normal testis and epididymis bilaterally.

Conclusion. Varicocele on the left.

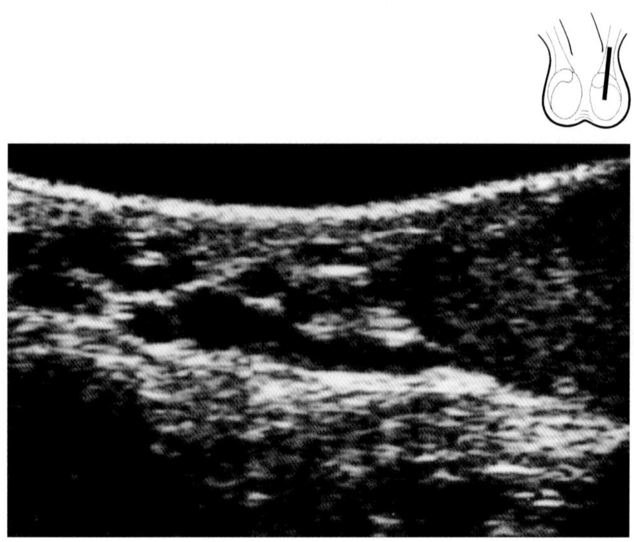

Case 15

A 33-year-old patient presents with a 6-month history of progressive, painless swelling of the left testis.

Physical Examination. The left testis is nodular, firm, and painless.

Ultrasound. Longitudinal scan showing part of the left testis (Fig. 15). The testis is enlarged and testicular tissue is replaced by large irregular cystic and solid portions. A rim of normal testicular parenchyma is seen posteriorly. A small amount of paratesticular fluid—hydrocele—can be seen. There is thickening of the scrotal skin.

Conclusion. Testicular tumor.

Histology. Malignant testicular tumor with elements of mature teratoma, embryonal carcinoma, and choriocarcinoma. No infiltration of the scrotal skin.

Notes. Intratesticular cystic lesions may be associated with a tumor (particularly teratoma). So-called secondary signs of inflammation, such as hydrocele or scrotal skin edema, sometimes also occur in conjunction with a testicular tumor.

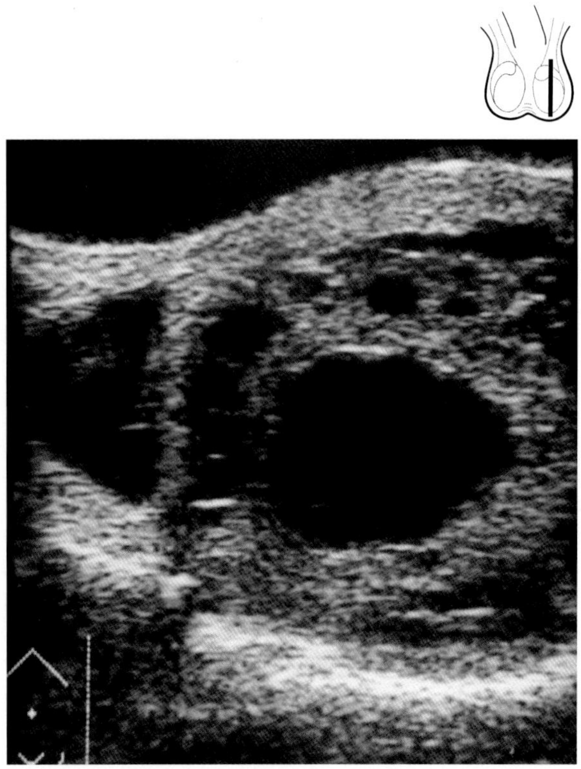

Case 16

A 43-year-old patient presents with a small lump at the upper pole of his right testis.

Physical Examination. A small, painless, firm mass can be palpated in the area of the right epididymal head. The right testis is normal to palpation. There is a hydrocele and no signs of inflammation.

Ultrasound. Longitudinal scan of the right testis (Fig. 16). Small, calcified foci can be identified in the head of the epididymis. The testis is of normal appearance. A moderately increased amount of fluid is seen superior to the testis.

Analysis. Although calcifications of the epididymis are rare, they may occur secondary to inflammatory processes or hemorrhages. On closer questioning, the patient reported that he had been a wrestler for several years and had experienced occasional scrotal trauma.

Conclusion. Calcifications of the epididymis (probably secondary to trauma). There is no evidence of a testicular tumor.

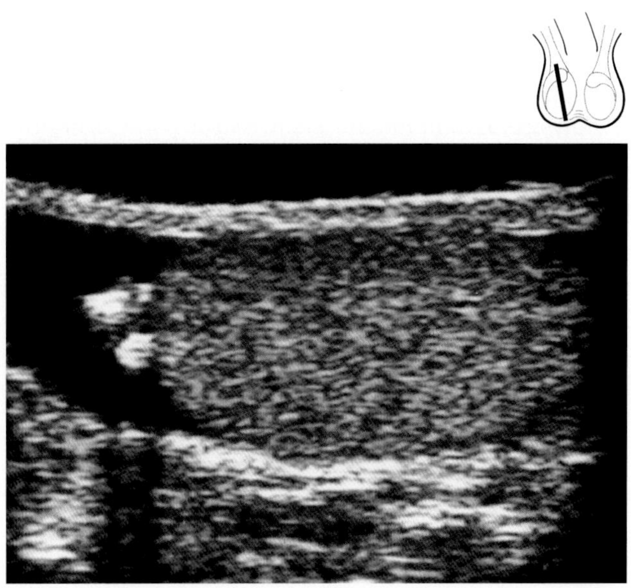

Case 17

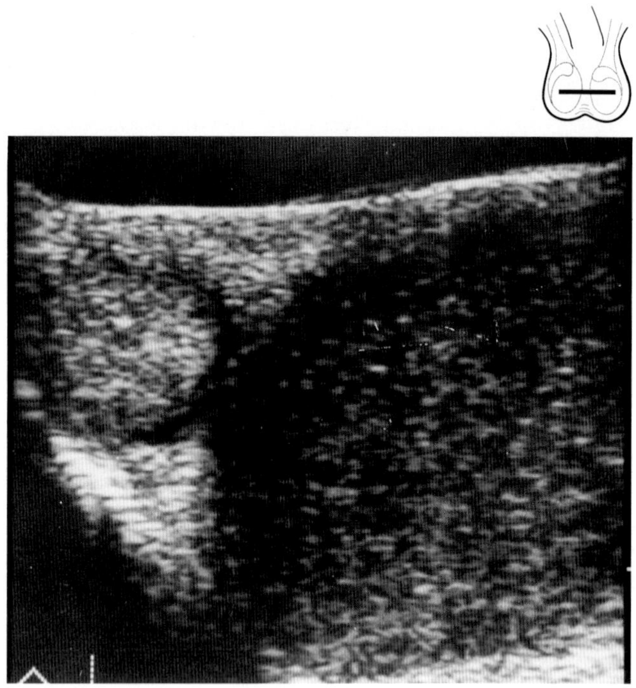

A 56-year-old patient presents with acute onset of slightly painful swelling of the left testis of 3 days' duration. Temperature of up to 40°C. Patient reports soft tissue swelling in the area of the left parotid gland 10 days prior to presentation.

Physical Examination. There is induration and pronounced swelling of the left testis with moderate tenderness.

Ultrasound. Transverse scan of both testes (Fig. 17). The left testis is markedly enlarged and hypoechoic.

Analysis. The rather painless and firm enlargement of the left testis in combination with the sonographic appearance suggests a testicular tumor. The elevated temperature suggests orchitis, probably mumps orchitis given the history of parotid gland swelling.

Conclusion. Suspicion of orchitis; no definite exclusion of a testicular tumor.

Clinical Course. Slow resolution of symptoms under conservative therapy. A subsequent biopsy demonstrated orchitis.

Case 18

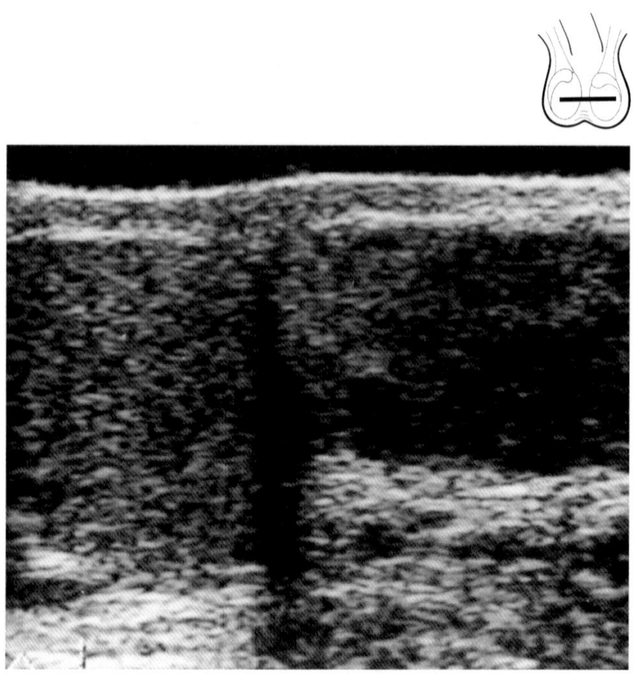

A 29-year-old patient presents with hardening of the left testis of 3 weeks' duration. There is no history of trauma or inflammation.

Physical Examination. There is firm, painless induration of the left testis, which is smaller than the contralateral testis.

Ultrasound. Transverse scan of both testes (Fig. 18). The left testis is small but the echotexture is inhomogeneous and echo-poor. Normal size and echogenicity of the right testis.

Conclusion. Left testicular tumor.

Histology. Seminoma.

Case 19

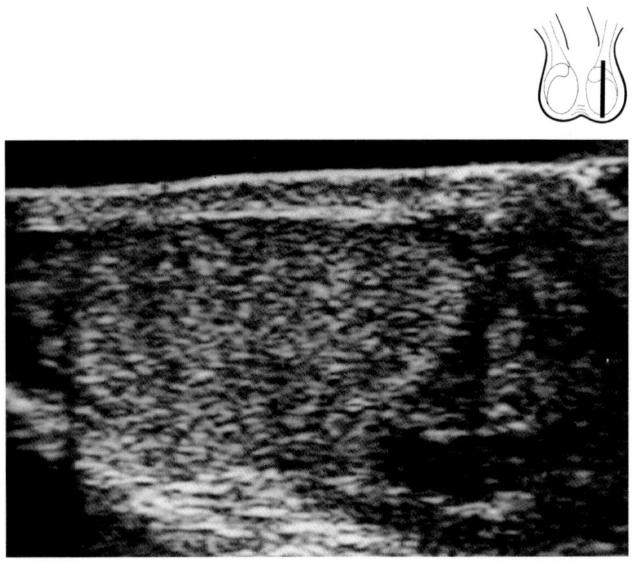

A 22-year-old patient presents with acute testicular swelling on the left and severe pain persisting for 2 days. He has been referred for suspected testicular torsion.

Physical Examination. There is very painful swelling and induration in the area of the lower pole of the left testis. The left epididymal head seems normal.

Ultrasound. Longitudinal scan of the left testis (Fig. 19). The testis appears normal, with a homogeneous echotexture of medium echogenicity. There is pronounced swelling, moderate inhomogeneity and hypoechoic appearance of the tail of epididymis; the head is unremarkable.

Analysis. The diagnosis of testicular torsion (initially indicated by the patient's age and the acute onset of pain) can be dismissed in view of the normal echotexture of the testis. A tumor in the area of the lower pole of the testis can likewise be excluded. Ultrasound examination clearly assigns the pathologic changes to the tail of the epididymis. Considering the clinical symptoms, epididymitis mainly affecting the tail appears to be the most likely diagnosis.

Conclusion. Left-sided epididymitis.

Clinical Course. Symptoms resolved with antibiotic treatment.

Case 20

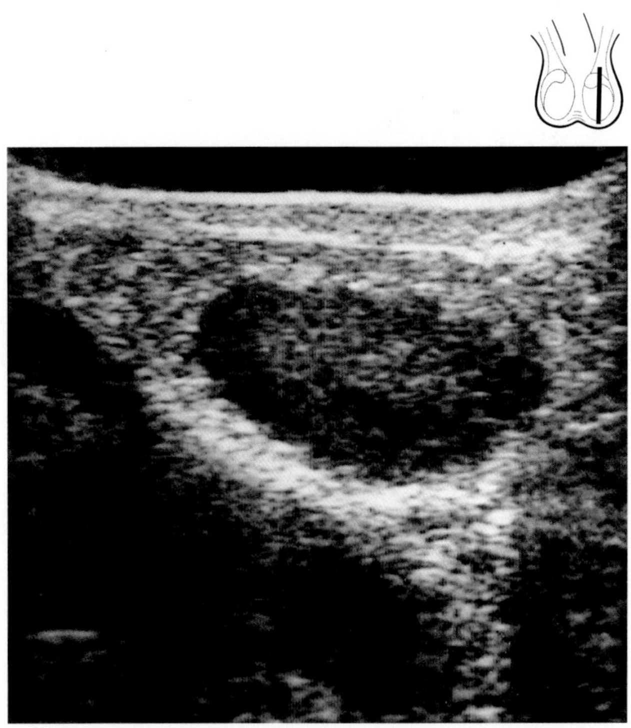

A 26-year-old patient presents for evaluation of a lump in the left testis discovered on self-examination.

Physical Examination. There is a painless, firm mass in the left testis.

Ultrasound. Longitudinal scan of the left testis (Fig. 20). A hypoechoic intratesticular lesion is surrounded by a thin rim of residual testicular parenchyma. The head of the epididymis is seen separately.

Conclusion. Left testicular tumor.

Histology. Seminoma.

Case 21

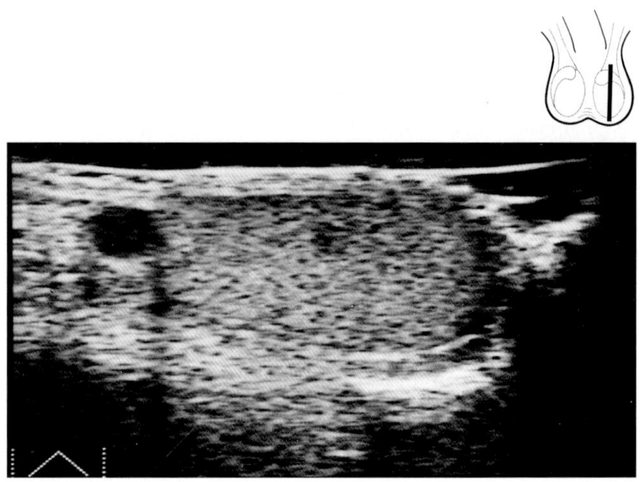

A 45-year-old patient presents with vague complaints related to the upper abdomen. Diagnostic tests demonstrate a large (approximately 11 cm in diameter) paraaortic mass. There is a history of left-sided mumps orchitis 8 years previously.

Physical Examination. Both testes are of normal shape, size, and consistency and there are no suspicious masses. A small, spherical mass in the area of the left epididymal head is suggestive of a spermatocele.

Ultrasound. Longitudinal scan of the left testis (Fig. 21). There is a very small (approximately 4 mm in diameter), hypoechoic intratesticular lesion with an otherwise normal testicular echotexture. A smoothly demarcated, cystic space in the epididymal head is clearly separate from the testis. The right testis (not shown) is unremarkable.

Analysis. The sonographic examination was performed to exclude a primary testicular cancer as the cause of the retroperitoneal mass. The findings, however (a focal intratesticular lesion in conjunction with a retroperitoneal mass), do suggest a testicular tumor, although it was not palpable.

Conclusion. High probability of a small testicular tumor on the left with extensive retroperitoneal metastases. A cyst in the head of the left epididymis is an incidental finding.

Histology. Seminoma.

Case 22

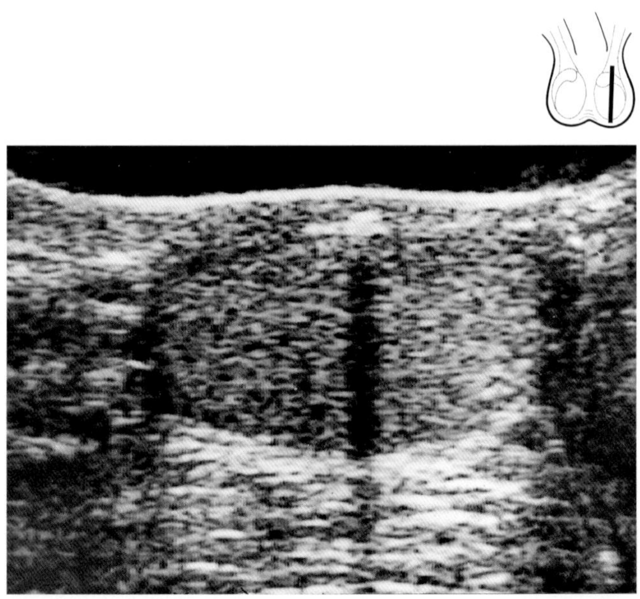

A 29-year-old patient presents for evaluation of a small lump in his left testis.

Physical Examination. The testes are of normal size. There is a firm, painless mass (approximately 5 mm in diameter) in the left testis.

Ultrasound. Longitudinal scan of the left testis (Fig. 22). A plaquelike calcification can be seen in the area of the tunica albuginea with posterior acoustic shadowing. Scanning of the left testis from a dorsal direction (not shown) demonstrates a normal, homogeneous echotexture of the testicular parenchyma adjacent to the calcified area.

Conclusion. Calcification of the tunica albuginea, no indication of tumor.

Clinical Course. Findings are unchanged at 6-month follow-up.

Case 23

A 35-year-old patient presents with azospermia and bilateral cryptorchidism.

Physical Examination. Both testes can be palpated in the superficial inguinal pouch.

Ultrasound. Longitudinal view of the left testis (Fig. 23). A small, elongated testicle of uniformly decreased echogenicity can be identified just outside the external inguinal ring. The right testis (not shown) has a similar appearance.

Conclusion. Bilateral hypoplastic undescended testis. There is no indication of tumor.

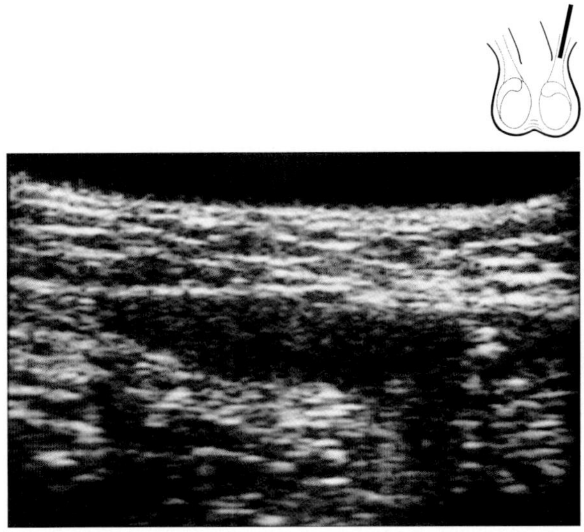

Case 24

A 26-year-old patient presents with painful swelling of the left hemiscrotum.

Physical Examination. There is painful induration of the left epididymal tail and induration along the spermatic cord. The testis is normal to palpation. Scrotal erythema and edema are apparent.

Ultrasound. Longitudinal scans showing the lower pole of the testis (Fig. 24A) and the spermatic cord (Fig. 24B) on the left.

Hypoechoic enlargement of the epididymal tail is identified. The testis is normal. There is a hypoechoic, bandlike structure in the area of the palpated induration along the spermatic cord.

Conclusion. Inflammation of the epididymal tail extending along the deferent duct.

Clinical Course. Urethral swab revealed gonococci, confirming gonorrheal epididymitis. Symptoms resolved with antibiotic treatment.

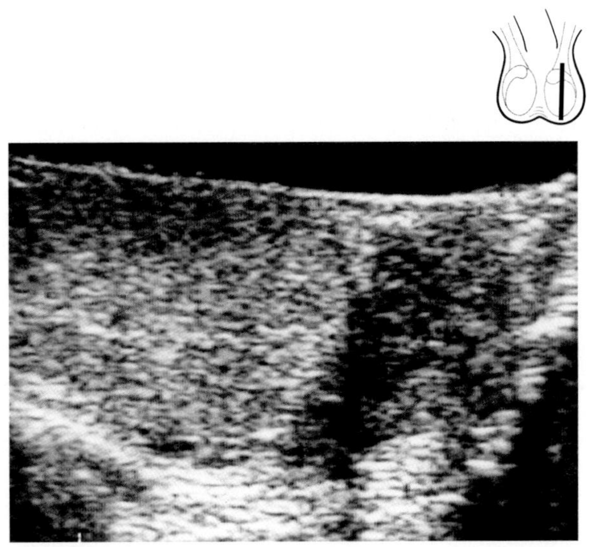

A

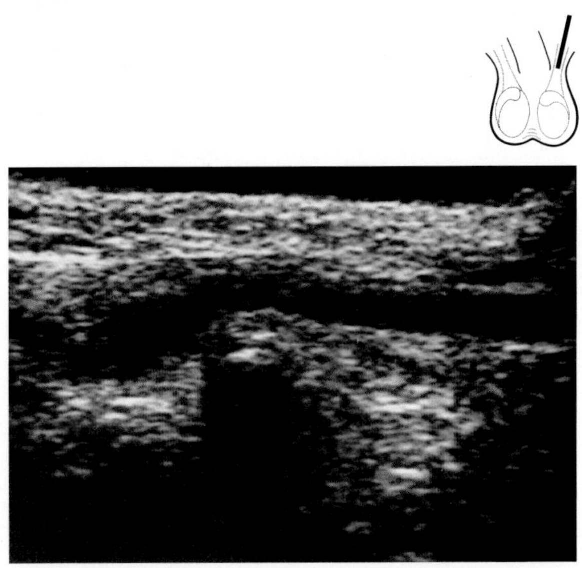

B

Case 25

A 37-year-old patient has noted a firm, nodular lump in his right hemiscrotum and presents for evaluation.

Physical Examination. There is a slightly tender mass (approximately 2 cm in diameter) in the area of the right epididymal head. The testis appears unremarkable to palpation.

Ultrasound. Longitudinal view of the upper pole of the right testis (Fig. 25). The testis is normal in appearance. Multiple, smoothly demarcated cystic spaces can be visualized in the area of the epididymal head.

Conclusion. Large, separate, multiple spermatoceles of the epididymal head on the right. No sign of testicular tumor.

Intraoperative Finding and Histology. Spermatoceles of the right epididymal head.

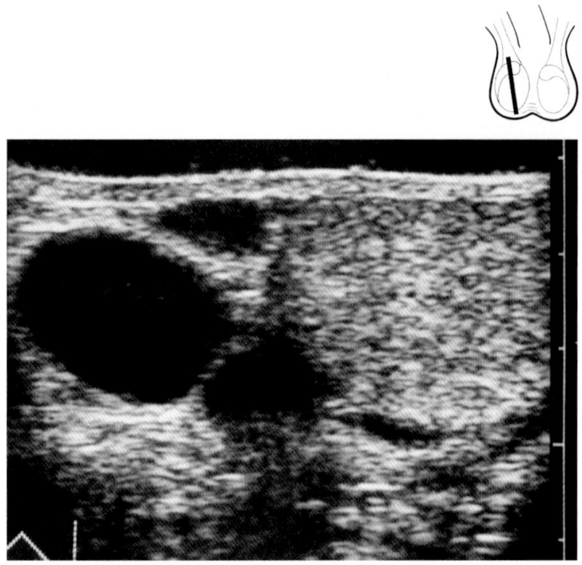

Case 26

A 20-year-old patient presents with acute left testicular pain of 4 days' duration. He has mild fever.

Physical Examination. The left hemiscrotum is very tender and palpation of the testis and epididymis is limited by pain.

Ultrasound. Longitudinal scan of the left testis (Fig. 26A). The left testis is normal in shape and size with uniformly decreased echogenicity. The head of the epididymis is enlarged and its echogenicity is similar to that of the testis.

Analysis. In view of the patient's age, a testicular tumor has to be considered. The palpation findings are of limited value because of considerable pain. However, the diffusely hypoechoic testis raises the possibility of infection.

Conclusion. Suspected epididymo-orchitis on the left.

Clinical Course. Symptoms improved with antibiotic treatment and at follow-up three months later palpation of the left testis was normal. A sonographic examination at this time (Fig. 26B) demonstrates multiple, poorly demarcated, hypoechoic testicular lesions corresponding to postinflammatory, irregular fibrotic changes.

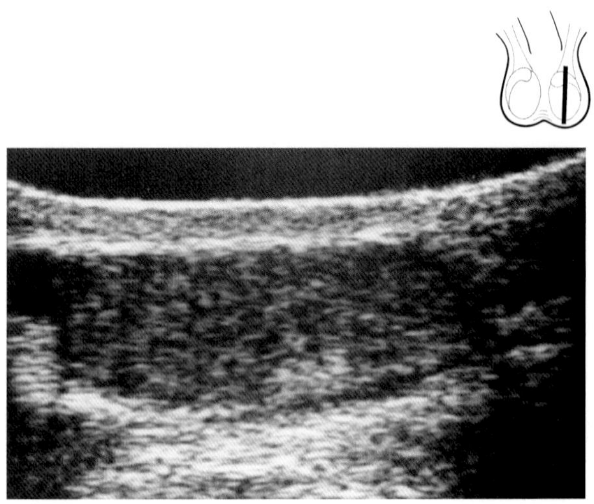

A

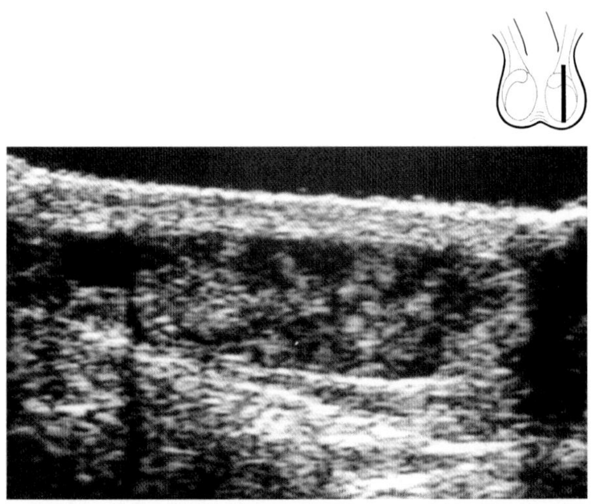

B

Case 27

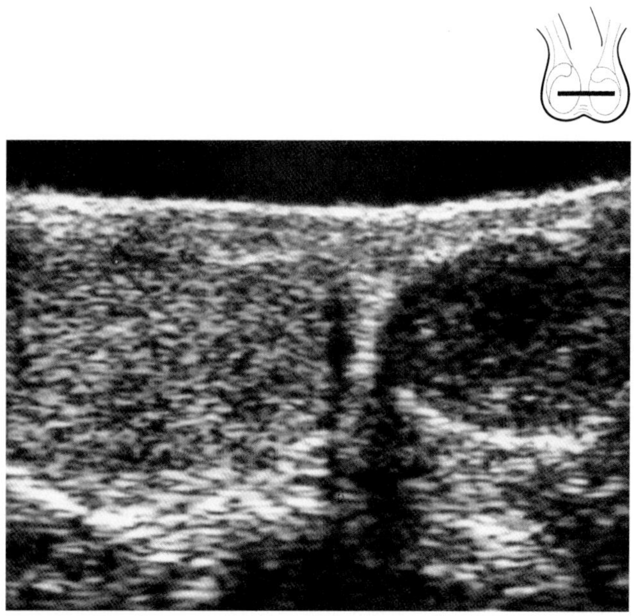

A 31-year-old asymptomatic patient with small left testis.

Physical Examination. The left testis is small and soft, the right hemiscrotum is normal to palpation.

Ultrasound. Transverse scan of both testes (Fig. 27). The left testis is small and hypoechoic.

Conclusion. Atrophy of the left testis (biopsy proven). Tumor, however, cannot be entirely excluded.

Notes. Combined findings from physical examination and ultrasound, fortified by a later given history of mumps infection, suggest testicular atrophy, but biopsy was still performed.

Case 28

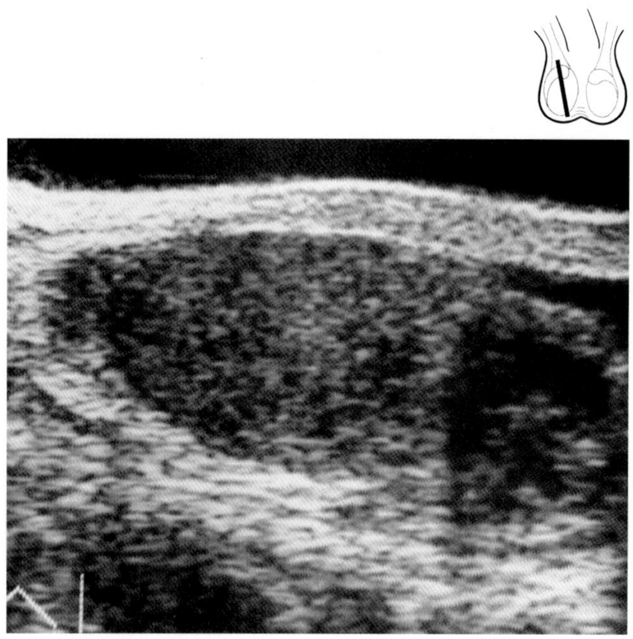

A 50-year-old patient presents with a painful right scrotal swelling of 12 days' duration.

Physical Examination. There is tender swelling and induration of the right scrotal contents. The lower pole of the testis and the epididymal tail cannot be delineated confidently. There is scrotal skin edema, and the hemiscrotum does not transilluminate.

Ultrasound. Longitudinal scan of the right testis (Fig. 28). There is enlargement of the epididymal tail, which contains several anechoic areas. The testis is slightly enlarged and hypoechoic (compared to the contralateral side) with preservation of the homogeneous echotexture of the testicular tissue. The lower pole of the testis is compressed by the mass in the area of the epididymal tail. A small fluid collection can be seen around the tail of the epididymis. There is thickening of the scrotal skin.

Analysis. The clinical findings alone do not permit reliable distinction between epididymitis (pain and scrotal skin edema) and a tumor (induration). The ultrasound examination permits differentiation of the testis from the enlarged epididymal tail. The anechoic areas in the tail portion suggest abscess formation. The homogeneously decreased echogenicity of the testis is consistent with concomitant orchitis and does not suggest tumor.

Conclusion. Epididymo-orchitis with abscess formation in the tail of the epididymis.

Clinical Course. Symptoms resolve with antibiotic treatment. There is no fluctuation palpable in the area of the epididymal tail at follow-up.

Case 29

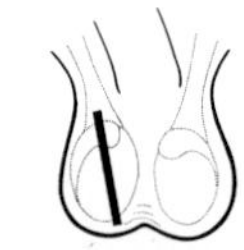

A 30-year-old patient presents with right testicular swelling, first noted 2 weeks earlier.

Physical Examination. There is a firm, slightly tender mass of the right testis. There are no signs of inflammation and the hemiscrotum does not transilluminate.

Ultrasound. Longitudinal scan of the right testis (Fig. 29). The right testis is completely replaced by a large, inhomogeneous mass containing small cystic spaces. The epididymal head can be seen separate from the testis and is of normal homogeneous echotexture.

Conclusion. Right testicular tumor.

Histology. Teratocarcinoma (embryonal carcinoma and teratoma).

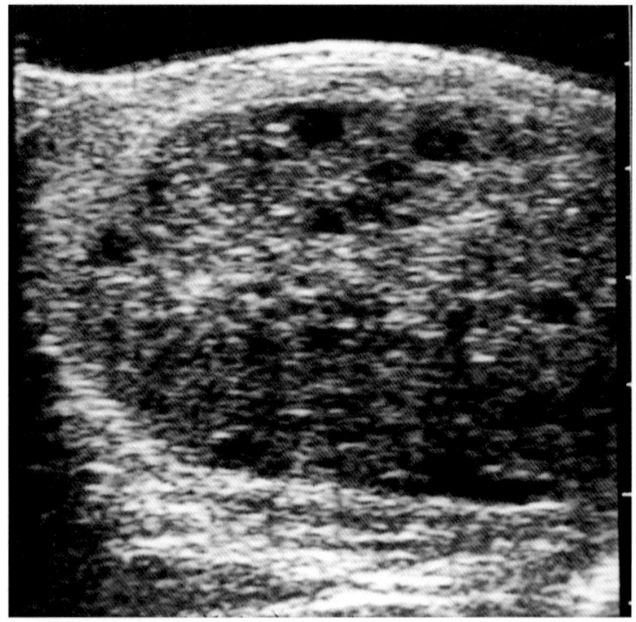

Case 30

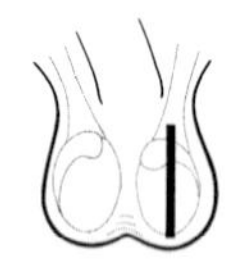

A 51-year-old patient presents with a 2-month history of recurrent epididymitis.

Physical Examination. There is painful swelling and erythema of the left scrotum with enlargement of the testis and epididymis. The patient is afebrile.

Ultrasound. Longitudinal scan of the left testis (Fig. 30). The testis is enlarged and homogeneously hypoechoic (primarily in the upper pole). The epididymis is also enlarged and separate from the testis. The scrotal skin is thickened.

Conclusion. Epididymo-orchitis without suspicion of tumor.

Clinical Course. Resolution of symptoms with antibiotic treatment.

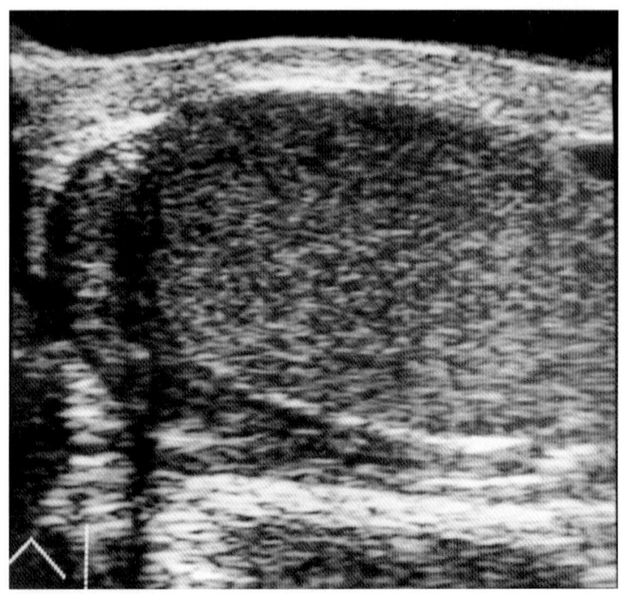

Case 31

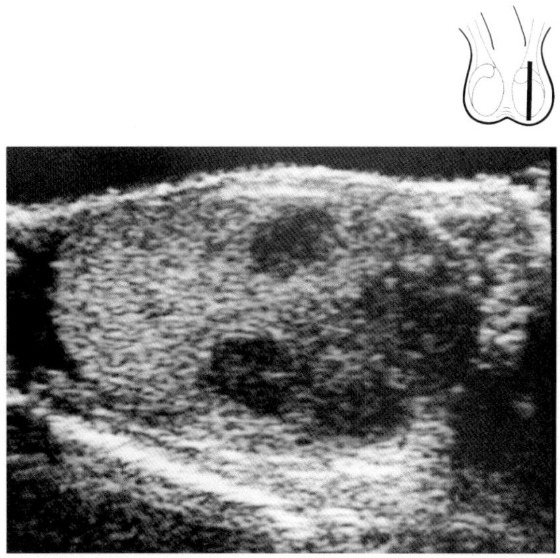

A 29-year-old patient presents with hard, painless left testicular enlargement of about 1 week duration.

Physical Examination. There is a firm, nodular, painless mass of the left testis and no signs of inflammation.

Ultrasound. Longitudinal scan of the left testis (Fig. 31). Ultrasound demonstrates multiple, hypoechoic lesions in the testis. The epididymis is normal.

Conclusion. Left testicular tumor with multiple intratesticular foci.

Histology. Seminoma.

Notes. Testicular tumors (in particular seminomas) occasionally show multiple intratesticular manifestations.

Case 32

A 75-year-old patient presents with a painless swelling of the right hemiscrotum of about 1-year duration.

Physical Examination. There is a large, firm, painless swelling of the right testis. The hemiscrotum does not transilluminate. There are no signs of inflammation.

Ultrasound. Longitudinal scans of the right (Fig. 32A) and left (Fig. 32B) testis. The right testis is markedly enlarged and almost entirely replaced by a solid, inhomogeneous mass. (Compare with the normal left testis.)

Analysis. Despite the patient's advanced age, the firm, solid mass strongly suggests the presence of a tumor.

Conclusion. Right testicular tumor.

Histology. Non-Hodgkin lymphoma (primary testicular manifestation).

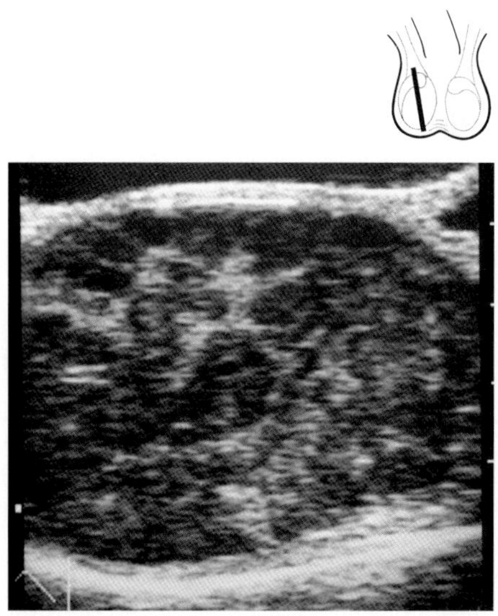

A

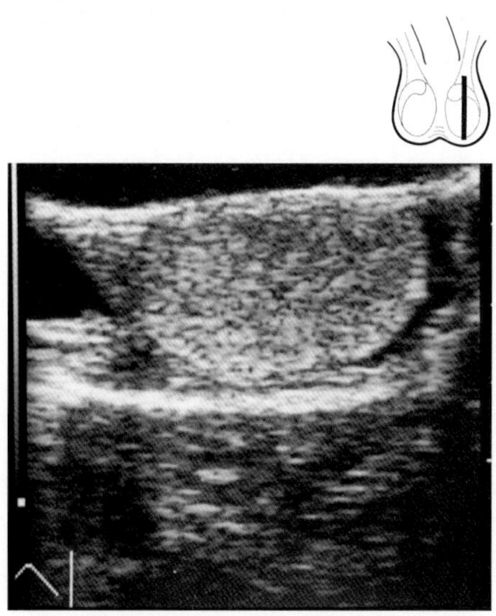

B

Case 33

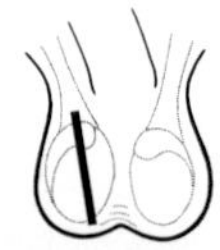

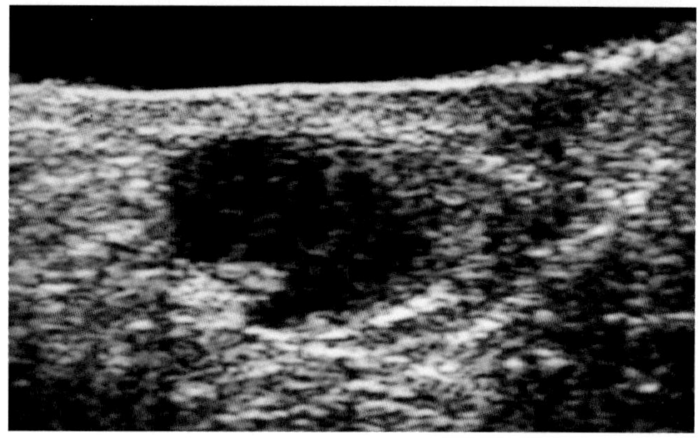

A 26-year-old patient seeks medical advice because of a smaller testis on the right than on the left. The patient underwent surgery for an undescended right testis during childhood.

Physical Examination. There is a cryptorchid right testis at the base of the scrotum. The testis is small and indurated. There are no signs of inflammation. The left hemiscrotum is normal to palpation.

Ultrasound. Longitudinal view of the right testis (Fig. 33). The small, oval-shaped testis is visualized. The normal echogenicity is preserved only in the area of the lower pole. The rest of the testis shows alteration of parenchymal echotexture with hypoechoic mass seen in the upper pole.

Analysis. Induration of the undescended right testis on palpation and the sonographically demonstrated irregularity of testicular texture suggest a tumor.

Conclusion. Right testicular tumor.

Histology. Seminoma.

Notes. There is a much higher risk of malignancy arising in a cryptorchid testis.

Case 34

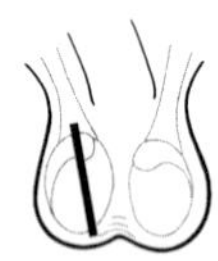

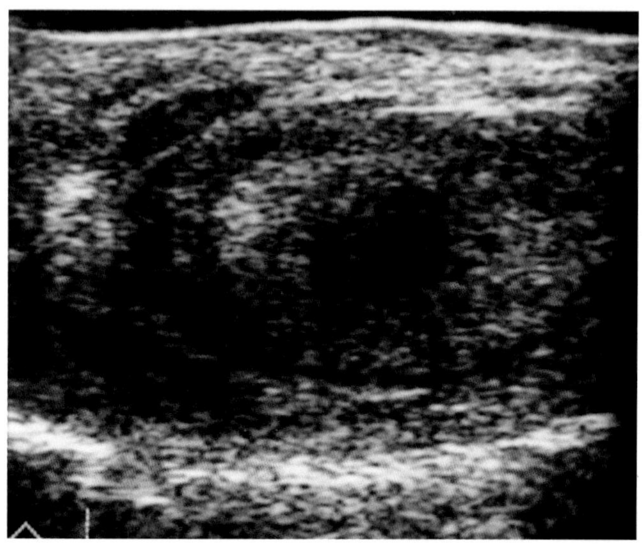

A 28-year-old patient presents with painful swelling of the right testis following testicular biopsy 10 days previously.

Physical Examination. There is tender swelling of the right hemiscrotum, and the testis and epididymis are difficult to differentiate. There is no transillumination and no fluctuant area is palpable. Fever and leukocytosis are present.

Ultrasound. Longitudinal scan of the right testis (Fig. 34). The right testis is of normal size and shape. A hypoechoic, focal lesion with poorly defined borders can be visualized. Enlargement of the epididymis and "onion peel" thickening of the paratesticular tissue are also present, and there is edema of the scrotal skin.

Analysis. The sonographic demonstration of a circumscribed intratesticular lesion might suggest a testicular tumor, but epididymo-orchitis with testicular abscess formation is more likely in view of the patient's preceding operation and the clinical and sonographic signs of inflammation.

Conclusion. Epididymo-orchitis with testicular abscess.

Clinical Course. Symptoms resolved with antibiotic treatment.

Case 35

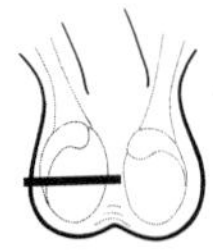

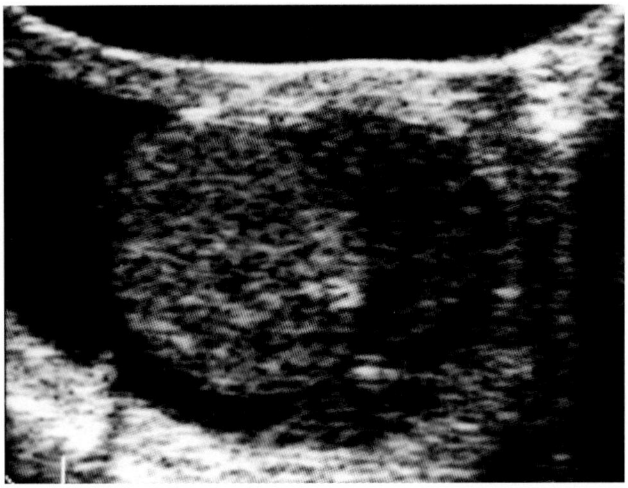

A 58-year-old patient presents with a tense, moderately painful swelling of the right hemiscrotum and mild fever.

Physical Examination. There is a very tender, tense right scrotal swelling. The testis and epididymis cannot be delineated confidently. The hemiscrotum transilluminates.

Ultrasound. Transverse scan of the right testis (Fig. 35). The epididymis is markedly enlarged and hypoechoic (the sonogram shows the area of the epididymal body). The testis is unremarkable (the small, marginally displayed, echo-dense structure is the mediastinum testis). Anechoic fluid can be seen surrounding the testis.

Conclusion. Right-sided epididymitis with a reactive hydrocele. There is no evidence of a testicular tumor.

Clinical Course. Resolution of symptoms with antibiotic treatment.

Case 36

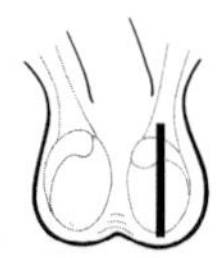

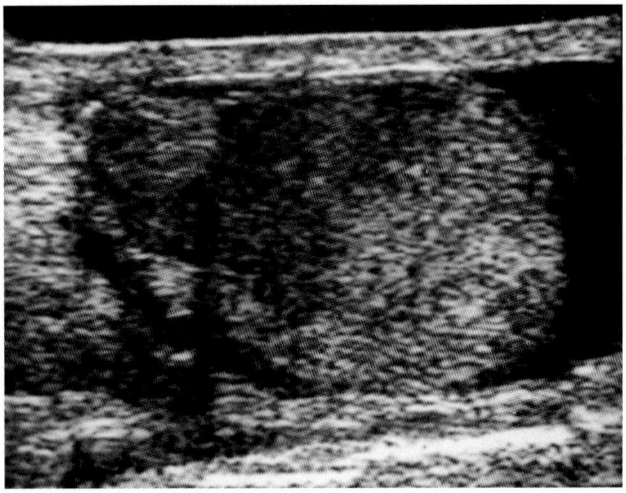

A 69-year-old patient presents with an acute swelling of the left testis, pain of 3-day duration, and fever.

Physical Examination. The epididymis is enlarged and very painful, which limits examination. To the extent it can be assessed, the testis appears to be of normal shape and consistency.

Ultrasound. Longitudinal scan of the left testis (Fig. 36). The head of the markedly enlarged, hypoechoic epididymis is displayed. The upper pole of the testis demonstrates homogeneous, decreased echogenicity. A moderately increased amount of fluid can be seen inferiorly.

Analysis. The clinical findings clearly point to epididymitis. The sonographically abnormal area of the testis has to be interpreted as inflammatory involvement because its pattern is homogeneous and there is also enlargement of the epididymis.

Conclusion. Epididymitis with concomitant orchitis and a reactive hydrocele.

Clinical Course. The patient's recovery was uneventful with antibiotic treatment.

Case 37

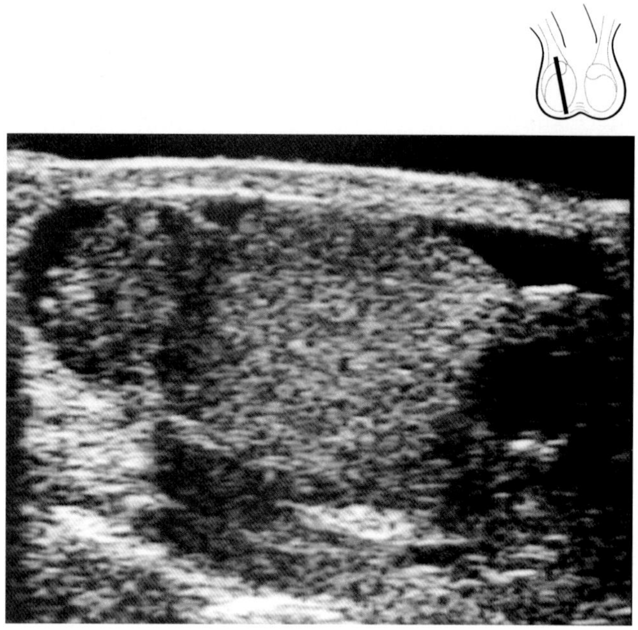

An 85-year-old patient presents with a painful swelling of the right hemiscrotum of 1 week's duration.

Physical Examination. There is painful induration of the right hemiscrotum, most likely related to the epididymis. The testis and epididymis cannot be reliably differentiated. The right hemiscrotum does transilluminate. A Foley catheter is placed for obstructive symptoms of benign prostatic hyperplasia (BPH).

Ultrasound. Longitudinal scan of the right testis (Fig. 37). The entire epididymis is enlarged (only the epididymal head and tail are visualized). An echo-poor lesion measuring about 12 mm in diameter is seen in the epididymal tail. The echotexture of the testicular tissue is normal, and a small fluid collection can be seen surrounding the testis and epididymis.

Conclusion. Acute epididymitis and suspected abscess formation in the tail of the epididymis. Small, reactive hydrocele.

Clinical Course. Symptoms resolved with antibiotic treatment and there was no fluctuation palpable in the area of the epididymal tail on follow-up.

Case 38

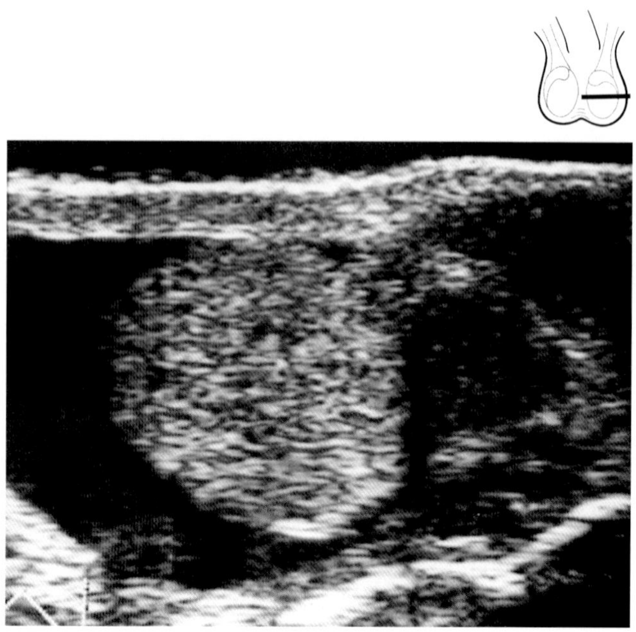

A 43-year-old patient presents with a slightly painful swelling of the left testis.

Physical Examination. There is a slightly tender, fluctuant swelling adjacent to the left testis. The testis itself, to the extent pain permits palpation, appears normal, but the testis and epididymis are fixed to the overlying scrotal skin. There is no fever.

Ultrasound. Transverse scan of the left testis (Fig. 38). The testis appears normal, but there is considerable enlargement of the epididymis. Hypoechoic areas are visualized not only in the epididymis but also in the scrotal skin. A fluid collection can be seen surrounding the testis.

Analysis. Despite only moderate pain, the clinical and sonographic findings in the epididymis and paratesticular tissue suggest an abscess-forming epididymitis. A testicular tumor can be excluded.

Conclusion. Epididymitis with abscess formation extending into the scrotal skin.

Treatment and Histology. A left epididymectomy was performed. There was extensive confluent and caseating necroses, and acid-fast rods consistent with florid tuberculosis of the epididymis were found.

Case 39

A 42-year-old patient presents with a 4-month history of left testicular enlargement.

Physical Examination. The left hemiscrotum is swollen with minimal transillumination. The left testis cannot be delineated.

Ultrasound. Transverse scan of the left testis (Fig. 39A). The left testis is very large with irregular, partly cystic alteration of normal echotexture. A moderately increased amount of fluid can be seen surrounding it.

Conclusion. Left testicular tumor and reactive hydrocele.

Histology. Seminoma, with extensive, partly liquified necroses (Fig. 39B is a surgical specimen).

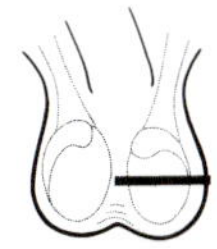

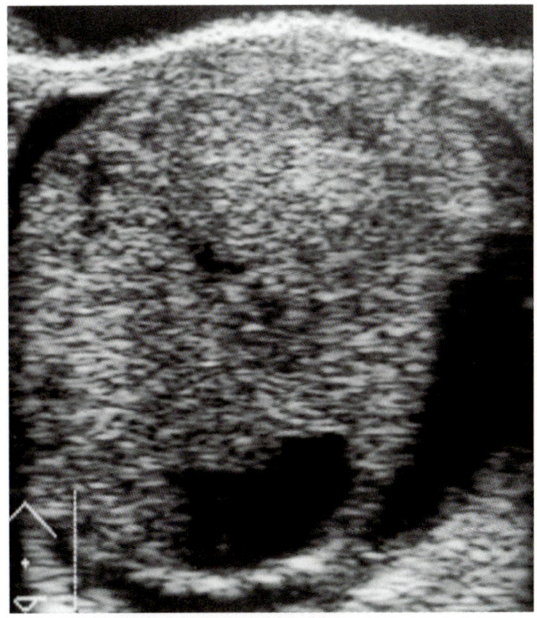

A

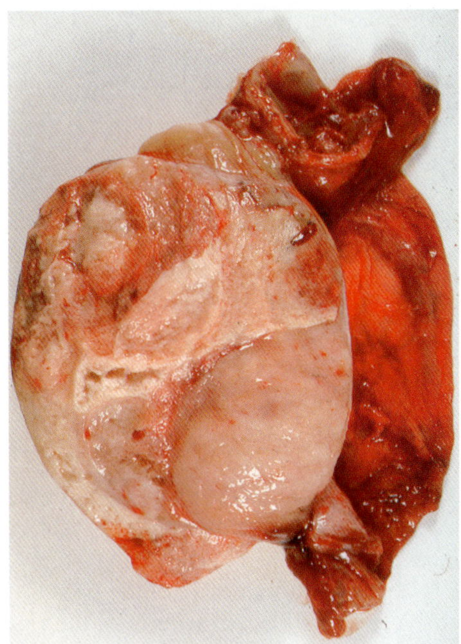

B

Case 40

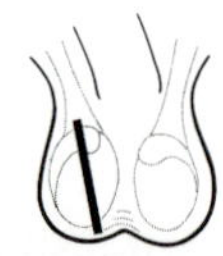

A 53-year-old patient presents with a history of recurrent scrotal pain.

Physical Examination. Findings on palpation are normal.

Ultrasound. Longitudinal scan of the right testis (Fig. 40A). There is an anechoic, sharply demarcated lesion in the right testis that cannot be palpated as a mass even by specific examination during scanning. The epididymis can be visualized and appears normal. There were no abnormalities in the left testis.

Conclusion. Simple testicular cyst in the right testis.

Histology. Simple intratesticular cyst; no sign of tumor (Fig. 40B is a surgical specimen).

Notes. In contradistinction to cystic areas in a tumor, simple testicular cysts cannot be palpated as a mass.

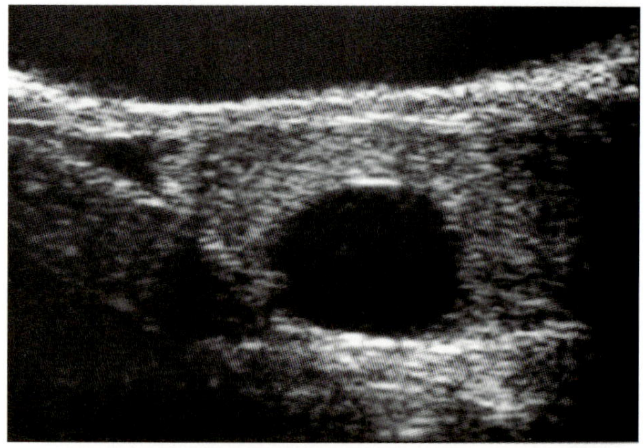

A

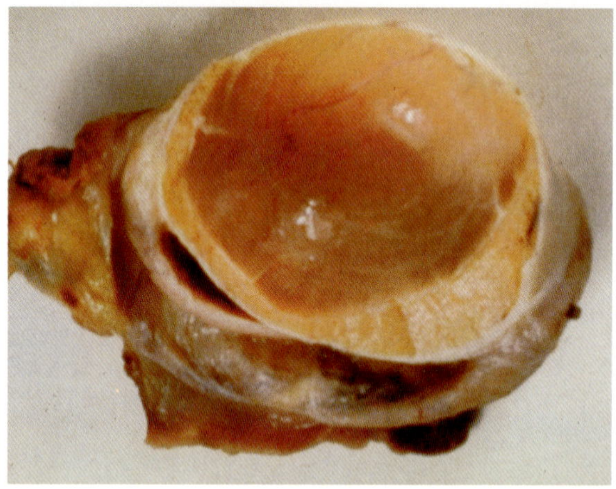

B

Case 41

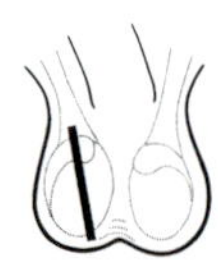

A 54-year-old patient presents with a right testicular induration that had not changed in size for several months.

Physical Examination. There is a circumscribed, nodular, and painless mass of the right testis, without signs of inflammation.

Ultrasound. Longitudinal scan of the right testis (Fig. 41). Extensive plaquelike calcification of the right testis is seen in the area of the tunica albuginea with posterior acoustic shadowing. Lateral scanning (not shown) demonstrates a normal, homogeneous echotexture of the testicular tissue. The epididymis is unremarkable.

Analysis. Despite palpation of a suspicious mass, a diagnosis of calcification of the tunica albuginea unrelated to a tumorous process may be made on the basis of the normal sonographic appearance of the testicular parenchyma. This diagnosis is substantiated by the patient reporting an unchanging lesion size over a relatively long period of time.

Conclusion. Extensive plaquelike calcification of the tunica albuginea.

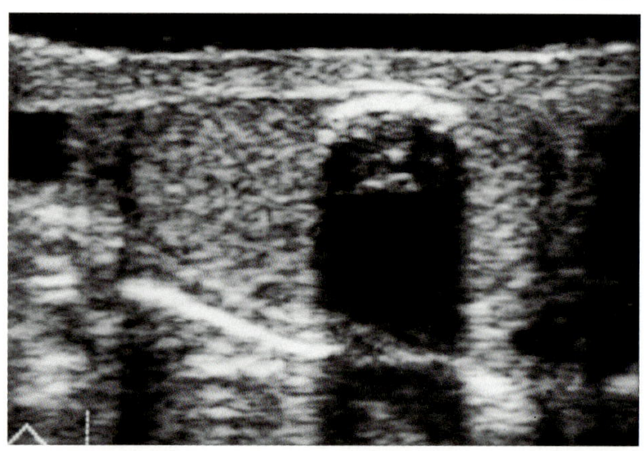

Case 42

A 30-year-old patient presents with development of gynecomastia.

Physical Examination. There is bilateral gynecomastia and a slightly tender mass of the upper pole at the left testis.

Ultrasound. Longitudinal scan of the left testis (Fig. 42A) and transverse scan of both testes (Fig. 42B). A hypoechoic intratesticular mass is seen in the upper pole of the left testis. The mass is separate from the epididymal head.

Conclusion. Left testicular tumor. The presence of gynecomastia suggests a hormonally active Leydig's cell tumor or NSGCT that produces HCG.

Histology. Leydig's cell tumor.

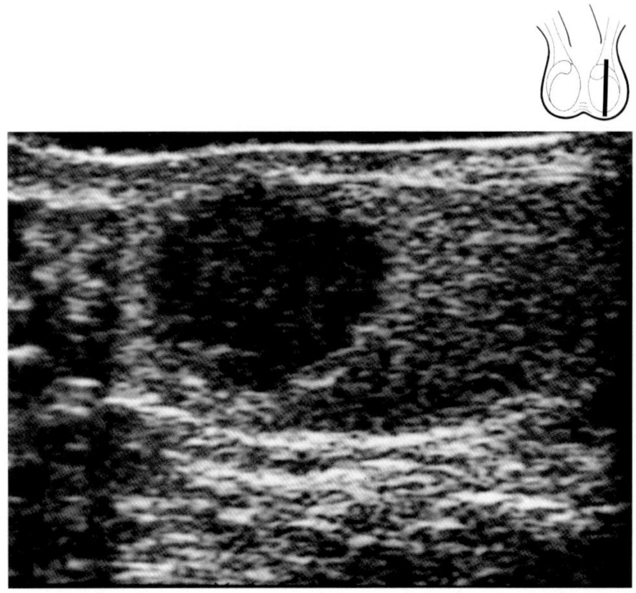

A

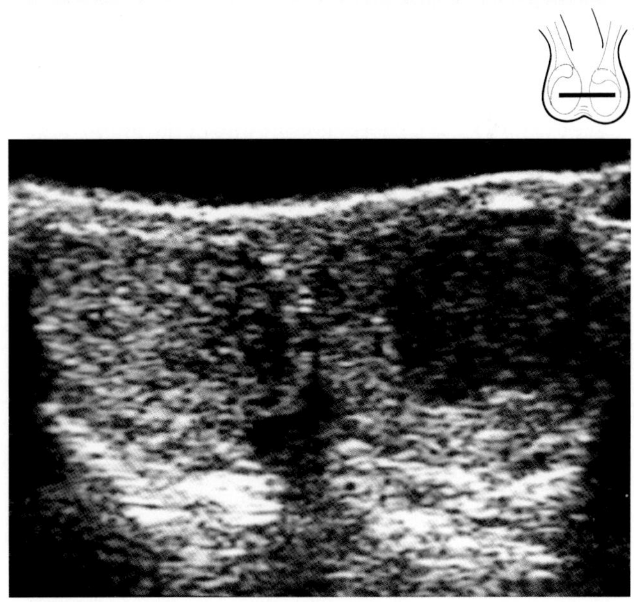

B

Cases 43 to 45

In these three cases the patients presented with a similar set of symptoms. In cases 43 and 44 the patients presented with a firm, painless mass in the area of the tail of the epididymis. There were no signs of inflammation. In case 45 the mass was firm, but moderately tender, and related to the lower pole of the testis or the epididymal tail.

Physical Examination. There was a firm mass in the tail of the epididymis in all three patients. There was tenderness of the palpable mass in case 45. The testis and epididymis were clearly delineated in all three cases.

Ultrasound. Longitudinal sonograms (Figs. 43 to 45). A circumscribed, hypoechoic lesion can be seen in the area of the epididymal tail in all three cases. There is good delineation of the testis and in case 45 the mediastinum testis can be seen.

Conclusion. Solid mass of the epididymal tail in all three patients.

Histology and Clinical Course. Case 43 was shown to have an adenomatoid tumor of the epididymis. Case 44 was shown to have a sperm granuloma of the epididymis. In case 45 the swelling of the epididymis subsided with antibiotic treatment, indicating granulomatous epididymitis.

Notes. These three cases illustrate good sonographic differentiation of the testis and epididymis, but also show the limits of ultrasound in distinguishing a tumor from other lesions.

Case 43

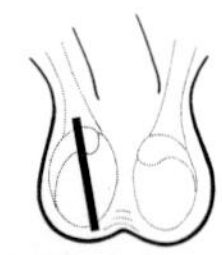

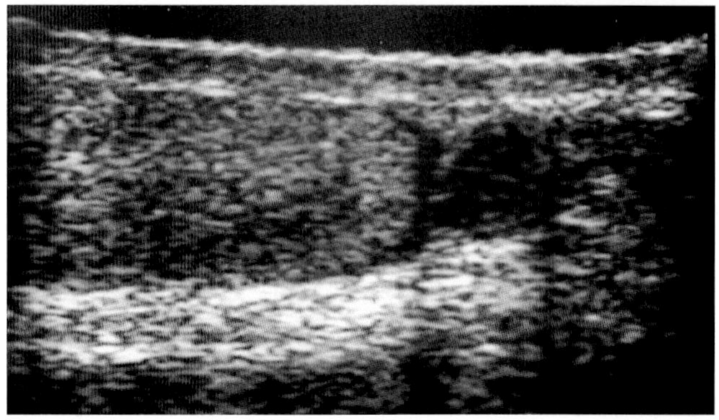

Case 44

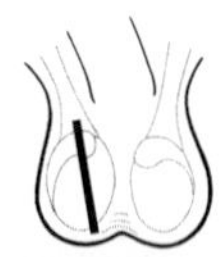

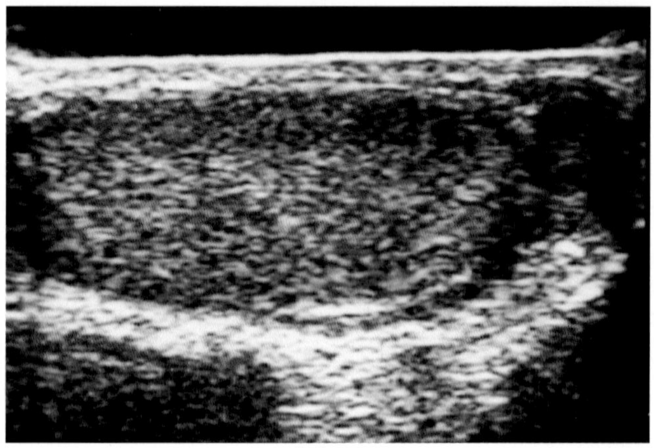

Case 45

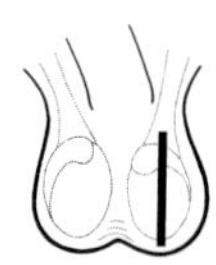

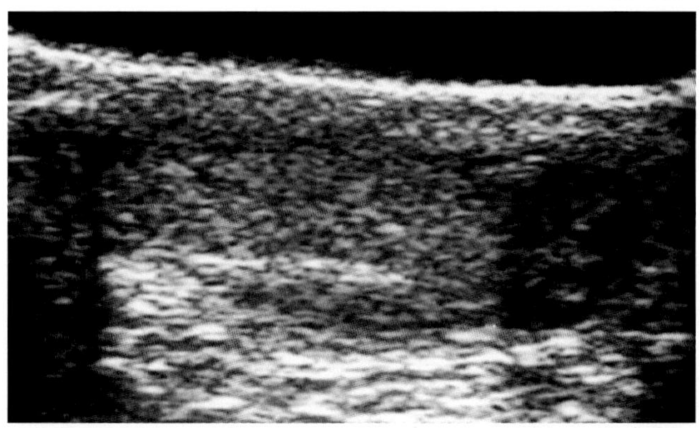

Case 46

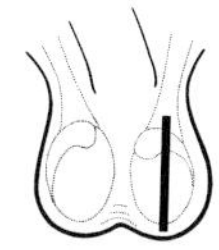

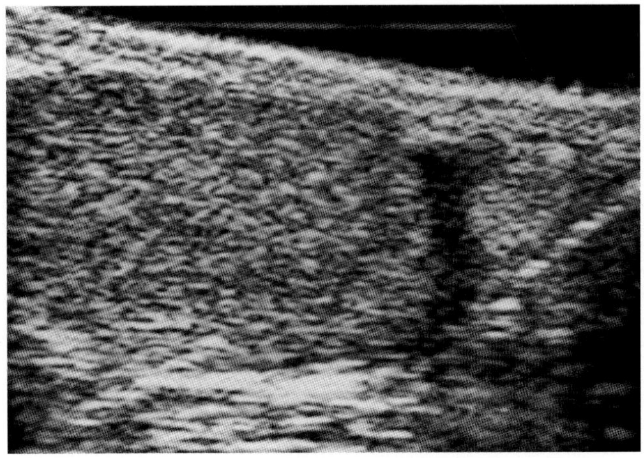

A 56-year-old patient presents with a roundish 1-cm mass at the lower pole of the left testis. The mass had not increased in size since first noted at least 3 months previously. There is no fever.

Physical Examination. A firm, painless mass can be palpated in the area of the lower pole of the left testis. It can apparently be moved independently of the testis. There are no signs of inflammation.

Ultrasound. Longitudinal scan of the left testis (Fig. 46). The left testis is normal, but a solid echo-dense, roundish lesion about 1 cm in diameter can be seen in the tail of the epididymis. There is good delineation of testicular and epididymal structures.

Conclusion. Suspected adenomatoid tumor of the epididymis.

Histology. Adenomatoid tumor of the epididymis.

Notes. In adenomatoid tumors echogenicity may be either increased or decreased as compared with the normal epididymal echotexture.

Case 47

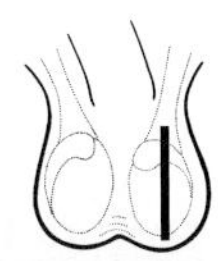

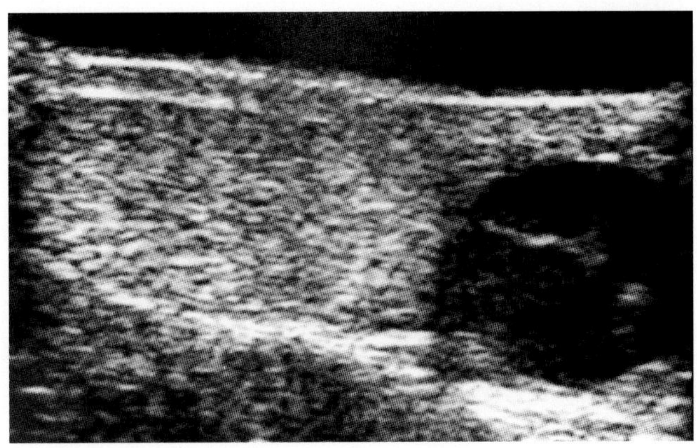

A 25-year-old patient presents with a nodular induration in the left scrotum. The patient experienced blunt trauma to the scrotum 3 weeks before presentation.

Physical Examination. There is an isolated, firm, slightly tender, and mobile mass below the left testis. The testis is normal to palpation. There are no signs of inflammation.

Ultrasound. Longitudinal view of the left testis (Fig. 47). The left testis is unremarkable. There is a smoothly demarcated, markedly hypoechoic mass traversed by septationlike structures in the area of the epididymal tail. Otherwise the epididymis (not shown) appears normal.

Analysis. It is possible to definitely exclude testicular tumor and isolated epididymal abscess (because there is no inflammatory swelling of the epididymis and absence of clinical signs of inflammation). The patient's history suggests a posttraumatic alteration.

Conclusion. An old, encapsulated hematoma secondary to trauma in the area of the epididymal tail

Intraoperative Findings and Histology. Blood-containing spermatocele.

Case 48

A 41-year-old patient with carcinophobia.

Physical Examination. Unremarkable.

Ultrasound. Longitudinal scan of the left testis (Fig. 48). An anechoic, well-defined, intratesticular lesion can be seen in a subcapsular location. There is no mass on repeated palpation during scanning.

Analysis. Despite the rather small diameter (5 mm), a tumor in a subcapsular position would be palpable as a circumscribed mass. Therefore, the diagnosis of a simple testicular cyst can be made (not palpable, cystic appearance on ultrasound without any abnormalities of the adjacent testicular tissue).

Conclusion. Simple cyst of the testis.

Intraoperative Finding. Subcapsular cystic lesion that, at open exploration of the testis, is identified only by transillumination with a fiber optic light. Local excision.

Histology. Simple cyst lined by a single layer of epithelial cells.

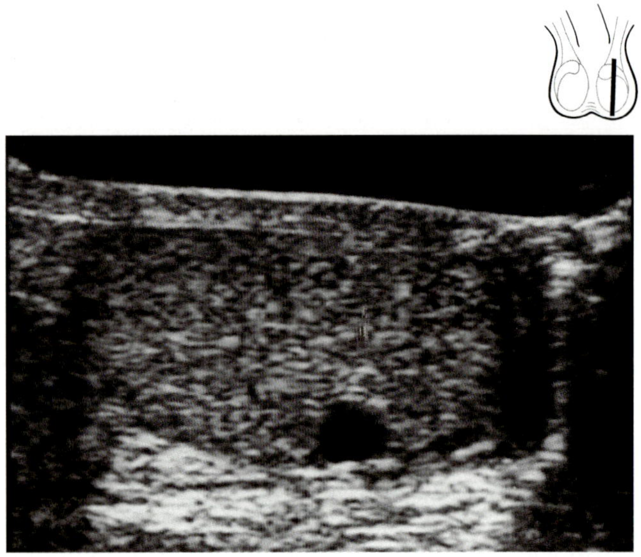

Case 49

A 22-year-old patient presents with a painless lump in his right testis of several years' duration.

Physical Examination. There is a circumscribed, firm, intratesticular mass.

Ultrasound. Longitudinal scan of the right testis (Fig. 49A). There is an intratesticular, echo-poor lesion with hyperechoic ventral and dorsal margins.

Analysis. The diagnosis of epidermoid cyst is suggested by the "cystlike" sonographic appearance of the intratesticular lesion and its reported persistence for several years.

Conclusion. Suspected epidermoid cyst.

Histology. Epidermoid cyst (Fig. 49B is a surgical specimen).

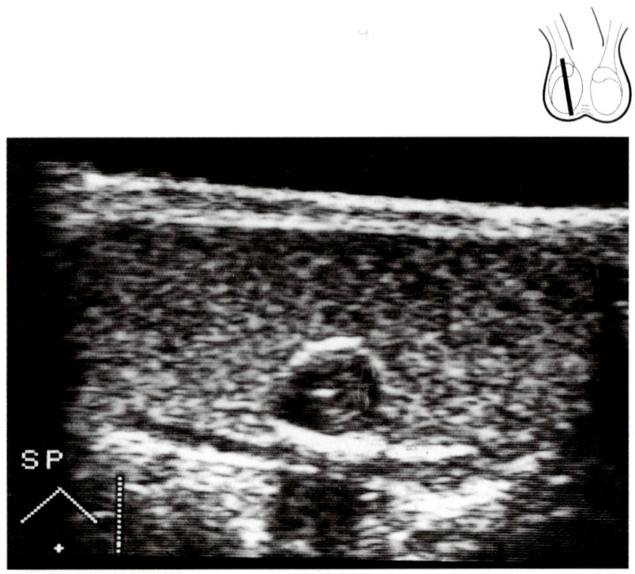

A

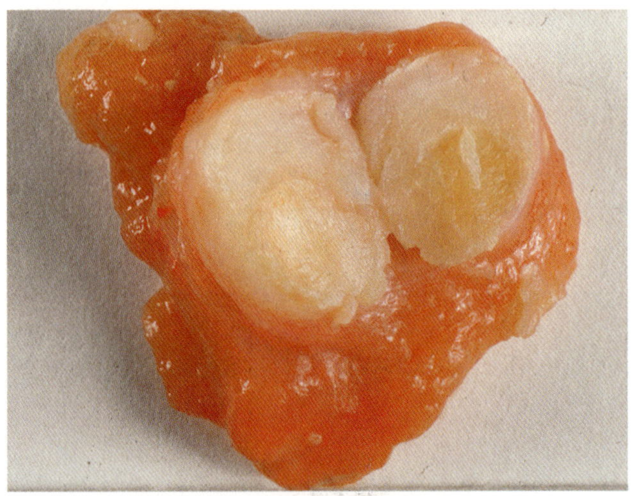

B

Case 50

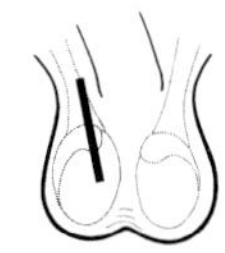

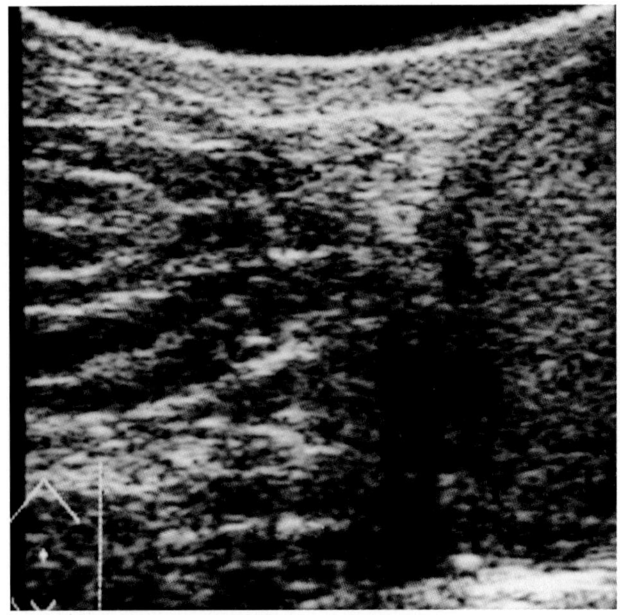

A 73-year-old patient presents with a swollen scrotum.

Physical Examination. A moderately tender mass is located superior to the right testis. The testis and epididymis are unremarkable.

Ultrasound. Longitudinal view of the upper scrotal compartment on the right (Fig. 50). The normal right testis can be seen at the right margin of the figure. Garlandlike structures can be seen cranial to the testis and along the entire inguinal canal. There is restricted mobility during the Valsalva maneuver.

Conclusion. Right-sided inguinal hernia with protrusion of bowel loops.

Case 51

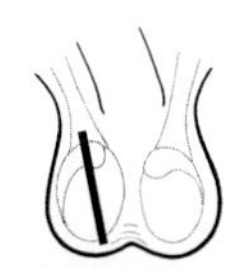

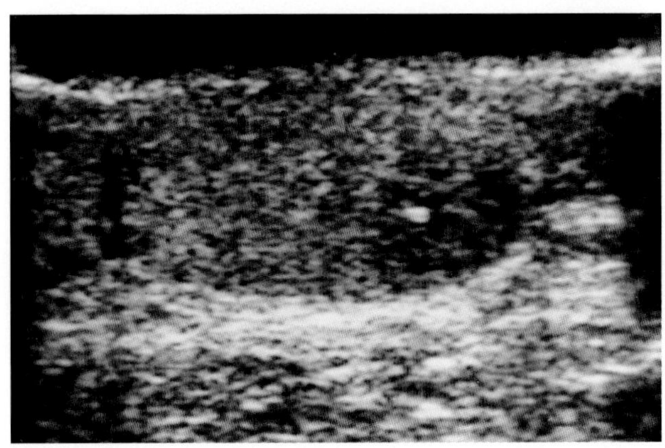

A 38-year-old patient presents with a painful swelling in the area of the right testis. The patient underwent a left-sided orchiectomy, radiotherapy, and chemotherapy for metastatic embryonal carcinoma 10 years previously. He has been in complete remission since then.

Physical Examination. There is a circumscribed, moderately painful mass in the right testis. There are no signs of inflammation and no fever.

Ultrasound. Longitudinal scan of the right testis (Fig. 51). A focal, intratesticular lesion is seen in the lower pole of the testis. The lesion is slightly hypoechoic, has poorly defined borders, and contains individual, small, echogenic foci. The epididymis is normal.

Analysis. Despite the presence of pain, the clearly intratesticular location of the lesion strongly suggests a tumor.

Conclusion. A second tumor is strongly suspected.

Histology. Malignant teratoma.

Notes. Dense echogenic areas in a tumor may correspond to fibrotic foci, calcifications, or cartilaginous structures. Patients with a testicular tumor are at an increased risk of developing a second tumor in the remaining testis.

Case 52

A 28-year-old patient presents with reported weight loss and exhaustion. There has been ultrasound demonstration of para-aortic lymphadenopathy and a presumptive clinical diagnosis of malignant lymphoma.

Physical Examination. Normal right testis, atrophic left testis.

Ultrasound. Transverse scan of both testes (Fig. 52A) and longitudinal scan of the left testis (Fig. 52B). The left testis is atrophic compared with the contralateral side. Multiple hypoechoic lesions and multiple small, echogenic lesions can be seen in the left testis (compare with the homogeneous echotexture of the right testis).

Analysis. The sonographic abnormality demonstrated in the testis and the presence of retroperitoneal lymphadenopathy suggest a testicular tumor. Atrophy of the tumorous testis is explained by cryptorchidism in childhood (related by the patient after repeated questioning). The multiple, small, echo-dense foci may correspond to calcifications or regressive changes (scars).

Conclusion. Tumor of the left testis (status postcryptorchidism) with lymphatic metastases.

Histology. Seminoma (Fig. 52C) in an atrophic left testicle. Multiple, small, intratesticular foci containing regressive calcifications and scars.

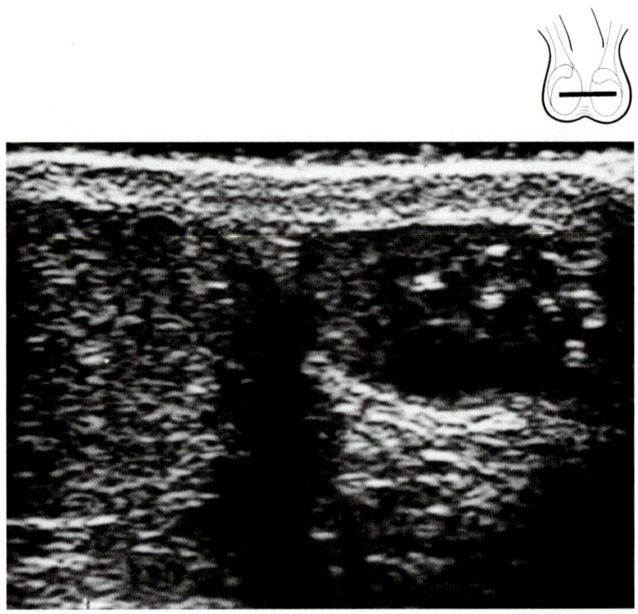

A

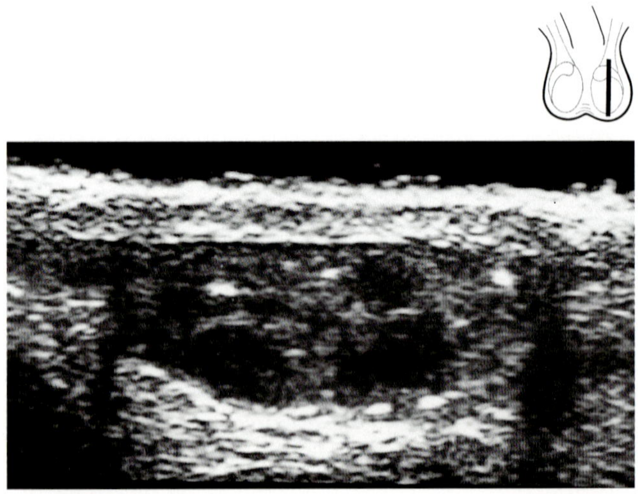

B

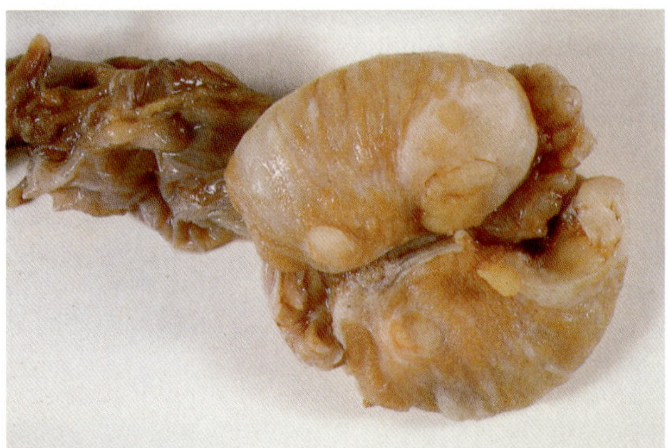

C

Case 53

A 34-year-old patient presents with a firm, painless swelling of the right hemiscrotum of several months' duration.

Physical Examination. The right testis is markedly enlarged and is palpated as a firm, nontender mass. There is nodular induration of the right spermatic cord. The right hemiscrotum does not transilluminate and there are no signs of inflammation.

Ultrasound. Longitudinal scan showing the upper pole of the testis and the lower segment of the spermatic cord on the right (Fig. 53A). There is a large, hypoechoic, and inhomogeneous lesion of the right testis with complete destruction of normal parenchyma. There are additional hypoechoic masses in the caudal segment of the spermatic cord.

Analysis. The sonographic appearance of the right testis indicates a tumor, although swelling of the ipsilateral spermatic cord is atypical. An inflammatory process (e.g., tuberculosis with beaded thickening of the spermatic cord) is very unlikely in the light of the palpation findings, the sonographic appearance, and the absence of clinical signs of inflammation. The diagnosis of a testicular tumor is substantiated by the sonographic detection of extensive retroperitoneal lymphadenopathy.

Conclusion. Right testicular tumor with invasion of the spermatic cord.

Histology. Embryonal carcinoma of the testis infiltrating the epididymis and spermatic cord (Fig. 53B).

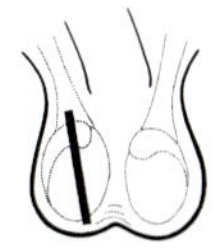

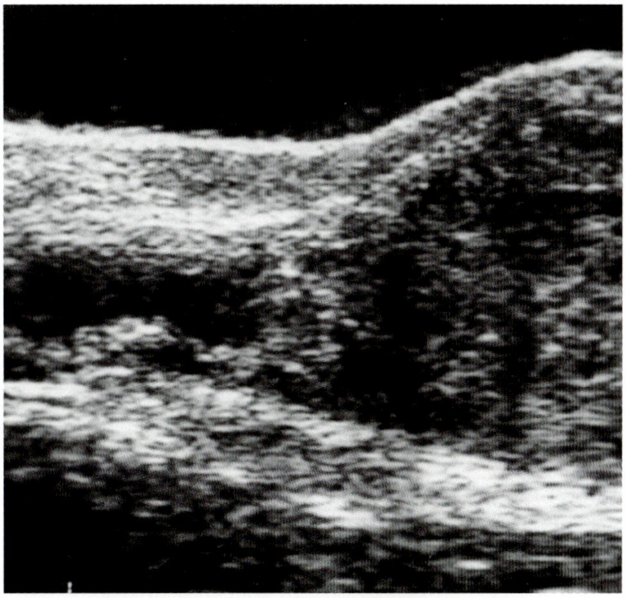

A

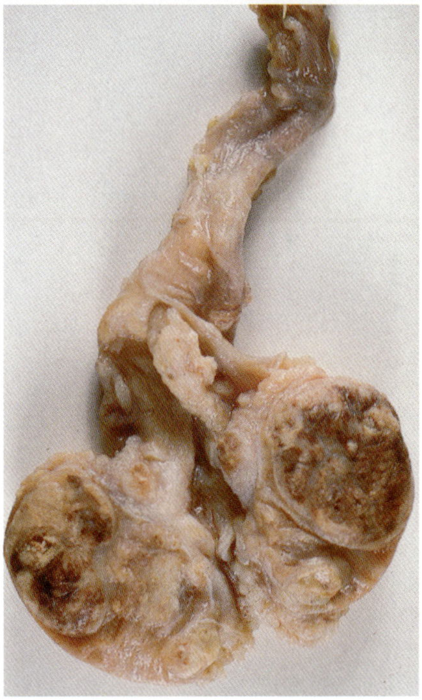

B

Case 54

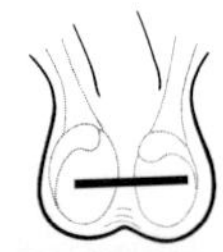

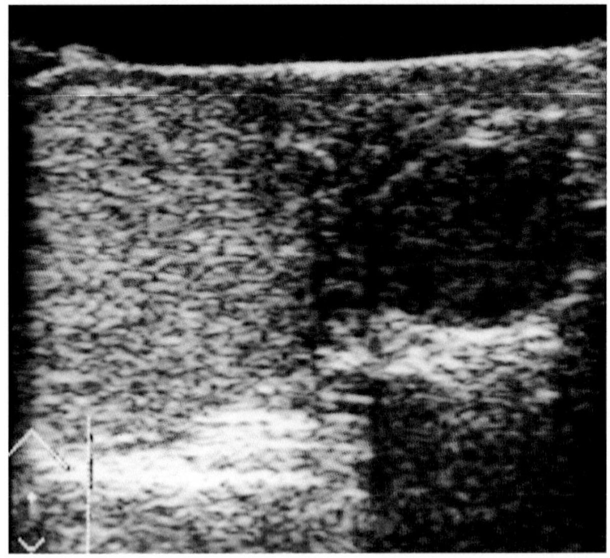

A 16-year-old patient presents with a small, painless, and indurated left testis. He has a history of an undescended testis. Approximately 6 months prior to presentation, he had an episode of acute pain on the left without fever. No treatment was instituted.

Physical Examination. The left testis is small and markedly indurated without tenderness. There are no signs of inflammation.

Ultrasound. Transverse scan of both testes (Fig. 54). The left testis is small, homogeneous, and hypoechoic. The para-aortic region (not shown) is normal.

Analysis. The size of the gonad could be attributed to cryptorchidism. The firm, painless mass on clinical examination suggests a testicular tumor. The homogeneous texture of the hypoechoic testis, the absence of retroperitoneal lymphadenopathy, and the reported episode of severe acute pain 6 months earlier raise other differential diagnoses.

Conclusion. Testicular atrophy on the left.

Histology. Old atrophy of the testis.

Notes. Testicular atrophy in this case may be attributed to testicular torsion 6 months earlier.

Case 55

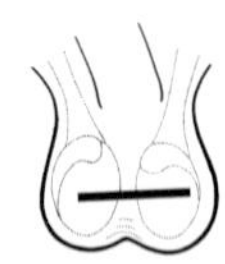

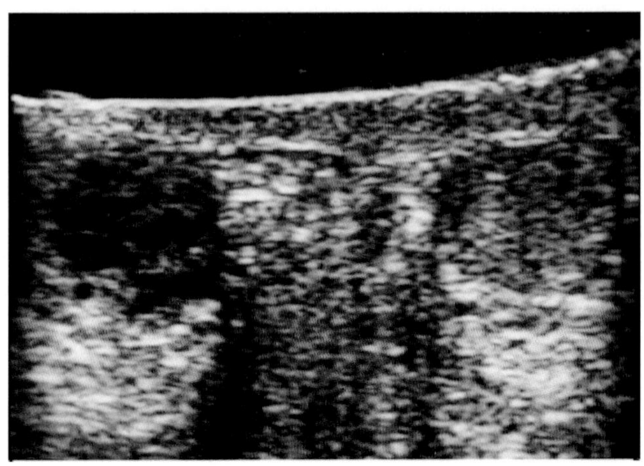

A 67-year-old patient presents with a painless, firm mass of the right testis, noted during a routine physical examination.

Physical Examination. Both testes are relatively small and there is marked induration on the right. There are no signs of inflammation.

Ultrasound. Transverse scan of both testes (Fig. 55). Compared with the left, the right testis is hypoechoic and has an inhomogeneous echotexture. There is no enlargement of the right testis. There are echogenic foci in the left testis.

Conclusion. Testicular tumor on the right. Testicular microlithiasis, left testis.

Histology. Seminoma, right testis.

Case 56

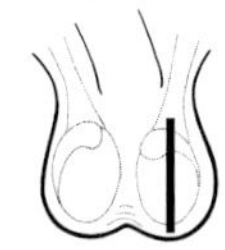

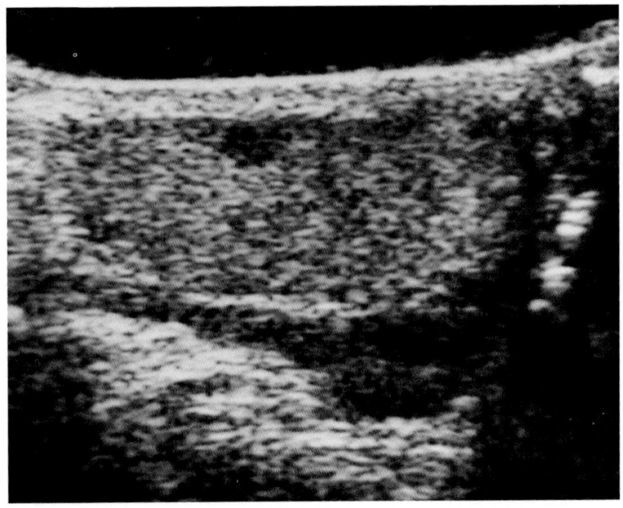

A 22-year-old patient presents with a small nodule on the left testis.

Physical Examination. There is a small, circumscribed mass of the left testis.

Ultrasound. Longitudinal scan of the left testis (Fig. 56). A small, hypoechoic, subcapsular lesion of the testis is seen in the area of the palpated mass.

Conclusion. Suspected small testicular tumor.

Histology. Leydig's cell tumor.

Notes. It is not possible to differentiate a Leydig's cell tumor from a malignant germ cell tumor on the basis of the sonographic appearance.

Case 57

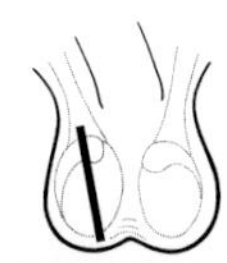

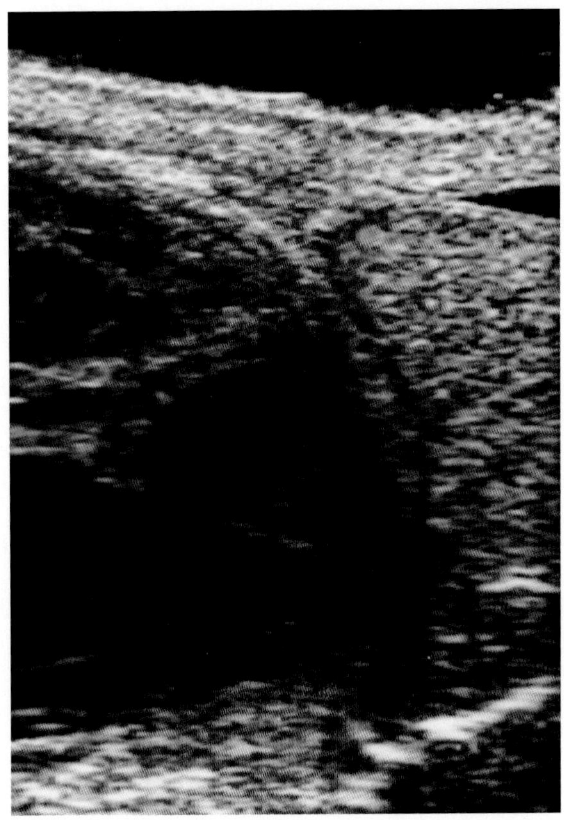

An 80-year-old patient presents with marked swelling of the right scrotum following hydrocele aspiration 10 days previously.

Physical Examination. There is a large, tense, and moderately tender swelling of the right hemiscrotum. The testis and epididymis cannot be delineated. The scrotal skin is thickened and erythematous. There is no transillumination.

Ultrasound. Longitudinal view of the right hemiscrotum (Fig. 57). A crescent-shaped deformity of the compressed right testis can be seen at the base of the right hemiscrotum. The echotexture of the testis is homogeneous. A large, septated fluid collection can be seen in the scrotal compartment. There is scrotal skin edema.

Analysis. The diagnoses of epididymitis or orchitis with pronounced enlargement of the testis can be excluded on the basis of the sonographic appearance. In the light of the patient's history, the septated fluid collection might be interpreted as a hematocele although swelling did not occur immediately after the puncture. It might also be an infected hydrocele that became a pyocele, accounting for the signs of inflammation.

Conclusion. Suspected pyocele on the right.

Intraoperative Finding and Histology. Pyocele on the right.

Case 58

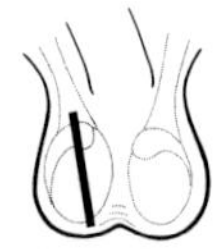

A 74-year-old patient presents with slow, progressive enlargement of the right hemiscrotum over several years. The patient reports no pain.

Physical Examination. The right hemiscrotum is markedly enlarged and tense. The testis and epididymis are not palpable. The hemiscrotum transilluminates.

Ultrasound. Longitudinal scan of the right hemiscrotum (Fig. 58). There is a large fluid collection surrounding the testis. The testis and epididymis are normal. The cystlike lesion in the epididymis is actually an extension of the hydrocele.

Conclusion. Large hydrocele. There are no signs of testicular tumor.

Notes. With ultrasound it is possible to evaluate the testis and epididymis rendered impalpable by a large surrounding hydrocele.

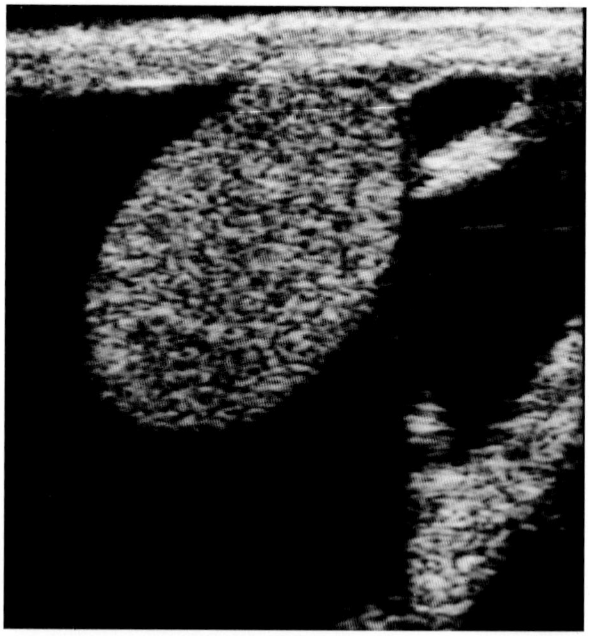

Case 59

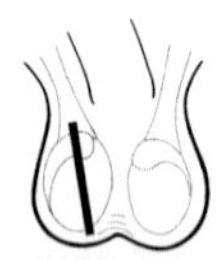

A 23-year-old patient presents with a firm swelling of the right testis noticed after a minor trauma some weeks previously.

Physical Examination. There is a firm, barely tender mass at the upper pole of the right testis. Patient does not have leukocytosis.

Ultrasound. Longitudinal scan of the right testis (Fig. 59). An irregular, partly hypoechoic, solid mass can be seen adjacent to the upper pole of the testis, probably related to the epididymal head. The mass is distinctly separate from the testis. The testis is normal.

Analysis. Although the clinical findings (a firm mass and the age of the patient) strongly suggest a testicular tumor, the sonographic examination demonstrates a solid, paratesticular mass without evidence of testicular tumor.

Conclusion. There is a solid mass in the area of the epididymal head. The differential diagnosis is organized hematoma, granulomatous inflammation, or epididymal tumor (rare).

Histology. Chronic granulomatous epididymitis.

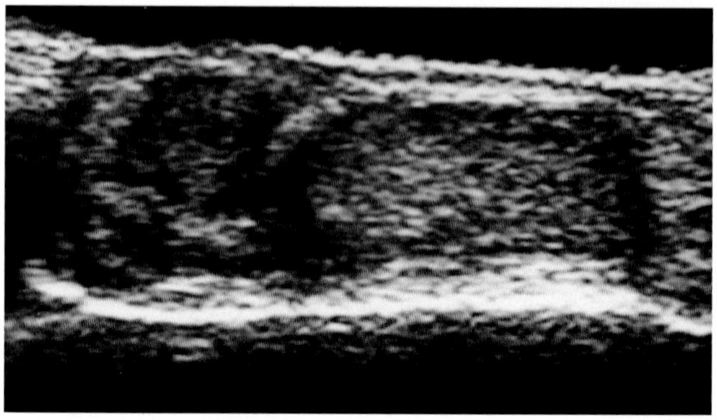

Case 60

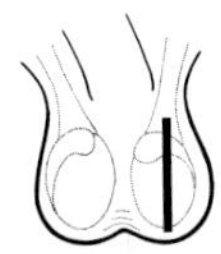

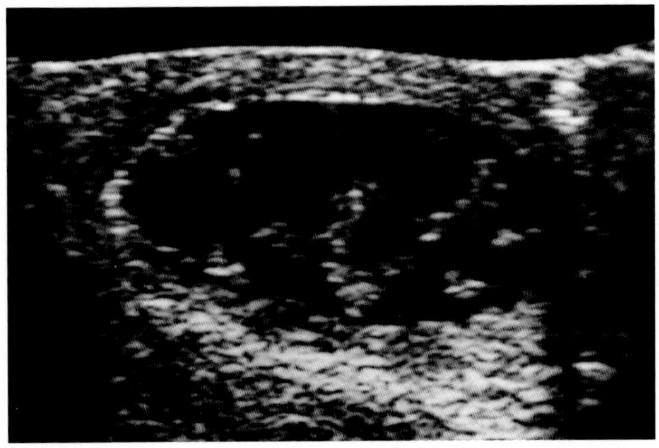

A 32-year-old patient presents with persistent left-sided scrotal swelling following ipsilateral orchiectomy (for carcinoma) 5 days previously. There is no fever.

Physical Examination. The left hemiscrotum is swollen, markedly indurated, and moderately tender. There is a suggestion of fluctuation. Scrotal skin edema is noted.

Ultrasound. Longitudinal scan of the left scrotum (Fig. 60). A smoothly demarcated, partly septated, intrascrotal fluid collection can be visualized.

Analysis. It is difficult to make a diagnosis based on the sonographic demonstration of a septated, intrascrotal fluid collection, since this sonographic appearance may be seen in abscess formation, a pyocele, or a liquified hematoma. However, the patient's history and the physical findings make an inflammatory condition less likely.

Conclusion. Suspected postoperative hematoma or possible abscess.

Aspiration. Liquified hematoma.

Case 61

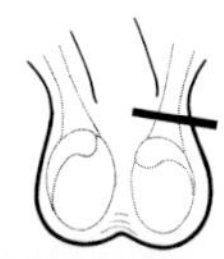

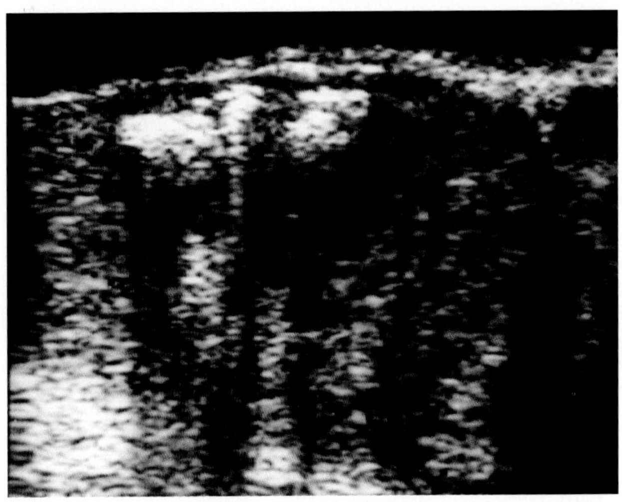

A 19-year-old patient, who underwent hydrocele surgery on the left 12 days earlier, presents with a hematoma and a temperature elevated to 39°C.

Physical Examination. The left hemiscrotum is very tender, firm, swollen, and nonfluctuant, with scrotal skin erythema and edema. Leukocytosis is present.

Ultrasound. Transverse scan of the left hemiscrotum cranial to the testis (Fig. 61). There is an intrascrotal fluid collection with poorly defined borders. Echogenic foci can be seen in the anterior part of the fluid collection with associated irregular acoustic shadowing. There is swelling of the remaining soft tissue.

Analysis. The echogenic foci correspond to air pockets.

Conclusion. Intrascrotal abscess formation secondary to an infected postoperative hematoma.

Intraoperative Finding. Abscess.

Case 62

A 24-year-old patient presents with a swollen left hemiscrotum.

Physical Examination. There is a paratesticular, nontender swelling extending along the spermatic cord. The testes are unremarkable.

Ultrasound. Transverse scan of both testes (Fig. 62A) and a longitudinal view of the left spermatic cord (Fig. 62B). Both testes appear normal. An abnormal paratesticular tissue, relatively hyperechoic, is surrounding the left testis and is extending into the inguinal canal. No fluid can be demonstrated.

Analysis. The clinical findings suggest a hydrocele extending into the spermatic cord, whereas the sonographic appearance provides evidence of the solid character of the lesion. The soft consistency and varying shape argue against a malignant tumor.

Conclusion. Lipomatosis of the left spermatic cord. Differential diagnoses include lipoma and inguinal hernia with protrusion of omental fat.

Intraoperative Finding and Histology. Lipomatosis of the left spermatic cord extending into the scrotum.

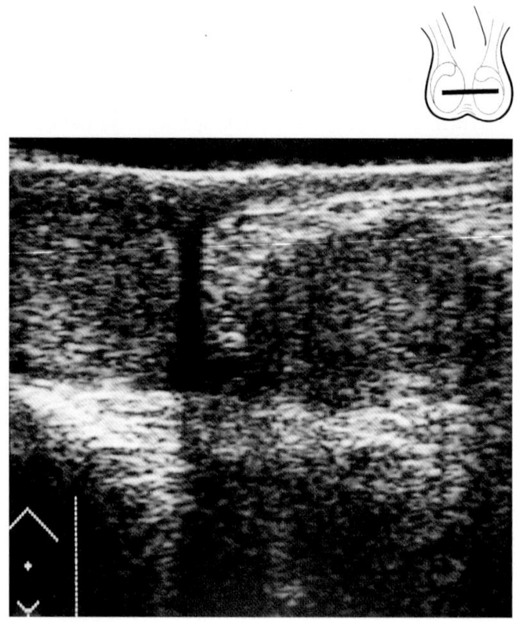

A

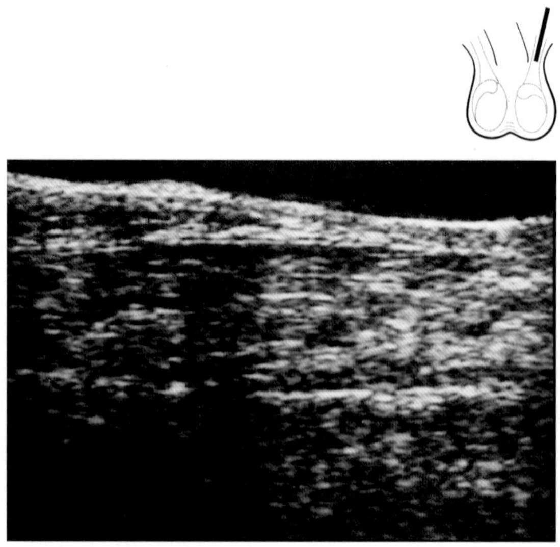

B

Case 63

A 12-year-old boy presents with a firm mass of the left testis discovered during a screening examination at school.

Physical Examination. There is a firm, slightly painful mass and enlargement of the left testis.

Ultrasound. Longitudinal scan of the left testis (Fig. 63). A solid, echogenic, well-delineated mass can be seen in the testis.

Conclusion. Testicular tumor.

Histology. Epidermoid cyst.

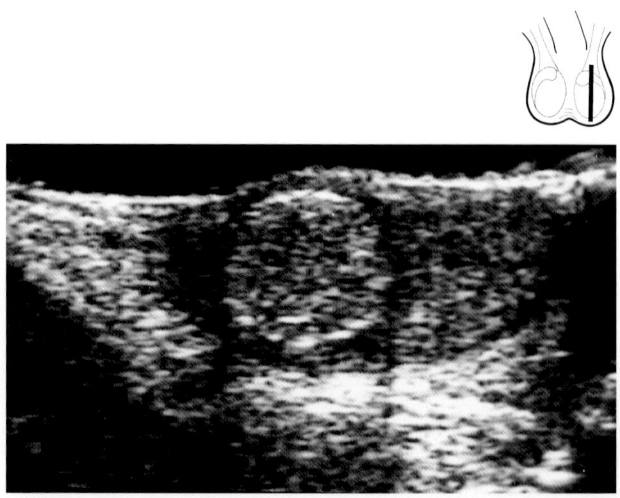

Case 64

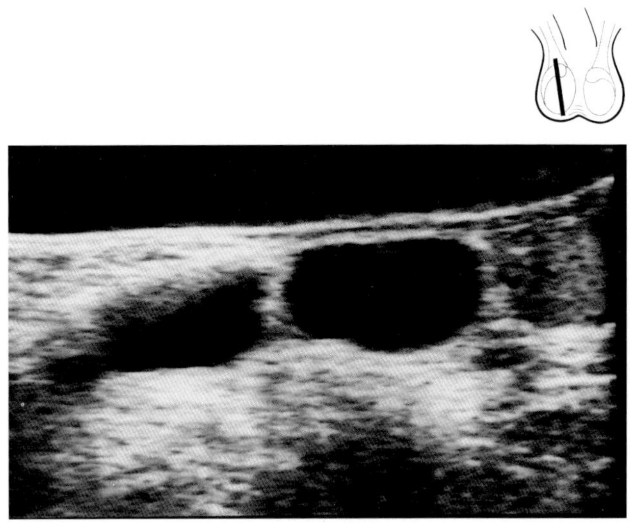

An 11-month-old infant presents with a swollen right hemiscrotum reported by the mother. There is no fever.

Physical Examination. There are several palpable nodules in the right scrotum extending to the inguinal canal. There is no pain and there are no signs of inflammation.

Ultrasound. Longitudinal scan of the right hemiscrotum (Fig. 64). The normal small right testis can be seen at the right margin of the figure. Multiple, smoothly demarcated, anechoic lesions are visualized along the spermatic cord.

Analysis. The sonographic demonstration of multiple circumscribed fluid collections in the area of the spermatic cord rules out a solid tumor (e.g., childhood rhabdomyosarcoma of the spermatic cord).

Conclusion. Funiculocele.

Clinical Course. Spontaneous regression after several weeks.

Case 65

A 6-month old infant presents with a lump in the right hemiscrotum noticed by his mother. There was no prior episode of acute pain indicative of testicular torsion.

Physical Examination. There is a firm, painless lump in the right scrotum. There is a normal small testis on the left. Transillumination findings are inconclusive.

Ultrasound. Longitudinal scans of the right (Fig. 65A) and left (Fig. 65B) testis. The enlarged right testis demonstrates heterogeneous echotexture with solid and cystic areas. Compare with the normal-sized and homogeneous echotexture of the left testis.

Analysis. Although testicular tumors are rare in childhood, the absence of signs suggesting earlier testicular torsion (e.g., a high-riding testicle) should alert the examiner to this possibility.

Conclusion. Right testicular tumor.

Histology. Mature teratoma.

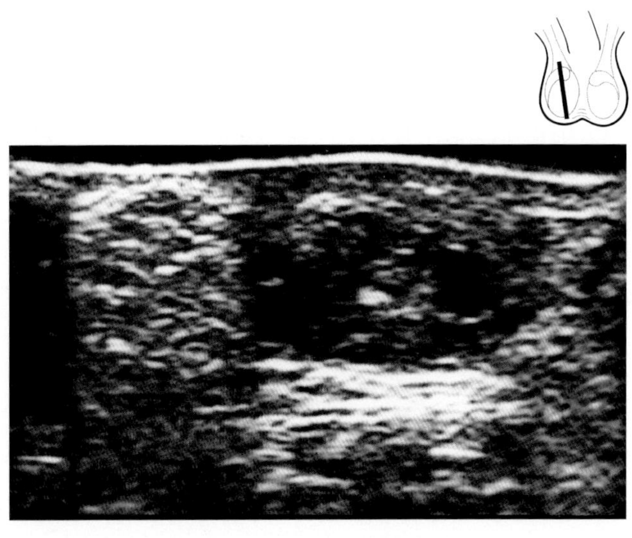

A

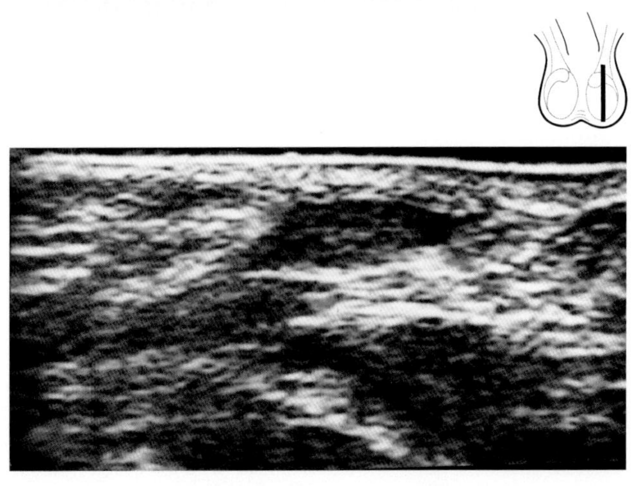

B

Case 66

A 21-year-old patient presents with a painful swelling of the lower pole of the right testis of 5 days' duration.

Physical Examination. There is a very painful swelling in the area of the epididymal tail on the right. No fluctuation is palpable; there is leukocytosis.

Ultrasound. Longitudinal scan of the right testis (Fig. 66). The tail of the epididymis is enlarged and demonstrates heterogeneous decreased echogenicity. The epididymal head (not shown) is unremarkable. The echotexture of the testis is normal, except for a hyperechoic, intratesticular band.

Conclusion. Right-sided epididymitis, mainly affecting the tail.

Clinical Course. Resolution of symptoms with antibiotic treatment.

Notes. The hyperechoic, intratesticular band corresponds to the mediastinum testis (unusually prominent).

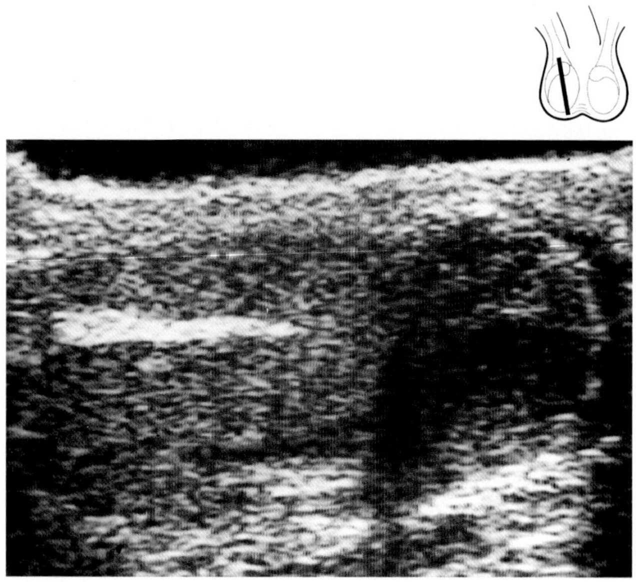

Case 67

A 30-year-old patient presents with increasing lumbar pain. Bulky disease in the para-aortic region has been demonstrated by computed tomography and there is a tentative diagnosis of malignant lymphoma.

Physical Examination. The scrotal contents are normal to palpation, but the left testis is slightly smaller than the right.

Ultrasound. Longitudinal scan of the left testis (Fig. 67A) and transverse scan of both testes (Fig. 67B). The testis on the left is smaller than that on the right. The echotexture of both testes is normal, except for focal, hyperechoic areas (some of which demonstrate acoustic shadowing) around the lower pole of the left testis.

Analysis. Focal testicular alteration in conjunction with the presence of retroperitoneal lymphadenopathy is strongly suggestive of a tumor. The echogenic foci might represent the scars and calcifications of a burned-out testicular tumor.

Conclusion. There is a high probability of a tumorous process in the left testis, possibly a burned-out testicular tumor.

Histology. There is focal fibrosis with calcifications and hemorrhagic residues, compatible with a so-called burned-out testicular tumor.

Notes. Small, intratesticular, echogenic scars or calcifications not related to a tumor are occasionally seen after trauma or surgery or in cases of microlithiasis. It is not possible to differentiate these from a small or a burned-out testicular tumor with sonography alone. The diagnosis is suggested by simultaneous evaluation of the retroperitoneal lymph nodes.

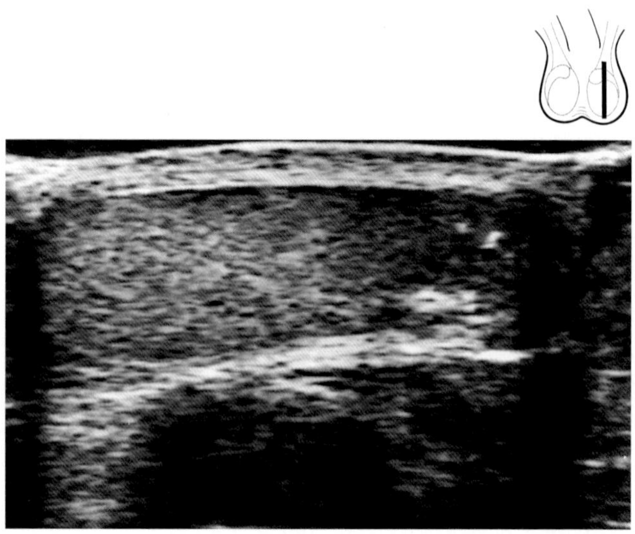

A

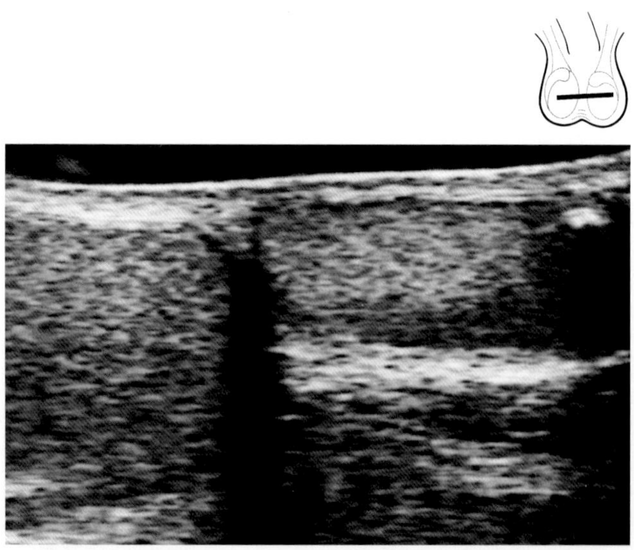

B

Case 68

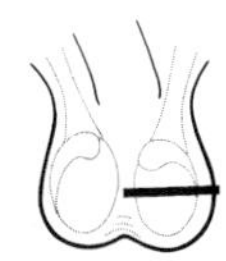

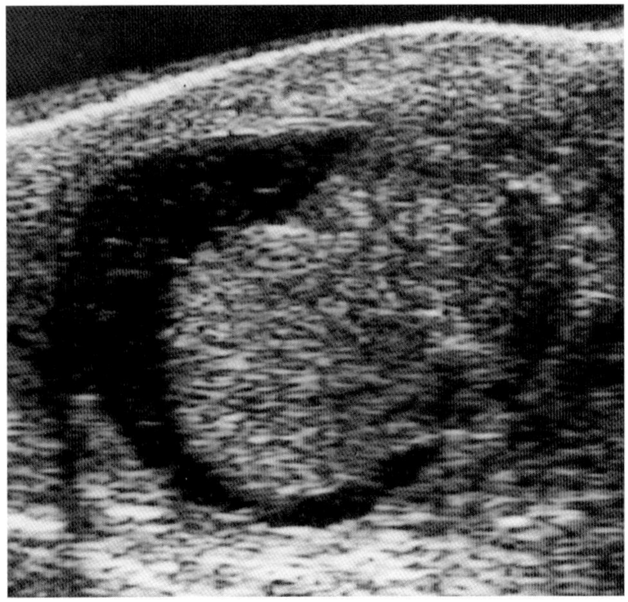

A 30-year-old patient presents with a 7-day history of painful swelling of the left testis and a fever.

Physical Examination. There is swelling and erythema of the left hemiscrotum, which has a tense, partly fluctuant consistency. The testis and epididymis cannot be delineated and the transillumination findings are equivocal

Ultrasound. Transverse view of the left testis (Fig. 68). There is pronounced enlargement of the epididymis and swelling of the paratesticular tissue. A crescent-shaped fluid collection with internal echoes can be seen surrounding the testis. The testis is unremarkable, without focal lesions. There is scrotal skin edema.

Analysis. Although the clinical findings (fluctuation noted on palpation) indicate an abscess, an underlying tumor should be excluded. Sonography demonstrates neither abscess formation nor suspicious focal lesions in the testis or epididymis. The fluctuation in this case is caused by the hydrocele.

Conclusion. Acute epididymitis with a reactive hydrocele.

Clinical Course. Resolution of symptoms with antibiotic treatment.

Case 69

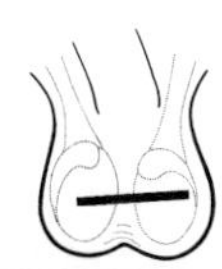

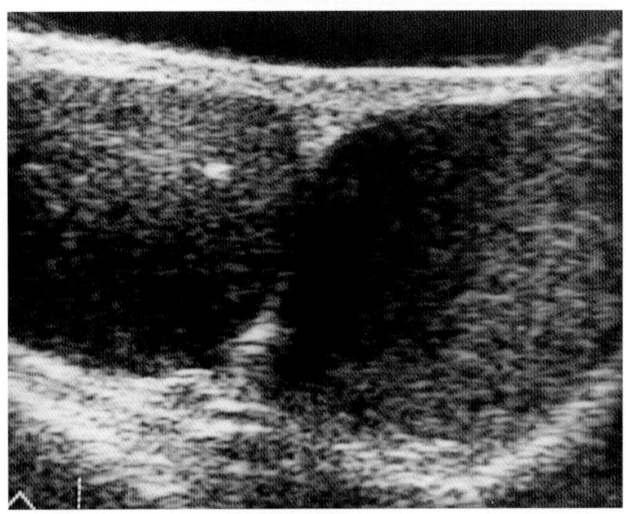

A 36-year-old patient with acute lymphocytic leukemia presents with swelling and possible leukemic infiltration of the left testis.

Physical Examination. There is moderate enlargement of the left testis compared with the right. The consistency of both testes is normal.

Ultrasound. Transverse view of both testes (Fig. 69). There are hypoechoic, poorly demarcated areas in both testes. Partially preserved testicular tissue of normal echogenicity is also seen bilaterally. In addition, a small echogenic focus can be seen in the right testis.

Conclusion. Bilateral testicular manifestations of acute lymphocytic leukemia. The small echogenic focus in the right testis might represent a regressive scar or calcification.

Clinical Course. There was regression of the hypoechoic testicular areas after irradiation with 12 Gy and three cycles of chemotherapy.

Case 70

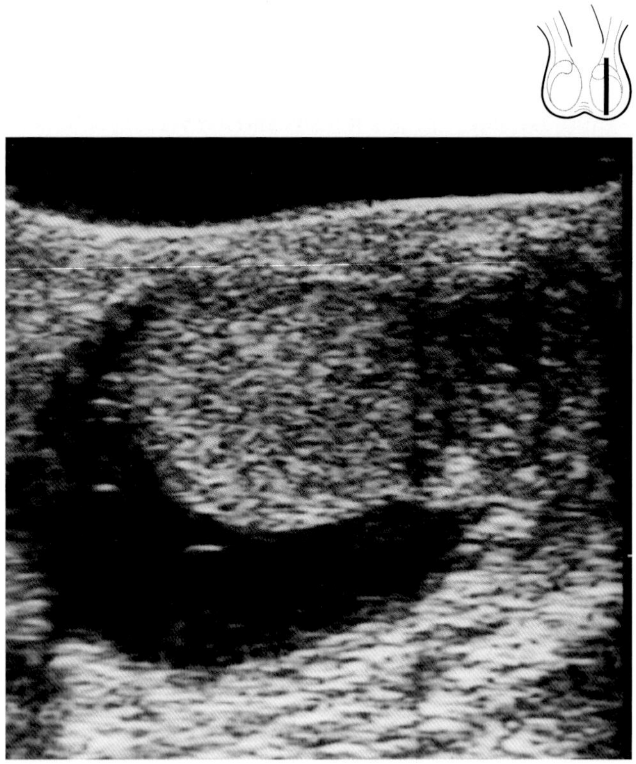

A 77-year-old patient presents with swelling and acute pain of the left scrotum of 4 days' duration. The patient has experienced repeated episodes of epididymitis.

Physical Examination. There is tense swelling of the left hemiscrotum limiting examination. A tender induration and enlargement of the epididymis, however, can be palpated. There is also scrotal skin edema and leukocytosis.

Ultrasound. Longitudinal scan of the left testis (Fig. 70). There is enlargement of the tail of the left epididymis with an additional small doughnut-shaped hypoechoic lesion. The testis appears normal and is differentiated from the epididymis. An increased amount of fluid with internal echoes can be seen.

Conclusion. Left-sided epididymitis with a reactive, inflammatory hydrocele and scrotal skin edema. There may also be a small abscess in the epididymal tail, but there is no evidence of a testicular tumor.

Clinical Course and Histology. Because of recurrent inflammation, orchiectomy was performed. The histologic examination revealed a severe, suppurative epididymitis with abscess formation.

Notes. Hydroceles occurring in conjunction with inflammatory processes frequently display internal echoes. Eventually, they may become septated and persistent.

Case 71

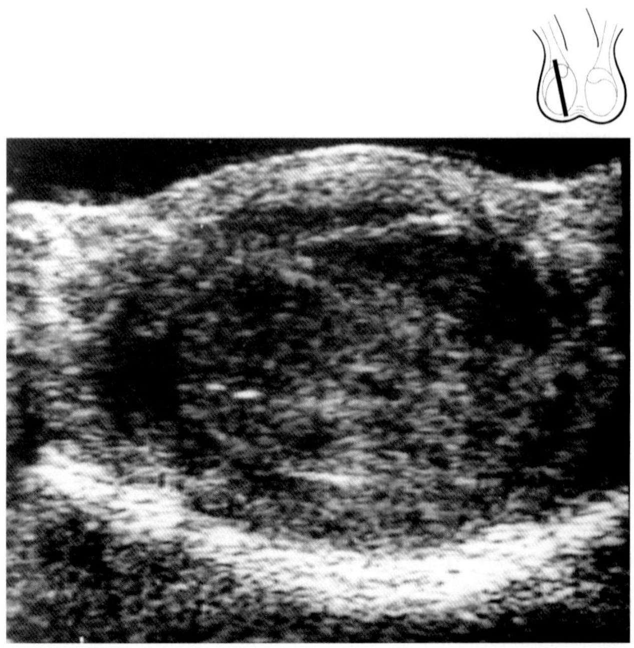

A 52-year-old patient presents with a 2-week history of a very painful, swollen right testis that has shown only slight improvement with antibiotic treatment. The patient underwent a kidney transplant 5 months earlier.

Physical Examination. There is a very painful, swollen, and indurated right hemiscrotum. The testis and epididymis cannot be delineated and there is erythema and edema of the scrotal skin. There is no transillumination.

Ultrasound. Longitudinal scan of the right testis (Fig. 71). The testis is enlarged, with irregularly decreased echogenicity throughout. The epididymis (not completely seen) is also enlarged. A small fluid collection and edema of the paratesticular tissue are also present.

Analysis. Given the clinical picture of inflammation, the sonographically demonstrated inhomogeneous, hypoechoic echotexture of the entire testis and enlargement of the epididymis strongly suggest an abscess-forming process.

Conclusion. Epididymo-orchitis with suspected intratesticular abscess formation.

Histology. Severe granulomatous orchitis with abscess formation.

Case 72

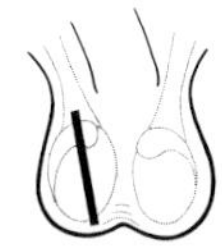

A 20-year-old patient presents with acute scrotal swelling after a motorcycle accident.

Physical Examination. There is a very painful, tense swelling of the right hemiscrotum. The testis cannot be delineated.

Ultrasound. Longitudinal view of the right scrotum (Fig. 72). The testis is inhomogeneously structured with a distorted contour. A fluid collection with internal echoes can be seen.

Analysis. The inhomogeneous texture of the testis in conjunction with a hematocele strongly suggests testicular rupture.

Conclusion. Right testicular rupture with hematocele.

Findings at Surgery. Right testicular rupture with hematocele.

Notes. In patients with scrotal trauma ultrasound examination can demonstrate or exclude testicular rupture, the finding of which indicates whether surgery is needed.

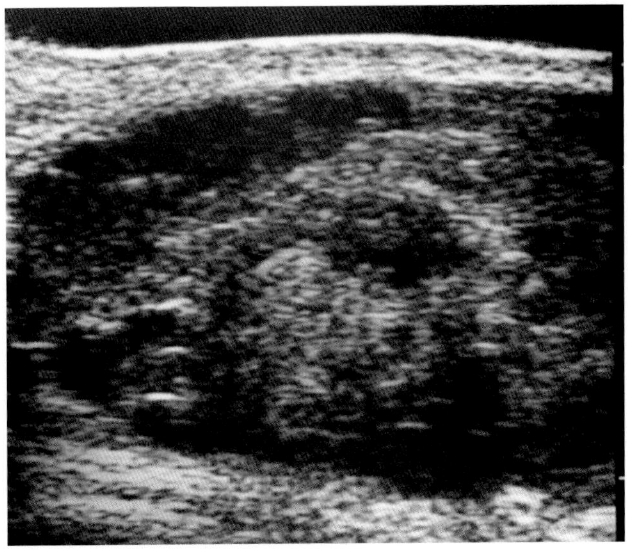

Case 73

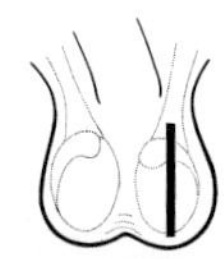

A 35-year-old patient with scrotal trauma presents with livid swelling after a fall from a scaffold.

Physical Examination. Palpation is not possible because of tense swelling of the entire scrotum.

Ultrasound. Longitudinal view of the left hemiscrotum (Fig. 73). The left testis is not identified. The enlarged scrotum contains poorly demarcated solid areas within the fluid. The fluid contains numerous internal echoes. The right testis (not shown) is normal.

Conclusion. Scrotal trauma with fragmentation of the left testis and hematocele.

Findings at Surgery. Testicular rupture and fragmentation on the left.

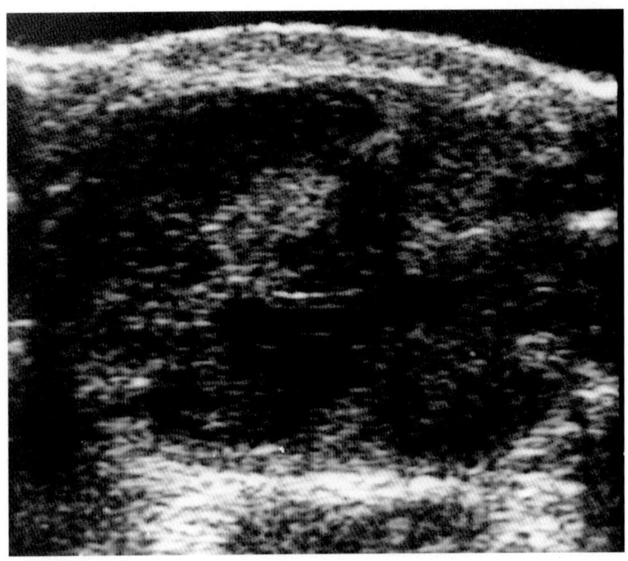

Case 74

A 65-year-old patient presents with a painless, swollen right testis. He experienced right-sided epididymitis 1 year previously.

Physical Examination. There is a painless, firm enlargement of the right testis and a moderately enlarged ipsilateral epididymis. There is no transillumination and there are no signs of inflammation.

Ultrasound. Transverse scan of both testes (Fig. 74A). The right testis is enlarged with homogeneously decreased echogenicity.

Analysis. Findings of a firm, palpable mass in combination with the sonographically demonstrated hypoechoic echotexture of the testicular parenchyma (although homogeneous) strongly suggests a testicular tumor.

Conclusion. High probability of a right testicular tumor.

Histology. Chronic fibrotic orchitis (Fig. 74B is a surgical specimen).

Notes. It is not always possible to differentiate chronic fibrotic or chronic granulomatous orchitis from a testicular tumor based on clinical presentation and sonographic appearance.

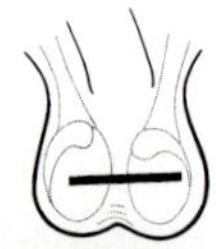

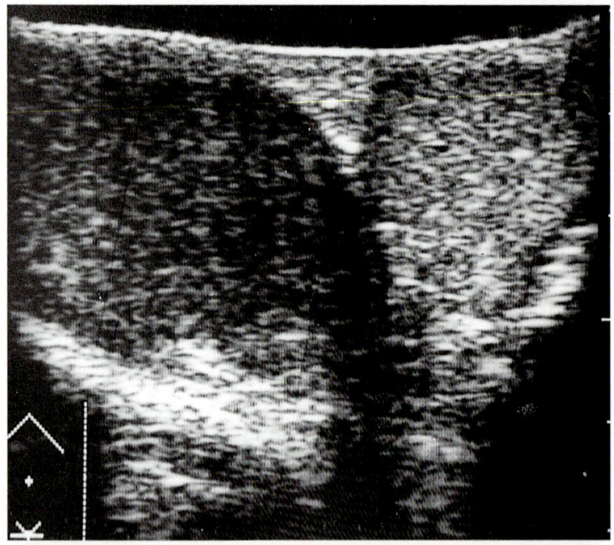

A

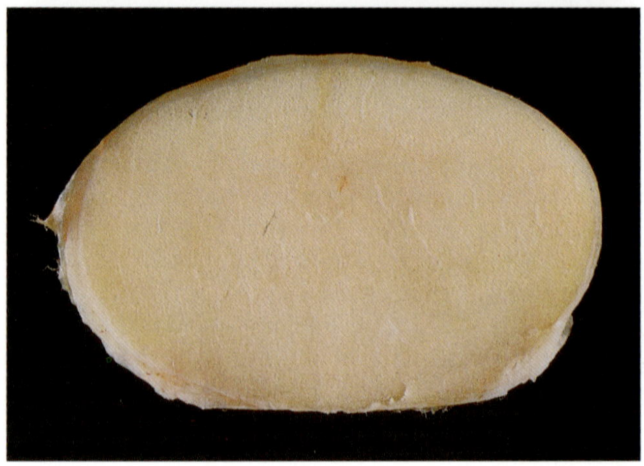

B

Case 75

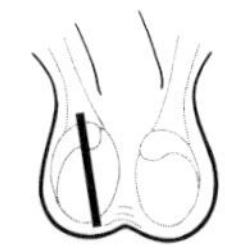

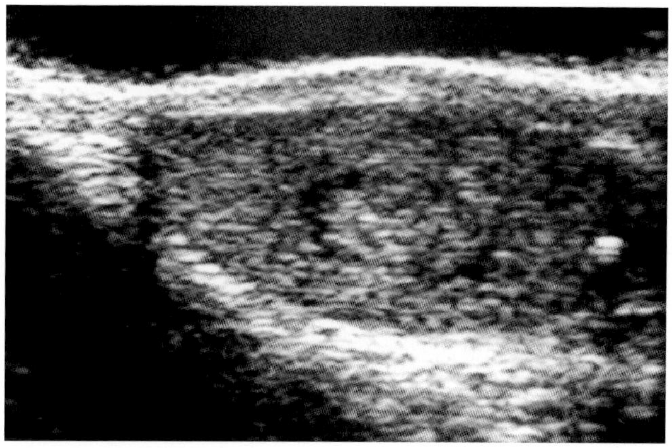

A 37-year-old patient presents with a hardening of the right testis.

Physical Examination. There is a firm induration of the normal-sized right testis.

Ultrasound. Longitudinal scan of the right testis (Fig. 75). There is a nearly isoechoic mass with an irregular, hypoechoic rim in the middle and lower third of the testis. In addition, there is calcification at the lower pole of the testis.

Analysis. At first glance the sonographic appearance is nearly normal. In view of the physical findings, however, the intratesticular tumor should not escape detection.

Conclusion. Right testicular tumor.

Histology. Teratoma.

Notes. In rare cases, testicular tumors (particularly teratomas) may be isoechoic with respect to the surrounding testicular parenchyma. In these cases, the clinical examination is the cornerstone of diagnosis.

Case 76

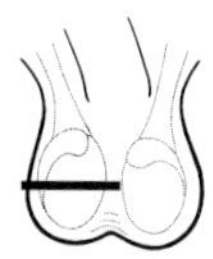

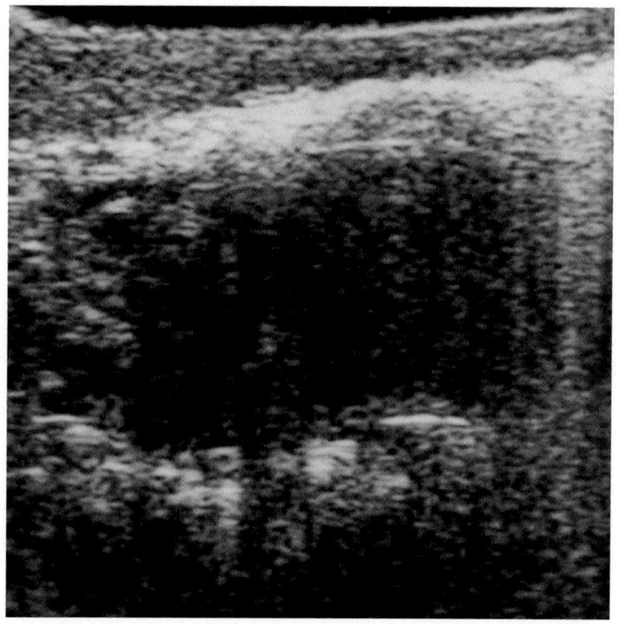

A 73-year-old patient presents with severe inflammatory swelling of the entire scrotum, a large perianal abscess, and a high fever.

Physical Examination. The entire scrotum is enormously swollen. The testis and epididymis are not palpable on either side. There is erythema and pronounced edema of the scrotal skin and leukocytosis.

Ultrasound. Transverse scan of the right scrotal compartment (Fig. 76). There is a large intrascrotal fluid collection. Extensive air pockets presenting as dense echogenic areas with distal "dirty" acoustic shadowing are also visualized. Further examination reveals bilaterally normal-sized testis and epididymis (not shown), but the examination is limited by interfering air.

Conclusion. Large scrotal abscess.

Surgical Findings. Large abscess requiring extensive drainage and debridement.

Case 77

A 72-year-old patient presents with firm induration of both testes. There is no pain and no fever.

Physical Examination. There is firm, nontender induration of both testes, more marked on the left. Neither epididymis can be delineated. There are no signs of inflammation.

Ultrasound. Transverse scan of both testes (Fig. 77A) and longitudinal scan of the left testis (Fig. 77B). The testes are normal, with a homogeneous echotexture. They are surrounded by a hypoechoic, partly calcified rim of varying thickness. Neither epididymis can be delineated.

Analysis. Clinical findings are strongly suggestive of bilateral testicular tumor, which can be ruled out by the sonographic demonstration of homogeneous echotexture of the testes. The palpably suspicious induration is produced by the rimlike thickening of the paratesticular tissue with focal calcified areas. The patient had an indwelling urinary bladder catheter inserted 1 1/2 years previously and had been suffering from recurrent urinary tract infections since.

Conclusion. Extensive, chronic periorchitis with bilateral calcifications. No evidence of a testicular tumor.

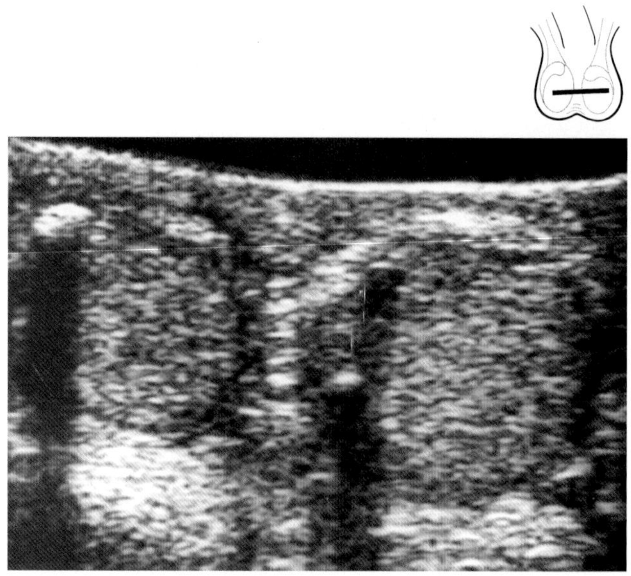
A

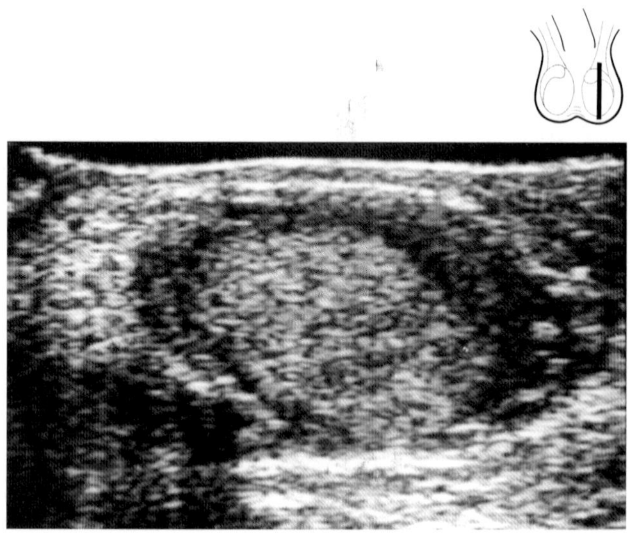
B

Case 78

A 16-year-old patient who has noticed a painless lump in his right testis. The patient has previously received hormone therapy for right-sided cryptorchidism.

Physical Examination. Testicles are of equal size but palpation reveals a circumscribed, painless, firm mass in the lower pole of the right testis. There are no signs of inflammation.

Ultrasound. Longitudinal scan of the right testis (Fig. 78) demonstrates a focal, hypoechoic lesion in the lower pole of the testis.

Conclusion. Right testicular tumor.

Histology. Teratocarcinoma of the testis (embryonal carcinoma and immature teratoma).

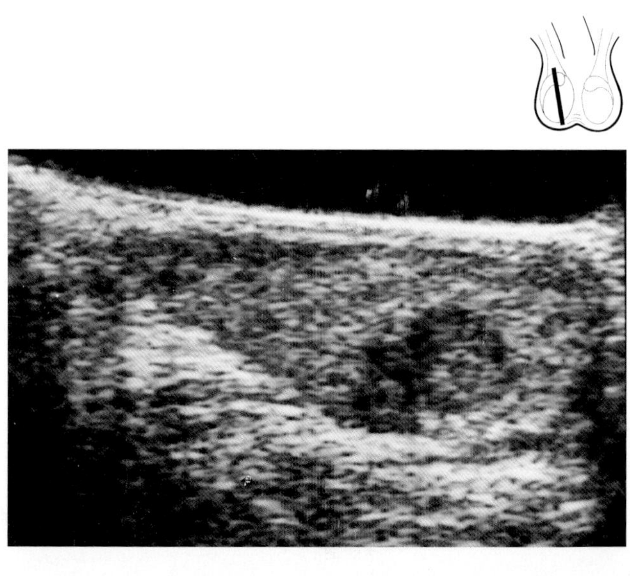

Case 79

A 36-year-old patient presents with a very painful, swollen left hemiscrotum and a high fever. He underwent urethrotomy and placement of a transurethral catheter 7 days previously.

Physical Examination. There is a very painful, swollen left hemiscrotum and the testis and epididymis cannot be delineated. There is erythema and edema of the scrotal skin and no transillumination.

Ultrasound. Longitudinal scan of the left testis (Fig. 79A) and transverse scan of both testes (Fig. 79B). The left testis and epididymis are markedly enlarged and hypoechoic. There is "onion peel" edematous appearance of the paratesticular tissue (compare with the contralateral side) and there is scrotal skin edema on the left.

Conclusion. Extensive epididymo-orchitis on the left.

Clinical Course and Histology. The patient deteriorated during a course of antibiotic treatment, therefore a left-sided orchiectomy was performed. Abscess-forming epididymo-orchitis was confirmed histologically.

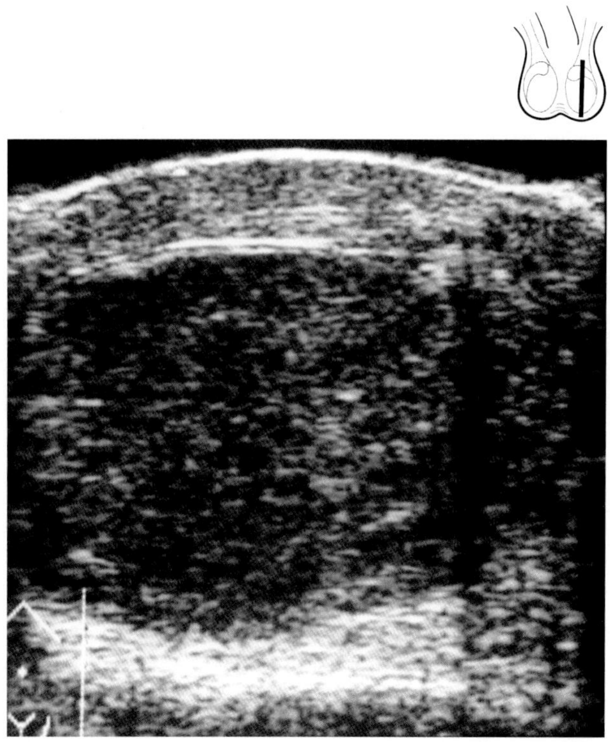

A

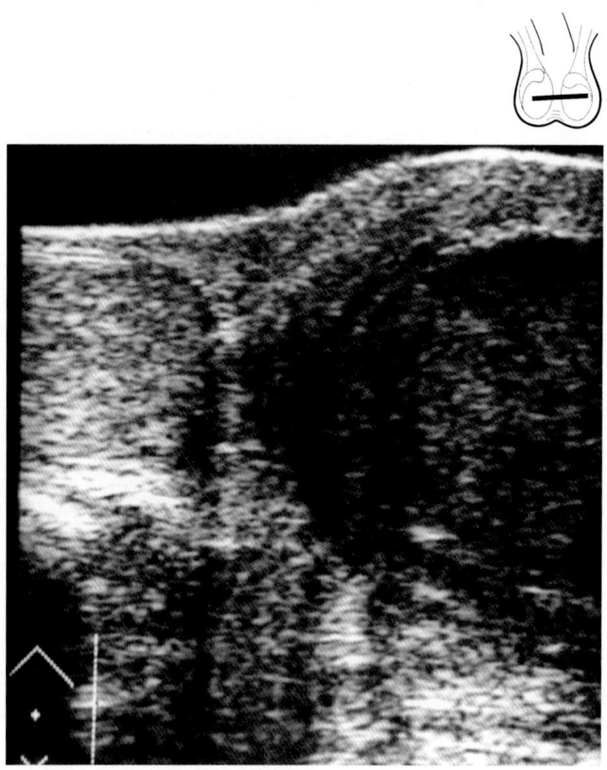

B

Case 80

An 11-year-old patient presents with acute onset of right testicular pain 4 days prior to presentation and subsequent progressive swelling.

Physical Examination. The right epididymis is moderately tender and considerably enlarged. There is moderate induration of the testis, scrotal skin edema, but no fever.

Ultrasound. Longitudinal view of the right testis (Fig. 80A). The normal-sized testis is of homogeneously decreased echogenicity. The epididymis is enlarged, inhomogeneous, and echogenic. A small fluid collection with internal echoes can be seen. There is swelling of the paratesticular tissue and scrotal skin. Color-coded duplex ultrasound (Fig. 80B) shows no blood flow in the testis and increased blood flow in the paratesticular tissue and scrotal skin.

Analysis. The sonographic appearance alone is not specific. The most likely differential diagnoses are epididymo-orchitis and testicular torsion of longer duration (acute pain, no fever). Hemorrhage into the epididymis often results in an increased echogenicity.

Conclusion. Testicular torsion of longer duration.

Intraoperative Finding and Histology. Hemorrhagic necrosis of the testis and epididymis secondary to torsion.

Notes. The sonographic appearance of testicular torsion is nonspecific. Color-coded duplex ultrasound adds specificity to gray-scale findings.

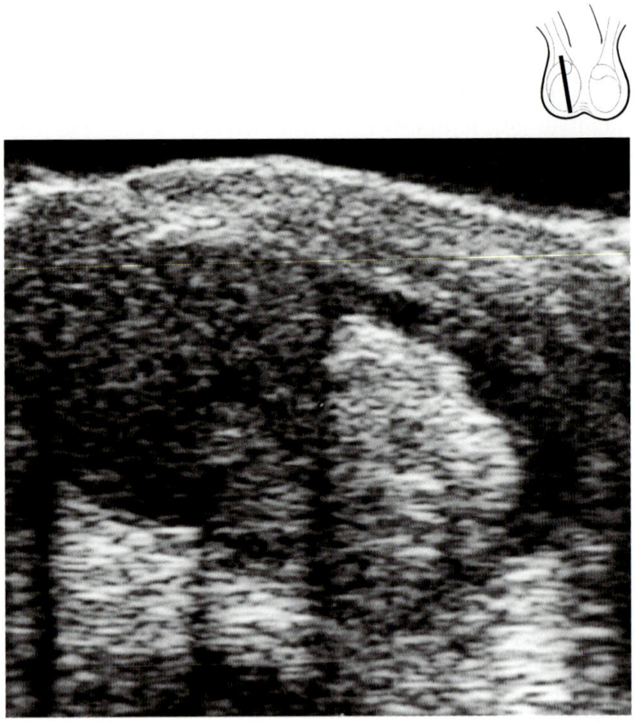

A

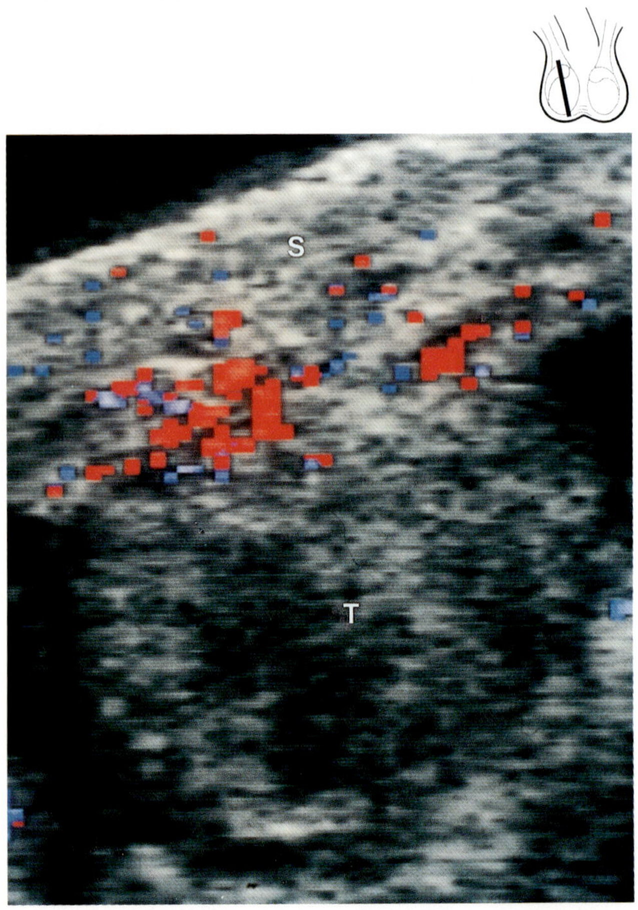

B

Case 81

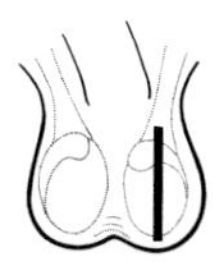

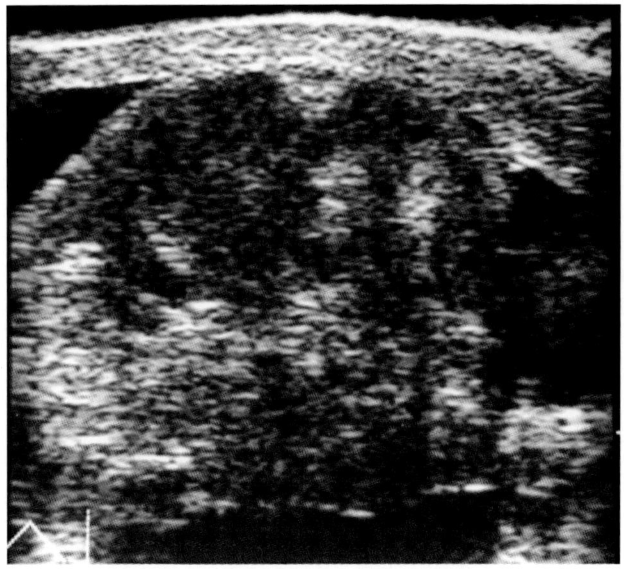

A 40-year-old patient presents with sudden, severely painful enlargement of the left testis of 6-days' duration.

Physical Examination. There is a large, indurated mass of the testis, and the testis and epididymis are difficult to differentiate. There is erythema and edema of the scrotal skin, but no fever.

Ultrasound. Longitudinal scan of the left testis (Fig. 81). The markedly enlarged testis demonstrates heterogeneous echotexture with areas of decreased and increased echogenicity. The epididymis is likewise enlarged and of increased echogenicity. A moderately increased amount of fluid is seen.

Analysis. The sonographic appearance of inhomogeneous echotexture and enlargement of the testis are suggestive of a tumor. However, since the patient convincingly claimed that the testis had been completely normal some days previously, the diagnosis of a tumor appears to be unlikely. The presence of pain and erythema of the scrotal skin associated with enlargement of the epididymis suggests a severe epididymo-orchitis, although the absence of fever is contradictory.

Conclusion. Suspicion of severe epididymo-orchitis on the left, possibly associated with hemorrhage.

Intraoperative Findings and Histology. Hemorrhagic testicular and epididymal necrosis secondary to torsion.

Notes. The gray scale sonographic appearance of testicular torsion is nonspecific. Even though it is rare, torsion can occur after puberty.

Case 82

A 29-year-old patient presents with a large, painless, swollen left testis.

Physical Examination. There is a large, firm, painless mass in the left testis. The right testis is of normal size and there are no signs of inflammation.

Ultrasound. Longitudinal scans of the right (Fig. 82A) and left (Fig. 82B) testis and transverse scan of both testes (Fig. 82C). The left testis is enlarged and diffusely abnormal in echogenicity. The normal-sized right testis shows an echo-poor, fairly well demarcated area with only a thin rim of normal testicular tissue detectable at the lower pole.

Analysis. The clinical findings alone suggest the diagnosis of a testicular tumor on the left. Sonographic examination demonstrates an additional tumor in the right testis, which also feels indurated on repeated palpation. This finding was missed in the initial clinical examination because of the obvious testicular tumor on the left.

Conclusion. Bilateral testicular tumor.

Histology. Seminoma of both testes (Fig. 82D is a surgical specimen).

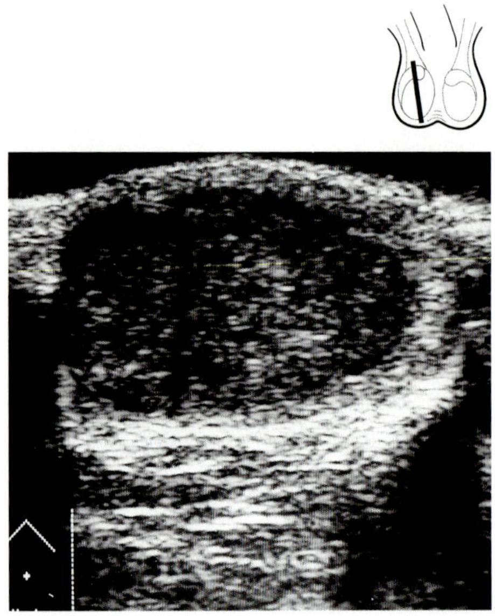

A

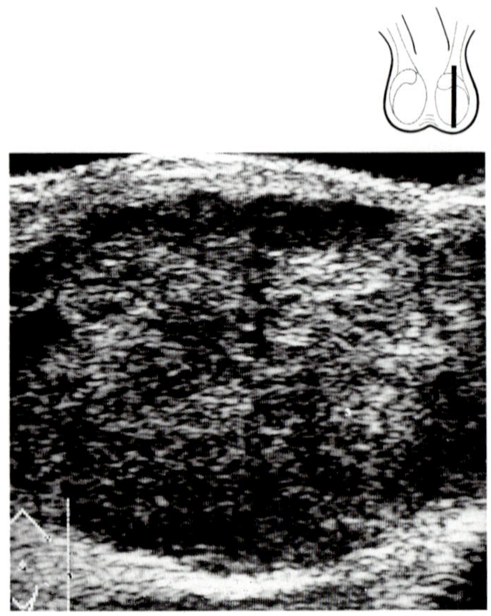

B

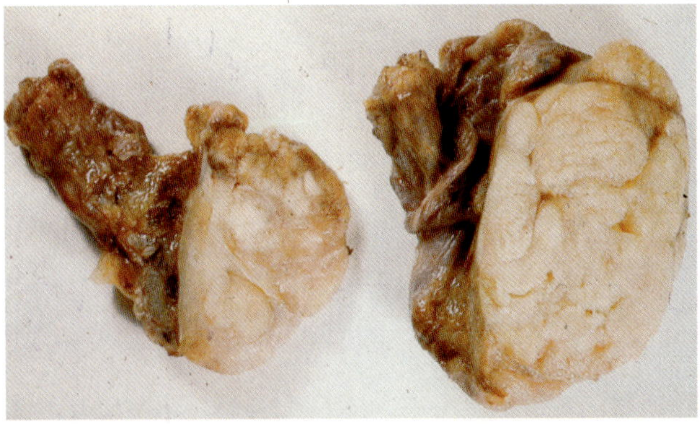

D

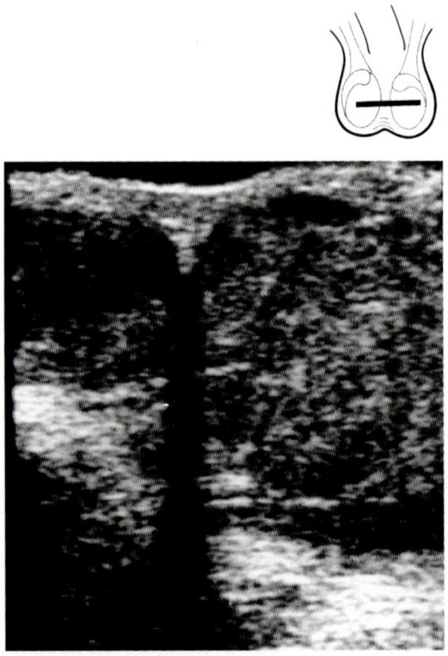

C

Case 83

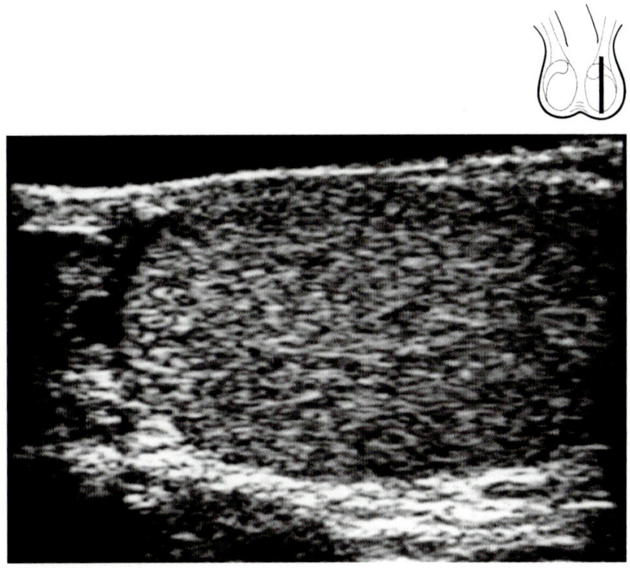

A 34-year-old patient presents with vague, left-sided pain. There is no fever.

Physical Examination. Unremarkable.

Ultrasound. Longitudinal scan of the left testis (Fig. 83). There is good differentiation between the testis and epididymis. A small cyst (about 5 mm in diameter) is seen in the head of the epididymis. The testis is normal.

Conclusion. Small epididymal cyst of the head of the left epididymis as an incidental finding.

Case 84

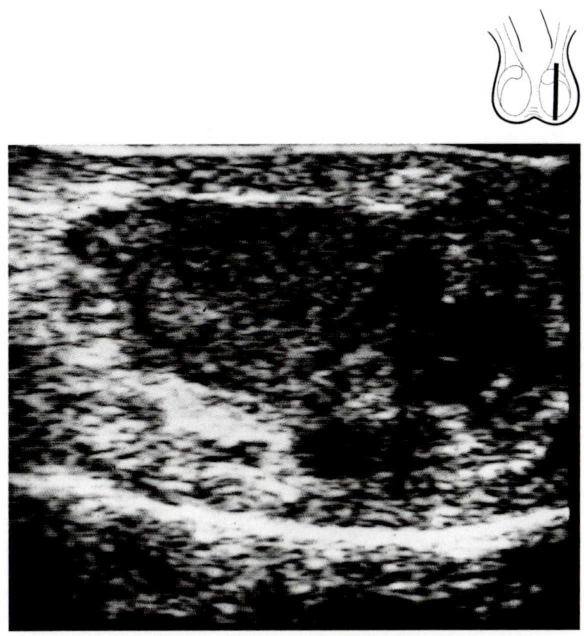

A

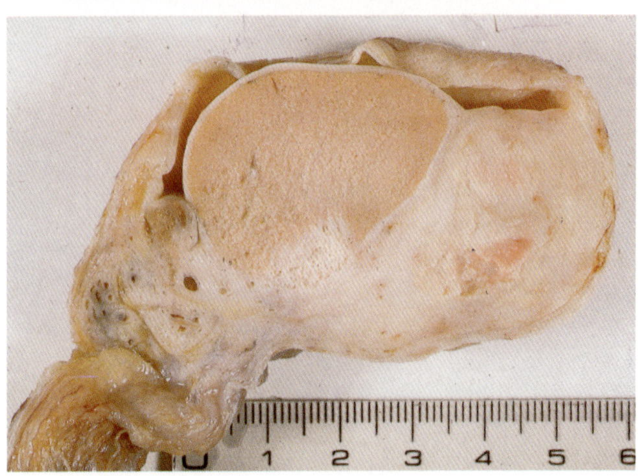

B

A 74-year-old patient presents with a moderately painful swelling of the left hemiscrotum of several weeks' duration. There is no fever.

Physical Examination. There is a firm, moderately tender swelling in the area of the lower pole of the testis. The testis and epididymis cannot be differentiated.

Ultrasound. Longitudinal scan of the left testis (Fig. 84A). There is an inhomogeneous, partly hypoechoic mass adjacent to the lower pole of the testis, more likely related to the epididymis. The lower pole of the testis is deformed and cannot be separated from the epididymal tail. The testicular echotexture is homogeneous.

Analysis. The palpation findings suggest a neoplasm despite pain, a suspicion that cannot be definitely ruled out by the sonographic appearance (solid lesion, no reliable differentiation of the enlarged epididymis from the lower pole of the testis, absence of scrotal skin edema).

Conclusion. Solid mass in the area of the epididymal tail, possibly extending to the lower pole of the testis. The differential diagnosis is chronic inflammation or tumor.

Surgical Findings and Histology. Chronic abscess-forming epididymitis with extensive fibrosis and deformity of the lower pole of the testis (Fig. 84B is a surgical specimen).

Case 85

A 28-year-old patient presents with a firm, painless, enlarged right testis.

Physical Examination. The right testis is nodular, indurated, and moderately enlarged, without tenderness. There is possible induration of the left testis. There are no signs of inflammation.

Ultrasound. Longitudinal scans of the right (Fig. 85A) and left (Fig. 85B) testis. The right testis is enlarged. Multiple, hypoechoic, focal lesions are seen in both testes. The epididymal head on the right also appears slightly enlarged.

Analysis. The incongruous findings on palpation (indicating a testicular tumor on the right) versus ultrasound (hypoechoic multiple lesions in both testes) do not permit a definite diagnosis. Such findings may be caused by bilateral tumor (e.g., lymphoma) manifestation, which is rare, or by a granulomatous inflammatory alteration.

Conclusion. Tumorous or granulomatous lesions of both testes.

Histology. Intratesticular gummas (right-sided biopsy).

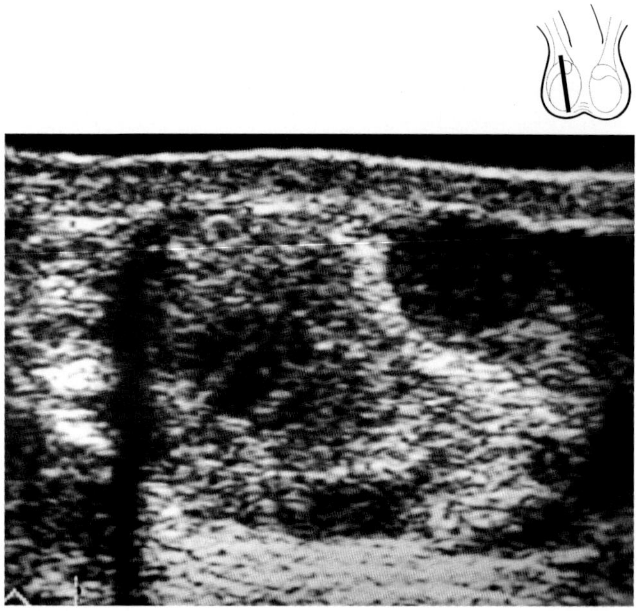

A

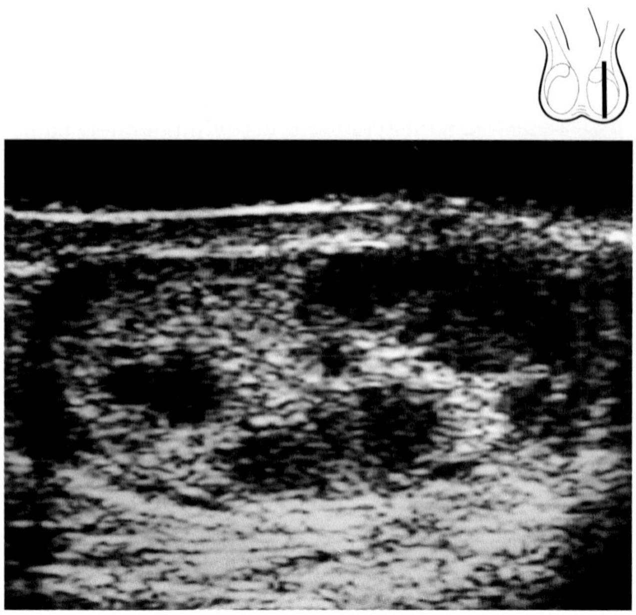

B

Case 86

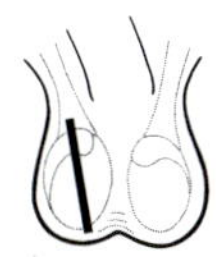

A 37-year-old soldier presents with a mass of the right testis incidentally found on clinical examination for severe osteomyelitis developing after an open lower leg injury 2 months earlier.

Physical Examination. There is a firm, nearly painless mass at the lower pole of the right testis. There are no signs of inflammation or trauma.

Ultrasound. Longitudinal scan of the right testis (Fig. 86A). There is a large crescent-shaped, hypoechoic lesion in the middle and lower testis. There is a second small, hypoechoic lesion identified separately. The epididymis is unremarkable (only the head is visualized).

Conclusion. Strong likelihood of a tumor in the right testis.

Intraoperative Findings and Histology. There is an old, partly liquified paratesticular hematoma with marginal fibroses and small subcapsular intratesticular hematoma (Fig. 86B is a surgical specimen).

Notes. The clinical and sonographic findings strongly suggest a testicular tumor. This is contradicted only by the pronounced hypoechogenicity of the lesions, although the smaller lesion is definitely intratesticular in location. It was not possible to obtain a sufficiently detailed history, which might have yielded decisive information about earlier scrotal trauma.

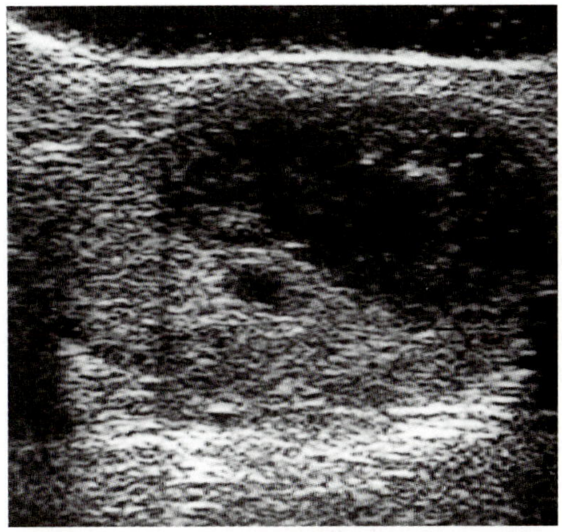

A

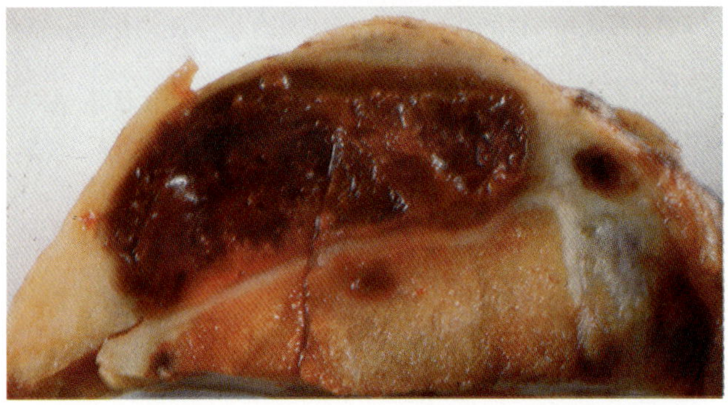

B

Case 87

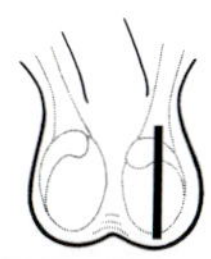

A 28-year-old patient presents with recurrence of a retroperitoneal tumor after surgical removal of a teratoma 14 months previously. The patient underwent orchiopexy during childhood.

Physical Examination. Both testes are normal to palpation.

Ultrasound. Longitudinal scan of the left testis (Fig. 87). There are isolated, intratesticular, echogenic foci in the lower pole. Otherwise the echotexture of the testis is normal. No mass can be felt during repeated clinical examination.

Conclusion. Intratesticular scars in the area of the lower pole of the left testis after childhood orchiopexy.

Histology. Small, mature teratoma of the left testis containing scars and hyaline cartilage.

Notes. A testicular lesion in the presence of a retroperitoneal tumor always suggests a tumor, even if the palpation findings are normal or if the patient's history suggests other possible causes.

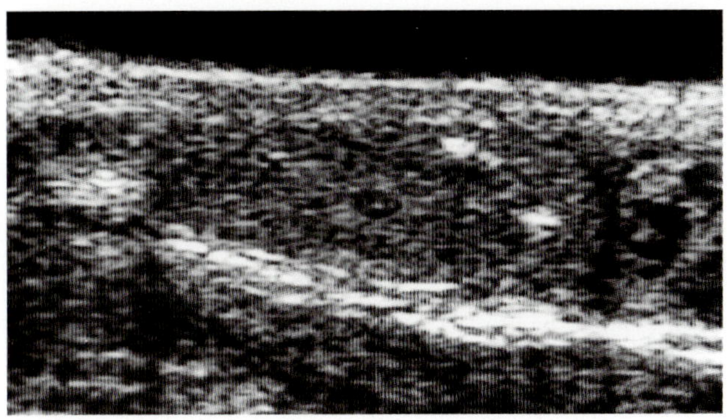

Case 88

A 54-year-old patient presents with an enlarged, painless right testis following right-sided epididymitis 5 weeks previously.

Physical Examination. The right testis is moderately enlarged, nontender, and firm. The testis and epididymis cannot be separated. There are no signs of inflammation and no leukocytosis.

Ultrasound. Longitudinal scans of the right (Fig. 88A) and left (Fig. 88B) testis. The right testis is mildly enlarged (as compared with the contralateral side), is hypoechoic, and has heterogeneous echotexture. There is no reliable identification of the right epididymis. On the left, the testis and epididymis are normal.

Analysis. The clinical and sonographic findings strongly suggest a right-sided testicular tumor. This suspicion cannot be refuted by the patient's report of a previous epididymitis because there might be a concealed tumor with concomitant inflammation.

Conclusion. High probability of a right testicular tumor.

Histology. Chronic granulomatous orchitis (Fig. 88C is a surgical specimen).

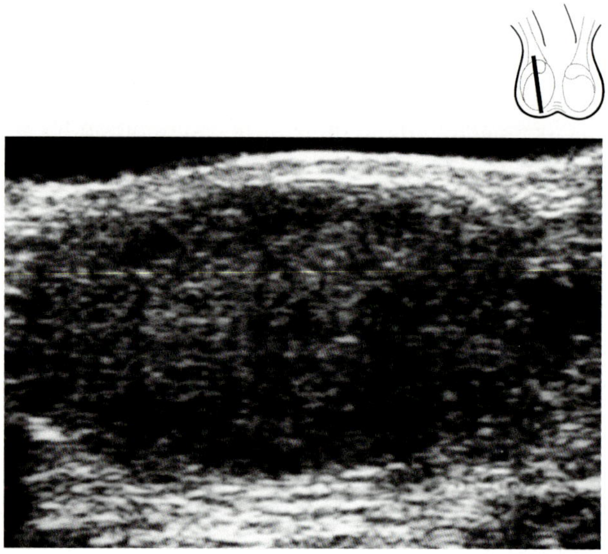

A

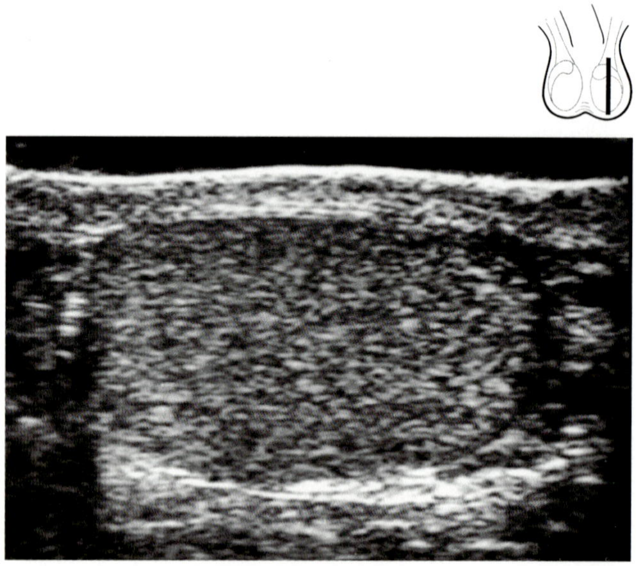

B

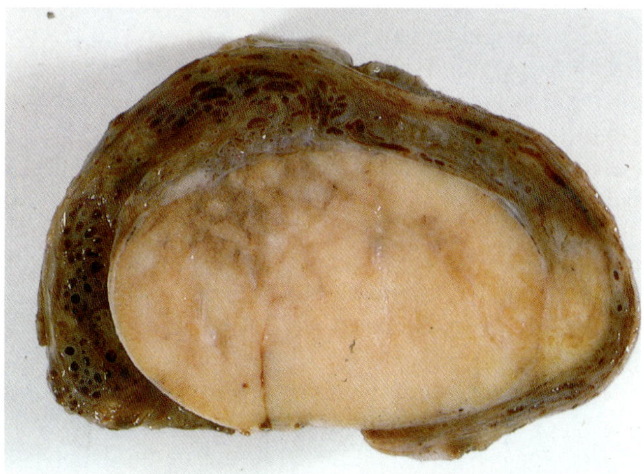

C

Case 92

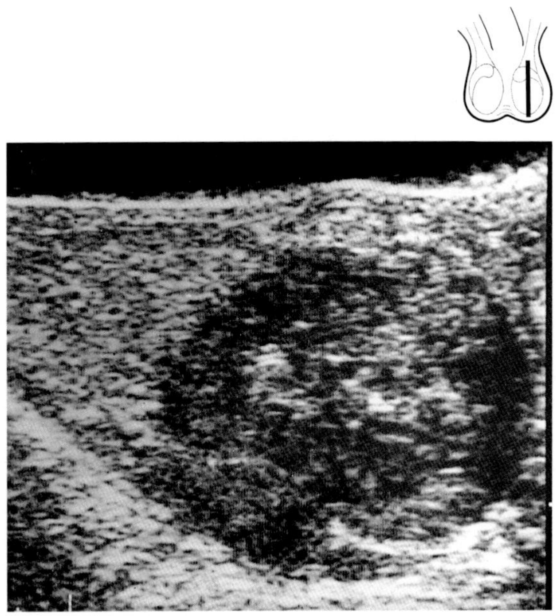

A 75-year-old patient presents with a firm lump in the left testicle. There is no history of inflammatory scrotal disease.

Physical Examination. There is a firm, slightly tender induration in the lower pole of the left testis. The testis and epididymis cannot be separated, there are no signs of inflammation, and there is no transillumination.

Ultrasound. Longitudinal scan of the left testis (Fig. 92). There is a large, echo-poor, and inhomogeneous mass. The lower pole of the testis is involved in this process or is compressed and deformed by the mass. The upper pole testicular parenchyma appears normal.

Analysis. The clinical picture indicates tumor. The ultrasound examination confirms presence of a solid mass primarily extratesticular in location, but does not permit definite exclusion of testicular involvement. The patient's history makes a chronic granulomatous inflammatory process of the epididymis very unlikely.

Conclusion. A malignant, extratesticular tumor of unclear origin is strongly suspected.

Histology. Paratesticular lymphosarcoma.

Case 93

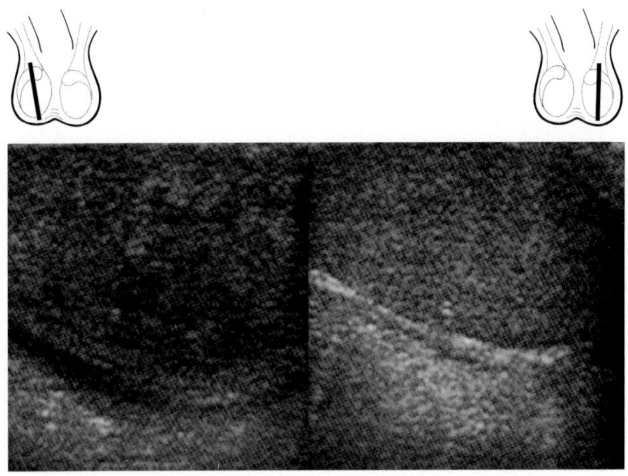

A

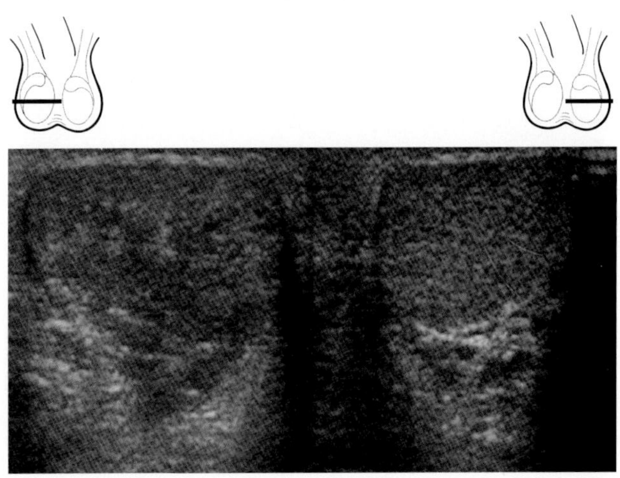

B

A 25-year-old patient presents with acute pain and swelling of the right hemiscrotum, which were first misdiagnosed as epididymitis.

Physical Examination. Severe pain and tenderness in the right side of the scrotum prohibit a thorough examination. No fever or leukocytosis was present.

Ultrasound. Longitudinal (Fig. 93A) and transverse (Fig. 93B) sonograms performed 5 days after the onset of symptoms show enlargement of the right testis and a poorly marginated focal hypoechoic intratesticular lesion.

Conclusion. A typical history of acute-onset scrotal pain and absence of fever and leukocytosis suggest the diagnosis of torsion of the spermatic cord. However, orchitis with abscess or even testicular tumor cannot be differentiated by ultrasound findings alone.

Histology. Surgery was done and a histologic diagnosis of torsion gangrene was made.

Case 94

A 26-year-old patient presents with acute scrotal pain and swelling after a motor vehicle accident.

Physical Examination. Moderately enlarged right hemiscrotum. Palpation was not possible because of severe pain and tenderness.

Ultrasound. Two adjacent longitudinal sonograms (Figs. 94A and B) demonstrate irregular contour defect in upper pole of right testis with disruption of the tunica albuginea and hematocele. Several hypoechoic areas are seen in testicular parenchyma.

Conclusion. Given the history of recent trauma, these findings represent rupture of right testis with associated hematocele.

Histology. Orchiectomy was done. At operation, rupture of the tunica albuginea and accompanying hematocele was confirmed. On histopathology, intratesticular hemorrhage and multifocal infarction were found.

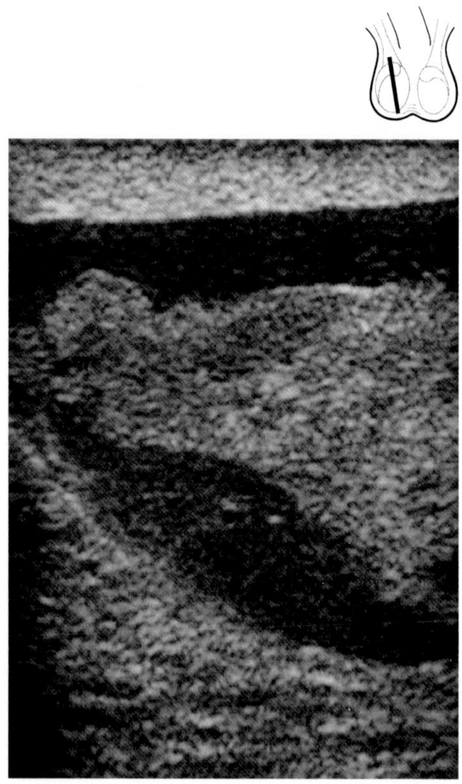

A

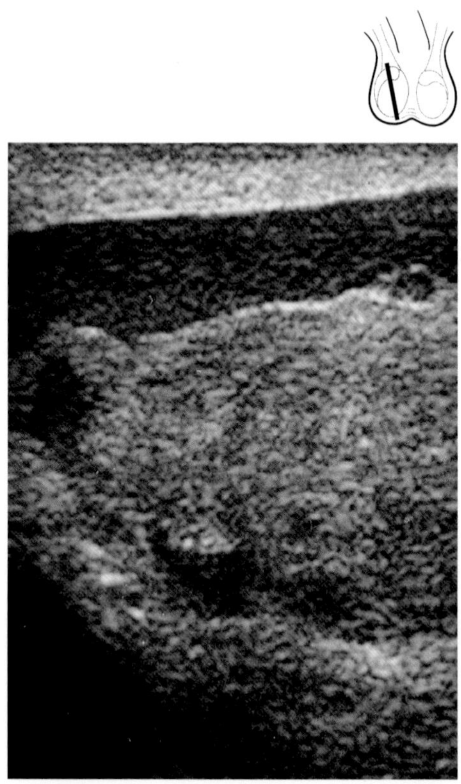

B

Cases 95–100

The following cases have been selected to illustrate the risk of making a diagnosis based on sonographic appearance, without considering the history and physical findings. For these cases the ultrasound scan is presented first, with its likely interpretation. Additional clinical information is presented subsequently, to aid in achieving the correct diagnosis.

Cases 95 and 96

Case 95 is a 28-year-old patient and case 96 is a 36-year-old patient.

Ultrasound. Longitudinal scans (Figs. 95 and 96). A focal, hypoechoic mass is seen at the upper pole of the testis in both patients. Based on sonographic appearance alone, the diagnosis of probable testicular tumor is raised in both cases.

History and Physical Examination. In case 95 the patient noticed a painless lump in the testis, and palpation confirmed a firm, painless mass in the area of the upper pole of the testis. There are no signs of inflammation. In case 96 the testis and epididymis are normal to palpation and there are no signs of inflammation. The patient experienced an episode of epididymitis 2 months earlier, but is now asymptomatic.

Conclusion and Histology. Considering all information, the probable diagnosis in case 95 is testicular tumor. Histologic examination confirmed choriocarcinoma, embryonal carcinoma, and seminoma. In case 96 the probable diagnosis is postinflammatory changes in the upper pole of the testis. The patient was placed on antibiotic therapy, and the subsequent clinical course was unremarkable.

Case 95

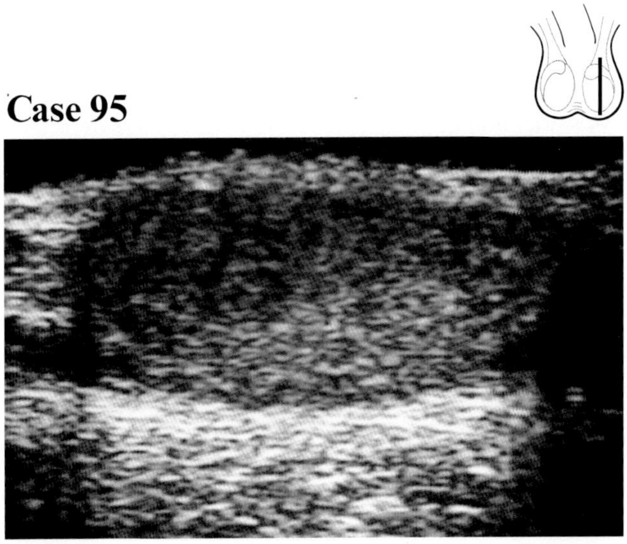

Case 96

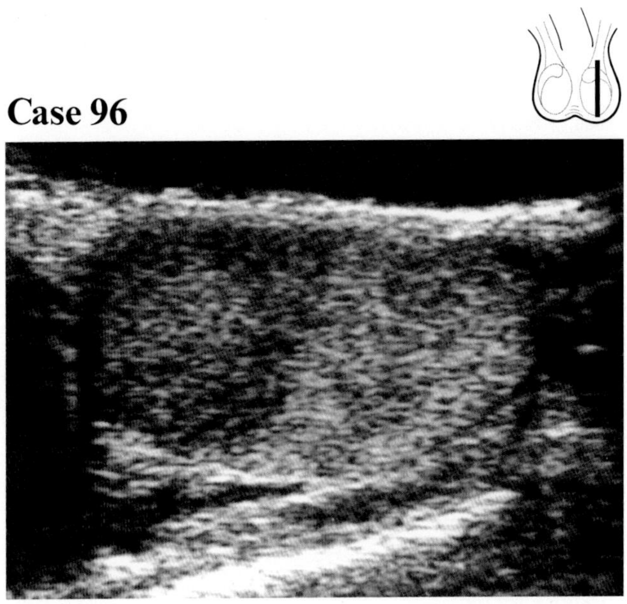

Cases 97 and 98

Case 97 is a 31-year-old patient and case 98 is a 25-year-old patient.

Ultrasound. Longitudinal scans (Figs. 97 and 98). In both cases there is a focal, hypoechoic intratesticular lesion and a normal-appearing epididymis. Based on ultrasound alone, the diagnosis would be testicular tumor in both patients.

History and Physical Examination. In case 97 the patient reported a dragging pain in the affected scrotal compartment of 2 weeks' duration. On palpation the testis was tender and of normal size, and no mass was detected (even on repeated palpation during scanning). Symptoms resolved with subsequent antibiotic treatment In case 98 the patient had undergone testicular biopsy 7 days earlier. Physical examination revealed a painful, moderately enlarged testis, no fever, and no leukocytosis.

Conclusion and Histology. The patient in case 97 was shown (by biopsy and histology) to have an inflammatory, lymphocytic infiltration of the testis. In case 98 the diagnosis was postbiopsy complications, and the clinical follow-up was unremarkable.

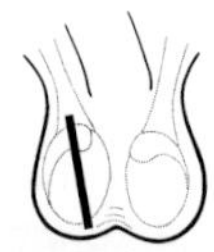

Case 97

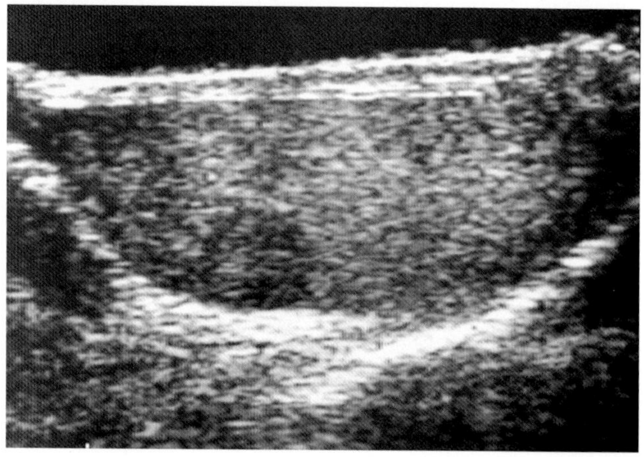

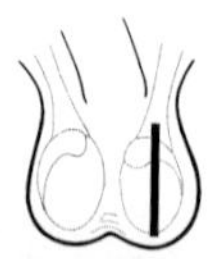

Case 98

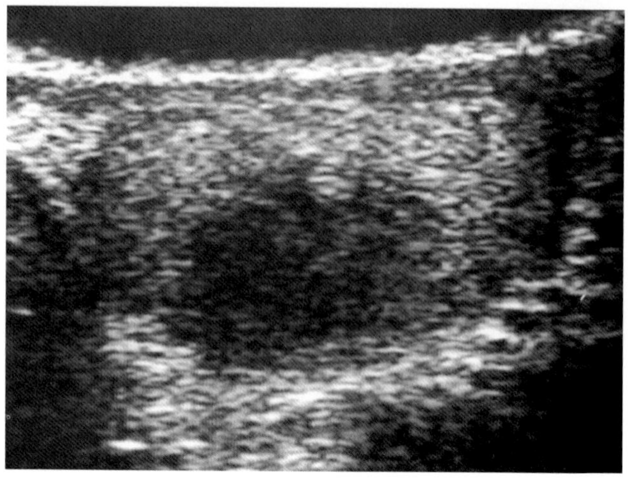

Cases 99 and 100

Case 99 is a 29-year-old patient and case 100 is a 51-year-old patient.

Ultrasound. Longitudinal scans (Figs. 99 and 100). In both cases there is inhomogeneous, hypoechoic destruction of the testicular parenchyma and a normal-appearing epididymis. When the sonograms alone are considered, the diagnosis is testicular tumor—in both patients.

History and Physical Examination. In case 99 the patient noted a painless hardening of the testis. At physical examination a painless, firm mass of the testis could be palpated. The patient in case 100 had undergone unilateral nephrectomy for renal tuberculosis 6 months previously. At that time he was treated for painless testicular swelling, which improved with tuberculostatic therapy. Physical examination now reveals a small, painless testis of soft consistency.

Conclusion and Histology/Clinical Course. In case 99 the diagnosis was testicular tumor, which histologic examination showed to be a seminoma. In case 100 the diagnosis was postinflammatory change of the testis. Clinical follow-up in this case was unremarkable.

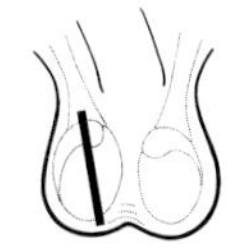

Case 99

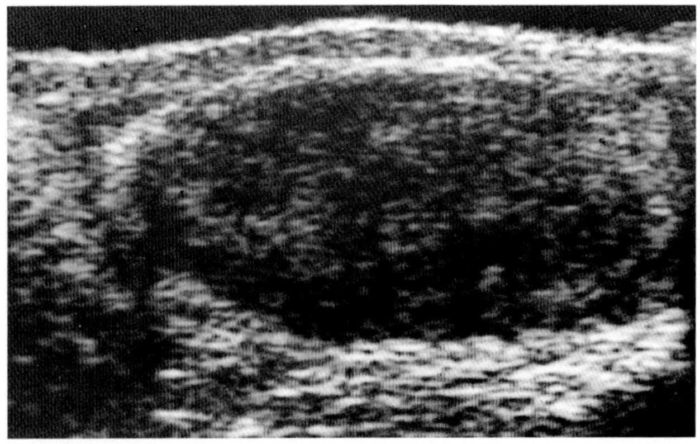

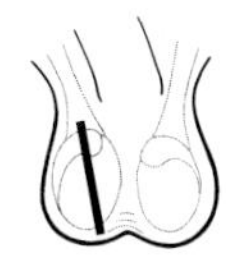

Case 100

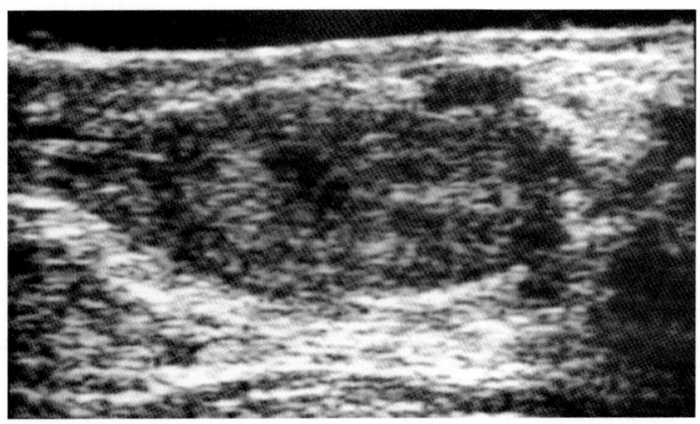

Case 101

A 50-year-old patient presents with dull pain and enlargement of the right hemiscrotum.

Physical Examination. The right hemiscrotum is enlarged and tender to palpation. The scrotal skin is unremarkable. Some transillumination is present.

Ultrasound. Oblique sonogram through the upper part of the right hemiscrotum (Fig. 101) demonstrated a cystic lesion in the region of the epididymal head. Within the testis there are tubular cystic structures in the vicinity of the mediastinum testis.

Conclusion. Spermatocele and tubular ectasia of the rete testis.

Analysis. The localized fluid collection in the head of the epididymis indicates the diagnosis of epididymal cyst or spermatocele. Because of the large size of the lesion, spermatocele is a more likely diagnosis. As a result of obstruction by the spermatocele, the rete testes are dilated. The diagnosis is based on a specific location as well as tubular configuration.

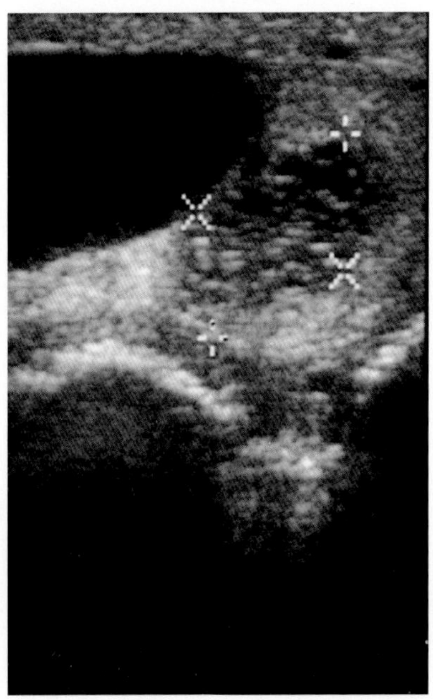

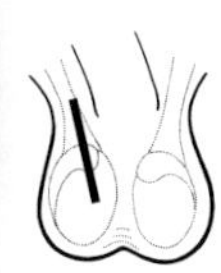

Case 102

A 27-year-old patient presents with acute painful swelling of the left hemiscrotum.

Physical Examination. The left hemiscrotum is enlarged and painful to palpation. No redness of the skin is detected. The findings of transillumination are equivocal. There is no evidence of leukocytosis and no fever is present.

Sonogram. Gray-scale (Fig. 102A) and color-coded Doppler sonograms (Fig. 102B) of the left testis. The testis is markedly enlarged and of heterogeneous echotexture. Heterogeneous vascularity is detected as well. There is associated hydrocele.

Analysis. Although, based on clinical findings, epididymitis or orchitis was suspected, the heterogeneous appearance of the testis is considered to indicate a malignant neoplasm unless proven otherwise. The epididymis was not enlarged. Reactive hydrocele can be seen in conjunction with testicular tumors as well.

Conclusion. Testicular tumor.

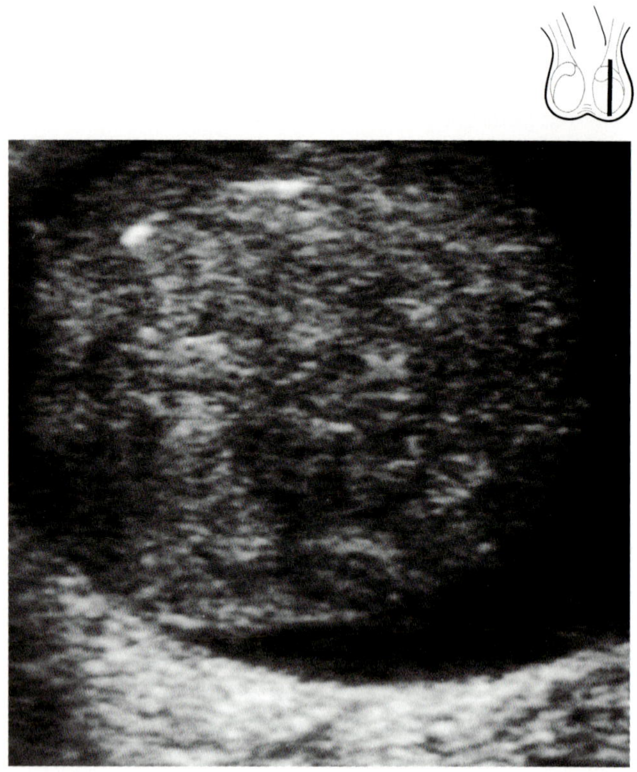

A

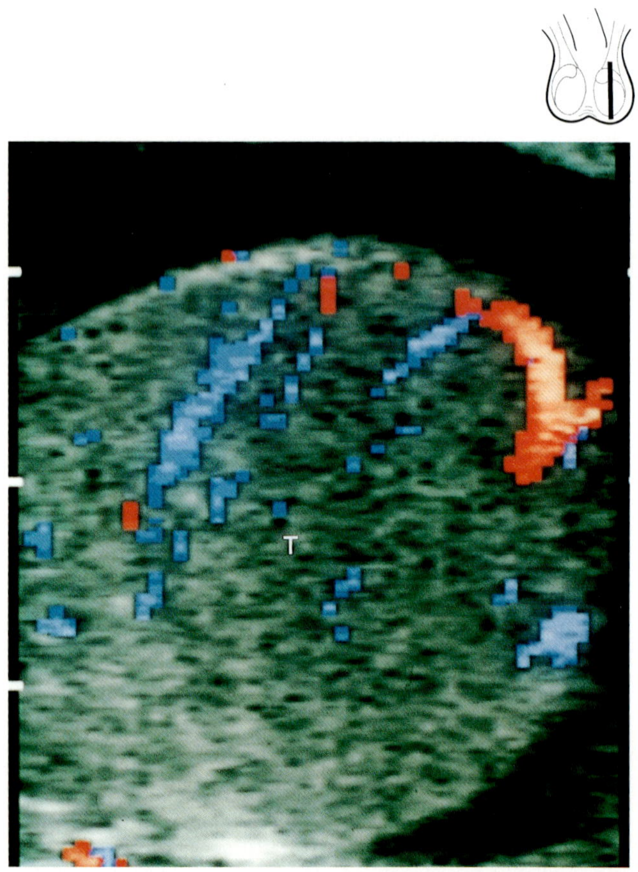

B

Case 103

A 72-year-old patient presents with marked swelling of the right hemiscrotum and high fever. There is a history of recurrent cystitis.

Physical Examination. There is severe fluctuant swelling of the right hemiscrotum. The scrotal skin is erythematous and markedly swollen. The testis and epididymis cannot be palpated.

Ultrasound. A transverse ultrasound image through the right testis (Fig. 103A) shows that the normal homogeneous echotexture of the testis is replaced by a lesion of mixed echogenicity. The outer margin of the testis is indistinct and the paratesticular structures are not differentiated from the testis. Echogenic foci with posterior reverberation artifacts suggest the presence of air within the mass.

Magnetic Resonance Imaging. Transaxial T2-weighted MR image (Fig. 103B) demonstrates an irregular amorphous predominantly high-signal-intensity mass replacing the entire testis. The low-signal-intensity foci indicate air collections. Marked thickening of the scrotal skin is also seen.

Conclusion. Right scrotal abscess.

Surgical Findings. Extensive right scrotal abscess.

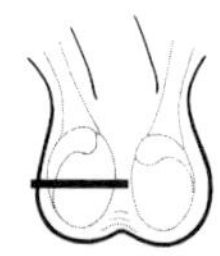

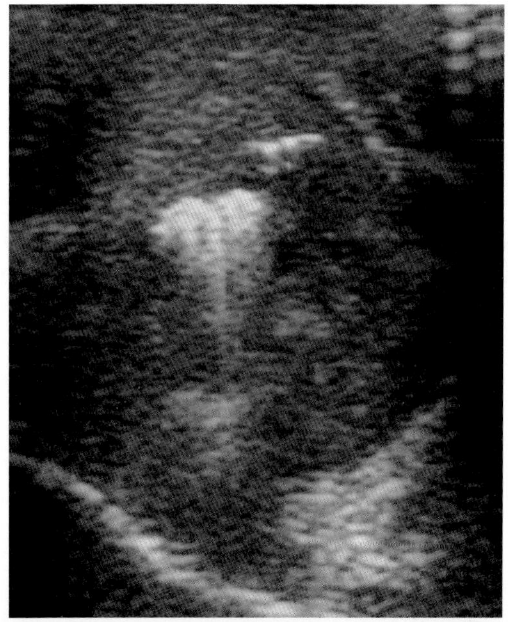

A

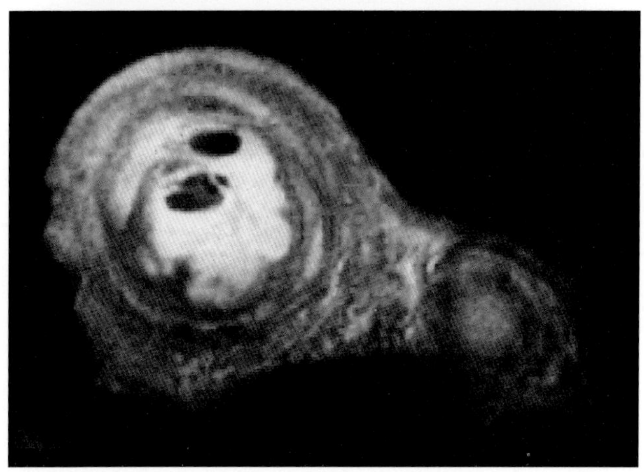

B

Case 104

A 34-year-old patient presents with mild fever and acute painful swelling of the left hemiscrotum.

Physical Examination. The scrotal skin is swollen, erythematous, and tender to palpation. The left spermatic cord is thickened and tender. Because of the extreme pain, an examination of the left testis could not be performed.

Magnetic Resonance Imaging. Two consecutive coronal T2-weighted images (Figs. 104A and 104B). The left epididymis is markedly enlarged and demonstrated a high signal intensity similar to the signal intensity of the testis. Both testes appear normal with homogeneous high signal intensity. The skin on the left hemiscrotum is mildly thickened and is increased in signal intensity.

Analysis. Because of the severe tenderness of the involved hemiscrotum, physical examination and ultrasonography were difficult to perform. Clinical features (e.g., fever) merely suggested the possibility of epididymitis. MRI confirmed the diagnosis of epididymitis and demonstrated the lack of testicular involvement

Conclusion. Acute epididymitis.

Clinical Course. Symptoms resolved with antibiotic treatment.

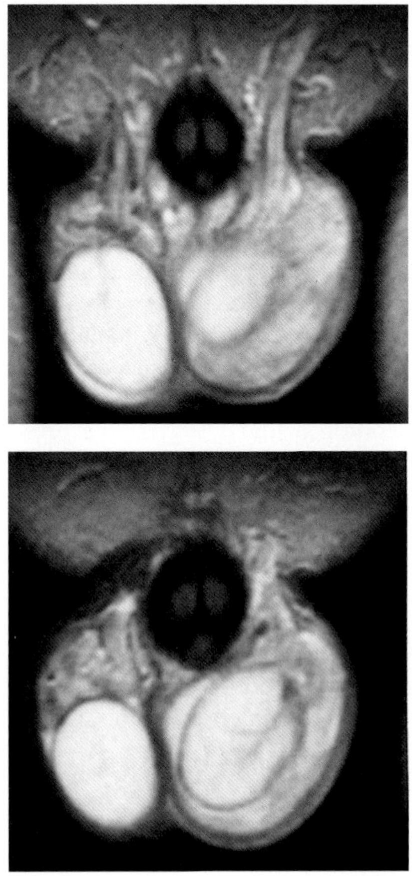

A

B

Case 105

A 35-year-old patient presents with a small lump in his left testis. Both serum AFP and hCG are elevated.

Physical Examination. The testes are normal in size. There is a firm, nontender nodule approximately 1 cm in diameter in the left testis.

Magnetic Resonance Imaging. A heterogeneous low-intensity mass is seen in the left testis surrounded by normal high-intensity testicular parenchyma. The tumor extends anterolaterally to the tunica albuginea.

Conclusion and Histology. Embryonal carcinoma of the left testis with invasion of the tunica albuginea.

Notes. Embryonal carcinoma is the most invasive tumor in the testis, and often it demonstrates early invasion of the tunica albuginea. This commonly results in bulging and distortion of the testicular contour.

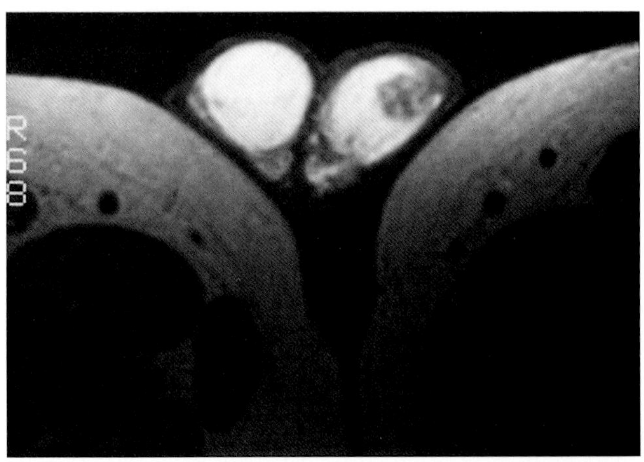

Case 106

A 22-year-old patient presents with left-sided cryptorchidism. The patient status is post–right orchiectomy.

Physical Examination. The right testis is absent. On the left, a small testis is palpable in the superficial inguinal pouch.

Magnetic Resonance Imaging. Proton density (Fig. 106A) and T2-weighted images (Fig. 106B). A small soft tissue mass at the level of the left external inguinal ring demonstrates low signal intensity on both proton density and T2-weighted images. A smaller lesion of similar signal intensity is seen in the right superficial inguinal pouch mimicking an undescended testis. Since the right testis has already been removed, this probably represents postoperative changes.

Conclusion. Left hypoplastic undescended testis at the level of the external ring.

Notes. Undescended testes often demonstrate the typical signal intensities of normal testes (i.e., low on T1-weighted images and high on T2-weighted images). Atrophic testes, however, demonstrate low signal intensity on T2-weighted images. The signal intensity of the atrophic testis and granulation tissue can be similar, and the diagnosis is based on morphologic findings of lesion, e.g., shape (round vs. irregular) and size.

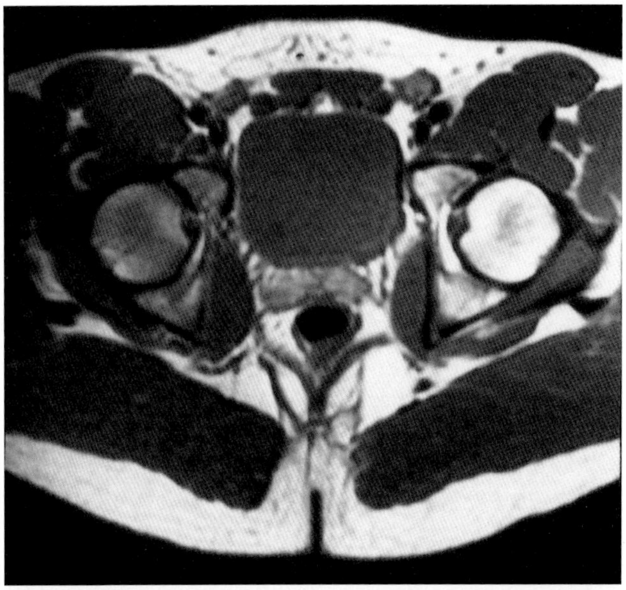

A

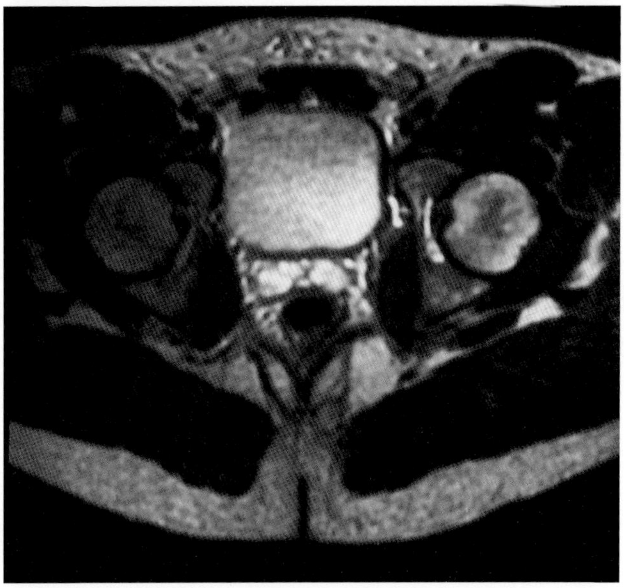

B

Case 107

A 30-year-old patient presents with marked swelling of the left hemiscrotum and mild, dull scrotal pain. The patient is negative for serum tumor markers (AFP and hCG).

Physical Examination. The left testis is markedly enlarged with a firm, nontender mass. The hemiscrotum does not transilluminate.

Magnetic Resonance Imaging. Sagittal T1-weighted image (Fig. 107A) and coronal T2-weighted image (Fig. 107B). The testis is markedly enlarged. There are multiple fine septa within the tumor. It demonstrates high signal intensity on T1-weighted image and medium signal intensity (similar to the normal right testis) on T2-weighted image. Also seen is a small amount of fluid within the scrotal sac.

Conclusion. Left testicular tumor with intratumoral hemorrhage.

Histology. Seminoma.

Notes. Seminomas are usually homogeneous and isointense with normal testes on T1-weighted images and hypointense on T2-weighted images. Some seminomas, as in this case, demonstrate high signal intensity on T1-weighted images and medium signal intensity on T2-weighted images.

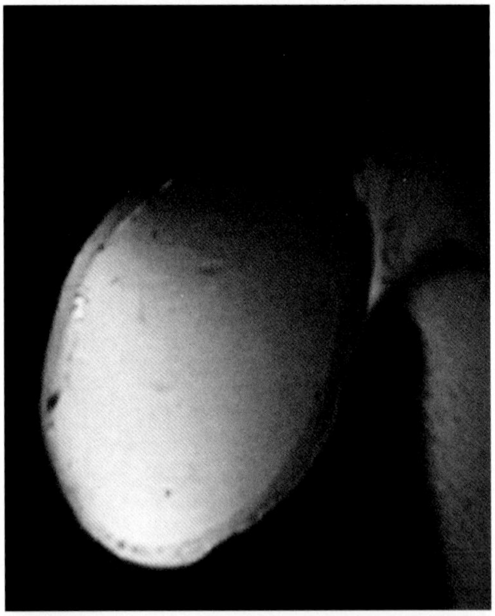

A

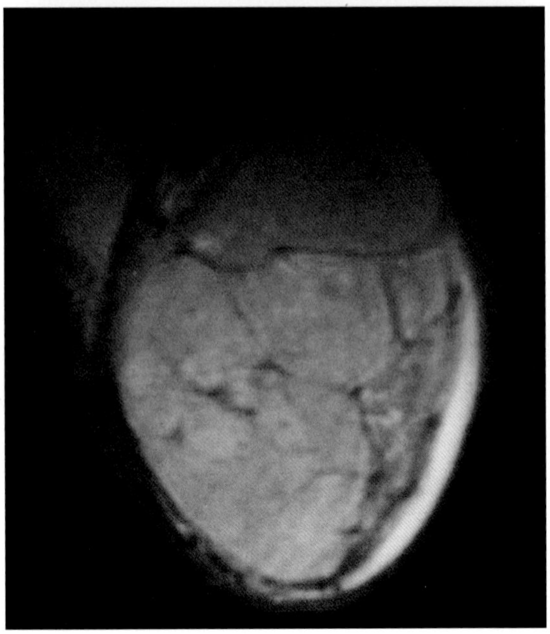

B

Case 108

A 34-year-old patient with prior scrotal surgery for mesothelioma presents with progressive swelling of the left hemiscrotum.

Physical Examination. There is a surgical deformity of the right hemiscrotum and moderate swelling of the left hemiscrotum.

Magnetic Resonance Imaging. Sagittal T1-weighted image through the left hemiscrotum (Fig. 108A), coronal T2-weighted (Fig. 108B), and contrast-enhanced T1-weighted images (Fig. 108C) of the scrotum. There is surgical deformity of the right hemiscrotum. The left spermatic cord is thickened, demonstrates medium signal intensity on T1-weighted image, and shows enhancement following contrast injection. There is also thickening and enhancement of the right spermatic cord. The left testis is unremarkable. The differentiation between the higher-signal-intensity testis and lower-signal-intensity epididymis is seen best on the T2-weighted image. There is a small left-side hydrocele.

Conclusion and Histology. Mesothelioma of the left spermatic cord and residual mesothelioma of the right spermatic cord.

Notes. Metastatic mesothelioma involving the peritoneum may spread through the spermatic cord and processus vaginalis to involve the scrotum. In this patient, there is a bilateral abnormality within the spermatic cord. No diagnosis of mesothelioma indicates tumor extension to that region. However, because similar MRI findings can be seen in diffuse inflammatory disease, a clinical history is needed.

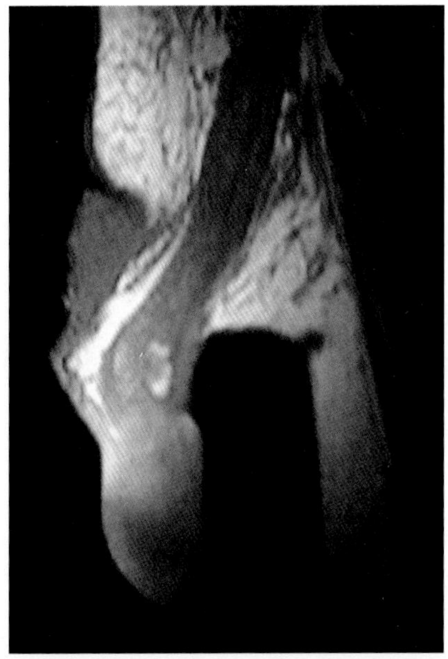

A

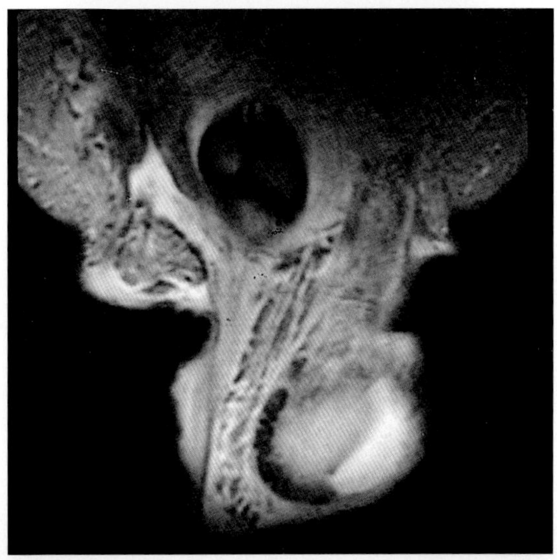

B

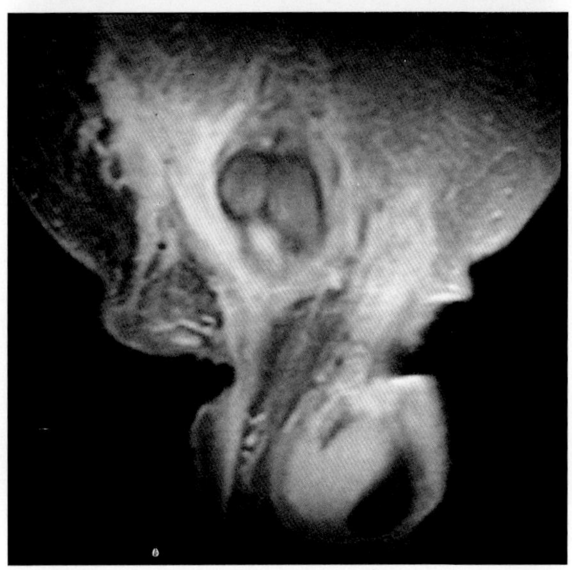

C

Case 109

A 27-year-old patient who had right-side orchiectomy for seminoma 12 months earlier. Now he is seen with swelling of the lower extremities.

Physical Examination. Both lower extremities are swollen and there is suggestion of a mass in the midline and right abdomen. Tumor markers are not elevated.

Magnetic Resonance Imaging. T1-weighted image (Fig. 109A), T2-weighted image (Fig. 109B), contrast-enhanced T1-weighted image (Fig. 109C), and GRE image (Fig. 109D). All presented images are at the same anatomical level. There is a large retroperitoneal mass invading and displacing the right kidney, showing extrinsic compression on the right psoas muscle and engulfing the aorta. Mass shows heterogeneous signal intensity with area of necrosis on postcontrast study. The inferior vena cava is not identified, and complete thrombosis of the inferior vena cava is confirmed on gradient-recalled echo image.

Conclusion. Large retroperitoneal adenopathy with obstruction of the inferior vena cava.

Histology. Mixed germ cell tumor (seminoma, embryonal cell carcinoma, and teratoma).

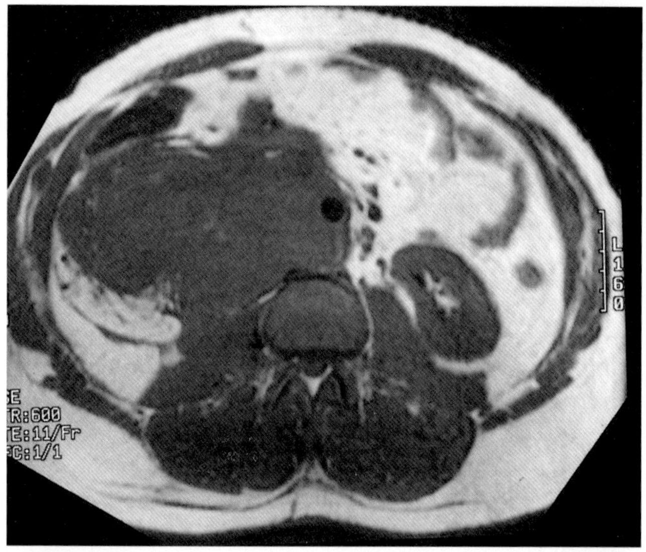

A

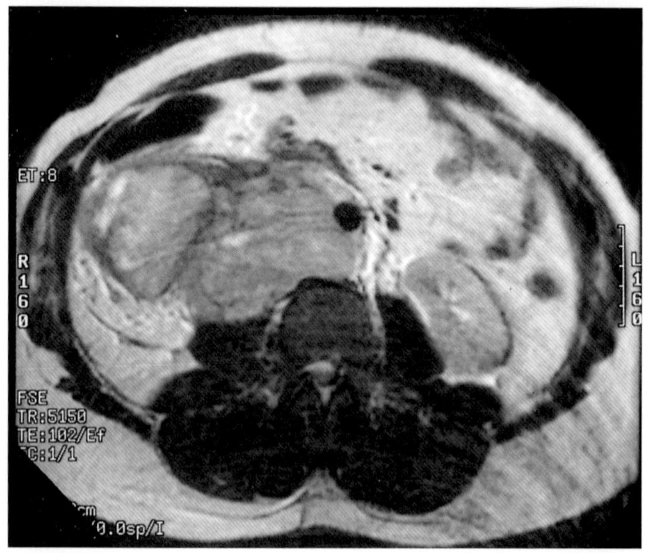

B

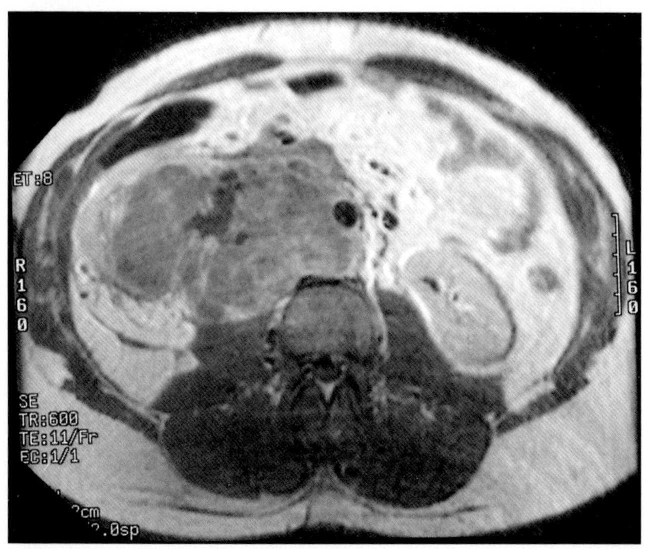

C

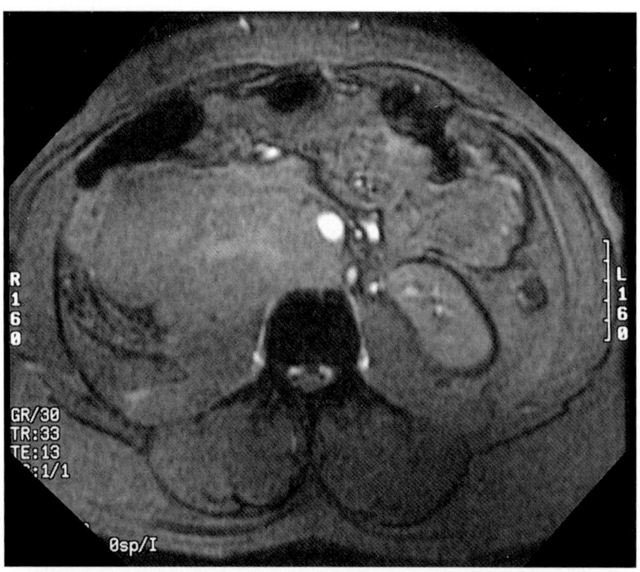

D

Case 110

A 68-year-old patient with known bladder cancer, status post–transurethral resection, presents with a long history of intermittent bulging of the right groin and scrotum bilaterally.

Physical Examination. Bilateral scrotal masses are present during Valsalva's maneuver. On rectal examination, the prostate gland is found to be enlarged.

Magnetic Resonance Imaging. Transaxial T2-weighted image (Fig. 110). Herniated small bowel on the right and mesenteric fat on the left are seen anterolateral to the symphysis pubis. A Foley catheter is located within the urethra.

Conclusion and Surgical Findings. Bilateral indirect inguinal hernias. Bowel is herniated on the right, and mesenteric fat is herniated on the left.

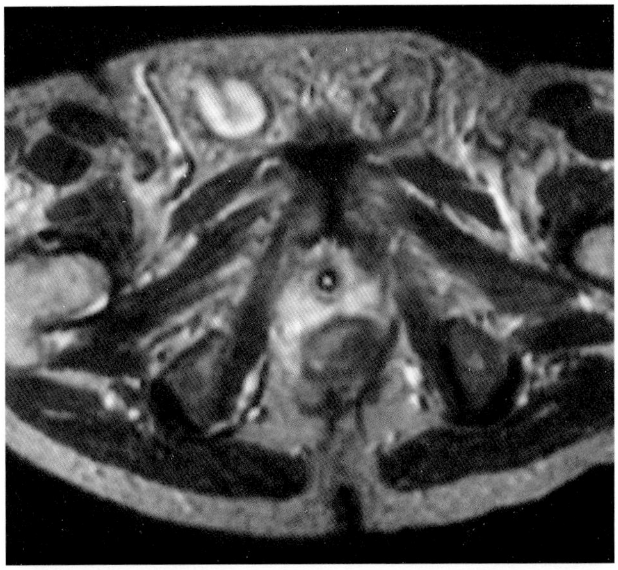

Case 111

A 26-year-old patient presents with fever and painful swelling of the left hemiscrotum.

Physical Examination. The left epididymis and testis are swollen, tender, and palpated as a single ill-defined mass.

Magnetic Resonance Imaging. Transaxial T2-weighted image (Fig. 111). The left epididymis is enlarged and shows slightly higher signal intensity than the contralateral side. The signal intensity of the left testis is lower than that of the right testis, and a reactive left hydrocele is present. In addition, the left scrotal skin is thickened and demonstrates high signal intensity.

Conclusion. Epididymo-orchitis with reactive hydrocele.

Clinical Course. With antibiotic treatment, the clinical course was uneventful.

Note. Orchitis, as with infiltrative neoplasm, can demonstrate diffuse low signal intensity on the testis on T2-weighted images. Therefore, based on signal intensity alone, the differentiation between orchitis and cancer can be difficult and MRI, similar to ultrasound, often relies on indirect signs of scrotal skin thickening and enlargement of the epididymis, and clinical presentation.

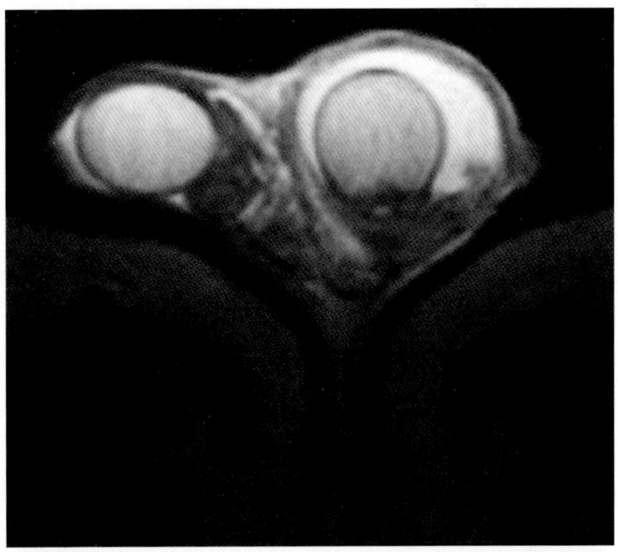

Case 112

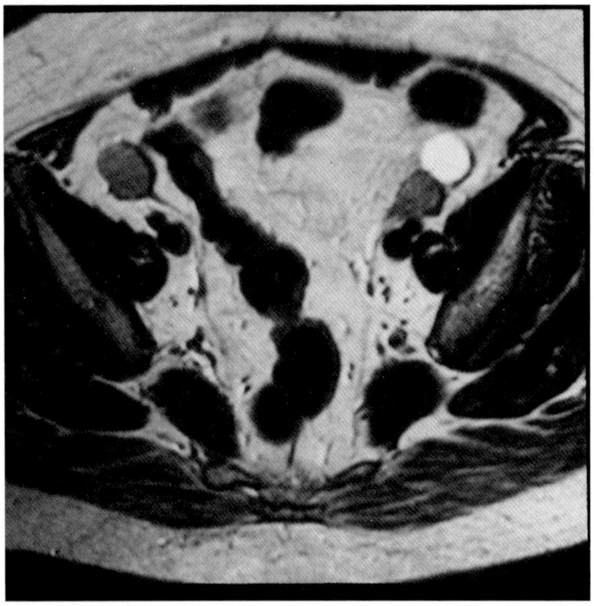

A 40-year-old woman presents with infertility work-up.

Physical Examination. The vagina is hypoplastic, and the uterus cannot be palpated. Subsequent hormonal analysis demonstrates the 46 XY chromosomal pattern indicating testicular feminization.

Magnetic Resonance Imaging. There are bilateral, solid lesions of low signal intensity on T2-weighted image (Fig. 112). In addition, there is a cystic lesion seen adjacent to the left solid mass.

Conclusion. Bilateral, intra-abdominal undescended testes. This was proven on subsequent surgery.

Case 113

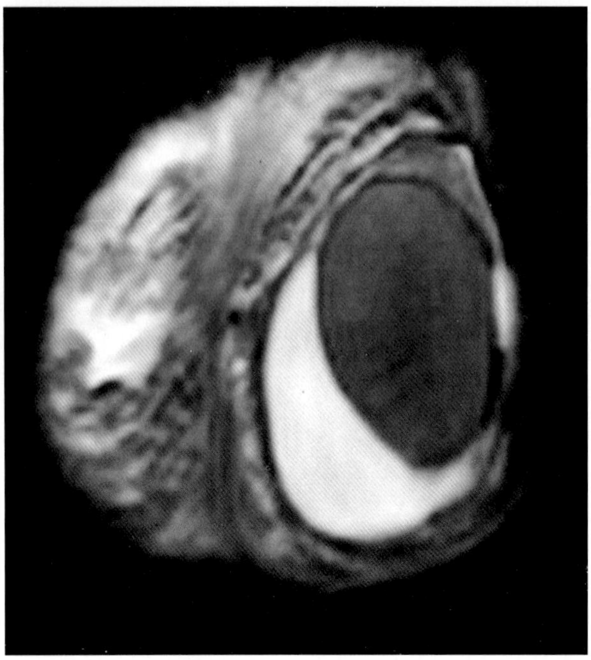

A 7-year-old boy presents with pubertas praecox.

Physical Examination. The external genitalia are fully developed and enlarged for the patient's chronological age. There is also hair growth, including beard and hair on the chest. The left hemiscrotum is larger than the right.

Magnetic Resonance Imaging. Coronal plane, T2-weighted image (Fig. 113). The left testis is large for the patient's age and demonstrates homogeneous low signal intensity. The signal intensity of the testis is similar to that of the head of the epididymis. There is evidence of hydrocele. Findings in the testis indicate diffuse infiltrative disease.

Conclusion. Left testicular tumor, most likely Leydig cell tumor. The diagnosis is based on combined clinical and MRI evaluation. Findings subsequently proven in surgery.

Case 114

A 62-year-old patient presents with acute left inguinal pain and swelling.

Physical Examination. A testis is not identified in either the right or left scrotum. Both scrotal sacs are hypoplastic. An undescended testis is palpated in the superficial inguinal pouch on the right side. In the left superficial inguinal pouch, there is a painful swelling. The overlying skin is erythematous. The patient has a fever and leukocytosis.

Magnetic Resonance Imaging. Coronal plane T1-weighted image (Fig. 114A) and contrast-enhanced T1-weighted image (Fig. 114B). Both testes are undescended. Undescended testis in a high scrotal position is identified on the right side. There is also evidence of hydrocele distending the spermatic cord. On the left side, the testis is enlarged, showing marked enhancement and infiltrative irregular margin. Diffuse infiltrative disease is suspected.

Conclusion. Epididymo-orchitis in the left undescended testis.

Clinical Course. Resolution of symptoms with antibiotic treatment.

Notes. In view of the clinical history of pain, fever, and swelling and of indirect signs of enlargement of the entire spermatic cord with a diffuse infiltrative margin, the diagnosis of inflammatory disease is most likely, although underlying tumor cannot be entirely excluded.

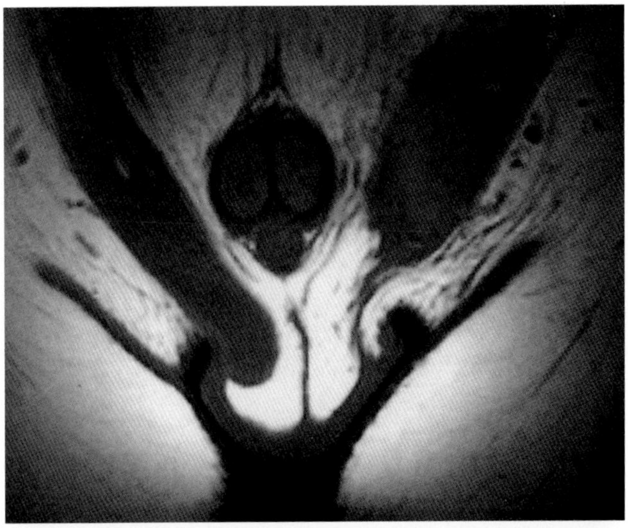
A

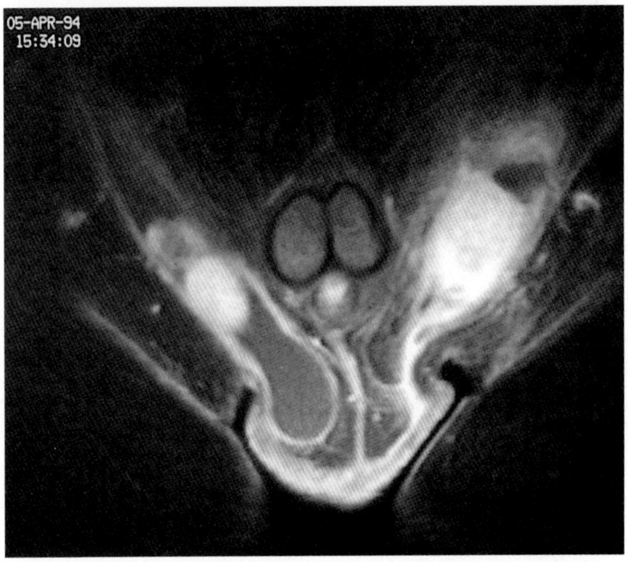

B

Case 115

A 6-year-old patient presents with right-sided cryptorchidism.

Physical Examination. The right hemiscrotum is empty, and the right testis can be palpated in the high scrotal region (superficial inguinal pouch).

Computed Tomography. An undescended right testis is located in the right high scrotal region. The normal left spermatic cord can be seen (Fig. 115).

Conclusion and Surgical Treatment/Findings. Undescended testis. A right orchiopexy was performed.

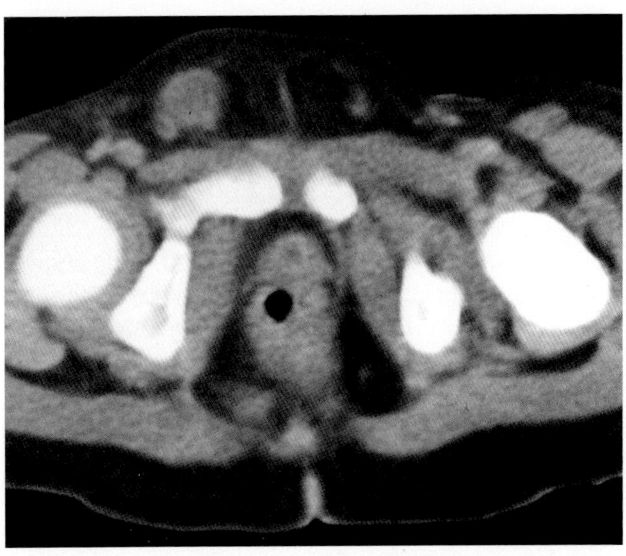

Case 116

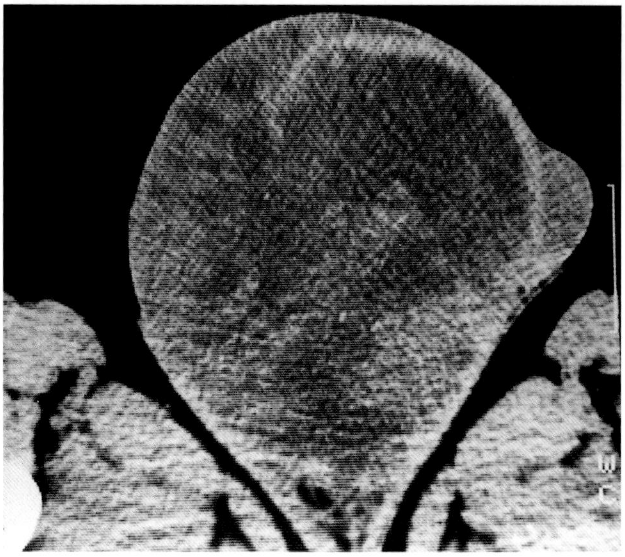

A 31-year-old patient presents with marked right scrotal enlargement. Serum tumor markers (AFP and hCG) are elevated.

Physical Examination. A large firm mass that does not transilluminate is present in the right hemiscrotum.

Computed Tomography. A large testicular mass can be seen within the right hemiscrotum (Fig. 116). The mass demonstrates heterogeneous low-attenuation value. The normal-sized left testis is identified.

Conclusion and Histology. Right testicular teratoma.

Notes. Because of their fatty component, teratomas tend to demonstrate low attenuation at both primary and metastatic sites.

Case 117

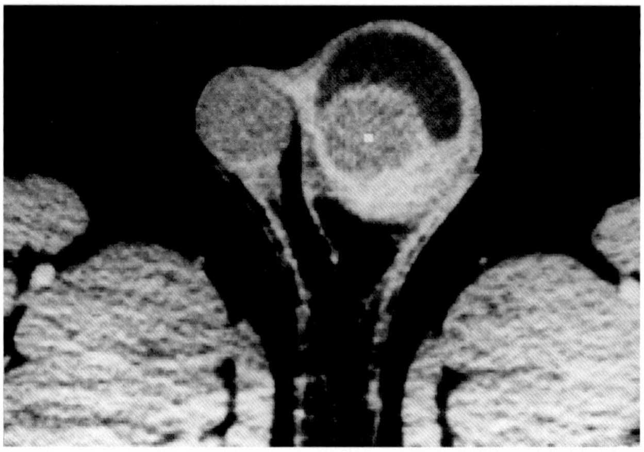

A 40-year-old patient presents with acute left scrotal pain.

Physical Examination. The left hemiscrotum is tender, swollen, and erythematous.

Computed Tomography. The left epididymis is enlarged and demonstrates marked contrast enhancement (Fig. 117). The scrotal wall is thickened and a reactive hydrocele is present. Both testes appear normal; however, there is thickening of the tunica albuginea of the left testis.

Conclusion. Left epididymitis with a reactive hydrocele.

Clinical Course. Symptoms resolved with antibiotic treatment.

Case 118

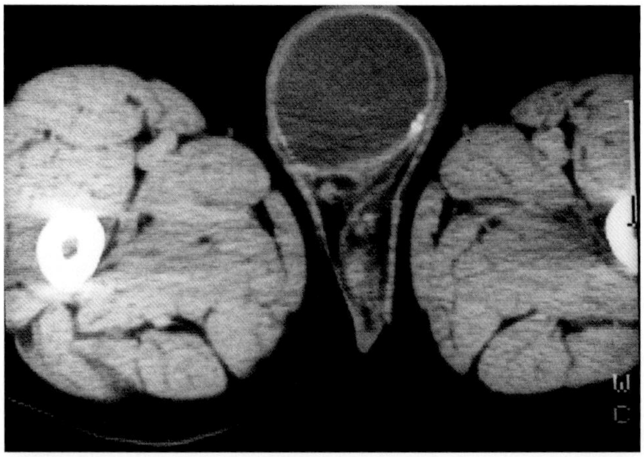

A 22-year-old patient with prior history of scrotal trauma (previous 7 months) presents with a right scrotal mass.

Physical Examination. The right hemiscrotum is enlarged and has a firm consistency. There is no transillumination. The testis and epididymis cannot be palpated. No signs of active inflammation are present.

Computed Tomography. A large, round, fairly homogeneous low-attenuation lesion is seen occupying the entire right scrotum (Fig. 118). There is enhancement of the outer rim, and small nodular calcifications can be identified in the posterolateral aspect of the lesion.

Conclusion and Surgical Finding. Organized intratesticular hematoma.

Case 119

A 13-year-old patient presents with a 3-day history of scrotal pain. The pain was acute at onset and radiates to the lower abdomen. The patient is afebrile and the urinalysis is normal.

Physical Examination. The right hemiscrotum is enlarged and does not transilluminate. The testis and epididymis cannot be palpated as separate entities.

Computed Tomography. The right hemiscrotum is enlarged and demonstrates an area of medium and low attenuation and heterogeneous value (Fig. 119). The scrotal skin is thickened and shows marked enhancement.

Conclusion and Surgical Treatment/Findings. Torsion of the spermatic cord. The patient underwent surgical exploration and orchiectomy. Torsion of the spermatic cord with extensive testicular necrosis was confirmed. The high-attenuation area seen on the CT scan corresponds to viable testicular tissue, and the low-attenuation regions likely correspond to area of necrosis. The enhancing outer rim probably represents the edematous testicular capsule and scrotal wall.

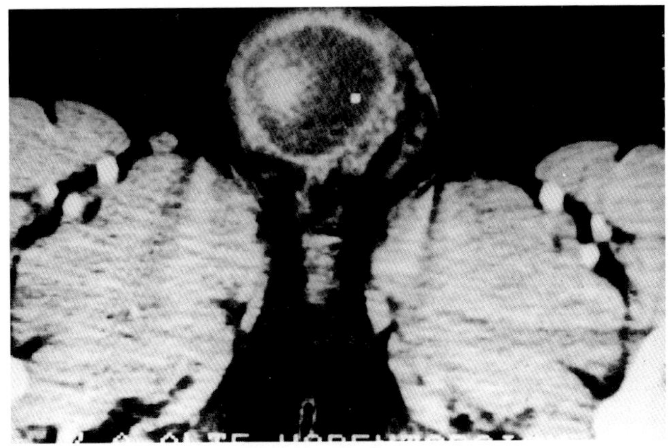

Case 120

A 35-year-old patient presents with a history of right testicular seminoma (stage T1). He had been treated by orchiectomy and surveillance.

Physical Examination. The examination is unremarkable except for identification of a right testicular prosthesis. Serum tumor markers (AFP and hCG) are negative.

Computed Tomography. A large, low-attenuation mass can be seen posterior to the pancreatic head (Fig. 120). The pancreatic head, the right kidney, and the hilum are anteriorly displaced by this lesion. There is dilation of the right renal pelvis due to compression and relative obstruction of the ureter by the mass. The aorta and the left diaphragmatic crus can also be identified.

Conclusion. Testicular seminoma with retroperitoneal lymph node metastasis.

Clinical Course. Chemotherapy markedly reduced the tumor size on follow-up CT examination.

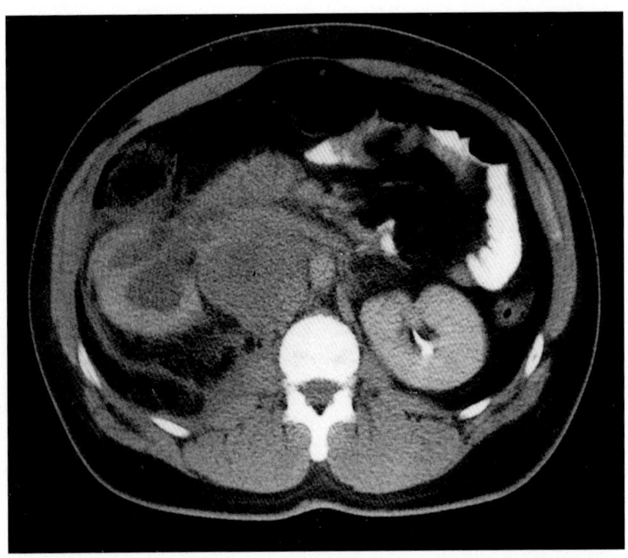

Case 121

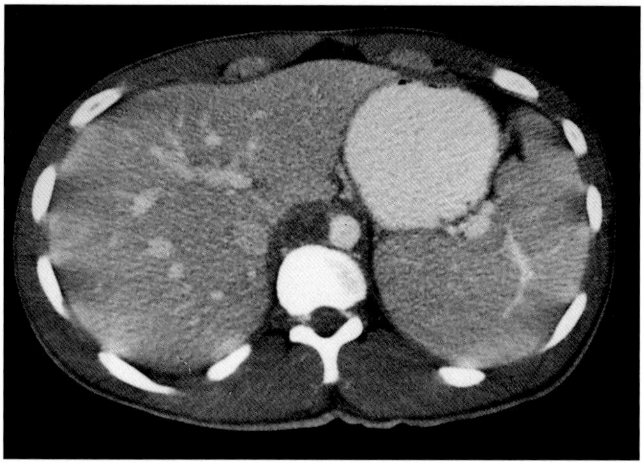

A 26-year-old patient presents with a painless right testicular mass. Serum tumor markers (AFP and hCG) are elevated.

Physical Examination. There is a mildly enlarged right testis with a palpable mass.

Computed Tomography. A round, low-attenuation mass is seen in the retrocrural region, just to the right of the aorta (Fig. 121). This lesion could be mistaken for a thrombosed inferior vena cava; however, the inferior vena cava is seen within the liver, lateral to this lesion. The crura of the diaphragm demonstrate low attenuation, similar to the lesion.

Conclusion and Treatment. Right testicular tumor with retrocrural lymph node metastasis. Right orchiectomy and retroperitoneal lymph node dissection were performed.

Histology. Mixed germ cell tumor of the testis and metastatic teratoma in retrocrural lymph nodes.

Notes. It is not uncommon for a mixed germ cell tumor, which has teratoma components, to metastasize as a pure teratoma. Because of the presence of fat in the tumor, it tends to demonstrate low attenuation on CT.

Case 122

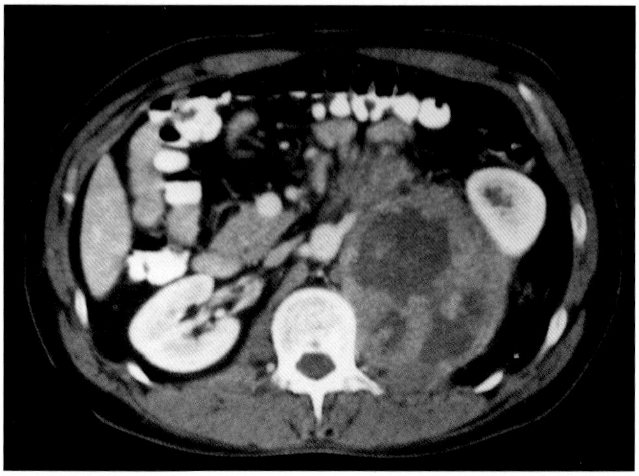

A 29-year-old patient presents with a painless left testicular mass. Serum tumor markers (AFP and hCG) are elevated.

Physical Examination. There is a large, firm mass palpable in the left upper quadrant of the abdomen.

Computed Tomography. A large, heterogeneous mass can be seen in the medial aspect of the left renal fossa (Fig. 122). The left kidney is anterolaterally displaced, and the left renal artery is seen draped along the anterior aspect of the mass. The aorta can also be seen.

Conclusion and Treatment. Metastatic testicular tumor involving the lymph nodes of the left renal hilum. Chemotherapy is the recommended treatment.

Case 123

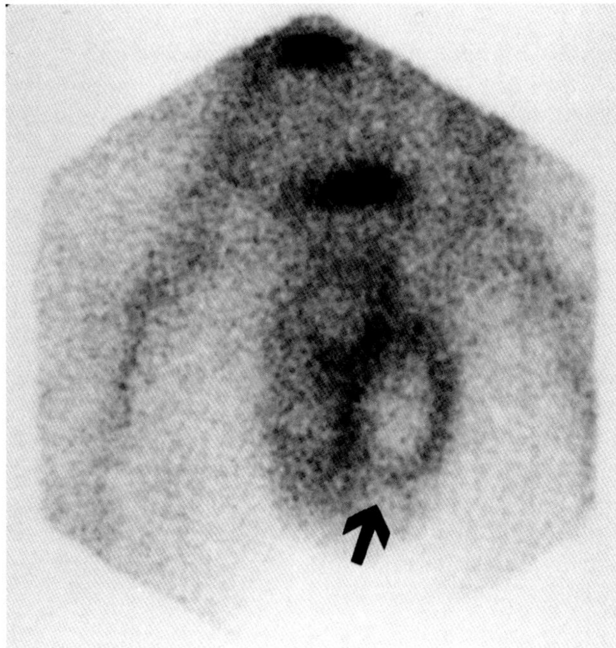

The patient is a 52-year-old man who presents with a 5-day history of increasing pain and swelling in the left scrotum.

Physical Examination. The left hemiscrotum is enlarged, tender, and warm. The patient has a low-grade fever and mild leukocytosis.

Nuclear Medicine. A Tc-99m pertechnetate testicular scan is performed. No flow study is available because of photographic problems. Immediately after the flow sequence, the static image (Fig. 123) shows markedly increased activity around the left scrotum. The scrotal contents show enlargement (edema) and a "cold" central defect (arrow).

Conclusion. Late torsion of the left testis.

Note. At surgery, a large infarcted left testis was found, rotated on itself at least 360°. The infarcted left testis was removed, and a right orchiopexy was performed.

Case 124

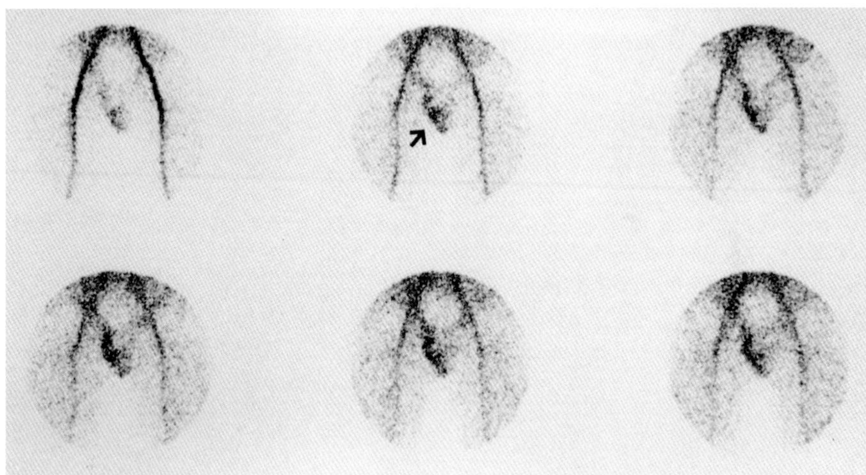

A

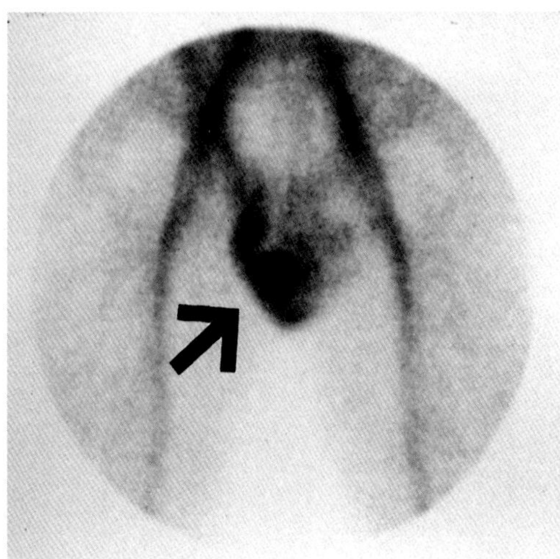

B

A young male patient presents with fever and acute painful swelling of the right scrotum of 1 1/2- to 2-hours duration.

Physical Examination. The right hemiscrotum is considerably swollen, erythematous, and quite tender to palpation.

Nuclear Medicine. Testicular flow sequence after intravenous injection of Tc-99m pertechnetate, with 3-second flow images (Fig. 124A). There is marked increase in flow to the right spermatic cord and scrotum (arrow). The immediate postflow static image (Fig. 124B) also shows markedly increased activity in the cord, epididymis, and testis on the right (arrow).

Conclusion. Epididymo-orchitis.

Note. Lack of a discrete cold center is more characteristic of epididymo-orchitis than of torsion.

Case 125

A young man presents with acute pain and tenderness of the right scrotum of several hours in duration.

Physical Examination. The right scrotum is considerably enlarged and tender, but shows definite transillumination. Mild leukocytosis and low-grade fever are noted.

Nuclear Medicine. After intravenous injection of Tc-99m pertechnetate, 3-second flow images (Fig. 125A) demonstrate a distinct increase in vascularity to the right spermatic cord and scrotum. In the immediate postflow static image (Fig. 125B), the right testis is markedly swollen and diffusely increased in activity. The testicular outline appears to cross the midline because the right scrotum is so swollen. A crescent-shaped cold defect is noted within the medial aspect of the right testis (arrow).

Conclusion. Epididymitis with associated hydrocele.

Note. The finding of a small or moderate-sized hydrocele with epididymitis or epididymo-orchitis is not uncommon and can be misinterpreted as testicular torsion or testicular abscess.

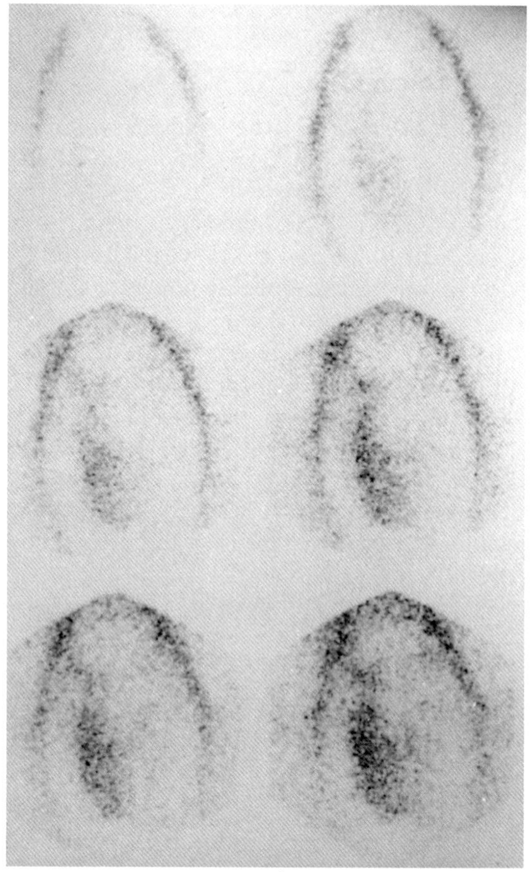

A

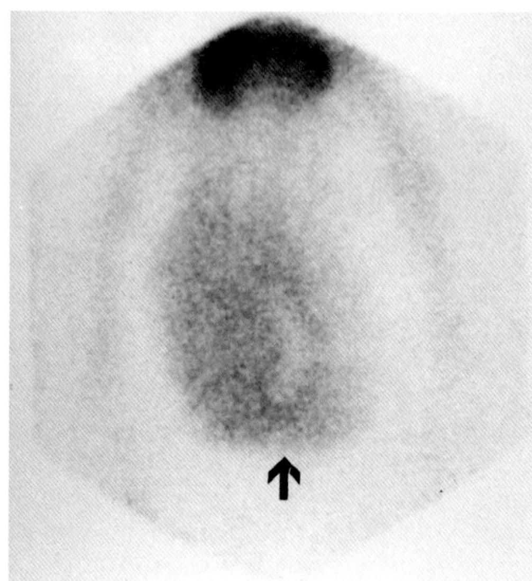

B

Case 126

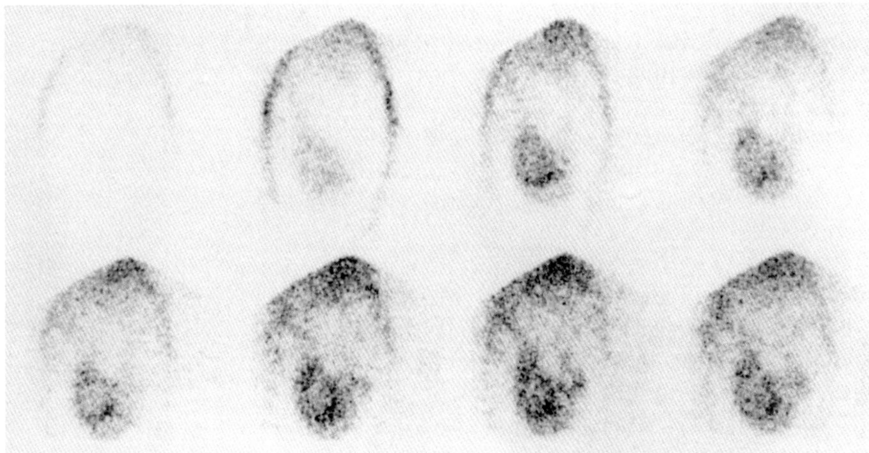

A

A young male patient was admitted with several days of increasing right testicular pain and swelling associated with fever and night sweats.

Physical Examination. The right testis is considerably swollen, tense, somewhat irregular to palpation, and acutely tender. The patient has a low-grade fever and leukocytosis.

Nuclear Medicine. After Tc-99m pertechnetate injection, the dynamic flow study (Fig. 126A) shows increased vascularity to the right testis with an irregular cold center. The postflow static image (Fig. 126B) demonstrates multiple areas of decreased activity within the hot right testis (arrow).

Conclusion. Testicular abscess.

Note. Multiple abscesses were drained at surgery. The marked irregularity to the cold center of this lesion makes testicular torsion and epididymitis with hydrocele very unlikely.

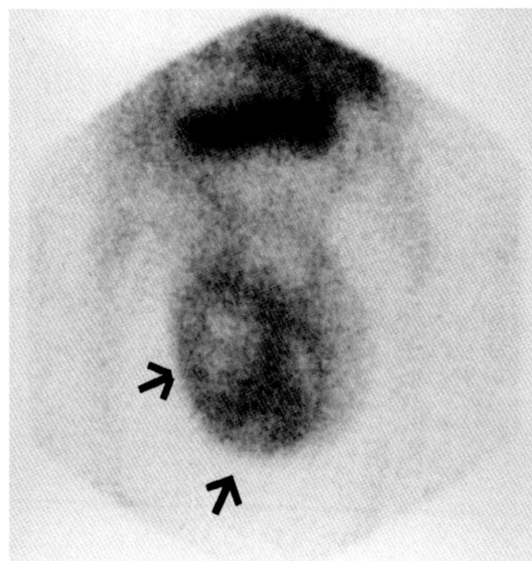

B

Case 127

A young male patient presents with a history of gradually increasing painless enlargement of the left testis over several months with no systemic symptoms of illness.

Physical Examination. The left testis is considerably enlarged, firm and smooth, nontender and with no erythema. Temperature and white blood cell count are normal.

Nuclear Medicine. An anterior scintiphoto performed 48 hours after intravenous injection of 5 mCi Ga-67 citrate (Fig. 127A) demonstrates normal bowel and pelvic marrow activity and an intense focus of uptake associated with the palpable swelling (arrow).

Conclusion. Testicular seminoma.

Nuclear Medicine. A repeat gallium scan performed several months later (Fig. 127B) shows a definite focus in the right iliac region due to a new lymph node metastasis (arrow). Note the cold defect in the left scrotum from the testicular prosthesis placed since the first study. A Ga-67 image of the neck (Fig. 127C) shows an additional metastasis to a left supraclavicular lymph node.

Note. Seminomas are tumors with a high likelihood of positive uptake of Ga-67. Consequently, a gallium scan can be particularly helpful in evaluating for metastatic disease.

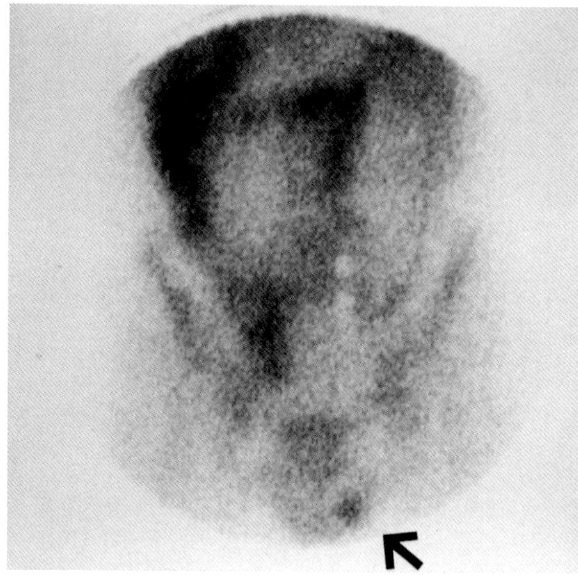

A

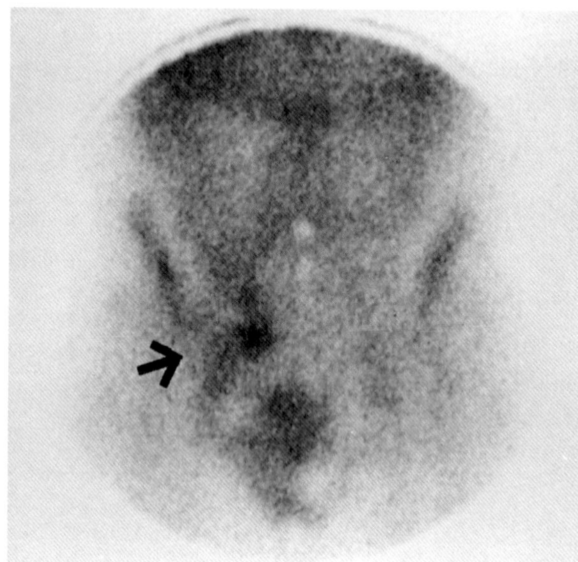

B

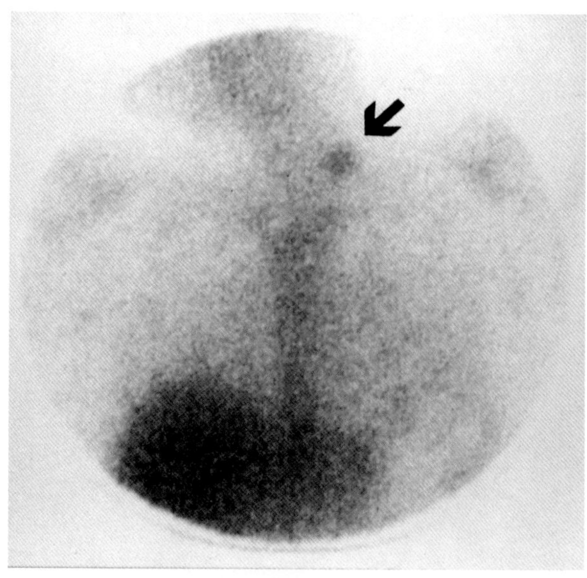

C

Case 128

The patient is a young man with a history of transient left scrotal pain following micturition for several years, neither worsening nor improving over recent time.

Nuclear Medicine. The initial Tc-99m pertechnetate flow and postflow dynamic images are completely normal. The late anterior pelvic image (Fig. 128A) shown, however, obtained immediately after painful micturition demonstrates unexpected reflux of Tc-99m labeled urine above the left testis in the region of the vas deferens (large arrow). The smaller arrows indicate the base of the penis (upper, midline) and activity in the urinal (below). A later postvoid image (Fig. 128B) shows disappearance of the activity in the region of the left scrotum. The patient's pain at this time has resolved.

Conclusion. Urine reflux on micturition into the left vas deferens.

Note. This is a very unusual, probably unique finding kindly provided by LTC Michael McBiles, Chief, Nuclear Medicine Section, Department of Radiology, Fitzsimons Army Medical Center, Aurora, Colorado.

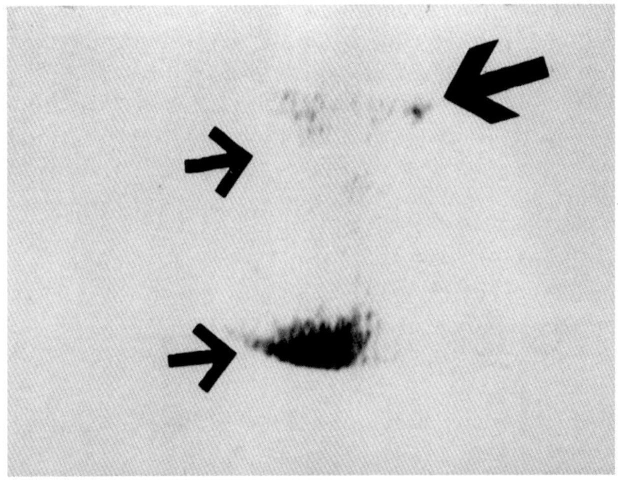

A

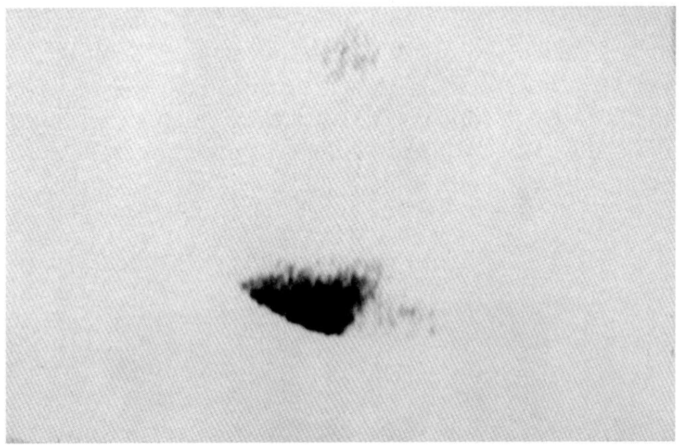

B

Case 129

A young male patient presents with a 48-hour history of gradually increasing right testicular pain and swelling associated with low-grade fevers and night sweats.

Physical Examination. The right testis is markedly swollen, tense, and tender.

Nuclear Medicine. After injection of Tc-99m pertechnetate, the dynamic flow sequence (Fig. 129A) demonstrates markedly increased vascularity in the right spermatic cord and testis, with evidence of reduced flow laterally. The immediate postflow static image (Fig. 129B) shows increased activity in the right cord and testis with a large associated cold defect laterally (open arrow).

Conclusion. Epididymitis with a large associated hydrocele.

Note. This pattern can be misinterpreted as a missed torsion, a vascular neoplasm with a necrotic center, or even a testicular abscess. The finding of a semilunar cold defect within the scrotum with normal or increased testicular activity should lead one to the diagnosis of epididymitis with hydrocele. Clinical correlation with the scintigraphic images is essential!

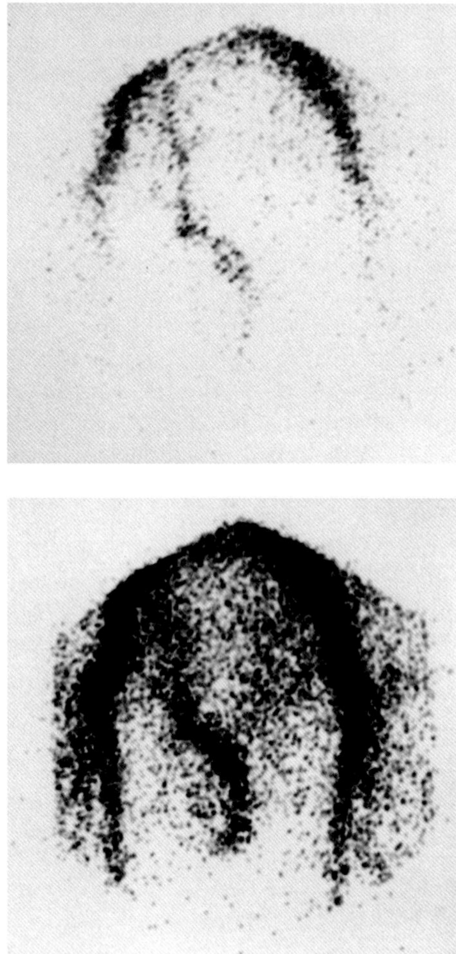

A

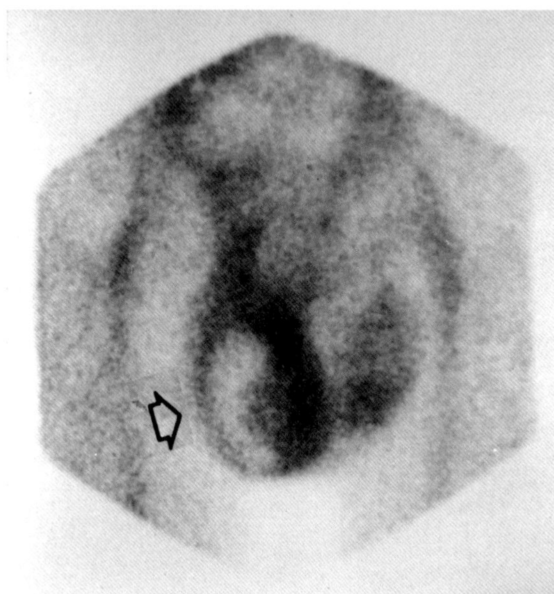

B

Case 130

A 15-year-old male patient was admitted with a 4-day history of intermittent left testicular pain and tenderness.

Physical Examination. The left testis is slightly swollen, red, and exquisitely tender.

Nuclear Medicine. After intravenous injection of Tc-99m pertechnetate, this arterial phase dynamic image (Fig. 130A) demonstrates a "nubbin" sign at the proximal end of the spermatic cord (open arrow) with mild hyperemia developing around the left testis (small closed arrow). The large closed arrow is an external marker in the right inguinal region. The postflow static image (Fig. 130B) shows the characteristic pattern of mild increased activity around a relatively cold left testis.

Conclusion. Early missed torsion of the left testis.

Note. At surgery, the left testis and epididymis were found to be infarcted and hemorrhagic. This study was provided through the courtesy of Col. Fredric A. Conte, Chief of Radiology and Maj. Rhonda A. Wyatt, Chief of Nuclear Medicine, David Grant USAF Medical Center, Travis AFB, Travis, California.

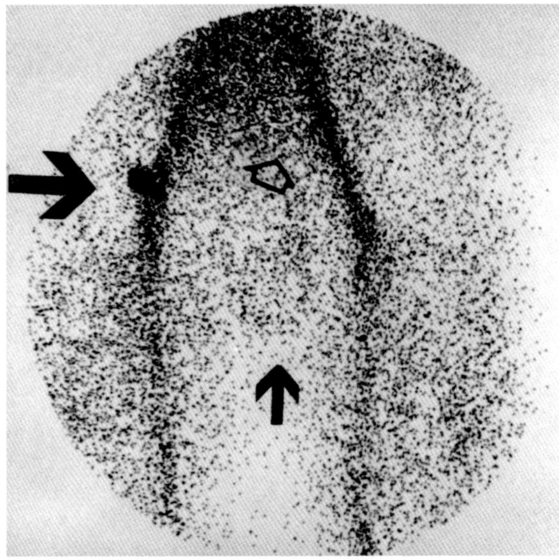

A

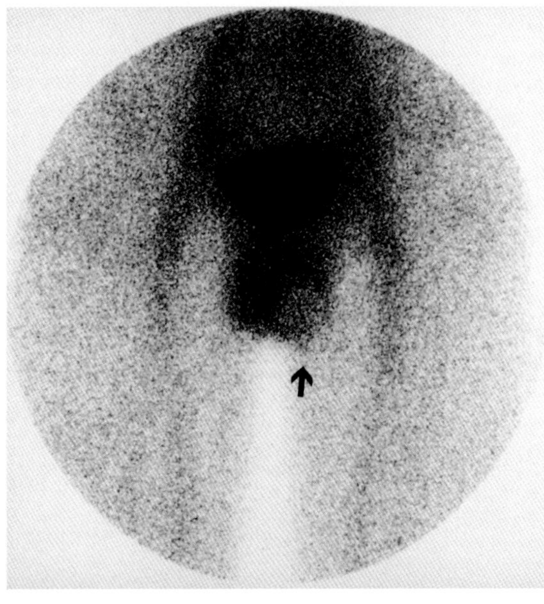

B

Subject Index

Subject Index

Page numbers in italic refer to illustrations.

U

V